HANDBOOK OF CRITICAL CARE

HANDBOOK OF CRITICAL CARE

SECOND EDITION

EDITED BY

James L. Berk, M.D.

Professor of Surgery, Case Western Reserve University School of Medicine, Cleveland, Ohio

James E. Sampliner, M.D.

Assistant Clinical Professor, Case Western Reserve University School of Medicine; Co-Director of the Intensive Care Unit, Hillcrest Hospital; and Assistant Visiting Surgeon, Mount Sinai Hospital, Cleveland, Ohio

FOREWORD BY

Francis D. Moore, M.D.

Moseley Professor of Surgery Emeritus, Harvard Medical School; Surgeon-in-Chief Emeritus, Peter Bent Brigham Hospital, Boston, Massachusetts

Little, Brown and Company
Boston

Library of Congress Catalog Card No. 81-82380

ISBN 0-316-09171-5

Printed in the United States of America

HAL

CONTRIBUTING AUTHORS

Stephen M. Ayres, M.D.

Professor and Chairman, Department of Internal Medicine, St. Louis University School of Medicine; Professor and Chairman, Department of Internal Medicine, St. Louis University Hospitals, St. Louis, Missouri

Robert L. Berger, M.D.

Professor of Surgery, Boston University School of Medicine; Director, Thoracic Surgical Service, and Director, Department of Cardiothoracic Surgery, University Hospital, Boston, Massachusetts

James L. Berk, M.D.

Professor of Surgery, Case Western Reserve University School of Medicine, Cleveland, Ohio

John E. Brimm, M.D.

Assistant Professor of Surgery and Pathology in Residence, University of California, San Diego, School of Medicine, La Jolla, California

Christopher W. Bryan-Brown, M.D.

Professor of Anesthesiology and Surgery, University of Texas Health Science Center, Houston, Texas

Kanu Chatterjee, M.B. (M.D.)

Professor of Medicine, University of California, San Francisco, School of Medicine; Chief, Coronary Care Unit and Associate Chief, Cardiovascular Division of the Department of Medicine, Herbert C. Moffitt Hospital, San Francisco, California

Nathan P. Couch, M.D.

Associate Professor of Surgery, Harvard Medical School; Surgeon, Brigham and Women's Hospital, Boston, Massachusetts

Robert A. Danielson, M.D.

Staff Surgeon, French Hospital of Los Angeles, Los Angeles, California

Jan R. Dmochowski, M.D.

Associate Professor of Surgery, University of Massachusetts Medical School; Surgical Coordinator, St. Vincent's Hospital, Worcester, Massachusetts

Hillary F. Don, M.D.

Associate Professor of Anesthesia, University of California,
San Francisco, School of Medicine; Director, Intensive Care Unit,
Herbert C. Moffitt Hospital, San Francisco, California

Josef E. Fischer, M.D.

Professor and Chairman, Department of Surgery, University of
Cincinnati College of Medicine; Surgeon-in-Chief, University
of Cincinnati Medical Center, Cincinnati, Ohio

Frank E. Gump, M.D.

Professor of Surgery, Columbia University College of Physicians and Surgeons;
Attending Surgeon, Presbyterian Hospital, New York, New York

J. Höper, M.D.

Research Fellow, Institut für Physiologie und Kardiologie,
University of Erlangen-Nürnberg, Nürnberg, West Germany

Donald Kapsch, M.D.

Resident in Surgery, Department of Surgery, University of
Missouri-Columbia School of Medicine, Columbia, Missouri

Manfred Kessler, M.D.

Professor of Physiology and Director, Institut für Physiologie und
Kardiologie, University of Erlangen-Nürnberg, Nürnberg, West Germany

John M. Kinney, M.D.

Professor of Surgery, Columbia University College of Physicians and Surgeons;
Attending Surgeon, Presbyterian Hospital, New York, New York

George I. Litman, M.D.

Associate Professor of Medicine, Northeastern Ohio Universities
College of Medicine; Chief of Cardiology, Akron General Medical Center,
Akron, Ohio

Dwight L. Makoff, M.D.

Associate Clinical Professor of Medicine, UCLA School of Medicine
(University of California, Los Angeles); Attending Physician,
Cedars-Sinai Medical Center, Los Angeles, California

William J. Mandel, M.D.

Associate Professor of Medicine, UCLA School of Medicine (University of
California, Los Angeles); Director, Clinical Electrocardiography, Department
of Cardiology, Cedars-Sinai Medical Center, Los Angeles, California

W. Scott McDougal, M.D.

Associate Professor of Surgery and Urology, Dartmouth Medical School;
Attending Surgeon, Division of Urology, Dartmouth-Hitchcock Medical Center,
Hanover, New Hampshire

Gideon Merin, M.D.

Associate Professor of Cardiothoracic Surgery, Hebrew University;
Principal Surgeon, Department of Cardiothoracic Surgery,
Hadassah University Hospital, Jerusalem, Israel

Konrad Messmer, M.D.

Professor of Experimental Surgery, Institute for Surgical Research,
University of Munich, Munich, West Germany

Joel D. Mittleman, M.D.

Clinical Instructor in Medicine, UCLA School of Medicine
(University of California, Los Angeles); Associate Physician,
Cedars-Sinai Medical Center, Los Angeles, California

Kazi Mobin-Uddin, M.B.B.S. (M.D.)

Associate Clinical Professor of Thoracic Surgery, The Ohio State University
College of Medicine, Columbus, Ohio; Attending Surgeon and Director,
Department of Cardiovascular Surgery, Frederick C. Smith Clinic, Marion, Ohio

Harold C. Neu, M.D.

Professor of Medicine and Pharmacology, and Chief, Division of
Infectious Diseases, Columbia University College of Physicians
and Surgeons; Attending Physician and Hospital Epidemiologist,
Presbyterian Hospital, New York, New York

Richard M. Peters, M.D.

Professor of Surgery and Bioengineering, University of California,
San Diego, School of Medicine, La Jolla, California; Co-Head,
Division of Cardiothoracic Surgery, University of California Medical
Center, San Diego, California

Howard C. Pitluk, M.D.

Clinical Instructor of Surgery, Case Western Reserve University
School of Medicine; Assistant Visiting Surgeon, Mount Sinai Hospital,
Cleveland, Ohio

U. Pohl, M.D.

Research Fellow, Institut für Physiologie und Kardiologie,
University of Erlangen-Nürnberg, Nürnberg, West Germany

Samuel R. Powers, Jr., M.D., D.Sc.(Med)†

Professor and Chairman, Department of Surgery, Albany Medical College
of Union University; Surgeon in Chief, Albany Medical Center Hospital,
Albany, New York

† Deceased

James E. Sampliner, M.D.

Assistant Clinical Professor, Case Western Reserve University
School of Medicine; Co-Director of the Intensive Care Unit, Hillcrest
Hospital; Assistant Visiting Surgeon, Mount Sinai Hospital, Cleveland, Ohio

William C. Shoemaker, M.D.

Professor of Surgery, UCLA School of Medicine (University of California,
Los Angeles); Surgeon, Harbor General Hospital, Torrance, California

John H. Siegel, M.D.

Professor of Surgery and Research Professor of Biophysical Sciences,
State University of New York at Buffalo School of Medicine;
Chief of Surgery, Buffalo General Hospital, Buffalo, New York

Donald Silver, M.D.

Professor and Chairman, Department of Surgery, University of
Missouri-Columbia School of Medicine, Columbia, Missouri

Robert L. Smith, R.R.T., R-C.P.T.

Technical Director, Pulmonary Function Laboratory, Cleveland
Metropolitan General Hospital, Cleveland, Ohio

Herbert J. Weiss, M.D.

Associate Clinical Professor of Psychiatry, Case Western Reserve
University School of Medicine; Associate Psychiatrist, University Hospitals;
Chief, Division of Psychiatry, Mount Sinai Hospital, Cleveland, Ohio

Martin H. Weiss, M.D.

Professor and Chairman, Department of Neurosurgery, University
of Southern California School of Medicine; Chief of Neurosurgery,
LAC-USC Medical Center, Los Angeles, California

Warren M. Zapol, M.D.

Associate Professor of Anesthesia, Harvard Medical School; Assistant
Anesthetist, Massachusetts General Hospital, Boston, Massachusetts

FOREWORD

In considering the "acute abdomen," it has been said that the term *acute* refers not so much to the speed of the pathologic process or its urgency but rather to the acuteness of judgment that the surgeon must bring to bear if he is to handle the patient correctly. Possibly it is time to make the same statement about critical care medicine. The patient may seem to be past the stage of critical illness, and there may be no immediate crisis; yet each small segment of treatment that the physician or surgeon carries out is of critical importance to the patient's recovery.

The two statements have a common thread. The pathologic causes of the acute abdomen are numerous and diverse, stemming from many unrelated sources; the illnesses encountered in critical care medicine are equally numerous and varied and include diseases of the heart, lungs, circulation, brain, and viscera.

Two developments of the past 25 years have rendered the medical and surgical care of critically ill patients a new and distinct field of hospital administration and departmental organization. The first is the improvement in the overall management of life-endangering illness through more intelligent use of blood transfusion, antibiotics, hemodialysis, and the host of techniques of metabolic care that daily are called into play for the dangerously ill person. The second development, which occurred rapidly after the advent of open heart surgery in about 1960, is the improvement in, and simplification of, respiratory assistance devices.

Most critical care units in this country today are tied together not so much by the disease entity involved, nor even by the host of details in metabolic management, but rather availability of respiratory assistance devices, together with a team of physicians and therapists expert in the minute-by-minute management of the critically ill patient for days or weeks at a time.

Many physicians of my generation remember seeing whole wards filled with poliomyelitis patients being "carried through" respiratory failure by the iron lung (the Drinker respirator). A device of such great weight, power demands, and bulk would be unthinkable today. Manipulation of the patient within the respiratory chamber was virtually impossible because the cyclic alteration in ambient pressure was thereby lost. Yet the lives of thousands of young people were saved by this device. For today's generation of students and residents, the development of direct endotracheal respiratory care devices seems to be part of ancient history because such devices are so widespread in their application and so relatively simple to use. Although they are easily moved about, are relatively inexpensive, and can produce a whole variety of pressure-flow patterns in the airway, present-day respiratory assist devices also have negative aspects. They can still be the source of sepsis if poorly sterilized and can produce pneumothorax, atelectasis, or anoxic arrest if one small dial is turned to the wrong setting.

The summation of these developments in treatment has made it possible for many young people, with their lives still ahead of them, to survive illnesses to which they formerly would have succumbed. Many patients are kept alive in such units over prolonged periods, although the mortality for some types of patients may be very high, as for patients with a combination of burns and renal failure or a combination of pulmonary insufficiency and gram-negative bacteremia. The prolonged presence of these patients in the hospital has rendered it essential to isolate an increasingly large number of beds for such care. Pathogeneses in these patients may be as remotely related as a severe burn is to an early postoperative mitral valvuloplasty, or a drug suicide attempt to a septic abortion, and yet there are surprisingly many common denominators in their care.

The editors, Drs. Berk and Sampliner, have put together a book that is a practical, handy reference for the student and practitioner and is equally useful to the nurse, respiratory therapist, and physician's assistant involved in critical care medicine.

Much of the *Handbook of Critical Care* focuses on "pattern recognition" rather than on conventional pathologic diagnosis. The pathophysiologic patterns of respiratory alkalosis with unconsciousness, paradoxical aciduria with gastric juice loss and hypovolemia, and pulmonary arteriovenous admixture are examples of the patterns that the critical care therapist comes to recognize and learns to treat.

The intensive care therapist must always keep a sharp eye to the basic diagnosis and to the pathologic problem at hand. The therapist should avoid the error of wasting the scarce resources of society on the very feeble elderly or the hopelessly ill patient with terminal cancer. The therapist often holds the key to long-range survival and success.

It is a pleasure to make even this small contribution to such a book. We can cheer the reader on with the thought that while modern medicine often seems to be a matter of gadgets and superspecialization—"high technology"—the care of the critically ill patient truly restores the physician's primary role: to look after the welfare of the *whole* patient. In critical care no physiologic system or body organ function can be spared from consideration, and through it all the intensive care provider must keep in mind the emotional adjustment of the patient, the drive to recovery, the need for a frequent word of encouragement, and an abiding concern for, and understanding of, the anxiety felt by the patient's family.

Francis D. Moore

PREFACE
TO THE SECOND EDITION

This book is intended to be a practical guide for physicians as well as for medical students, nurses, and allied health personnel involved in the care of critically ill patients. The need for such a guide was recognized by the house officers and students at Case Western Reserve University School of Medicine.

Because an understanding of underlying theory and basic science is essential for the successful application of the various techniques and modes of therapy described, basic concepts have been included and correlated with the practical portions.

This book does not pretend to include everything that may be considered to be part of the large and rapidly expanding field of critical care medicine. It is intended that the text, references, and selected readings will serve as a basic source of practical information for use in the intensive care setting as well as a foundation on which students and physicians can build.

To keep pace with the advances in critical care medicine, this edition of the *Handbook* has been completely revised. All chapters have been updated. Seven new chapters have been added, which include discussions of multiple organ failure, noninvasive diagnostic techniques, oxygen administration, the neurosurgical patient, monitoring PO_2 in skeletal muscle, blood substitutes, and mass spectrometry. The chapter on circulatory assistance with intra-aortic balloon counterpulsation has been expanded to include the left ventricular assist device. The chapter on circulatory assistance with external counterpulsation has been deleted because this mode of therapy has not continued to gain acceptance as a useful tool.

The editors wish to thank Lin Richter, Editor-in-Chief of the Medical Division, Little, Brown and Company, and Beverly Taylor of Cleveland Metropolitan General Hospital for a great deal of help in preparation of the manuscript.

J. L. B.
J. E. S.

CONTENTS

To

William D. Holden, M.D. *Former Oliver Payne Professor and Chairman, Department of Surgery, Case Western Reserve University School of Medicine, who by his exemplary care of the critically ill, combining the scientific approach with compassion and wisdom, has added immeasurably to the care of critically ill patients everywhere through his teaching of more than a generation of students and house officers.*

Francis D. Moore, M.D. *Moseley Professor of Surgery Emeritus, Harvard Medical School; Surgeon-in-Chief Emeritus, Peter Bent Brigham Hospital. A surgeon's surgeon, physiologist, teacher, scholar, and friend, who by his application of physiology and metabolism to clinical care, has had a major and lasting influence on the care of critically ill patients.*

I / CRITICAL CARE MANAGEMENT

Notice

The indications and dosages of all drugs in this book have been recommended in the medical literature and conform to the practices of the general medical community. The medications described do not necessarily have specific approval by the Food and Drug Administration for use in the disease and dosages for which they are recommended. The package insert for each drug should be consulted for use and dosage as approved by the FDA. Because standards for usage change, it is advisable to keep abreast of revised recommendations, particularly those concerning new drugs.

James L. Berk / 1. MULTIPLE ORGAN FAILURE

The reader may wonder why the chapter on multiple organ failure appears at the beginning of the book rather than near the end. Multiple organ failure occurs late in the course of a critical illness, often marking the terminal phase, and, as such, might logically appear after the chapters dealing with specific organ systems. However, I believe that multiple organ failure frequently results from specific, identifiable causes that lead insidiously to a vicious cycle of progressively failing systems and that may be prevented in many instances by meticulous attention to details early in the illness. It is my intent that by presenting this chapter early on, the reader will gain an understanding of the common factors in the pathogenesis of multiple organ failure and the effects of one failing organ on others. With this understanding, the ensuing chapters will be more closely interrelated and thus more meaningful.

Advances in medicine have permitted the prolonged survival of critically ill patients, creating the syndrome called multiple organ failure. This syndrome most commonly follows trauma or surgery but may be associated with any serious illness, such as gastrointestinal hemorrhage, pancreatitis, diverticulitis, or shock from any cause.

During the 1930s and early 1940s, cardiovascular collapse or shock was the major limitation to survival. An understanding of the role of blood loss in shock and the introduction of blood banking techniques permitted the survival of many patients with massive blood loss. By the end of World War II, acute renal failure following trauma had become the condition that limited survival; the subsequent use of dialysis permitted the survival of many patients with established renal failure. During the Vietnam conflict, rapid evacuation and prompt fluid replacement resulted in survival from previously fatal injuries, and acute respiratory failure, "shock lung," became recognized. Thus, the successful treatment of one failing organ system has permitted survival and the subsequent failure of other systems.

To prevent multiple organ failure one must identify the factors that contribute to organ failure, including those specific for single organs and those common to all organs, so that they may be prevented or, if that is not possible, corrected promptly. Failure of an organ that has not been or can no longer be corrected may affect other organs and set up a cycle of failing organs—a physiologic domino effect. Finally, a stage is reached when the treatment of one failing organ results in failure of other organs, making survival unlikely.

Trauma may affect organ function directly, as in a myocardial contusion, or indirectly, through circulatory or respiratory failure. Prompt resuscitation with establishment of an airway, adequate ventilation, and fluid replacement, followed by required surgery—which may include hemostasis, débridement of devitalized tissues, repair of damaged viscera, or stabilization of fractures—may prevent multiple organ failure later.

Following major surgery or trauma and associated with critical illness, there is an increased energy requirement and a negative nitrogen balance. Both are greatly increased by sepsis. Caloric requirements may approach 40 to 70 Cal/kg/day or 5000 Cal/day. Three liters of 5% D/W will supply 600 Cal. In a patient receiving no dietary protein, protein losses may approach 250 g per day. Additional protein losses of 10 to 50 g per day may occur with hemorrhage, intestinal obstruction, and wound exudates (burns, pancreatitis, and generalized peritonitis). Critically ill posttraumatic patients can lose more than 3 lb of muscle tissue or its equivalent per day. Studies in surgical patients have shown that an acute loss of 30 percent of body weight in 30 days is uniformly fatal. Therefore, critically ill patients with alimentary tract dysfunction, which is common in these patients, should receive early total parenteral nutrition to supply the increased energy required for fuel and the proteins needed to make essential enzymes and to maintain cellular structure. Malnutrition is a major factor contributing to multiple organ failure and must be prevented. In seriously ill patients who cannot be expected with certainty to take and absorb adequate nutrition orally within 5 to 7 days, parenteral hyperalimentation should be begun as soon as the patient is hemodynamically stable. Withholding total parenteral nutrition (TPN) because of its possible risks and because it is hoped that the patient will be able to eat "in a few days" frequently results in malnutrition and, in turn, in multiple organ failure. (See Chapter 17.)

Injured, postsurgical, and critically ill patients may have an altered immune response and decreased resistance to infection. This altered response can be an important factor in the development of sepsis from contamination or in the inability of the patient to combat an established septic process. The degree of suppression is related to the magnitude of stress. Additional factors that contribute to the decreased immune response are anesthesia, shock, blood loss, sepsis, malnutrition, liver disease, and drugs (e.g., corticosteroids and azathioprine). Depressed neutrophil antibacterial activity and depressed lymphocyte function have been demonstrated in patients following trauma and elective surgery. A deficiency of opsonins, serum proteins that interact with organisms to increase cellular recognition and removal by phagocytosis, has also been demonstrated in patients following trauma. Systemic reticuloendothelial (RE) system depression occurs after trauma and in a variety of shock states. With contamination bacteremia is more likely to occur and, in turn, bacteremia may cause further impairment of the RE system. In addition, many seriously ill patients show no skin reaction when antigens are injected into the skin. This anergy or depression of the delayed hypersensitivity response has been correlated with depressed neutrophil function and is associated with an increased incidence of infection, septicemia, and death related to the infection. Erosion of body cell mass has been correlated with the anergic state. Adequate nutrition and aggressive surgical drainage of the infection will restore the delayed hypersensitivity response, improve abnormal cellular and serum components of host defense, and increase chances of survival. Providing nutrition after the development of septic complications may be too late to correct contracture of body cell mass and the anergic state. Thus, stress, trauma, drugs, inadequate nutrition, and infection itself can alter the host's immune response and defense against infection, which, once established, can result directly in multiple organ failure.

Acute respiratory failure in critically ill patients (see Chapter 6) plays a major role in the pathogenesis of multiple organ failure. The large number of descriptive names for the syndrome (see Table 1-1) reflects a lack of understanding of the pathophysiology; consequently, there are many theories concerning the etiology. Some physicians believe that the respiratory distress syndrome (RDS)—the most popular name for acute respiratory failure in critically ill patients—is a specific entity. When it "arrives," they believe themselves scholarly to have recognized it and know that respiratory failure is progressive, and that death is usually inevitable. They give therapeutic doses of corticosteroids around the clock. Of one thing I am certain: this theory is incorrect.

I believe that RDS is caused by specific, often unrecognized, entities occurring alone or in combination (see Table 1-2). Fluid overload and left heart failure contribute significantly to acute respiratory failure in 80 to 90 percent of surgical patients. The respiratory failure of sepsis is frequent if the PaO_2 is evaluated in relation to the fraction of inspired oxygen. Because the low PaO_2 in septic patients results in part from interstitial edema owing to increased capillary permeability, it is easy to understand why septic patients are particularly vulnerable to a fluid overload or left heart failure. In critically ill patients with unexplained tachypnea and respiratory alkalosis and an inappropriately low PaO_2, suspect sepsis. Often the pulse, temperature, and white blood count are increased, but not always. The source of sepsis may not be obvious and must be actively sought not only by careful physical examination but by x-ray films, ultrasound, gallium scans, and computed tomography (CT) (see Chapter 4). Adequate treatment of the infection, including drainage of an abscess, can reverse progressive respiratory failure and prevent multiple organ failure. Conversely, survival is unlikely, regardless of all other medical care, if the abscess is not drained. Usually the respiratory failure from specific identifiable causes, other than

TABLE 1-1. Synonyms for Acute Respiratory Failure in the Critically Ill Patient

Shock lung
Posttraumatic pulmonary insufficiency
Respiratory distress syndrome (RDS)
Respiratory distress syndromes (RDS)
Acute respiratory distress syndrome (ARDS)
Adult respiratory distress syndrome (ARDS)
Acute respiratory failure
Congestive atelectasis
Da Nang lung
Hemorrhagic atelectasis
Pump lung
Posttransfusion lung
Progressive pulmonary consolidation
Respiratory lung
Stiff lung syndrome
Traumatic lung
Transplant lung
White lung syndrome
Adult hyaline membrane disease
Pulmonary hyaline membrane disease
Noncardiac pulmonary edema
Wet lung of trauma
Respiratory insufficiency syndrome
Progressive respiratory distress
Progressive pulmonary consolidation
Hemorrhagic lung syndrome
Bronchopulmonary dysplasia

sepsis, occurs early in the course of the illness, and that from advanced sepsis later, but any of the causes can and do occur at any time and are additive. All are made worse by preexisting lung disease. Hypoxemia resulting from respiratory failure, often unrecognized, is a major cause of multiple organ failure even if present for only a short time. Because of the key role of respiratory failure in the pathogenesis of multiple organ failure, the treatment of acute respiratory failure will be described in some detail.

Prevention is the best treatment for acute respiratory failure. Early attention to detail can prevent progressive pulmonary insufficiency from occurring several days later. Avoid overhydration following resuscitation

TABLE 1-2. Causes of Acute Respiratory Failure in the Critically Ill Patient

Fluid overload
Left heart failure
Trauma: fractured ribs, flail chest, pneumohemothorax, contusion of
    lung and heart
Sepsis
Shock
Atelectasis
Inadequate tracheobronchial toilet
Thromboembolism
Fat embolism
Aspiration pneumonia
Bacterial pneumonia
Viral pneumonia
Abdominal distention
Multiple blood transfusions—particulate matter
Oxygen toxicity
Ventilator injury
Cardiopulmonary bypass
Humoral substances
    Pancreatitis
    Endotoxin
    Vasoactive drugs
    Kinins
    Myocardial depressant factor
    Histamine
    Prostaglandins
Transfusion reactions
Head injuries
Burns
Drug abuse—heroin pulmonary edema
Anaphylaxis
Metabolic, e.g., hypophosphatemia
Preexisting lung disease

from shock. If high-output renal failure is not present, urine output greater that 50 ml per hour suggest overhydration and set the stage for pulmonary failure 2 or 3 days later. Overhydration is not uncommon in small, critically ill patients in an antidiuretic state who are receiving intravenous fluids for prolonged periods. A patient may require no more than 1,000 to 1,200 ml per day maintenance yet may receive 2,000 to 3,000 ml per day for several days. Patients particularly vulnerable to overhydration are the elderly and those with congestive heart failure, chronic pulmonary disease, advanced sepsis, and lung trauma. Accurate measurement of intake, output, and daily weight is essential to prevent fluid overloading. Remember that a patient can become overhydrated and develop pulmonary insufficiency without an elevated central venous or pulmonary capillary wedge pressure. Once detected, overhydration should be treated vigorously by fluid restriction and diuretics as necessary.

In critically ill patients, deep breathing, coughing, turning, and early ambulation are essential to prevent mucous plugs, which can lead to ventilation-perfusion inequalities, alveolar collapse, and pneumonia. Patients can sit in a chair and even walk if they are on a ventilator. Chest physical therapy and postural drainage will help avoid mucous plugs. Oversedation permits patients to lie flat on their backs for long periods without moving or coughing and can set the stage for pulmonary problems later. Adequate humidity must be provided to prevent inspissated secretions and injury to the respiratory ciliary action. Tracheobronchial aspiration should be used as necessary.

Paralytic ileus is extremely common in critically ill patients. Abdominal distention causes elevation of the diaphragms, basilar atelectasis with shunting, and a decreased vital capacity. Nasogastric suction should be begun early. Premature oral feeding may result in additional abdominal distention and further compromise of pulmonary function. Aspiration pneumonia is not infrequent and often goes unrecognized as a cause of respiratory failure, particularly in obtunded, debilitated patients and in tube-fed patients.

Prolonged use of concentrations of oxygen above 50% may cause pulmonary damage (oxygen toxicity) and should be avoided. However, it is better to use 100% oxygen than to permit one minute of hypoxia. A PaO_2 greater than 70 to 80 torr is unnecessary. Positive end expiratory pressure (PEEP) should be considered early; remember that although PEEP may result in an increased PaO_2, the cardiac output may be decreased so that the oxygen transport may actually be decreased. Measurements of the cardiac output, blood gases, and hemoglobin concentration are essential (see Chapter 8).

In critically ill patients—particularly those with congestive heart failure, prolonged immobilization, or a malignancy—a high index of suspicion should be maintained for pulmonary emboli, another cause of respiratory failure. Not infrequently, the fall in PaO_2 is transient. Remember that a friction rub, hemoptysis, and a classical wedge-shaped shadow on the chest x-ray appear late and are signs of pulmonary infarction, not pulmonary embolism. If treatment is withheld until infarction is obvious, the patient may die of a subsequent embolus. The diagnosis should be suspected early in the appropriate clinical setting. Remember that the chest x-ray and electrocardiogram may or may not be abnormal. A lung scan may be diagnostic if there are no other abnormalities on the chest x-ray, but a pulmonary angiogram is definitive. (See Chapter 14.)

Embolization of particulate matter from multiple blood transfusions has been implicated in pulmonary insufficiency. If blood loss is excessive and transfusions exceed 4 units, blood filters should be used. Dacron-wool and polyester mesh of 25 to 40 microns appears to be effective and should be changed after every 3 units of blood.

Trauma can result directly or indirectly in respiratory failure. Fractured ribs and a flail chest may be obvious, but pulmonary or myocardial contusions may not be. A pneumothorax or hemothorax secondary to the fractured ribs may appear some time after admission. A subclavian venipuncture, particularly when it is followed by positive pressure anesthesia, use of a ventilator, or PEEP, may result in an unrecognized pneumothorax. Prompt adequate débridement of all devitalized tissue can prevent a nidus for infection and subsequent respiratory failure. Consider fat emboli in patients with long bone fractures following major trauma. Early fixation of fractures permits early mobilization with the attendant beneficial effects on cardiac, pulmonary, and gastrointestinal function and on nitrogen balance.

Vasoactive drugs can result in ventilation-perfusion inequalities by causing a redistribution of the pulmonary microcirculatory blood flow and can contribute to pulmonary insufficiency. These drugs should be used only when necessary and with appropriate monitoring of blood gases.

With the routine use of automated multi-channel blood chemical analyses, hypophosphatemia is now being recognized with increasing frequency as a cause of acute respiratory failure as well as multiple organ failure. The common clinical setting for hypophosphatemia is in the nutritionally depleted, critically ill patient receiving hyperalimentation (the phosphorus moves with glucose into the cells) and antacids (which bind phosphorus) who is being dialyzed (with a phosphate-poor bath). Alcoholic patients are particularly susceptible. Again, prevention is important: give additional phosphate in the hyperalimentation fluid when necessary. Once hypophosphatemia becomes established, intravenous phosphate may be lifesaving. (See Chapter 15.)

In summary, acute respiratory failure in critically ill patients results from one or more specific, frequently unrecognized causes. Attention to details can often prevent respiratory failure, but if it should occur, early detection and correction of the contributory problems can frequently still prevent acute, progressive respiratory failure—a major factor contributing to multiple organ failure.

Cardiac failure is not only a major cause of acute respiratory failure owing to pulmonary edema (backward failure), but also a major cause of multiple organ failure owing to decreased organ perfusion (forward failure). Backward failure usually precedes forward failure, but not always. Cardiac failure frequently occurs insidiously in critically ill patients, particularly those with preexisting heart disease, resulting from the increased circulatory requirements imposed by stress, trauma, and sepsis and the reduced coronary perfusion associated with low-flow states. Hypovolemic, septic, and cardiogenic (sometimes from a silent myocardial infarction) shock may be present and contribute to decreased coronary perfusion even though the classical signs of shock—low blood pressure and cold, clammy, pale skin—are absent. Fluid overload, hypoxemia from respiratory failure, acidosis, and electrolyte abnormalities may also contribute to cardiac failure. Pericardial tamponade or a myocardial contusion following trauma can also result in decreased cardiac function. In addition, a decreased cardiac output and hence decreased coronary flow can be caused by positive pressure ventilation, PEEP, and vasopressors, particularly in a failing heart. Left heart failure should be detected and treated long before frank pulmonary edema and hypotension occur. Remember that the PaO_2 falls before congestive heart failure can be detected clinically, that the central venous pressure may be normal in 30 to 50 percent of critically ill patients with significant left heart failure, and that even young, previously healthy, critically ill patients can develop left heart failure. A Swan-Ganz flow-directed catheter should be placed early. Critically ill patients have little tolerance for delays in diagnosis and in beginning definitive treatment. Diuretics may suffice, but depending on the hemodynamic findings, afterload-reducing drugs, inotropic agents, or mechanical circulatory support may be necessary. Cardiac failure is a major, often unrecognized, cause for multiple organ failure.

Acute renal failure (see Chapter 21) may follow low-flow states, including hypovolemic, cardiogenic, and septic shock. Remember, hypotension need not be present. Hypoxia resulting from acute respiratory failure, particularly if associated with decreased perfusion, is a common factor contributing to acute renal failure. In addition, advanced sepsis, such as an undrained abscess, appears to have a direct effect on the kidney in producing renal failure. Transfusion reactions, myoglobin from a crush injury, and increased bilirubin from any cause when associated with hypotension may result in renal failure. Nephrotoxic drugs—such as gentamicin, kanamycin, cephalosporins, methicillin, and methoxyflurane—are also common causes of renal failure. Renal failure may follow hepatic failure, the hepatorenal syndrome. Occlusion of the renal blood vessels occurs in disseminated intravascular coagulation, shock, and severe infections. Renal vaso-constriction from vasoactive drugs has been implicated in renal failure. Prompt fluid replacement, adequate respiratory and circulatory support, drainage of abscesses, and awareness of potentially nephrotoxic drugs may avoid renal failure in many instances. The treatment of established renal failure is dialysis.

Abnormalities of hepatic function frequently occur in critically ill patients. Within 2 to 4 days after trauma or operation, a mild, transient jaundice appears, resulting from multiple transfusions, hematoma resorption, drugs, and anesthesia. This transient jaundice has no prognostic significance. A larger increase in bilirubin plus an increase in liver enzymes may occur later, usually 1 to 3 weeks after injury. Severe infection is present in approximately 75 percent of the patients. Typically, the patient is in a hyperdynamic state and frequently has pulmonary and renal failure. There are several known causes of hepatic failure. Hypoperfusion resulting from traumatic and hypovolemic shock occurs early, and that resulting from cardiogenic and septic shock usually occurs later. Low-flow states may not be clinically obvious, and appropriate hemodynamic monitoring is essential for early detection. Damage to the hepatic parenchyma may occur early, with abnormal function appearing later, much like acute tubular necrosis. Hypoxia from acute respiratory failure plays an important role in the pathogenesis of liver failure. Hepatic vasoconstriction—either endogenous, related to stress, or exogenous, from vasoactive drugs—may contribute to hypoperfusion. Liver injury per se is not likely to cause liver failure unless a massive resection is accompanied by shock or sepsis. Sepsis has a direct effect on the Kupffer cells and hepatocytes, resulting in impairment of enzymatic function and bile transport. Malnutrition is also a major cause of liver failure. It results in failure of the liver to synthesize essential substances (e.g., decreased serum albumin and coagulation factors) and failure of energy-dependent mechanisms. Bile salt excretion into bile is energy dependent and can contribute to hepatic bile stasis. Impairment of hepatocellular sodium and potassium transport, also energy dependent, can result in increased intracellular water and cell swelling. Lastly, liver damage can result from anesthetics such as halothane and drugs such as tetracycline, chlorpromazine, and heroin.

Coagulopathies are common in the critically ill patient (see Chapter 19). Blood transfusions greater than 10 units in 24 hr will cause a decrease in platelets and factors 5 and 8, which are not stored in bank blood. To prevent this, 1 unit of fresh blood should be given for every 4 units of bank blood. Disseminated intravascular coagulation (DIC) follows severe trauma, sepsis, shock, and incompatible blood transfusions and may cause consumption of clotting factors, resulting in bleeding; or if fibrinolytic activity is insufficient, the microcirculation may become obstructed by thromboses, which can lead to cellular necrosis and multiple organ failure. Hyperfibrinolysis follows extensive trauma, acute hypoxia, and shock and can lead to excessive bleeding. Drugs such as chloramphenicol can depress the bone marrow and lead to thrombocytopenia and bleeding disorders. If given in amounts greater than 1.5 liter per day, or less if there are decreased platelets, dextran, 40 or 70, may cause decreased platelet adhesiveness and an increase in thrombus lysibility. Hepatic insufficiency causes a decreased synthesis of coagulation factors 5 and 7 to 10, increased fibrinolysis, and platelet dysfunction. Renal failure causes platelet dysfunction, which can be improved by dialysis. Sepsis, particularly gram-negative septicemia, results in decreased platelets owing either to chronic DIC or a primary effect. Again, prevention is the best treatment of coagulopathies. Otherwise, early treatment of causative factors and replacement of factors when possible may help prevent excessive bleeding, which, particularly if stress ulcers are present, can lead to hypovolemic shock and multiple organ failure.

Stress gastric bleeding usually occurs in critically ill patients with respiratory failure and sepsis. Such patients often have renal failure, hepatic dysfunction, and a coagulopathy; many have been ill for some time and are malnourished. Recent studies suggest that upper gastrointestinal bleeding occurs in approximately one-third of critically ill patients with septicemia. Usually there are multiple erosions in the body and fundus of the stomach, referred to as acute hemorrhagic gastritis. Less commonly, there is a single, acute peptic ulcer in the antrum or duodenum. The etiology of stress bleeding is controversial. Most authorities agree that acid is necessary, but they have found little correlation between acid hypersecretion and stress ulcers except following head injury. Back diffusion of acid owing to loss of the mucosal integrity may explain the lack of correlation and may result in cellular damage. Hypoperfusion of the mucosa, as seen in various types of shock, and hypoxia appear to play important roles in the pathogenesis of stress bleeding. Vasoactive drugs may cause vasoconstriction and add to the ischemia. High metabolic demands and rapid turnover of mucosal cells at a time of a deficiency of high-energy intermediates and protein substrates (malnutrition) appear to be major causes of cellular necrosis and stress bleeding. Aspirin and possibly corticosteroids can contribute to mucosal damage.

Factors involved in the pathogenesis of stress bleeding should be prevented or corrected early. An adequate blood volume along with satisfactory cardiac function, ventilation, and oxygenation should be maintained to prevent hypoperfusion and hypoxia. Sepsis should be prevented by early use of antibiotics, appropriate débridement of devitalized tissue, and prompt drainage of pus. Early total parenteral nutrition to prevent malnutrition in critically ill patients is essential. Installation of antacids to maintain the gastric pH greater than 3.5, or possibly greater than 6, appears to be beneficial. Although it will not prevent all stress ulcers, cimetidine appears to be effective and should be used together with antacids. Coagulation abnormalities should be looked for regularly and corrected, if possible, using plate-lets, fresh-frozen plasma, and vitamin K. If the bleeding cannot be controlled, surgery should be considered. Remember that regardless of treatment, if the stress is not removed—that is, infection is not adequately controlled—the patient most likely will not survive.

Often in critically ill patients, but not always, organ systems fail in a sequential pattern. Respiratory failure usually occurs first, followed in order by cardiac, renal, hepatic, hematologic, and gastrointestinal failure. This pattern results from the frequency of occurrence of causative factors that result in failure of specific organs; organ susceptibility to the common factors of low flow, hypoxia, malnutrition, and sepsis; preexisting organ disease; and the effect of failure of one organ on others.

Many factors contribute to pulmonary failure, so it occurs commonly in critically ill patients. The resultant hypoxia must be corrected promptly or it will contribute to failure of other organs.

Cardiac failure usually results from a combination of preexisting disease, low-flow states, hypoxia, and increased cardiac work owing to stress and sepsis. It often occurs insidiously and may not be recognized even though it is contributing to respiratory failure and decreased organ perfusion, both of which contribute to multiple organ failure. As tissue hypoxia and ischemia increase, anaerobic metabolism increases and lactic acidosis occurs, which, in turn, will tend to decrease cardiac function still more.

When pulmonary and cardiac failure occur simultaneously, particularly in association with continued sepsis, renal failure becomes likely. Of course, if the patient is receiving a nephrotoxic antibiotic, if a major transfusion reaction takes place, or if the patient has been in shock, renal failure can occur independently.

Following shock, if no other factors contributed to specific organ failure, renal and, later, hepatic failure would be most likely to occur because these organs are especially susceptible to low-flow states. The lungs, kidneys, liver, and coagulation factors, in that order, appear to be more susceptible to sepsis than is the heart.

As sepsis, malnutrition, hypoxia, or hypoperfusion continues, the liver begins to fail. Failure of protein synthesis for cell structure and essential substances leads to further multiple organ failure. The decreased plasma albumin concentration results in generalized edema, which can adversely affect the function of all organs. The decreased synthesis of clotting factors will contribute to a coagulopathy that is likely already to have begun to develop. Progressive hepatic failure will contribute to renal failure by way of the increased bile pigments and also by unknown humoral effects—the hepatorenal syndrome.

Coagulopathy usually begins after prolonged sepsis and starvation and progresses as renal and hepatic failure occur. A marrow-depressant drug, such as chloramphenicol, can cause a coagulopathy to occur earlier.

With continued sepsis, malnutrition, respiratory or cardiac failure, and often renal and hepatic failure, stress bleeding occurs. Bleeding will be worse if a coagulopathy is present or if the patient is being dialyzed and the heparin used regionally is not fully reversed—a not uncommon occurrence. It is likely that gastrointestinal bleeding will occur earlier if the patient has an ulcer diathesis, received ulcerogenic drugs, or did not receive adequate prophylactic ulcer therapy. If, as a result of gastrointestinal bleeding, hypoperfusion and shock occur, all organs will deteriorate even more rapidly.

As multiple organ failure progresses, a point is reached when a vicious cycle begins and the treatment of one failing organ makes the function of another worse. For example, in cardiac and pulmonary failure, mechanical ventilation or PEEP will improve oxygenation and ventilation but will tend to decrease further the output of a failing heart. Diuretics will decrease pulmonary edema and improve respiratory function, but frequently will decrease the output of a failing heart further by decreasing the required elevated pre-load. Conversely, by giving fluids to increase the pre-load of a failing heart to improve the cardiac output and tissue perfusion, pulmonary failure is made worse. In addition, inotropic agents required to increase the output of a failing heart will cause a redistribution of a pulmonary blood flow and increase the pulmonary shunt, causing still more hypoxia. Thus, when pulmonary and cardiac failure occur simultaneously, a point is reached when the treatment of one makes the other worse and progressive failure of both leads to rapid multiple organ failure.

Similarly, the treatment of cardiac and renal failure may not be compatible. The removal of water by dialysis may decrease the required pre-load of a failing heart and result in hypotension. Intravenous fluid and albumin given to reverse the hypotension associated with dialysis may mitigate some of the beneficial effect of dialysis. Vasopressors, also given to raise a falling blood pressure during dialysis, are likely to affect the failing heart adversely by increasing the afterload.

When cardiac, pulmonary, or renal failure are present, the volume of parenteral nutrition may be limited. When renal or hepatic failure occurs, volume and protein content of parenteral nutrition may be limited. As it progresses, malnutrition will result directly in failure of all organ systems and indirectly in failure as well, by contributing to decreased immune response and enhancing sepsis. As sepsis continues, antibiotics which might be beneficial in controlling the infection may have to be withheld because of toxic effects on failing kidneys, liver, or bone marrow.

In summary, the best treatment of multiple organ failure is prevention of the many causative factors or, if this is not possible, early detection and correction. Attention to details may prevent progressive multiple organ failure. Adequate perfusion, ventilation, and oxygenation should be maintained. Infection should be prevented by judicious use of antibiotics and appropriate surgery when necessary. Malnutrition should be prevented by early total parenteral nutrition. If failure of an organ is suspected, do not guess at the proper therapy, and then wait for hours to see if it is efficacious. Rather, make definitive measurements so that correct therapy can be begun promptly and maintained precisely. Critically ill patients have no tolerance for the wrong therapy or delay in the correct therapy. Failure of one organ affects the function of other organs; in time, a vicious cycle sets in, when treatment of one failing organ adversely affects the function of other organs. At this point, progressive multiple organ failure results, and survival becomes unlikely.

SELECTED READINGS

MULTIPLE ORGAN FAILURE

Baue, A. E.   Multiple, progressive, or sequential systems failure. *Arch. Surg.* 110:779, 1975.

Berk, J. L.   If you don't know. *Arch. Surg.* 112:17, 1977.

Eiseman, B., Beart, R., and Norton, L.   Multiple organ failure. *Surg. Gynecol. Obstet.* 144:323, 1977.

Moore, F. D.   Low flow states: Differences between trauma and sepsis. *Antibiot. Chemother.* 21:44, 1976.

SEPSIS AND IMMUNOSUPPRESSION

Alexander, J. W.   Emerging concepts in the control of surgical infections. *Surgery* 75:934, 1974.

Constantian, M. B., Menzoian, J. O., Nimberg, R. B., Schmidt, K., and Mannick, J. A.   Association of a circulating immunosuppressive polypeptide with operative and accidental trauma. *Ann. Surg.* 185:73, 1977.

Kaplan, J. E., Scovill, W. A., Bernard, H., and Saba, T. M.   Reticulo-endothelial phagocytic response to bacterial challenge after traumatic shock. *Circ. Shock* 4:1, 1977.

McLoughlin, G. A., Wu, A. V., Saporoschetz, A., Nimberg, R. B., and Mannick, J. A.   Correlation between anergy and a circulating immunosuppressive factor following major surgical trauma. *Ann. Surg.* 190:297, 1979.

Meakins, J. L., Pietsch, J. B., Bubenick, O., Kelly, R., Rode, H., Gordon, J., and MacLean, L. D.   Delayed hypersensitivity: Indicator or acquired failure of host defenses in sepsis and trauma. *Ann. Surg.* 186:241, 1977.

Schildt, B. E.   The present view of RES and shock. *Adv. Exp. Med. Biol.* 73:375, 1976.

Scovill, W. A., Saba, T. M., Caplain, J. E., Bernard, H. R., and Powers, S. R., Jr.   Disturbances in circulating opsonic activity in man after operative and blunt trauma. *J. Surg. Res.* 22:709, 1977.

METABOLISM AND NUTRITION

Bistrian, R. R., Blackburn, A. L., and Vitale, J. V.   Prevalence of malnutrition in general medical patients. *J.A.M.A.* 235:1567, 1967.

Border, J. R., Chenier, R., McMenamy, R. H., LaDuca, J., Seibel, R., Birkhahn, R., and Yu, L.   Multiple systems organ failure: Muscle fuel deficit with visceral protein malnutrition. *Surg. Clin. North Am.* 56:1147, 1976.

Cahill, G. F., Jr.   Starvation in man. *N. Engl. J. Med.* 282:668, 1970.

Duke, J. H., Jorgensen, S. B., and Broel, J. R.   Contributions of protein to caloric expenditure following injury. *Surgery* 68:168, 1970.

Fitzgerald, F.   Clinical hypophosphatemia. *Ann. Rev. Med.* 29:177, 1978.

Kinney, J. M. (Ed.).   *Proceedings of a Conference on Energy Metabolism and Body Fuel Utilization*. Cambridge: Harvard University Press, 1966.

Kinney, J. M., Long, C. L., and Gump, F. E.   Tissue composition of weight loss in surgical patients. *Ann. Surg.* 168:459, 1968.

Wilmore, D. W.   Hormonal responses and their effect on metabolism. *Surg. Gynecol. Obstet.* 56:999, 1976.

RESPIRATORY FAILURE

Berk, J. L.   The respiratory distress syndrome. *Primary Cardiol.* 6:69, 1980.

Collins, J. A.   The acute respiratory distress syndrome. *Adv. Surg.* 11:171, 1977.

Wilson, R. F.   Acute respiratory failure. *Crit. Care Med.* 4:79, 1976.

HEPATIC FAILURE

Champion, H. R., Jones, R. T., Trump, B. F., Decker, R., Wilson, S., Stega, M., Nolan, R., Crowley, R. A., and Gill, W.   Post-traumatic hepatic dysfunction as a major etiology in post-traumatic jaundice. *J. Trauma* 16:650, 1976.

Norton, L., Moore, G., and Eiseman, B.   Liver failure in the post-operative patient: The role of sepsis and immunologic deficiency. *Surgery* 78:6, 1975.

Nunes, G., Blaisdell, F. W., and Margaretten, W.   Mechanisms of hepatic dysfunction following shock and trauma. *Arch. Surg.* 100:546, 1970.

Sarfeh, I. J., and Balint, J. A.   Hepatic dysfunction following trauma: Experimental studies. *J. Surg. Res.* 22:370, 1977.

COAGULOPATHY

Bergentz, S.   On bleeding and clotting problems in the post-traumatic states. *Crit. Care Med.* 4:41, 1976.

John M. Kinney / 2. DESIGN OF THE INTENSIVE CARE UNIT

Intensive care is a concept as old as our knowledge of critically ill and injured patients, but the concept of specific hospital units for intensive care has emerged only in the past 20 years. Many factors have contributed to the evolution of intensive care units (ICUs), particularly the postanesthesia recovery room. In the United States, the recovery room did not gain widespread acceptance until the period 1948 to 1960. During a comparable period, 1960 to 1972, the integration of intensive care units into modern hospital practice took place. The major questions regarding units for intensive care no longer involve their acceptance in principle but, rather, learning to employ them most effectively within the economic restraints of hospital operation in the 1980s.

The concept of the ICU has had many and diverse origins. However, it is important to note that the rate of growth in intensive care depends in part on the degree to which the design of each unit is appropriate for the needs of that particular institution. The success of the multidisciplinary ICU in the community hospital was belatedly recognized and emulated by teaching hospitals. Then small (4–6 beds) to medium-sized (6–12 beds) units were organized to meet the needs of a single clinical service, such as cardiology, surgery, or pediatrics. Respiratory care units arose as the iron lung was superseded by more sophisticated bedside devices for mechanical ventilation. Renal dialysis, cardiac pacemakers, and other life support systems were developed and applied to the growing number of acute clinical problems. Complex hemodynamic and physiologic measurements began to be used more and more to analyze and evaluate therapy in shock and trauma patients with multiple injuries and perhaps failure of more than one vital organ system.

This growth has been followed by large integrated multidisciplinary critical care centers that include extensive laboratory and subspecialty support. Within such an organization, many kinds of intensive care are provided for different types of patients, but with a maximum effort to avoid unnecessary duplication of space, staff, and equipment.

The good ICU is the "hospital's hospital." It represents all the assets and advantages that a given institution should be able to mobilize for the management of the critically ill patient. It should represent none of its liabilities. Administrative or staff problems, problems in supporting services, and so on, which may be tolerated in ordinary hospital operation, become intolerable in the intensive care setting.

Probably no other field of medicine is more dynamic, more volatile, more diverse, and more creative than intensive care medicine. Part of the fascinating evolution of the ICU has involved the development of design. A creative design can do much to maximize the benefits accruing from the application of professional skill and technology to patient care; an improper or inflexible design can be a hindrance to the staff and may actually pose problems of safety for the patient.

Once the decision has been made that a particular hospital might benefit from developing a new ICU, a planning committee should be appointed. The committee should include a representative of the hospital administration, a member of the nursing staff, one member of each of the hospital professional services that might use the ICU, and the chief anesthesiologist or his delegate. The initial purpose of the committee should be to write the specific objectives of the proposed ICU, the types of patients to be admitted, and how the length of stay in the unit is to be determined. The committee should make an analysis of the number of potential patients, the most common diagnoses represented, and the estimated average length of stay in an ICU. The survey should cover a sufficiently long period to give representative data (usually 3–6 months).

Clarity of objectives and accuracy of information regarding potential demand for ICU care will greatly assist both staff and consultants in deciding between conflicting alternatives as to size, location, design, and staffing. At the present time, the field is too young and professional opinions too varied to expect an architect to produce the best design for an ICU with the same assurance that one would expect him to design more conventional areas of the hospital. The interested professional staff have a special obligation to study the matter themselves and to guide the architect toward the type of ICU they desire. Nowhere in hospital planning will detailed study by physicians yield greater dividends than with an ICU, where patient care, staff relations, and operating expenses are closely interconnected.

The planning committee for an ICU must represent breadth of background and interest but must *always remain patient-oriented*. This seemingly obvious phrase needs to be called to mind many times when compromises in the design or operation of an ICU are considered. Ironically, the ICU patient often can be forgotten in the preoccupation with elaborate equipment and emergency procedures. It is hard to preserve tranquility, courage, and kindness; but unless the patient is totally oblivious to his surroundings, the need for these qualities is nowhere greater than in an ICU.

BED CAPACITY OF AN INTENSIVE CARE UNIT

An ICU tends to have larger and more unpredictable fluctuations in patient census than any other area in the hospital. This emphasizes the importance of proper selection of the number of beds for a proposed ICU. A unit that is filled year round with patients needing intensive care would imply a significant number of additional patients who are denied intensive care because of the lack of accommodations. However, an ICU with enough beds to meet occasional peak demands has an unnecessarily high operational cost per bed resulting from the low average bed occupancy. Each institution must determine the number of ICU beds that represents an appropriate compromise between maximal bed occupancy and maximal hospital service. The process of achieving this compromise requires educating the professional staff to expect a few periods during the year when peak demands cannot be fully met, and educating the hospital administration to expect a lower average occupancy than elsewhere in the hospital. An ICU may have an average occupancy of less than 50 percent during the first year of operation, but it will rise gradually as the professional staff gains direct experience with the advantages of such a unit for the critically ill patient. A nursing unit of proper design for intensive care can function well for many less demanding types of medical care. Unfortunately, an attempt to provide true intensive care in a conventional area of the hospital is seldom successful.

One measure of the appropriate number of beds for an ICU is the total number of beds in the institution or portion of the institution that would supply patients to the ICU. Most estimates place the number of ICU beds at 3 to 6 percent of the total beds. It is usually not practical to develop the special nursing staff and facilities required for a separate ICU if the unit is to contain fewer than 4 beds. Thus, hospitals of less than 75 to 100 beds cannot ordinarily support an ICU. The opposite limit in size appears to be 12 to 15 beds, since more beds cause difficulty in providing intensive nursing care from a single nursing station. Institutions requiring more than 12 to 15 ICU beds should consider subdividing a single unit into two or more nursing areas.

The total need for ICU beds must take into account the expected average stay for the patient population to be served. Acutely ill postoperative patients have an average stay from 3 to 5 days, unless the postoperative period is complicated by major infection or specific organ failure. The average stay in the latter group is usually between 2 and 4 weeks.

A hospital organized for progressive patient care will have a larger intensive care section than that discussed previously, usually amounting to between 10 and 20 percent of the total institutional beds it serves. The level of professional care is usually geared to routine postoperative convalescence rather than to the occasional patient who represents a complicated therapeutic challenge.

RELATION TO SPECIAL AREAS AND SPECIAL DISORDERS

The proper location for a single ICU is determined by many factors. Among them are the types of local patients with greatest need for intensive care, the availability of space, and the particular interests of the physicians who will be responsible for the unit. Hospitals may elect to locate an ICU adjacent to a recovery room, an emergency ward, or wards already specializing in a particular type of clinical problem. The majority of hospitals have an ICU that is integrated to some degree with the recovery room. This is often the case because (1) the ICU has a large number of postoperative patients; (2) the ICU concept is considered to be an extension of recovery room care; or (3) the anesthesiologist is expected to assume responsibility for the ICU (as he often does for the recovery room), because of his special knowledge of ventilatory problems and inhalation therapy.

The relation of an ICU to the recovery room is partly a matter of the size of the institution. Hospitals of less than 75 beds usually keep intensive care patients in the recovery room facilities, using the same nurses and equipment. The ICUs in hospitals of 75 to 150 beds are often located adjacent to the recovery room, with certain of the nursing staff and equipment in common. Hospitals of intermediate size (150–300 beds) usually find their need for intensive care great enough and their interests broad enough to warrant building at least one ICU independent of the recovery room. The unit may still serve as a recovery room nights and weekends when the regular recovery room is not in operation. Larger hospitals (over 300 beds) may decide that requirements for intensive care are great enough and sufficiently diversified to justify the construction of several ICUs, each oriented around a particular type of patient. The advantages of sharing nurses and equipment when multiple units are located adjoining one another must be weighed against the more frequent visits of the medical staff to an ICU located closer to the area of their customary activities. Weil and Shubin [7] have pioneered in the concept of multiple ICUs grouped together as a center for critical care medicine.

Since not all smaller hospitals require a separate ICU, have space for it, or can afford it, it is important to consider carefully the advantages and disadvantages of a combined ICU–recovery room. The beds, utilities, resuscitative aids, monitoring devices, and so on are identical for the most part. Patient diseases may differ, but there are certain similarities in the nursing care that is required. The *advantages* of this combination for the smaller hospital are threefold: (1) economy of space, equipment, and personnel; (2) increased flexibility of operation—beds not needed for one phase may be utilized for the other; (3) availability of postanesthesia care on a 24-hour-a-day, seven-day-a-week basis, which is not practical for the recovery rooms of most smaller hospitals. For the anesthesiologist and surgeons, there is the added convenience of having a location near the operating room.

Unfortunately, the *disadvantages* of this combination are often not so carefully considered. It is obvious that there may be some interference with recovery room functions by intensive care requirements, and vice versa. Patients who might infect others cannot be treated in a combination ICU–recovery room, since the recovery room is technically a part of the operating room. This rule denies admittance to seriously ill patients who have infections, although they may require intensive care even more than other patients who are admitted. When there is a combined facility, the physical design is generally that of the single large room with curtained bed areas, dictated by the need for surveillance in a recovery room. Curtains are available for privacy in a recovery room, but they are seldom closed, since they obstruct nursing surveillance. Such a facility may be satisfactory when the patient spends a few hours recovering from anesthesia and when awareness and need for privacy are minimal. Some ICU patients are sick enough to be oblivious to their surroundings; others are conscious of their surroundings, and their fears are heightened by watching acutely ill patients around them. The lack of privacy and the extra apprehension that may be aroused in a patient residing in an open recovery room for many days can be a significant deterrent to recovery.

A new factor is now seen as relevant when choosing the proper location of an ICU within the hospital—namely, the availability of space for step-down beds. Step-down beds allow for transfer of patients who need continued monitoring or skilled care at a level less than that provided in the parent ICU. Many ICUs suffer from overcrowding and unnecessary pressure to admit more patients than they can properly care for, simply because there are no suitable hospital beds for this intermediate level of care that is necessary until the patient is ready for routine floor care in the hospital. It is important that step-down beds be located close to the parent ICU so that the professional staff of the intensive care unit can follow patients within the step-down unit, and also patients who are being monitored by electrocardiogram telemetry outside of the unit. Because of progressively more stringent financial limits being placed on hospital operations, nursing coverage on the ordinary floor tends to be marginal at best. Therefore, if step-down beds are not available, patients will be held in the ICU longer than might otherwise be necessary, leading to overcrowding and inefficient operation. The design requirements for step-down beds from the ICU will undoubtedly apply to more and more general care beds in future hospital designs.

Special considerations arise for units designed to provide intensive care for a special type of disorder. The premature nursery is a long-established specialized ICU. The evolution of mechanical ventilatory assistance has been followed by the appearance of special respiratory units. The particular skills required for the management of mechanical ventilators and tracheostomy patients necessitate detailed training for both nursing and medical staff. Special ICUs devoted to cardiac patients have arisen because of the particular usefulness of electronic monitoring of such patients and the need for equipment for electrical pacing of the heart as well as defibrillation. The recognition that a high proportion of deaths during convalescence from myocardial infarction occurs during the first 48 to 72 hours makes the continuous monitoring of the ECG during this period assume extra significance.

In addition to premature infants and cardiac patients, there are two categories of surgical patients for whom special skill and equipment are needed in the postoperative period, both in the recovery phase following anesthesia and during the first few days of convalescence: patients undergoing open heart surgery and those having neurosurgical procedures. In larger institutions, each service may develop a special area that functions as both recovery room and ICU.

The nature and complexity of the management of burn patients have stimulated interest in the design of specialized units or centers for the care of burns. Despite the special nature of the clinical problem, the same fundamental principles apply to the design and operation of a burn unit as to other ICUs.

THE DESIGN OF AVAILABLE SPACE

After the decision has been reached as to the appropriate location and number of beds for a proposed ICU, the problems of design must be faced. An ICU for a new building often may assume whatever shape is considered best: rectangular, square, or even circular. However, the majority of ICUs are built by reconstruction of existing hospital space, which is commonly an L-shaped or rectangular area in a wing of the hospital. An ICU built as a large, single room with curtained bed areas provides maximal surveillance with minimal floor space per bed and the poorest control of cross-infection. It exposes the patient to a high level of noise and activity, offering a minimum of privacy and opportunity for visitors. An ICU composed of individual patient rooms has the opposite advantages and disadvantages. Rigid-walled cubicles with floor-to-ceiling partitions on each side are often a reasonable compromise, with glass panels at an appropriate height (usually 48 in) on each side allowing the patient to be seen by a nurse but providing a visual barrier and a partial sound barrier between patients lying in adjacent beds.

The area devoted to each bed in a large open room is usually from 70 to 100 square feet, a rigid-walled cubicle requires 100 to 140 square feet, and separate rooms usually require 140 to 180 square feet per bed (plus approximately 50 square feet if a toilet is included). The total area of an ICU generally approximates two and one-half to three times the area allotted for beds alone. Thus, a 10-bed unit with 1,300 square feet allotted to bed space might require a total of 3,000 to 4,000 square feet for the complete unit.

The ideal ICU is designed to permit surveillance from the nurses' station to each bed area, while guaranteeing privacy for patients. Some surgical ICUs have been designed similarly to postanesthesia recovery rooms, which are large and open with curtained bed areas; the curtains in such rooms are usually drawn back to provide maximum surveillance from a single nurses' station. This arrangement is effective for its purpose, namely, to provide semiconscious patients a few hours of skilled care while they return to full consciousness. Such arrangements become progressively less desirable when patients remain for several days or weeks, during which they are exposed to critically ill patients. A standard rule of ICU design should be that "no patient's bed should remain exposed simply because it is necessary for surveillance to be maintained from the nurses' station to a more distant bed." Patients vary in the relative amount of surveillance or privacy appropriate for their level of consciousness, individual personality, and stage of convalescence. The optimum design of an ICU will be sufficiently flexible to allow any particular patient the proper balance between surveillance and privacy at any given time.

Studies of nurses preparing and administering drugs on a conventional hospital ward have shown that an average of 18 percent, or one medication in every six, was in error. Two major causes of medication errors are haste and interruptions. The nurses' station of an ICU is, of necessity, the focal point of a high-activity area. This increased chance of error is coupled with the greater seriousness of an error in some of the critically ill patients. Therefore, to minimize the chances for error, the medicine preparation area should be located where a nurse may be partially protected from the frequent interruptions at the nurses' station.

One of the crucial aspects of ICU design is allowing adequate space for all necessary functions thereby avoiding the inefficiency and frustration inherent to overcrowding. When there is inadequate space in an ICU, it is nearly always the nurses' station that suffers. Conferences about critically ill patients and teaching conferences for students are often held in the nurses' station. The medicine preparation area is often inappropriately placed in the busiest part of the nurses' station. Collection of laboratory data and entry into the hospital chart are often done in the nurses' station. If doctors have no other convenient location, they sit in the nurses' station to write progress notes. Extra supplies are often stored in the nurses' station. Obviously, the conventional nurses' station on any hospital floor is inadequate to accommodate the extra volume of activity in an ICU. The proper functions of the nurses' station should be considered in detail when the ICU is being designed and appropriate space should be designated for each task.

Before actual construction is begun on an ICU, it is extremely helpful to have a life-sized mock-up constructed of a standard bed area and the nurses' station. Physicians and nurses will take more interest in such a model than in blueprints, and thus it will elicit more suggestions and criticisms that should be considered while changes are relatively inexpensive.

There are obvious advantages to having the distance between nursing station and patient as short as possible. This contributes not only to nursing efficiency but sometimes also to a patient's sense of security. The size of the corridor around a central nurses' station must be a compromise between unnecessary distance to the patient and adequate space to accommodate the traffic of equipment, housekeeping sterile supplies, and so on, as well as the movement of medical personnel. Optimal ICU design involves provision for access of outside carts and bulky equipment to the utility and storage areas without interfering with traffic around the nurses' station.

Appropriate mechanical and electrical connections for each bed area will depend on the type of patient to be cared for. Two suction outlets are usually adequate, but three may occasionally be useful (e.g., for a patient with a chest tube and gastric suction who requires frequent tracheal suction). There are seldom too many wall electrical outlets near the bed; two duplex receptacles is the minimum required. One circuit should have a heavy amperage fuse for the operation of a cooling blanket. A portion of the total electrical outlets and lights should be connected to an emergency power system that is appropriately labeled. Conventional oxygen humidifiers are relatively inefficient, and heated humidifiers should be included as part of the standard ICU equipment.

The lighting of the ICU patient area requires extensive thought. The patient, the nurse, and the physician each requires a different level of illumination. Lighting levels required in the room range from a fraction of a footcandle for night-lighting up to 100 footcandles or more for examination or treatment. Several levels between these extremes are needed for patients' use and for routine nursing care. Central lighting should be arranged for appropriate intensity and color tones. Ceiling lighting above each bed should be designed to minimize the glare in a patient's eyes but still provide bright lighting promptly in an emergency. A dimmer can add flexibility and comfort to a standard lighting arrangement.

Controversy persists regarding the value of windows in an ICU. The issue is not a lack of ventilation or illumination (these are taken care of by air conditioning and artificial lighting) but, rather, the absence of visual stimulation. Wilson described the high incidence of postoperative delirium among patients deprived of windows. Keep emphasized that both patients and staff in ICUs showed evidence of stress caused by deprivation of visual stimuli from the outside world. Taylor has recently deplored the absence of windows in ICUs, noting that they are as important in a hospital as in an office or factory.

The floor plan of a 10-bed ICU shown in Figure 2-1 has been designed to fit into the wing of an existing hospital, using common outside dimensions and accommodating weight-bearing columns at 24-foot intervals. Approximately 65 percent of the space is devoted to the patient bed area and nursing station, with 35 percent for supporting functions that will allow the unit to function semiindependently from other wards in the hospital.

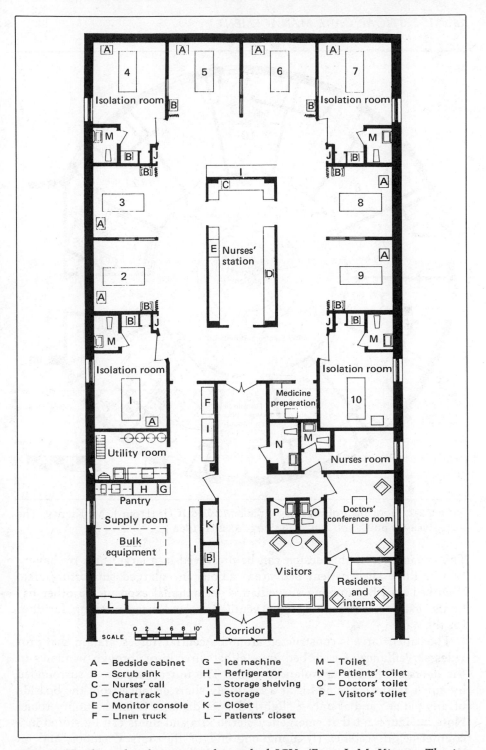

FIGURE 2-1. Floor plan for rectangular 10-bed ICU. (From J. M. Kinney, The intensive care unit. *Bull. Am. Coll. Surg.* 51:201, 1966.)

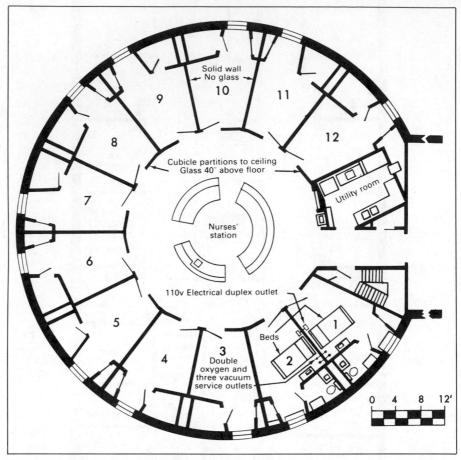

FIGURE 2-2. Floor plan of an early circular 12-bed ICU. (From J. M. Kinney, The intensive care unit. *Bull. Am. Coll. Surg.* 51:201, 1966.)

The advantages of this design can be preserved in a larger unit by having two or three such patient bed areas adjoin an enlarged supporting area. Each bed area has nursing surveillance yet minimal exposure to other patients, independent lighting and ventilation, and hand-washing facilities for the staff.

The patient area is constructed around a central nurses' station that provides surveillance of each bed area, either directly or through windows in the doors of the corner isolation rooms. The nurses' station is surrounded by ample traffic space and is at a relatively short distance from the bedside of any patient and at only a slightly longer distance from the utility room. Note in Figure 2-1 that emergency sterile kits and fluids can be stored in a counter-height cabinet (*I*) along one end of the nurses' station and on shelves of cabinets adjacent to the door of each patient room (*J*). The medicine preparation area has been removed from the nurses' station and placed in a separate but nearby location to reduce errors owing to preparing medications in the midst of other urgent activities.

The 10 beds are accommodated in six cubicles and four rooms, providing a basic set of utilities and services for each bed. The rooms are shown with permanent walls, but each pair of cubicles is divided by a removable floor-to-ceiling partition. The partition is composed of (1) a solid panel that provides privacy between the head ends of adjacent beds and (2) window panels between cubicles for surveillance by nurses while outside the nurses' station. There is ample floor area around each cubicle bed for immediate use of bulky equipment. However, if more extensive space is needed about a single bed, orderlies can promptly remove and store the three panels of the partition, leaving a single open area instead of any of the three pairs of cubicles. Conversion of each pair of cubicles would accommodate six extra stretchers for temporary care of multiple casualties.

The patients' toilet will accommodate a wheelchair and is separate from toilets for staff and visitors. A nurses' lounge, physicians' conference room, and residents' room are conveniently located, yet out of the high activity area. A visitors' area with toilet, adjoining the entry to the unit, is a small investment in space that yields big dividends in goodwill from patients' families. Outside traffic for supplies and disposal can reach the utility and storage area without entering the patient area.

Physicians who come to the ICU from outside the hospital often have no place for their coats and hats, which are then dropped on the first unoccupied bed. A coat closet, washbasin, and closet for white coats has therefore been placed just inside the door opposite the visitors' area.

The floor plan for a circular 12-bed ICU, designed by Ellerbe & Company and constructed at the Methodist Hospital, Rochester, Minnesota, is shown in Figure 2-2. It preserves the shortest radius of nursing travel for a number of beds, combined with the features available in private rooms. Extensive studies of nursing efficiency in a circular unit have been reported. The primary disadvantage is that circular buildings are uncommon, and such a design is thus usually practical only in a new building. The plan that is shown has minimal space for supporting function and storage; this could be provided at the expense of bed area or obtained in adjoining space if available. The need for ample traffic space about the nurses' station is the same for the circular design as for the rectangular unit shown in Figure 2-1.

Sometimes there is need for a small ICU when the only available space is a narrow rectangle. The floor plan in Figure 2-3 demonstrates a 5-bed unit within the restrictions of a narrow rectangle. The same basic principles of bed location and patient care that were noted for the rectangular unit are available in this smaller unit. Two isolation rooms and three cubicles are provided, with a nursing station that is approximately equidistant from each bed. However, it is evident that the smaller the bed capacity of

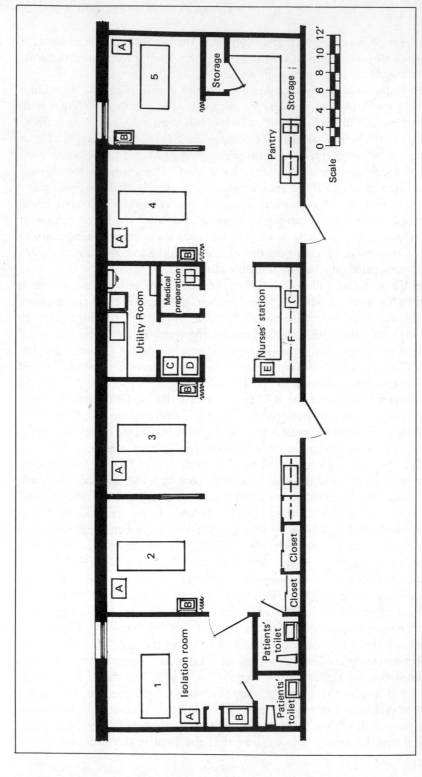

FIGURE 2-3. Floor plan for rectangular 5-bed ICU. (A) bedside cabinet; (B) scrub sink; (C) ice machine; (D) refrigerator; (E) nurses' call; (F) chart rack; (G) monitor console. (From J. M. Kinney, The intensive care unit. *Bull. Am. Coll. Surg.* 51:201, 1966.)

TABLE 2-1. Facilities and Space Provided by ICUs of Various Capacities

Area and Facility	12-Bed Circular Unit (sq ft)	10-Bed Rectangular Unit (sq ft)	5-Bed Rectangular Unit (sq ft)
Minimum cubicle	variable	126	126
Isolation room with toilet	176	235	195
Total area	3,846	4,655	1,440
Area per bed	321	465	288
Bed area plus nurses' station	3,520 est.	2,950	variable
Supporting area	variable	1,705	variable

an ICU, the more the unit will depend on the rest of the institution for supporting functions, such as equipment storage and facilities for staff.

Certain features of an ICU bed area require special attention. The ICU bed is a compromise that provides the comfort of a conventional hospital bed with a full-thickness mattress but is narrower than a standard bed and can be moved and positioned easily. There is ample floor space for a resuscitation team and bulky equipment around the bed. High-intensity emergency lighting is focused from the ceiling on the bed area. A movable lamp at the head of the bed provides a reading light and also low-intensity indirect lighting. Standard floor-mounted equipment and furniture are kept to a minimum. Wall panels behind the bed provide nurses' call and remote monitoring connections if desired. Three or four dual convenience receptacles provide adequate power; one is supplied by the hospital emergency power system. A minimum of two (preferably three) wall suction outlets should be available for patients with complex problems that might require separate suction for abdominal and chest tubes as well as airway suctioning. A heated humidifier supplies oxygen with approximately four times the water content per unit of gas as that supplied by the conventional cold humidifiers. Thus, it is important to mount the humidifier low enough so that water condensation in the tubing runs back to the humidifier and not onto the patient.

Excessive noise is now recognized as a health hazard, a form of pollution that harms physical and mental well-being. In the past, careful measurement of the noise levels in daily hospital operation has been neglected. A noise level of 75 decibels is considered an annoyance threshold prohibiting telephone conversation. A level of 65 decibels is the equivalent of listening to an electric typewriter 10 feet away. Some experts have recommended that the sound level in an ICU be held to 50 decibels, a sound level that allows normal conversation. The noise of daily activities in many hospitals exceeds this level at least part of the time. It is of interest that 35 decibels is considered the level that is appropriate for sleeping. The design of an ICU presents special problems because porous, sound-absorbent surfaces are difficult to sterilize, whereas smooth, hard-finish surfaces are easily cleaned with liquid germicide but have a high sound reflectant. Proper design criteria to reduce the noise levels of an ICU are not currently available; the development of such criteria is clearly needed. Also under study is the theory that soft music may be therapeutic for some patients.

ELECTRICAL MONITORING

There has been a rapid growth over recent years in electrical equipment designed for monitoring a patient in the operating room, recovery room, and ICU. Certain units are designed to present the information at a bedside unit; others send the information along cables to a central monitoring station at the nurses' desk. There, the information is usually presented on an oscilloscope that also has a device to record certain portions if desired. Most of this equipment has been used for continuous monitoring of the conventional vital signs (temperature, blood pressure, and cardiac electrical activity). Measurement of body temperature with a rectal probe is one of the most straightforward forms of electrical monitoring. However, this information is rarely of interest more often than every 4 hours. The production of an inexpensive, foolproof device for the automatic monitoring of blood pressure without arterial cannulation remains in the developmental stage. Information regarding heart rate is usually of secondary interest to more fundamental indications of circulation, such as central venous pressure and cardiac output. Pressures in a central vein or the pulmonary artery are commonly obtained as an intermittent bedside procedure, although by using catheters and strain gauges, continuous measurement is possible along with measurement of arterial pressure. Unfortunately, the monitoring of respiratory rate is largely an expensive tribute to tradition and offers little information on either minute or alveolar ventilation. Continuous ECG monitoring has been made more reliable by the introduction of new electrodes that reduce the artifacts associated with motion. Space research has hastened the application of telemetry to the transmission of physiologic monitoring signals. Thus, the patient of the future may be continuously monitored without the nuisance and restrictions of many wires and cords. Remote monitoring by telemetry, at its present stage of development, seems to offer the most benefit for the monitoring of cardiac patients.

Certain elaborate monitoring systems have been sold to hospitals as a result of the claim that the equipment would reduce the number of nurses required in the ICU. Our present understanding of physiologic disturbances in acutely ill patients is much too primitive to expect that such equipment can replace bedside nursing. *Electrical monitoring should be used to supplement nursing care, not to replace it!*

Since this field is developing rapidly and uncertainties remain about the best approach to monitoring, some ICUs are being constructed with large empty conduits between the nursing station and each bed area. Such arrangements depend on bedside monitoring now but will allow installation of future remote monitoring equipment if desired with a minimum of cost and disruption of the physical facilities.

ELECTRICAL HAZARDS

Patients in an ICU are often more vulnerable to electric shock than are healthy persons. Increased cardiac irritability results from hypoxia, electrolyte imbalance, and the effects of drugs. The increasing use of electrical devices for both monitoring and treating the patient, the use of two or more devices simultaneously on the patient, and the use of subcutaneous and intravascular electrodes have aroused increasing concern about the shock hazard to which a patient undergoing such treatment may be exposed. Unfortunately, the great majority of physicians are unaware of the extent of the hazards.

All equipment must be reliably grounded. Convenience receptacles throughout an ICU should accept three-pronged connections, and all electrical equipment used in an ICU should have sufficiently long cords with a three-pronged, or grounded, connector. Be sure that such connecting plugs are wired correctly, particularly if an amateur has replaced the plug. The cord and plug must have adequate current-carrying capacity. Never use cords that become hot when carrying current, and never use adaptors that permit the connection of nonmatching plugs and receptacles. Never use equipment with a two-pronged plug or extension cord without being aware of the lack of grounding.

Exposed plumbing has traditionally provided a pathway for grounding electrical equipment. Electric beds may also provide a contact between patient and ground, a hazard that is often overlooked. The dangers of operating electrical equipment while standing in the bathtub are well known, but few recognize the identical hazard for an incontinent patient when he tunes his radio while lying in a wet bed that is grounded through its power cord. Some authorities have recommended that electric beds not be used in intensive care units. Others have emphasized that doubly insulated electric beds can be used, permitting nursing staff the added convenience of electric power without electrical hazard to the patient.

Engineers have written building codes on the basis that electricity that cannot be felt is safe. Current building codes require that the current flowing through a grounded person touching an exposed metal part of electrical equipment be limited to 5 ma with a potential of only a few volts. Normal skin is a high-resistance barrier to the passage of electric current, but in ICU patients, a variety of transducers, electrodes, catheters, and probes penetrate the skin and thus allow current to be delivered directly to vital organs. It has become apparent to perceptive physicians that electrical currents too small to be sensed can precipitate ventricular fibrillation when delivered to the myocardium within the period of excitation. The amperages of these dangerous leakage currents are only a small percentage of that of current called "safe" by present building codes.

The combination of grounding and isolation affords the maximum safety that can be designed into equipment operated from the power line and intended for use on patients. Any electrical equipment can cause shock and death unless it is properly maintained and periodically tested. The most frequent hazard arises from simple and obvious things such as frayed cords and broken plugs. The following rules should regulate electrical usage in an ICU:

1. It must be assumed that patients are grounded and are thus liable to electric shock.
2. A single power source should be provided for the receptacles in each patient location.
3. The power distribution system must have an adequate ground system. The current in the ground bus must be checked daily.
4. All receptacles must be correctly connected and incorporate a connection for an equipment ground. Optimal conditions require a separate wire for the equipment ground running in the same conduit as the live conductor.
5. Electrical devices must have an integral three-wire cord long enough to provide the necessary mobility. The plug should match the receptacle. Adaptors and extension cords must not be used.
6. Electrical devices that are defective must never be used. The little shock felt by a nurse may be a lethal shock under other circumstances. The equipment cord and its plug must be physically intact.
7. Electrical devices that require the application of transducers or electrodes to the patient should have an isolation transformer in the power supply to minimize the exposure to electric faults in the distribution system and in other electrical appliances that are used simultaneously, as well as in the device itself.

ADMISSION OF INFECTED PATIENTS

Some institutions refuse admission of any infected patient to the ICU. Such a patient is then usually cared for by special nurses in a single room elsewhere in the hospital. The importance of being able to admit such patients to an ICU goes beyond the difficulty and expense of providing true intensive care outside the ICU. The no-admittance policy is often compromised by two factors: (1) the noninfected patient becomes infected while being cared for in the ICU, thus deserving intensive care even more; and (2) patients with borderline sepsis are tolerated in the ICU for various nonmedical reasons.

Isolation techniques in an ICU are similar (1) for containment of bacteria within the area occupied by a patient who disseminates bacteria and (2) for exclusion of bacteria from the premises occupied by a patient who is vulnerable to infection because of an endocrine, immunologic, or metabolic disturbance. Such isolation requires four interrelated objectives: definition of the patient care area, disinfection of the premises, control of exchange of bacteria, and removal of accumulating bacteria. The details of these techniques have been reviewed by Walter.

A poorly designed facility will defeat the best intentions to follow good isolation technique. The number and location of washbasins are important—"a distant basin is an unused basin." The floor and other horizontal surfaces should be designed to allow periodic cleaning with liquid germicide. Special items may represent unsuspected points of bacterial exchange (hand soap) or multiplication (the infrequently cleaned oxygen humidifier).

The ICU should be air-conditioned and its temperature maintained at approximately 75° F, with a relative humidity of 40 to 50 percent. The ICU should be maintained at a slight positive pressure relative to the outside corridor to prevent the infiltration of contaminated air. The significance of contact spread of bacteria is more readily accepted than that of airborne spread, yet a significant number of "contact" bacteria were airborne earlier in their movement about the ICU. A minimum ventilation of four air changes per hour is needed, and higher rates of ventilation will reduce the concentration of droplet nuclei and their associated bacteria. The ventilation system should be independent of other areas of the hospital, preferably with no recirculation. Each room and cubicle on the ICU should have an independent air inlet and exhaust, with the system balanced for equal pressure in the bed areas and elsewhere in the unit.

Because of the problems and expenses of providing an aseptic room or cubicle for an ICU patient, the utilization of clear, sterilizable plastic film is under investigation in several centers. Its uses include the construction of plastic walls with glove ports extending over the adjacent bed for nursing care, a sterile plastic enclosure around the patient and his mattress, and a ventilated sterile plastic bubble that allows the patient to maintain isolation while moving around in a wheelchair.

PSYCHIATRIC RESPONSE OF THE INTENSIVE CARE UNIT PATIENT

It is generally accepted that patients in a recovery room are unconcerned about the presence of other sick patients around them and often have amnesia for the hours immediately following their operations. This same lack of concern will certainly characterize some of the most severely ill patients in an ICU; however, many patients in an ICU not only are conscious but also are apprehensive. Therefore, it is of great importance that careless comments not be made in conversations between members of the ICU staff, since misinterpretation or exaggeration may cause needless worry for the patient. The undesirable effect on such a patient of watching a nearby patient have a convulsion or cardiac arrest is obvious. The most effective prevention of this needless stress to the ICU patient remains in the visual limits set for each patient by the ICU design.

The psychiatric evaluation of patients after open heart surgery has emphasized in another way the importance of the environment provided by the ICU. Many factors combine to produce sleeplessness and sensory deprivation, adding environmental stress to the acute medical and surgical problems at hand. Following such observations, Kornfeld has suggested the following environmental guidelines for the care of ICU patients:

1. Preserve the day-awake, night-asleep cycle whenever possible.
2. Provide individual rooms, to allow quiet and reduced lighting for sleep.
3. Keep all monitoring equipment away from the patient's view and hearing.
4. Eliminate constant, monotonous sounds (e.g., fans and blowers) if possible.
5. Provide a variety of stimuli, such as patient-controlled radio and television.
6. Provide a large clock and a calendar that are visible to each patient.

SELECTED READINGS

GENERAL DESIGN AND OPERATION

Beal, J. M., and Eckenhoff, J. E. (Eds.). *Intensive and Recovery Room Care.* London: Macmillan, 1969.

Burn, J. M. B. Design and staffing of an intensive care unit. *Lancet* 1:1040, 1970.

Burrell, L. O., and Burrell, Z. L. Intensive Care Unit: Physical Plan, Equipment and Policies. In *Intensive Nursing Care.* St. Louis: Mosby, 1973.

Collins, J. A., and Ballinger, W. F. The surgical intensive care unit. *Surgery* 66: 614, 1969.

Dornette, W. H. L. The Intensive Care Facility. I. Location, Capacity and Design. In *Anaesthesia Items and Inhalation Therapy Topics* 9(2), May 1963. Madison, Wis.: Ohio Chemical and Surgical Equipment Company.

Dornette, W. H. L. The Intensive Care Facility. II. Equipment, Staffing and Operation. In *Anaesthesia Items and Inhalation Therapy Topics* 9(3), August 1963. Madison, Wis.: Ohio Chemical and Surgical Equipment Company.

Goldin, M. D. (Ed.). *Intensive Care of the Surgical Patient.* Chicago: Wiley, 1974.

Kinney, J. M. National Academy of Sciences National Research Council, Committee on Anesthesia. In Workshop on Intensive Care Units. *Anesthesiology* 38:132, 1966.

Kinney, J. M. The intensive care unit. *Bull. Am. Coll. Surg.* 51:201, 1966.

Kinney, J. M., and Walter, C. W. The Design of an Intensive Care Unit. In J. M. Kinney, H. H. Bendixen, and S. R. Powers, Jr. (Eds.), *Manual of Surgical Intensive Care.* Philadelphia: Saunders, 1977.

The Planning and Operation of an Intensive Care Unit. Battle Creek, Mich.: W. K. Kellogg Foundation, 1961.

Robinson, J. S. The design and function of an intensive care unit. *Br. J. Anaesth.* 38:132, 1966.

Smith, R. W., et al. Evaluation of a Small Rural, Community Hospital Intensive Care Unit. In W. H. L. Dornette (Ed.), *Clinical Anesthesiology and Clinical Care.* Philadelphia: Davis, 1967.

Sturdavant, M., et al. *Comparison of Intensive Nursing Service in a Circular and Rectangular Unit.* Chicago: American Hospital Association, 1960.

U.S. Department of Health, Education and Welfare, Public Health Service, Division of Hospital and Medical Facilities. Elements of Progressive Care (Chap. 3, Part I). In *Intensive Care*. Washington, D.C., 1962.

Weil, M. H., and Shubin, H. Centralized Hospital Care for the Critically Ill. In P. Safar (Ed.), *Clinical Anesthesia*. Philadelphia: Davis, 1974.

Whalin, W. L., and van der Vliet, A. *Intensive Care*. London: Wiley, 1974.

Wiklund, P. E. Intensive care units: Design, location, staffing ancillary areas, equipment. *Anesthesiology* 31:122, 1969.

ELECTRICAL SAFETY

Aspinall, M. J. Guidelines for Electrical Safety (Appendix D). In *Nursing the Open-Heart Surgery Patient*. New York: McGraw-Hill, 1973.

Bruner, J. M. R. Hazards of electrical apparatus. *Anesthesiology* 28:2, 1967.

Phillips, D. F., and Peirson, P. S. NFPA approves new standards. *Hospitals* 47: 125, 1973.

Von der Mosel, H. A. Electrical safety and our hospitals. *J. Assoc. Adv. Med. Instrum.* 4:1, 1970.

Walter, C. W. Safe electric environment in the hospitals. *Bull. Am. Coll. Surg.* 54:4, 1969.

CROSS-INFECTION

Burke, J. F. A Bacterial Controlled Nursing Unit and Individual Patient Isolation Facility. In *Proceedings of International Conference on Nosocomial Infection. Center for Disease Control*. Chicago: American Hospital Association, 1971.

Davies, W. L., et al. Environmental control with laminar flow. *Hosp. Pharm.* 4:2, 1969.

Haynes, B. W., and Hench, M. E. Hospital isolation system for preventing cross-contamination by staphyloccocal and pseudomonas organisms in burn wounds. *Ann. Surg.* 162:641, 1965.

Walter, C. W. Isolation technique for containment or exclusion of bacteria for the prevention of cross-infection in hospitals. *Surg. Clin. North Am.* 43:897, 1963.

PSYCHOLOGICAL ASPECTS

Abram, H. S. Psychological aspects of the intensive care unit. *Hosp. Med.* 5:94, 1969.

Keep, P. J. Stimulus deprivation in windowless rooms. *Anesthesia* 32:598, 1977.

Kornfeld, D. S. Psychiatric view of the intensive care unit. *Br. Med. J.* 50:108, 1969.

Smith, J. S. Adverse Effects of Critical Care Units. In C. M. Huda, B. M. Gallo, and T. Lohr (Eds.), *Critical Care Nursing*. Philadelphia: Lippincott, 1973.

Taylor, L. The natural history of windows: A cautionary tale. *Br. Med. J.* 1:870, 1979.

Wilson, L. M. Intensive care delirium: The effect of outside deprivation in a windowless unit. *Arch Int. Med.* 130:225, 1972.

RESPIRATORY UNITS

Campbell, D., et al. Four years of respiratory intensive care. *Br. Med. J.* 4:255, 1967.

Petty, T. L., and Nett, L. M. The Respiratory Care Department. In *Intensive and Rehabilitative Respiratory Care* (2nd ed.). Philadelphia: Lea & Febiger, 1974.

CORONARY CARE UNITS

Church, G., and Biern, R. O. Intensive coronary care: A practical system for a small hospital without house staff. *N. Engl. J. Med.* 281:1155, 1969.

Killip, T., and Kimball, J. T. A survey of the coronary care unit: Concepts and results. *Prog. Cardiovasc. Dis.* 11:45, 1968.

Lown, B., et al. Coronary and pre-coronary care. *Am. J. Med.* 46:705, 1969.

NEONATAL UNITS

Gluck, L. The newborn special care unit; its role in the large medical center. *Hosp. Prac.* 3:33, 1968.

Gluck, L. Design of a perinatal center. *Pediatr. Clin. North Am.* 17:777, 1970.

Segal, S., and Pirie, G. E. Equipment and personnel for neonatal special care. *Pediatr. Clin. North Am.* 17:793, 1970.

BURN UNITS

Feller, I., and Crane, K. *Planning and Designing a Burn Care Facility.* Ann Arbor, Mich.: Institute for Burn Medicine, 1968.

Muir, I. F. K., and Barclay, T. L. (Eds.). Administrative Aspects of Burns. In *Burns and Their Treatment* (2nd ed.). Chicago: Year Book, 1974.

James E. Sampliner | 3. GENERAL CARE OF THE CRITICALLY ILL PATIENT

CARING FOR CRITICALLY ILL PATIENTS

The critically ill patient frequently comes to the intensive care unit (ICU) from the emergency room, from the operating room, or from another floor of the hospital and is often sedated or still unconscious from surgical anesthesia. When fully awake, he is confronted with unfamiliar surroundings and is often unable to talk because of an endotracheal tube or tracheostomy. In addition, the complex equipment and sophisticated monitoring techniques used in critical care units seem formidable. The patient is understandably confused and frightened. It is at this point that the physicians and staff must take the time to explain the situation to the patient. A well-informed patient is easier to care for and often requires less sedation than a bewildered one. Concern, compassion, and kindness help form a necessary base for the delivery of critical care and assist in easing patients' anxiety.

The ICU is also a stressful environment for the physicians and staff. Critically ill patients require constant attention, and their often total dependence on the staff intensifies the emotional strain placed on those responsible for the patients' care. Frequently, the ICU is filled, and the staff too busy to leave the unit during their shift. It is therefore helpful to provide the staff with a lounge where they can relax. Some units allow nurses and other staff members to rotate periodically out of the isolation and stress of the ICU to noncritical care floors. When feasible, this is probably a useful technique to employ. Also, there may be periods when the ICU will be relatively quiet. During these times, continuing education conferences can be held. In our institution, these conferences augment the daily patient teaching rounds. In addition, conferences should be held in which the members of the staff are allowed to verbalize their feelings toward patients.

The condition of critically ill patients changes rapidly, and at times a physician and nurse may have to remain at the patient's bedside almost continually. This type of situation emphasizes the need for precise patient management with attention to even the smallest detail. Aggressive investigation and therapy are often identified with the care of critically ill patients. Unfortunately, aggressiveness has a negative connotation to many physicians. In general, one need not institute therapy or change therapy in response to a single change in patient status; instead, one must investigate the cause of the change. To delay seeking the reason for a change in status because of the idea that the patient is doing well, or to ignore a single sign or symptom because one considers it spurious, can often prove disastrous. For example, hyperventilation is often encountered in critically ill patients. Many physicians assume that this reflects anxiety or pain, and undoubtedly sometimes this is the case; however, frequently hyperventilation and hypocapnia with respiratory alkalosis are signs of early sepsis [16, 17, 19]. When prompt therapy based on appropriate tests is instituted, one can often keep septic shock from occurring later in the course of the illness.

The goal of patient care in the ICU must be total body care, with attention to all of the body's organ systems. In this way, the morbidity and mortality associated with critical illness can be significantly reduced.

APPROACH TO THE CRITICALLY ILL PATIENT
GENERAL APPROACH
The management of critically ill patients presents a complex problem to the physicians responsible for their care. No one routine format will suffice for all ICU patients, but a general approach can be outlined that is useful with such patients [1]. Optimal management requires a multidisciplinary approach to the total patient—an integrated system of separate but interdependent subsystems, each requiring evaluation and appropriate therapy. One person must coordinate the efforts of all physicians caring for a given patient so that the best possible care can be delivered without conflict.

Because of the complex nature of critical illness, there is a tendency to treat the patient as an abstraction. To avoid this situation, the ICU physicians and staff should make special attempts to maintain physical contact with the patient and to communicate with the patient. The patients must be able to express their feelings to those responsible for their care; when the patient is on prolonged ventilatory assistance, this often requires special measures. In addition, the physicians and staff should explain procedures to be carried out to the patient and provide psychological support (see Chapter 22).

The patient's orientation as to time and place should be maintained. This can be done by the staff and by placing various aides (e.g., clocks, calendars, newspapers) at the bedside [15].

Frequently, physicians and staff stop to discuss a patient's case at the bedside. This is not a good practice, since the patient may overhear something that will cause him anxiety. It is important to remember that patients today know a great deal of medical terminology, which often leads to problems. The patient may understand only bits and pieces of a discussion and may arrive at an improper conclusion based on the words he has understood.

A physician should explain to the patient that a group of doctors and/or nurses will be coming by on rounds and that this is routine procedure. In addition, the patient should be told that a member of the medical staff will stop by following rounds to discuss any questions the patient might have. If these guidelines are followed, psychological stress can be minimized.

An effort should be made to arrange regular times for the physicians responsible for the patient's care to communicate with the family of the critically ill patient. In addition, the ICU staff should arrange a way to notify the family in the event of a change in the patient's condition.

Attention must be directed to organ systems that are not the cause of the patient's immediate problem. This avoids deterioration of another organ system or systems while intensive monitoring and therapy are directed to the current problem. In addition, it should be remembered that physiologic interrelationships and deterioration in one system may contribute to or precede the development of organ failure in another system.

Finally, it must be remembered that the ICU offers its facilities to those patients with a chance for survival [8]. On occasion, discontinuation of support may spare a patient and his family unduly prolonged suffering, both emotionally and financially. The dilemma of continuing aggressive therapeutic support versus offering only supportive care generates ethical and emotional problems for physicians, nursing staff, and patients' families. Solutions are not easy, but are necessary so as not to erode the care of the remaining critically ill patients and morale of the ICU.

Subsequent chapters in this handbook will provide specific information concerning each vital organ system. However, even in the care of the critically ill, a precise general care plan is necessary.

HISTORY AND PHYSICAL EXAMINATION

Obtain as much history as possible from either the patient or a family member. Particular attention should be paid to medications, allergies, bleeding disorders, and any other previous problems (particularly those relating to the current illness).

A rapid but thorough physical examination is essential, and particular attention should be paid to the cardiorespiratory system. The examination not only gives needed medical information but also provides physical contact between physician and patient.

BASELINE STUDIES

Simultaneously with the history and physical examination, baseline laboratory and physiologic measurements (e.g., vital signs, weight) should be obtained. In addition, the physician should note all indwelling lines and treatment agents being administered. In this way, he will have all necessary data available for his review shortly after the conclusion of the history and physical examination.

Before actually writing orders for the patient, the physician should enumerate the patient's problems and the goals of therapy and outline the plan of action that he will take.

WRITING THE ORDERS

The following are some general rules for writing physician's orders:

1. Orders should be written each morning and then reviewed throughout the day for changes that may be indicated by any change in the patient's condition.
2. The orders should be written clearly, so that misinterpretation is avoided.
3. The orders should be approached in a systematic, logical fashion. In this way, oversights in the orders will be avoided.

AMBULATION

While most critically ill patients will be confined to their beds, even patients on respirators can get out of bed. In addition, the patient should be turned in bed and encouraged to exercise his legs. The foot of the bed may be elevated when this is not contraindicated.

DIET

Diets of critically ill patients will vary, and specific nutritional considerations will be dealt with elsewhere. It is, however, important to give specific diet orders (e.g., amounts, concentrations, type, and route of administration).

INTRAVENOUS FLUIDS

The orders for intravenous fluids include the type of solution to be administered and the rate and route to be used (e.g., in patients with more than one intravenous line). The critically ill patient often presents a complicated fluid management problem. For this reason, it is probably desirable to write fluid orders for these patients every 8 hours, based on their intakes, outputs, temperatures, and chemical findings.

There is a tendency to replace abnormal losses (e.g., nasogastric suction, ileostomy drainage) with "standard solutions" (e.g., nasogastric suction is replaced milliliter for milliliter with normal saline). This, however, can lead to overreplacement or underreplacement in the critically ill patient. It is therefore desirable to collect aliquots of the drainage and have them analyzed. One then replaces the fluid loss with electrolyte solution or solutions, based on the electrolyte composition of the aliquots.

HYPONATREMIA. Hyponatremia is not an uncommon finding in critically ill patients. In most instances this is a reflection of water excess rather than of sodium depletion. The treatment therefore should include water restriction. Hyponatremia may also occur as a result of dilution (i.e., Na^+ and water losses replaced with water alone); it also may be due to inappropriate antidiuretic hormone secretion or to inability to dilute the urine (e.g., cirrhosis, congestive heart failure). Severe symptomatic hyponatremia rarely occurs until the serum Na^+ falls below 115 mEq/liter. In order to abolish symptoms, hypertonic saline (3% or 5%) can be used to correct the deficit. To calculate the Na^+ deficit:

(Desired Na^+ [mEq/L] − patient's Na^+ [mEq/L])
$$\times \text{ total body water (TBW) (liters)} = Na^+ \text{ deficit (mEq)}$$

Example
  Patient's weight = 70 kg
  TBW (in liters) = 0.6 × body weight
  Patient's TBW = 0.6 × 70 = 42 liters
  Desired serum Na^+ = 125 mEq/L
  Patient's serum Na^+ = 110 mEq/L
  Difference (125 − 110) = 15 mEq/L
  Deficit = 15 mEq/L × 42 = 630 mEq

The 630 mEq required is given carefully over a 24-hour period. It is best to use this calculation only as a guideline to sodium administration. In addition, the patient should be followed with serial serum sodium determinations.

The use of hypertonic sodium chloride may precipitate acute circulatory overload, and the patient must therefore be closely monitored (e.g., central venous pressure [CVP], or pulmonary artery and pulmonary capillary wedge pressures).

An alternative method of correcting hyponatremia using diuretics (e.g., furosemide) has been described [12]. This usually will correct the hyponatremia within 6 to 8 hours. The correction is based on replacement of urinary sodium and potassium losses, using 3% sodium chloride with supplemental potassium.

HYPOKALEMIA. Like hyperkalemia, hypokalemia is a potentially life-threatening situation. In severe hypokalemia (i.e., serum K^+ less than 2.5 mEq/liter with ECG abnormalities) KCl may be safely administered at a rate of up to 40 mEq/hr. A central vein should be used since KCl in this concentration will be too irritating for a peripheral vein.

SODIUM BICARBONATE. Acid-base imbalances are discussed in Chapter 16. However, metabolic acidosis is a subject that deserves added emphasis here.

When treating the patient with metabolic acidosis, the first priority must be the reestablishment of flow, to return tissue metabolism to an aerobic state. However, in certain situations it may be necessary to administer $NaHCO_3^-$ exogenously. Any attempt to assess bicarbonate deficit is fraught with difficulties, since one can only estimate extracellular deficits. The following is a useful formula that can serve as a guideline for $NaHCO_3^-$ administration:

$$mEq\ NaHCO_3^-\ deficit = base\ deficit \times 0.3 \times patient's\ weight\ (kg)$$

The deficit is replaced by administering one-half of the deficit and then re-calculating the deficit in 1 to 2 hours. In addition, one should remember that $NaHCO_3^-$ will lower serum K^+, and therefore one must pay close attention to serum K^+ when administering large amounts of $NaHCO_3^-$.

Example
  Patient's weight = 70 kg
  Base deficit = 18 mEq/L (as determined by blood gases)
  0.3 = extracellular $NaHCO_3^-$ space

$$NaHCO_3^-\ deficit\ (mEq) = 18 \times 0.3 \times 70 = 378\ mEq$$

The patient would be given 189 mEq (this is approximately 4 ampules, 45 mEq/amp) acutely, and the deficit would be calculated again in 1 to 2 hours.

Be careful not to create a metabolic alkalosis, with its detrimental effect on the oxyhemoglobin dissociation curve (see Chapter 24).

Intake and Output

The importance of strict intake and output records cannot be overemphasized. Each intake and output should be listed and totaled separately. In addition, the intake and output should be totaled every 8 hours and the cumulative and net fluid balances recorded. When conscientious fluid balance records are combined with daily weight measurements, the inadvertent overloading that often occurs in critically ill patients can be avoided.

Monitoring

The physician will record the parameters to be monitored and the frequency with which the monitoring is to be done. They include temperature, pulse, blood pressure, respirations, intravascular pressures (pulmonary artery and pulmonary capillary wedge pressure and CVP), mental status, and any other parameters that the physician wants to have monitored.

Laboratory Investigations

Included here are the tests required, the specific times they are to be obtained, and exact details (if the blood is to be drawn from an artery rather than a vein, this should be specified). These orders, like all the others, should be very specific, to avoid any possibility of misinterpretation or misreading.

osmolality. The determination of serum osmolality is frequently required in the care of critically ill patients. This can be done in the laboratory using freezing-point depression. However, one occasionally will be unable to determine osmolality in the clinical laboratory. In these situations the following formula may be used:

Osmolality (mOsm/kg) = 1.86 (Na) + BUN/2.8 + blood glucose/18

In most situations, the calculated serum osmolality will be 5 to 8 mOsm/kg less than that measured by the freezing-point depression method. The calculated osmolality should not be substituted for the actual measurement, since in some situations there will be a substantial discrepancy between the calculated and measured osmolalities (e.g., in uremia, hyperlipemia, and multiple myeloma).

MEDICATIONS
Each medication and its frequency of administration, dose, and route of administration should be specifically indicated. It should be remembered that intravenous medications often represent a significant additional fluid intake, and this should be taken into account when fluid restriction is important.

Critically ill patients often receive several drugs. One should therefore be familiar with the adverse reactions that may accompany the drugs being administered.

The possibility of drug interactions in patients receiving several medications should be kept in mind. Most physicians are aware of the recognized potentiation of certain drugs (e.g., kanamycin and curarelike drugs). There are also drugs that may antagonize one another. Many hospital pharmacies have set up a computerized drug surveillance program that will alert the physician to potential interactions. An excellent book on the subject, *Drug Interactions* [11], is available and should be kept in the ICU for reference.

DIAGNOSTIC PROCEDURES
Included in the orders for diagnostic procedures are ECGs, roentgenograms, and other procedures that may be requested (e.g., electroencephalograms, radionuclide scanning, and ultrasonography).

INSTRUCTIONS TO NURSING STAFF
The instructions to the nursing staff include orders pertaining to suctioning of the patient, irrigation of tubes (e.g., nasogastric, Cantor), turning of the patient, changing of dressings, caring for invasive lines and drains, and specific instruments to be kept at the bedside (e.g., tracheostomy sets, airways, Ambu bags).

NOTIFYING OF THE PHYSICIAN
Orders concerning notification of the physician should include detailed instructions covering situations that require that the physician be notified (e.g., changes in general condition, changes in blood pressure, vital signs, fever).

GENERAL MEASURES

The general measures in the orders relate to consideration of the patient's comfort (e.g., laxatives, sleep medications, psychological support).

SPECIAL CONSIDERATIONS

PATIENTS ON RESPIRATORS

Strict fluid balance recording and daily weights are of utmost importance in patients on respirators [20]. Because these patients are on ventilatory support, they have virtually no insensible losses, and careful attention to fluid balance is required to avoid further compromise of their respiratory status.

To obtain the maximum benefit from ventilatory assistance, the patient must be in phase with the ventilator. The patient who fights the ventilator not only interferes with oxygenation and ventilation but also increases his metabolic requirements. The patient on ventilatory assistance presents a complex problem to the physician; Chapter 6 deals with this subject in depth.

RENAL FAILURE PATIENTS

The problems of renal failure patients will be covered in Chapter 21. However, the following considerations are worthy of additional emphasis:

1. Medications. Because many drugs are excreted through the renal route, their dosages must be adjusted [5].
2. Fluid management. The rate of fluid administration in these patients must be determined by their urine output and other outputs (e.g., nasogastric tubes, chest tubes) and insensible losses. Consultation with the renal service, if available, is desirable for optimal management.
3. Antacids. The use of magaldrate (Riopan) is contraindicated in renal failure. Also, because of their high sodium content, preparations such as Maalox must be used cautiously.

GASTROINTESTINAL BLEEDING

In patients with gastrointestinal bleeding, the goal is to stabilize the patient hemodynamically and concomitantly to ascertain the site of bleeding. The incidence of upper gastrointestinal hemorrhage in critically ill patients appears to be reduced. The serious problem of stress ulcer with bleeding is less, especially when strict control of gastric acidity has been undertaken. Once bleeding occurs, rapid resuscitation and prompt diagnosis are important. Early esophagogastroduodenoscopy is vital. Methods of nonoperative control of bleeding include iced-saline lavage, intragastric or intraperitoneal levarterenol, selective intra-arterial pharmacologic control of embolization, intensive antacid therapy, and endoscopic electrocoagulation.

In critical illness, prevention of upper gastrointestinal bleeding is also important.

ANTACIDS. The use of an antacid preparation to maintain the gastric pH above 5 has been advocated to reduce the incidence of acute gastrointestinal bleeding [13]. Hourly gastric instillation of a volume of antacid determined by the amount needed to elevate the pH of gastric aspirate above 5 is carried out.

Special Diets. The use of enteral or parenteral hyperalimentation (see Chapter 17) has been thought by some to provide protection for the gastric mucosa. However, this conclusion is largely based on some preliminary animal studies and clinical impressions. If the enteral route is used for nutritional support, a feeding tube is inserted into the stomach and a continuous drip of an appropriate diet is started. The concentration and volume of feeding are increased on a daily basis. Feedings are given with the head of the bed elevated 30 degrees to prevent aspiration. Gastric residuals are checked every 4 hours. Urine spot-checks are done every 6 hours, and blood sugars and osmolalities are closely watched.

CIMETIDINE. A histamine H_2-receptor antagonist, cimetidine has recently been used in both the prevention and treatment of acute upper gastrointestinal bleeding [6]. While well-controlled, randomized prospective trials using cimetidine to control acute bleeding are not available, this drug can be used in the prevention and control of upper GI bleeding along with all currently accepted modalities. An initial dose schedule of 300 mg given IV piggyback every 6 hours can be tried.

COAGULATION TESTS. In patients with gastrointestinal bleeding, it is important to evaluate coagulation parameters to determine whether or not deficiencies exist. In some of these patients, the use of fresh frozen plasma, platelets, and/or fresh blood may be advisable (see Chapter 19 for details).

INTRA-ARTERIAL INFUSION OF POSTERIOR PITUITARY EXTRACT (VASOPRESSIN) IN GASTROINTESTINAL BLEEDING. Since operative intervention for control of bleeding is poorly tolerated in the critically ill, numerous nonsurgical therapeutic modalities have been introduced (see page 44). However, with the advent of selective angiography and concomitant intra-arterial drug therapy [4], an improved nonoperative method of control has been made available [3, 10]. Intra-arterial vasopressin perfusion has been found effective in gastric mucosal hemorrhage secondary to stress ulcer, erosive gastritis, Mallory-Weiss syndrome, esophageal varices, and bleeding diverticulosis.

Following esophagogastroduodenoscopy, and having decided upon the use of intra-arterial vasopressin for therapy, a nasogastric tube, arterial and central venous pressure lines, and a Foley catheter are inserted. The patient is then sent to the x-ray department with a constant infusion pump (e.g., Holter pump, or IVAC) for continuous intra-arterial infusion and with the following vasopressin mixtures: 100 units in 500 ml or 5% D/0.25% saline (0.2 units) and 200 units in 500 ml of 5% D/0.25% saline (0.4 units). In the x-ray department, a Seldinger catheter is inserted, and bleeding is demonstrated angiographically. Vasopressin is then perfused at 0.2 units/min for 20 minutes. A postinfusion angiogram is required to observe vasoconstriction of the distal branches of the perfused vessel, with flow into the capillary and venous phases without extravasation. (The infusion rate may then be raised or occasionally lowered to meet these criteria.)

After the angiography, the patient is transferred to the ICU for perfusion at the determined rate for 24 hours (0.4 units/ml/min in celiac or 0.2 units/ml/min in superior mesenteric artery [SMA], inferior mesenteric artery [IMA], or subselective branches if necessary). After clinical control of bleeding for 24 hours, the concentration is reduced to 0.1 units/min for 24 additional hours. This is followed with 12 to 24 hours of 5% D/0.25% saline perfusion before removing the catheter. In addition, the following should be done:

1. Monitoring of vital signs, including CVP, urinary output, and daily weight.
2. Daily KUB to check catheter position.
3. Irrigation of the nasogastric tube until it is clear; then antacid instillation to maintain the gastric pH above 5 should be begun. Cimetidine may also be used.
4. Careful observation for bradycardia, water intoxication, and postvasopressin diuresis.
5. Good catheter maintenance, including aseptic catheter puncture site, a close check of the distal pulses, and the curtailment of leg movement to prevent catheter displacement and possible arterial injury.

Following catheter removal, adequate pressure should be provided to control bleeding from the puncture site. Strict control of additional fluid administration should be maintained.

Recently, similar portal and systemic hemodynamic changes were noted with both intraarterial and intravenous vasopressin [2]. Because of the quickness and ease with which the intravenous route of therapy can be initiated, especially in the middle of the night, more use of continuous peripheral venous infusion is being made [7]. A dose schedule similar to the intraarterial one can be used.

FEVER

ETIOLOGY. Temperature elevations are common in critically ill patients. Because fever may produce adverse effects (e.g., tachycardia, increased oxygen requirements, increased fluid loss, convulsions), it is imperative that one attempt to identify the cause of the fever as soon as possible. Frequently, the source of the fever may be retained secretions in the lungs. This is especially common in patients only a few hours after operation and in patients who are intubated and on mechanical ventilatory assistance.

In general, one should not institute therapy for a fever without first determining its etiology (see Chapter 18). This, however, does not apply when the fever itself is endangering the patient's life. It is essential to obtain cultures (e.g., blood, wound, sputum, urine) before initiating or changing antibiotic therapy. In addition, when the patient is uncomfortable because of the fever, an antipyretic or sponge baths may make the patient more comfortable.

THERAPY

Hypothermia Blankets. The use of a hypothermia blanket (K-Thermia) is a common practice in many ICUs. Such blankets, however, are extremely uncomfortable, and often the patient may shiver so severely that it becomes a problem. The patient on a cooling blanket must be closely monitored. A rectal probe facilitates close monitoring and minimizes the problem associated with inserting thermometers frequently. However, the use of rectal probes is not advised in patients who are incontinent of feces or who are having frequent bowel movements. The K-Thermia is turned off when the patient's temperature reaches 101° F (39.9° C), since an additional drop in temperature will occur after the machine is turned off.

Alcohol Baths. Alcohol baths are somewhat effective in lowering fevers. However, the alcohol often so dries the skin that the skin becomes susceptible to breakdown and the subsequent development of decubitus ulcers.

Ice Packs. Placing several surgeon's gloves filled with crushed ice around the patient (e.g., in the groin area, under the axillae) may be helpful. However, these packs are almost as uncomfortable as hypothermia blankets.

Antipyretic Drugs. Administration of antipyretic drugs is by far the commonest treatment for fever and also is the treatment of choice. Acetaminophen (Tylenol) can be used in critically ill patients, since it does not affect platelet function. These drugs are available for both oral and rectal administration.

ANTICOAGULATION

The complications seen in the clinical thrombotic states (i.e., deep vein thrombosis, pulmonary embolism, acute arterial embolism) are not confined to the general medical-surgical patient, but are also present in the critically ill. Anticoagulation is not only vital for therapy in these states, but may have a prophylactic role as well.

THERAPEUTIC USE. Heparin and the concomitant administration (when the patient can tolerate oral intake) of an oral anticoagulant such as warfarin (Coumadin) form the basis of therapy. Once anticoagulation therapy is decided on, a baseline partial thromboplastin time (PTT) is determined [21], and if no intravenous line has been established, a 23-gauge butterfly heparin lock is placed. Heparin can be given by intermittent or continuous intravenous infusion to maintain the PTT at two to two and a half times control [22].

The recommended dose of heparin varies, depending on the institution, the body weight, and the associated problems of the patient. A maintenance intermittent dose schedule employs between 5,000 and 10,000 units (50–100 mg) given intravenously every 4 hours. A dose of 100 units/kg will usually provide an effective safe starting dose. One hour prior to the second dose of heparin, the PTT is checked. Once having determined the patient's response to heparin, it is not necessary to repeat the PTT unless a situation develops that would alter the dose schedule. An individual's response to heparin remains constant and predictable. If a continuous infusion schedule is used, a bolus of 5,000 to 10,000 units of heparin is given, followed by the administration of 1,000 units per hour through a continuous infusion pump. This dose is also adjusted by PTT monitoring.

Oral anticoagulants (e.g., Coumadin) should be started along with heparin as soon as the gastrointestinal tract is functional. During the initiation of Coumadin therapy, there is a disparity in the rate of suppression of the blood levels of the four vitamin K–dependent factors (factors VII, IX, X, and prothrombin) affected by Coumadin. Although the PT may be prolonged at 36 hours, a true antithrombotic effect may not be present for seven days [18].

Heparin is generally discontinued between the seventh and the tenth day. Therefore, to reduce the failure rate of anticoagulation by having an unprotected period, at least one week of simultaneous drug administration is necessary. Coumadin is started in a daily dose of 10 mg, adjusting the dose schedule to obtain a prolongation of the PT two to two and a half times control time. Oral anticoagulation can then be used for the appropriate time span for the thrombotic state under treatment. When adjusting the daily Coumadin dose, it is important to pay attention to the multitude of drugs that interact to increase anticoagulant action (e.g., antibiotics, salicylates, phenylbutazone, hepatotoxic drugs) and those that decrease it (e.g., corticosteroids, antihistamines, barbiturates).

PROPHYLACTIC USE. To prevent the development of venous thrombosis and subsequent pulmonary embolism is a difficult task. There has been some promise in the prophylactic use of low-dose heparin therapy if it is started early enough (i.e., preoperatively in the surgical patient and at the onset of illness in the medical patient [9, 14]). For the surgical patient, 5,000 units of heparin is given subcutaneously 2 hours preoperatively and then every 12 hours postoperatively. Medical patients must be started immediately on 5,000 units of heparin given subcutaneously every 12 hours (an alternate schedule would be every 8 hr). Conclusions about the real prophylactic

effectiveness of low-dose heparin have not been reached, but this form of therapy may have a role in prevention of thrombotic states in patients at high risk.

REFERENCES

1. Artz, J. S., et al.   Application of a critical care monitoring program in the diagnosis and management of critically ill patients in a community hospital. *Crit. Care Med.* 2:42, 1974.
2. Barr, J. W., et al.   Similarity of arterial and intravenous vasopressin on portal and systemic hemodynamics. *Gastroent.* 69:13, 1975.
3. Baum, S., et al.   Gastrointestinal hemorrhage: Angiographic diagnosis and control. *Adv. Surg.* 7:149, 1973.
4. Baum, S., and Nusbaum, M.   The control of gastrointestinal hemorrhage by selective mesenteric arterial infusion of vasopressin. *Radiology* 98:497, 1971.
5. Bennett, W. M., et al.   A guide to drug therapy in renal failure. *J.A.M.A.* 230:1544, 1974.
6. Bubrick, M. P., et al.   Control of acute gastroduodenal hemorrhage with cimetidine. *Surgery* 84:510, 1978.
7. Chojkier, M., et al.   Intra-arterial vs. intravenous vasopressin in the treatment of massive upper gastrointestinal hemorrhage. *Gastroent.* 75:958, 1978.
8. Clinical Care Committee of the Massachusetts General Hospital.   Optimum care for hopelessly ill patients. *N. Engl. J. Med.* 295:362, 1976.
9. Council on Thrombosis of the American Heart Association.   Prevention of venous thromboembolism in surgical patients by low-dose heparin. *Circulation* 55:423A, 1977.
10. Geronilla, D. R., and Sampliner, J. E.   Gastrointestinal bleeding: Treatment with intra-arterial vasopressin. *Am. Surg.* 41:321, 1975.
11. Hansten, P. D.   *Drug Interactions* (2nd ed.). Philadelphia: Lea & Febiger, 1973.
12. Hantman, D., et al.   Rapid correction of hyponatremia in the syndrome of inappropriate secretion of antidiuretic hormone. *Ann. Intern. Med.* 78:870, 1973.
13. Hastings, P. R., et al.   Antacid titration in the prevention of acute gastrointestinal bleeding. *N. Engl. J. Med.* 298:1041, 1978.
14. Kakkar, V. V., et al.   Low doses of heparin in prevention of deep-vein thrombosis. *Lancet* 2:669, 1971.
15. Kiely, W. F.   Psychiatric aspects of critical care. *Crit. Care Med.* 2:139, 1974.
16. MacLean, L. D., et al.   Alkalosis in septic shock. *Surgery* 62:655, 1967.
17. Mazzara, J. T., et al.   Extreme hypocapnia in the critically ill patient. *Am. J. Med.* 56:450, 1974.
18. Salzman, E. W., and Britten, A. B.   *Hemorrhage and Thrombosis.* Boston: Little, Brown, 1965.
19. Simmons, D. H., et al.   Hyperventilation and respiratory alkalosis as signs of gram-negative bacteremia. *J.A.M.A.* 174:2196, 1960.
20. Sladen, A., et al.   Pulmonary complications and water retention in prolonged mechanical ventilation. *N. Engl. J. Med.* 279:448, 1968.

21. Sussman, L. N. The clotting time—an enigma. *Am. J. Clin. Pathol.* 60:651, 1973.
22. Wilson, J. R., and Lampman, J. Heparin therapy: A randomized prospective study. *Am. Heart J.* 97:155, 1979.

SELECTED READINGS

Ayres, S. M., et al. *Care of the Critically Ill* (2nd ed.). New York: Appleton, 1974.

Ballinger, W. F., et al. *American College of Surgeons Manual of Surgical Nutrition.* Philadelphia: Saunders, 1975.

Behrendt, D. M., and Austin, W. G. *Patient Care in Cardiac Surgery* (2nd ed.). Boston: Little, Brown, 1976.

Boedeker, E. C., and Dauber, J. H. (Eds.). *Manual of Medical Therapeutics* (22nd ed.). Boston: Little, Brown, 1977.

Davenport, H. W. *The ABC of Acid-Base Chemistry* (6th ed.). Chicago: University of Chicago Press, 1974.

Gervin, A. S. Complications of heparin therapy. *Surg. Gynecol. Obstet.* 140: 789, 1975.

Goldberger, E. *A Primer of Water, Electrolyte and Acid-Base Syndromes* (5th ed.). Philadelphia: Lea & Febiger, 1975.

Goldin, M. D. (Ed.). *Intensive Care of the Surgical Patient.* Chicago: Year Book, 1971.

Graef, J. W., and Cone, T. E. (Eds.). *Manual of Pediatric Therapeutics* (2nd ed.). Boston: Little, Brown, 1978.

Harvey, A. M. *Principles and Practice of Medicine* (19th ed.). New York: Appleton, 1976.

Kinney, J. M., et al. *American College of Surgeons Manual of Preoperative and Postoperative Care* (2nd ed.). Philadelphia: Saunders, 1971.

Kinney, J. M., et al. *American College of Surgeons Manual of Surgical Intensive Care.* Philadelphia: Saunders, 1977.

Koch-Weser, J., and Sellors, E. M. Drug interactions with coumarin anticoagulants. *N. Engl. J. Med.* 285:487, 1971.

Masoro, E. J., and Siegel, P. D. *Acid-Base Regulation: Its Physiology and Pathophysiology.* Philadelphia: Saunders, 1978.

Massachusetts General Hospital Department of Nursing. *Massachusetts General Hospital Manual of Nursing Procedures.* Boston: Little, Brown, 1975.

Maxwell, M. H., and Kleeman, C. R. (Eds.). *Clinical Disorders of Fluid and Electrolyte Metabolism* (2nd ed.). New York: McGraw-Hill, 1972.

Moore, F. D. *Metabolic Care of the Surgical Patient.* Philadelphia: Saunders, 1959.

Papper, S. *Clinical Nephrology* (2nd ed.). Boston: Little, Brown, 1978.

Pitts, R. F. *Physiology of the Kidney and Body Fluids* (3rd ed.). Chicago: Year Book, 1974.

Safar, P., and Grenvik, A. Critical care medicine: Organizing and staffing intensive care units. *Chest* 59:535, 1971.

Skillman, J. J. *Intensive Care.* Boston: Little, Brown, 1975.

Sodeman, W. A., Jr., and Sodeman, W. A. *Pathologic Physiology* (5th ed.). Philadelphia: Saunders, 1974.

Valtin, H. *Renal Function: Mechanisms Preserving Fluid and Solute Balance in Health.* Boston: Little, Brown, 1973.

Weil, M. H., and Shubin, H. The new practice of critical care medicine. *Chest* 59:473, 1971.

Wilson, R. F. *Fluids, Electrolytes and Metabolism.* Springfield, Ill.: Thomas, 1973.

Winters, R. W. (Ed.). *The Body Fluids in Pediatrics: Medical, Surgical, and Neonatal Disorders of Acid-Base Status, Hydration, and Oxygenation.* Boston: Little, Brown, 1973.

George I. Litman / # 4. NONINVASIVE DIAGNOSTIC TECH- NIQUES IN CRITICAL CARE

Noninvasive diagnostic procedures involve no cutting or puncturing of the skin and therefore result in few, if any, complications. Radioisotopic studies do use intravenous injection, but are otherwise noninvasive, as are computed tomography and echocardiography. With portable gamma cameras and ultrasound units, these techniques can be taken to the bedside of even the most critically ill patient. The purpose of this chapter is to introduce these noninvasive procedures and relate them to specific critical care problems.

ECHOCARDIOGRAPHY

Echocardiography employs ultrasound to produce images of the heart and adjacent structures. Ultrasound has a frequency of greater than 20,000 cycles per second (Hertz or Hz). Medical sonography employs frequencies between 1 and 20 Hz. These high frequencies are produced by subjecting a special ceramic material, a piezoelectric crystal, to a short voltage spike. The piezoelectric crystal acts as both transmitter and receiver of high frequency pulses of very short duration, which travel through the body tissues at a known velocity. The echoes reflected from blood-tissue interfaces are detected by the transducer, amplified, and then displayed on an oscilloscope or a strip-chart recorder. Displayed against time, the reflected ultrasound yields a detailed picture of the motion of the structures of the heart and great vessels during the cardiac cycle.

The standard method, termed M mode, employs a single, narrowly focused beam of ultrasound. This widely used technique, providing excellent diagnostic information without risk or discomfort, may be performed at the bedside. Disadvantages include the expense of the equipment and the amount of professional time and skill needed to obtain and interpret high-quality echocardiograms. Even proficient personnel may not obtain complete information from a particular study, since chest wall deformities create difficulty in obtaining adequate tracings and an acutely ill patient may be restless and uncooperative or may have hyperinflated lungs owing to mechanical ventilation, making it impossible to obtain satisfactory echo-cardiograms.

Although the two-dimensional sector scanning technique of echocardiography is becoming more available, its high cost and small advantage over M mode preclude further discussion [4, 9, 27, 32].

PERICARDIAL EFFUSION

Echocardiography is currently the most sensitive and specific procedure for the diagnosis of pericardial effusion. The detection and serial follow-up of the presence and approximate amount of pericardial fluid are more accurate than with any other method [12].

A pericardial effusion appears as an echo-free space behind the epicardial surface of the posterior wall and in front of the pericardium [10, 11, 17]. Where a small effusion exists, this echo-free space will be small, and the epicardial-pericardial separation will occur primarily during systole. As the effusion becomes larger, this separation is increased and is present during both systole and diastole. With a larger effusion, an echo-free space is also seen in front of the right ventricular wall.

When a large pericardial effusion is present, the heart may swing like a pendulum in the pericardial sac with each cardiac cycle. The echocardiogram will detect the abnormal motion of all the cardiac walls, including the septum, moving in the same direction with each heart beat [41] (Fig. 4-1). The abnormal wall and valve configurations may be confused with other valvular lesions [20]. Electrical alternans is often seen on the electrocardiogram in this situation. As the heart swings anteriorly, there is a larger R wave, and conversely, as the heart moves posteriorly, a smaller R wave.

A negative echocardiogram may not rule out a pericardial effusion. There is evidence that clotted blood may have an echo reflectance similar to that of the myocardium. Therefore, a blood clot in the posterior pericardium may not be detected as fluid by echocardiography [18]. This is clearly a disadvantage, especially in the trauma patient.

CARDIAC TAMPONADE

Cardiac tamponade is a clinical syndrome defined on the basis of physical and hemodynamic findings. The hemodynamic significance of a pericardial effusion is not determined by the volume of fluid alone. For this reason, echocardiography has not been helpful in establishing the diagnosis of tamponade. It is of value in distinguishing the patient with a large left ventricle owing to left ventricular failure from the patient with a large pericardial effusion causing cardiac tamponade, since either of these patients may present with severe hemodynamic compromise.

AORTIC DISSECTION

Acute dissection of the thoracic aorta is among the most lethal of all medical emergencies. In a review of 425 cases by Hirst et al., 21 percent of pa-

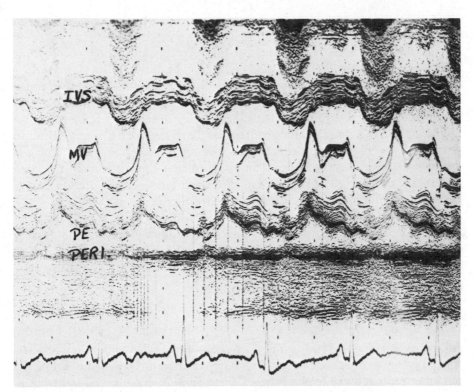

FIGURE 4-1. Echocardiogram demonstrating significant pericardial effusion. IVS = intraventricular septum; MV = mitral valve; PE = pericardial effusion; PERI = pericardium.

tients were dead within 24 hours, and 49 percent died within four days of the onset of symptoms [16]. The early diagnosis and aggressive treatment of these patients may prolong survival and allow time for potentially definitive surgery.

Echocardiography can be valuable in the diagnosis of proximal aortic dissection by demonstrating the separation of the aortic layers, and the presence or absence of aortic valve regurgitation [24]. Nanda et al. first reported the echocardiographic findings of the demonstration of a false lumen, dilation of the aortic root, widening of both anterior and posterior aortic walls, and preservation of normal aortic valve motion [25]. These criteria were later refined by Brown, Papp, and Kloster, who used the following as diagnostic of proximal aortic dissection: (1) a clinical history suggestive of dissection, (2) the anterior aortic wall is equal to or greater than 16 mm, (3) the aorta is dilated to 42 mm or less, and (4) parallel aortic root echoes are maintained throughout systole and diastole [2].

In spite of these recent advances, the diagnosis of dissecting aortic aneurysm and the definition of its origin and extent must be established by contrast angiography.

ACUTE AORTIC VALVE REGURGITATION

Acute aortic valve regurgitation may occur as a result of infective endocarditis or acute traumatic rupture. Echocardiography provides much useful information. The regurgitant jet itself produces fine fluttering of the anterior leaflet of the mitral valve in diastole. That the aortic regurgitation is acute and severe is supported by the finding of early coaptation of the mitral leaflets in diastole, before the QRS on the simultaneously recorded electrocardiogram [23]. In contrast to chronic aortic regurgitation, exaggerated wall motion and a markedly dilated ventricle are not seen.

The echocardiogram may also assist in elucidating the cause. Dense, irregular echoes from one or more valve leaflets may represent the vegetations of endocarditis [31, 43]. These are usually best seen in diastole. A flail leaflet prolapsing into the left ventricular outflow tract in diastole suggests valve disruption.

NUCLEAR MEDICINE

LUNG SCANNING

Following intravenous injection of technetium-labeled albumin particles, special gamma-counting cameras can be used to scan the distribution of the resulting radioactivity in the lungs. This technique has proved valuable in detecting the presence of pulmonary arterial emboli.

PULMONARY EMBOLISM

Pulmonary embolism is a common, recurrent, age-related phenomenon that can occur without warning in its most lethal form. It accounts for 50,000 to 100,000 deaths each year in the United States. Pulmonary embolism must be considered in the differential diagnosis of every acute cardiorespiratory disorder.

The lungs lend themselves well to the study of regional function with radioactive tracer techniques [13, 14]. This method accurately reflects the distribution and severity of perfusion abnormalities from any cause [40]. Because of its relatively noninvasive nature, the perfusion lung scan has become the principal screening procedure for patients suspected of suffering a pulmonary embolus.

When multiple views are obtained, a normal lung scan essentially excludes any clinically detectable pulmonary embolism. When the scan is abnormal, the likelihood of embolic phenomena can be determined from the nature of the observed defects. Lung scans with a high probability of pulmonary embolism demonstrate multiple wedge-shaped or concave defects which follow a segmental vascular distribution. Low probability scans show nonsegmental and nonvascular distributions of perfusion defects.

A chest x-ray obtained in conjunction with the lung scan enhances its diagnostic specificity. A concave peripheral perfusion defect in the presence of a normal chest roentgenogram is likely to be caused by an embolus.

In a recent study, 75 percent of scans with high probability for embolus were confirmed by pulmonary angiography. With a normal scan, the angiogram was also normal [13]. In the Urokinase Pulmonary Embolism Trial, among 10 patients with a large embolus in the proximal main pulmonary artery, none of the lung scans were normal [40]. False positive tests are encountered in a variety of pulmonary and cardiac conditions, such as neoplasms, pneumonia, atelectasis, chronic bronchitis, and chronic obstructive pulmonary disease. These can usually be identified on chest x-ray.

In combination with a normal Xenon 133 ventilation study, an abnormal lung scan is virtually diagnostic of pulmonary embolism. On the other hand, in a patient with an abnormal perfusion lung scan and a matching abnormal ventilation study, the presence of pulmonary embolism is less likely, but cannot be absolutely excluded [22]. With the increased specificity attainable by combining ventilation and perfusion scans, it is possible to limit pulmonary angiography to patients who do not meet these criteria, or who have coexisting pulmonary embolism and chronic obstructive pulmonary disease.

CARDIAC ISOTOPE IMAGING

The use of radioisotopes in clinical cardiology is an exciting advance in nuclear medicine. These noninvasive techniques permit easy evaluation of the size and function of the cardiac chambers, and allow visualization of the physiologic adequacy of blood flow to the myocardium. Maximum information is obtained when a combination of Thallium 201 (^{201}Tl) and Technetium 99 pyrophosphate (^{99m}Tc PYP) is used in addition to dynamic ventriculography with ^{99m}Tc-labeled albumin or red cells.

When ^{99m}Tc is bound to human albumin and injected intravenously, ^{99m}Tc displays the dimensions of the great vessels and chambers of the heart. It is thus used to calculate the size and functional capabilities of the heart, expressed as cardiac output or systolic ejection fraction. In addition, ^{99m}Tc albumin can detect intracardiac shunts and abnormal wall motion [28], and ^{99m}Tc PYP reveals the blood flow distribution in the myocardium, but is eventually concentrated in regions of acute myocardial ischemia and infarction.

The myocardial blood flow is also demonstrated by ^{201}Tl, the agent of choice for perfusion scanning [35, 36]. After intravenous injection, ^{201}Tl uptake will be seen in the normally perfused left ventricular myocardium of the resting patient. Since the right ventricular muscle mass is much less than that of the left, visualization of the right ventricle is usually abnormal. Areas with decreased or absent flow are identified as cold spots. An area with compromised circulation only during exercise is ischemic, whereas an area with a consistent perfusion defect at rest exhibits the scar of a previous infarction. A hypertrophied area of myocardium may show greater than normal uptake. Therefore, the evaluation of a ^{201}Tl scan permits: (1) determination of the size, shape, and position of the heart; (2) definition of areas of ischemia or infarct; (3) visualization of an abnormal right ventricle; and (4) measurement of the thickness of the myocardium in some cases.

The future of myocardial imaging may well lie with three-dimensional image reconstruction [19]. Ter-Pogossian and his colleagues have accomplished this with a positron-emitting tracer and positron-tomographic cameras [39]. However, a positron-based technique requires the availability of a cyclotron and expensive detection equipment, formidable requirements which place these techniques beyond the reach of the average institution.

ACUTE MYOCARDIAL INFARCTION

When employed within 6 to 8 hours after the onset of symptoms, ^{201}Tl is most sensitive for the indication of an acute myocardial infarction [30]. When used in evaluating over 1,600 patients with recent episodes of chest pain, ^{201}Tl scintigraphy was helpful in identifying those with infarcts [42]. However, the most common cause of focal defects in ^{201}Tl scanning in nonsymptomatic patients at rest is scar tissue from old myocardial infarction.

If radioisotopic imaging is delayed, ^{99m}Tc PYP becomes the agent of choice because it is selectively taken up by infarcted cardiac cells and appears as a hot spot on the scintigram, delineating the site and extent of the damaged area [1, 3, 29]. The ^{99m}Tc PYP scan becomes positive 10 to 12 hours after infarction, and then becomes increasingly positive for 24 to 72 hours. Therefore, it is suggested that the ^{99m}Tc PYP scintigram be obtained within 48 hours after suspected infarction, and repeated 48 hours later if the initial scan was equivocal or negative in the face of high clinical suspicion. Repeat studies are also beneficial in determining whether there was extension of infarcted areas [45, 46].

These new noninvasive techniques are particularly advantageous when other diagnostic methods are inadequate. The distinction between subendocardial ischemia and infarction is impossible based on electrocardiogram findings alone. Intraventricular conduction defects, such as left bundle branch block, obscure the electrocardiogram changes of an acute myocardial infarction. No history is available from patients who arrive at the hospital comatose, and serum enzyme measurements may not be positive in patients who present hours or days after the onset of symptoms. In the perioperative and postoperative periods, especially following coronary artery revascularization, patients may have chest pain and elevated serum enzymes, obscuring the diagnosis of a new infarct. With portable gamma cameras now available, these studies can be performed in the intensive care setting.

MYOCARDIAL CONTUSION

More patients survive transport to an emergency medical facility following severe blunt chest injury and penetrating wounds of the heart as a result of improved on-the-scene resuscitative techniques. Standard evaluation begins with a thorough physical examination, including special attention to the structural integrity of the bony thorax, the adequacy of respiration and circulation, and the peripheral pulses [15]. Despite chest x-ray and electrocardiogram data, myocardial contusion is easily overlooked, and may present formidable complications during the recovery period [21].

Regardless of etiology, ^{99m}Tc PYP will identify myocardial necrosis if some blood flow is present and a critical mass of tissue is involved [29, 46]. A scintigram should be obtained for any victim of major blunt chest trauma, even without suggestive electrocardiographic findings such as premature ventricular contractions or minor intraventricular conduction disturbances [47]. The timing of the scan is the same as for an acute myocardial infarction. If the scan is positive, the patient must be monitored closely for arrhythmias, congestive failure, and other complications of acute infarcts.

MYOCARDIAL FUNCTION AND SHUNT DETERMINATIONS

Radioisotopic angiography can be performed using ^{99m}Tc-labeled human albumin or red cells. These studies have been improved by computer technology that enables one to evaluate ventricular wall motion, cardiac output, and systolic ejection fractions. It is now possible to determine cardiac function noninvasively in the critically ill patient.

In addition, radioisotopic angiography permits detection and calculation of intracardiac shunts. Shunts, such as ventricular septal defects, may be congenital or the result of myocardial infarction or blunt chest trauma.

COMPUTED TOMOGRAPHY

The operation of computed tomography scanners involves the axial rotation of an x-ray beam around the patient with detectors opposite the x-ray source. These detectors measure the attenuation of the x-rays after they have passed through the tissue. After the data are collected in multiple projections, a computer calculates the attenuation coefficient of each point of a matrix, thus producing an image of the scanned sections. This image is stored and may be recorded photographically [37, 38].

Computed tomography (CT) differs from conventional shadow radiography and tomography because the x-ray beam is thinly collimated to reduce the effect of scatter; the detector system (sodium iodide crystal or xenon gas) has greater response capability than a conventional photographic plate; and a computer is used that resolves the summed x-ray projection data perceived by the detector into discrete linear attenuation coefficients [44].

The field of computed tomography is changing more rapidly than any other area in radiology. Its usefulness as a diagnostic tool shows overwhelming promise. It is said to provide more diagnostic information in the spectrum of intracranial disease than any other single neuroradiologic examination [6, 8]. It is also fulfilling a role as a low-risk, painless, and noninvasive method for evaluation of the abdominal cavity.

CENTRAL NERVOUS SYSTEM: INTRACRANIAL LESIONS

Computed tomography is estimated to be 90 to 98 percent accurate in the imaging of intracranial lesions and is thus one of the most effective medical detection systems available [5]. It is generally sufficient alone as a diagnostic procedure for victims of acute head trauma [7, 48]. Intracranial hematomas, subdural hematomas, cerebral infarctions, and traumatic edema are easily recognized. CT can also identify blood in the subarachnoid space, intraventricular hematomas, and the thrombosed portion of a giant aneurysm. However, angiography is still necessary to visualize the base of an aneurysm and its relation to adjacent vessels and vascular spasm, as well as to delineate vessel lacerations, traumatic fistulas, and isodural (balanced) subdural hematomas [7, 26].

If a patient with suspected intracranial bleeding demonstrates altered mentation, papilledema, or focal neurologic findings, a CT scan should be the initial procedure. A lumbar puncture may precipitate transtentorial herniation if the bleeding is a result of a mass lesion or a ruptured aneurysm. The CT scan visualizes the bleeding and may indicate the need for emergency angiography [44].

ABDOMINAL COMPUTED TOMOGRAPHY

Although it is generally agreed that CT scanning of the head has become indispensable for patients with suspected intracranial disease, the situation with regard to CT of the rest of the body is less clear. There is less clinical experience with CT body scanning as compared with head scanning. Because all body organs can be examined, the number of disease processes that remain to be studied with CT is vast, and the data will be amassed slowly.

PANCREAS

Computed tomography appears to be more reliable in the demonstration of the normal and abnormal pancreas than almost any other procedure. Abdominal CT scanning is worthwhile in the evaluation of pancreatic carcinoma and pancreatitis, especially with abscesses, pseudocysts, or phlegmon [33].

JAUNDICE

Computed tomography has been shown to be practical and accurate in the distinction of obstructive and nonobstructive jaundice. Normal intrahepatic ducts are usually not identifiable on scans. Dilated intrahepatic bile ducts appear as linear branching or circular, low-density structures that are less dense than the adjacent portal vein branches [33].

RETROPERITONEAL SPACE
The retroperitoneal space is one of the most inaccessible areas of the body to conventional radiography, yet is readily visualized with CT scanning. Location and identification of abscesses, hemorrhage, and mass lesions are possible and practical.

Hemorrhage is seen as a more or less diffuse mass. Retroperitoneal hemorrhage can occur as a result of external trauma, internal trauma to vessels cannulated for various reasons, a leaking aortic aneurysm, bleeding diathesis, anticoagulation, or certain neoplasms [34].

CONCLUSIONS
Noninvasive diagnostic procedures, increasingly available and safe, have demonstrated unique potential in the evaluation of the critically ill patient. Echocardiography is the procedure of choice for diagnosis of pericardial effusion and acute aortic valve regurgitation. It is helpful in the evaluation of proximal aortic root dissection or possible cardiac tamponade.

Techniques of nuclear medicine aid the diagnosis of pulmonary embolism, acute myocardial infarction, and acute myocardial contusion. In addition, myocardial function may be examined with radioisotopic angiography, which permits shunt detection, observation of ventricular wall motion, and the computation of cardiac output and left ventricular systolic ejection fractions.

Computed tomography is a radiologic procedure that detects and distinguishes intracranial tumors, hemorrhages, infarcts, and hematomas. Abdominal computed tomography clearly visualizes pancreatic processes, aids in the separation of obstructive and nonobstructive jaundice, and demonstrates the retroperitoneal space.

REFERENCES
1. Buja, L. M., Tofe, A. J., Kulkarni, P. V., et al. Sites and mechanisms of localization of technetium-99m phosphorous radiopharmaceuticals in acute myocardial infarcts and other tissues. *J. Clin. Invest.* 60:724, 1977.
2. Brown, O. R., Popp, R. L., and Kloster, F. E. Echocardiographic criteria for aortic root dissection. *Am. J. Cardiol.* 36:17, 1975.
3. Burno, F. P., Cobb, F. R., Rivas, F., and Goodrich, J. K. Evaluation of 99m technetium stannous pyrophosphate as an imaging agent in acute myocardial infarction. *Circulation* 54:71, 1976.
4. Christensen, E. E., Curry, T. S., and Dowdey, J. E. *An Introduction to the Physics of Radiology.* Philadelphia: Lea & Febiger, 1978. Pp. 361–394.
5. Davis, D. O. CT in the diagnosis of supratentorial tumors. *Semin. Roentgenol.* 12:97, 1977.

6. Davis, K. R., Poletti, C. E., Roberson, G. H., Tadmor, R., and Kjellberg, R. N. Complementary role of computed tomography and other neuroradiologic procedures. *Surg. Neurol.* 8:437, 1977.

7. Davis, K. R., Taveras, J. M., Roberson, G. H., Ackerman, R. H., and Dreesball, J. N. Computed tomography in head trauma. *Semin. Roentgenol.* 12:53, 1978.

8. Evens, R. G. New frontiers for radiology; computed tomography. *A.J.R.* 126:1117, 1976.

9. Feigenbaum, H. *Echocardiography* (2nd ed.). Philadelphia: Lea & Febiger, 1976. Pp. 5–53.

10. Feigenbaum, H., Waldhausen, J. A., and Hyde, L. P. Ultrasound diagnosis of pericardial effusion. *J.A.M.A.* 191:107, 1965.

11. Feigenbaum, H., Zaky, A., and Waldhausen, J. A. Use of ultrasound in the diagnosis of pericardial effusion. *Ann. Intern. Med.* 65:443, 1966.

12. Felner, J. M. Echocardiography: Pericardial Disease. In J. W. Hurst (Ed.), *The Heart* (4th ed.). New York: McGraw-Hill, 1978. P. 473.

13. Gilday, D. L., Poulore, K. P., and DeLand, F. H. Accuracy of detection of pulmonary embolism by lung scanning correlated with pulmonary angiography. *A.J.R.* 115:732, 1972.

14. Greenspan, R. H. Does a normal isotope perfusion scan exclude pulmonary embolism? *Invest. Radiol.* 9:44, 1974.

15. Hipona, F. A., and Paredes, S. The radiologic evaluation of patients with chest trauma. *Med. Clin. North Am.* 59:65, 1975.

16. Hirst, A. E., Johns, V. J., Jr., and Kime, S., Jr. Dissecting aneurysms of the aorta: A review. *Medicine* 37:217, 1958.

17. Horowitz, M. S., Schultz, C. S., Stinson, E. B., Harrison, D. C., and Popp, R. L. Sensitivity and specificity of echocardiographic diagnosis of pericardial effusion. *Circulation* 50:239, 1974.

18. Kerber, R. E., and Payvandi, M. N. Echocardiography in acute hemopericardium: Production of false negative echocardiograms of pericardial clots. *Circulation* 56(Suppl. 3):III–24, 1977.

19. Kuhl, D. E., and Edwards, R. Q. Cylindrical and section radioisotope scanning of the liver and brain. *Radiology* 83:926, 1964.

20. Levisman, J. A., and Abbasi, A. A. Abnormal motion of the mitral valve with pericardial effusion: Pseudo prolapse of the mitral valve. *Am. Heart J.* 91:18, 1976.

21. Levitsky, S. New insights in cardiac trauma. *Surg. Clin. North Am.* 55:43, 1975.

22. McNeil, B. J., Holman, B. L., and Adelstein, S. J. The scintigraphic definition of pulmonary embolism. *J.A.M.A.* 227:753, 1974.

23. Mann, T., McLaurin, L., Grossman, W., et al. Assessing the hemodynamic severity of acute aortic regurgitation due to infective endocarditis. *N. Engl. J. Med.* 293:108, 1975.

24. Moothart, R. W., Spangler, R. D., and Blount, S. G., Jr. Echocardiography in aortic root dissection and dilatation. *Am. J. Cardiol.* 36:11, 1975.

25. Nanda, C., Gramiak, R., and Shah, P. M. Diagnosis of aortic root dissection by echocardiography. *Circulation* 48:506, 1973.

26. Osborn, A. G. Computer tomography in neurologic diagnosis. *Ann. Rev. Med.* 30:189, 1978.
27. Parisi, A. F., and Tow, D. E. *Noninvasive Approaches to Cardiovascular Diagnosis.* New York: Appleton, 1979.
28. Parkey, R. W., Bonte, F. J., Buja, M. L., and Willenson, J. T. *Clinical Nuclear Cardiology.* New York: Appleton, 1979.
29. Perez, L. A. Clinical experience: Technetium 99 labeled phosphate myocardial imaging. *Clin. Nucl. Med.* 1:2, 1976.
30. Pohost, G. M., Zir, L. M., Moore, R. H., et al. Differentiation of transient ischemia from infarcted myocardium by serial imaging after a single dose of thallium 201. *Circulation* 55:294, 1977.
31. Roy, P., Tajik, A. J., Giuliani, E. R., et al. Spectrum of echocardiographic findings in bacterial endocarditis. *Circulation* 53:474, 1976.
32. Salcedo, E. E. *Atlas of Echocardiography.* Philadelphia: Saunders, 1978.
33. Sheedy, P. F., Stephens, D. H., Hattery, R. R., Brown, L. R., and MacCarty, R. L. Computed tomography of the abdominal organs. *Adv. Intern. Med.* 24:455, 1979.
34. Stephens, P. H., Williamson, B., Sheedy, P. F., Hattery, R. R., and Miller, W. E. Computed tomography of the retroperitoneal space. *Radiol. Clin. North Am.* 15:377, 1977.
35. Strauss, H. W., Harrison, K., Langan, J. K., Lebowitz, E., and Pitt, B. Thallium 201 for myocardial imaging—relation of thallium 201 to regional perfusion. *Circulation* 51:641, 1975.
36. Strauss, H. W., and Pitt, B. Thallium 201 as a myocardial imaging agent. *Semin. Nucl. Med.* 7:49, 1977.
37. Ter-Pogossian, M. M. Computerized cranial tomography: Equipment and physics. *Semin. Roentgenol.* 12:13, 1977.
38. Ter-Pogossian, M. M., Phelps, M. E., Brownell, G. L., et al. *Reconstruction Tomography in Diagnostic Radiology and Nuclear Medicine.* Baltimore, Md.: University Park Press, 1977.
39. Ter-Pogossian, M. M., Phelps, M. E., Hoffman, E. J., and Mullani, N. A. Position-emission transaxial tomograph for nuclear imaging (PETT). *Radiology* 114:89, 1975.
40. Tow, D. E., and Simon, A. L. Comparison of lung scanning and pulmonary angiography in the detection and follow-up of pulmonary embolism: The urokinase pulmonary embolism trial experience. *Prog. Cardiovasc. Dis.* 17:239, 1975.
41. Usher, B. W., and Popp, R. L. Electrical alternans: Mechanisms of pericardial effusion. *Am. Heart J.* 83:459, 1972.
42. Wackers, F. J. T., Becker, A. E., Samson, G., et al. Location and size of acute transmural myocardial infarction estimated from thallium 201 scintiscan: A clinicopathological study. *Circulation* 56:72, 1977.
43. Wann, L. S., Dillon, J. C., Weyman, A. E., et al. Echocardiography in bacterial endocarditis. *N. Engl. J. Med.* 295:135, 1976.
44. Weisberg, L. A. Computed tomography in the diagnosis of intracranial disease. *Ann. Intern. Med.* 91:87, 1979.
45. Willerson, J. T., Parkey, R. W., Bonte, F. J., Meyer, S. L., and Stokely, E. M.

Acute subendocardial myocardial infarction in patients; its detection by Tc-99m stannous pyrophosphate myocardial scintigrams. *Circulation* 51:436, 1975.

46. Willerson, J. T., Parkey, R. W., Bonte, F. J., Stokely, E. M., and Breja, L. M. Technetium stannous pyrophosphate myocardial scintigraphy: A new method of proven value for the diagnosis and localization of acute myocardial infarcts and for the detection of infarct extension in patients. *Tex. Med.* 72:51, 1976.

47. Willerson, J. T., Parkey, R. W., Buja, L. M., Lewis, S. E., and Bonte, F. J. Causes of necrosis other than infarction; myocardial trauma. In R. W. Parkey (Ed.), *Clinical Nuclear Cardiology*. New York: Appleton, 1979. Pp. 209–224.

48. Zimmerman, R. A., Bilaniuk, L. A., Genneralli, T., Bruce, D., Dolinskas, C., and Uzell, B. Cranial computed tomography in diagnosis and management of acute head trauma. *A.J.R.* 131:27, 1978.

James E. Sampliner
Howard C. Pitluk 5. HEMODYNAMIC
AND RESPIRATORY
MONITORING

The goal of therapy in the critically ill patient is to restore normal physiologic function of all vital organ systems. A patient's hemodynamic and respiratory profile, developed from monitoring the cardiopulmonary system as an interrelated unit, provides a scientific basis for the early detection and ongoing therapy of critical illness.

HEMODYNAMIC MONITORING
Hemodynamic monitoring includes parameters that are monitored directly (e.g., arterial blood pressure) and those that are calculated from other measurements (e.g., systemic vascular resistance, ventricular stroke work).

The decision to institute hemodynamic monitoring in the critically ill patient must be made early in the course of disease in order to detect clinically unrecognizable organ dysfunction and to begin appropriate, aggressive therapy. Patients who show circulatory instability, have fluid management problems, or have deteriorating cardiac or pulmonary function will benefit from invasive monitoring techniques. Advantages of invasive monitoring techniques must be weighed against possible complications, but the latter are now infrequent on intensive care units with monitoring experience.

PRESSURE MONITORING
TRANSDUCERS
There are two primary techniques for determining intravascular pressure. The first is the water manometer, in which the pressure in the vessel supports a column of water, the height of the column being equal to the pressure. The second is the transducer (strain gauge), in which the pressure from the vessel is transmitted to the diaphragm of the transducer, where the pressure is read as an electrical signal; this, in turn, is converted to a reading in millimeters of mercury or centimeters of water. The accuracy of the measurement is dependent both on proper calibration of the transducer and on the use of the appropriate reference point.

REFERENCE LEVEL (ZERO) FOR PRESSURE MEASUREMENT
Among anatomic landmarks used as the zero point for pressure monitoring are: (1) a point 5 cm below the sternal angle, (2) the midchest, and (3) the

sternal angle. A reference point is required to establish the level at which the venae cavae enter the heart. Of these three reference points, the second is probably the most reliable.

Above all, a standard routine must be employed when measuring pressures. It is useless to compare measurements that are made with the patient in different positions. In addition, when a patient is on a respirator, the measurement should be made with the patient off the ventilator. If this is not possible, *all* measurements should be made without interrupting ventilator support; otherwise, the comparative value of the determinations is lost. Only when measurements are made properly and consistently can the true value of individual determinations be obtained.

ARTERIAL PRESSURE

Arterial blood pressure has been one of the cornerstones of hemodynamic monitoring. Unfortunately, there are many misconceptions regarding arterial blood pressure. An exhaustive discussion of the measurement and interpretation of arterial blood pressure is beyond the scope of this chapter and can be found elsewhere [4, 12, 21, 23]. However, it cannot be overemphasized that arterial blood pressure is not the sine qua non of shock and should not be used as the sole criterion of the effectiveness of therapy for shock. In addition, it must also be emphasized that pressure is not synonymous with flow, but rather, the two are related by the following equation:

Pressure = flow × resistance

or

Arterial pressure = cardiac output × systemic vascular resistance

MEASUREMENT

Blood pressure can be measured in a variety of ways, which can be divided into two categories—direct and indirect methods. Direct methods include any measurements that are made by inserting an intra-arterial catheter, whether this be merely a short catheter or a longer line that is advanced to the central aortic region. Indirect methods include the use of the sphygmomanometer, ultrasonic blood pressure monitors, and Doppler techniques.

The measurement of blood pressure in the critically ill is vital, and therefore the use of indwelling intra-arterial lines is desirable. Cuff pressures for shock patients are frequently inaccurate. Moreover, the intra-arterial monitoring of blood pressure allows the simultaneous display of the arterial waveform [31], which can provide useful physical and technical information.

PLACEMENT OF INTRA-ARTERIAL LINES

SITE. Intra-arterial lines should preferably be inserted in sites where thrombosis would not endanger the limb or where the site itself would not be exposed to the possibility of contamination (e.g., the femoral artery). In keeping with these proscriptions, the radial artery is the preferred site, provided the ulnar artery is patent by palpation or Doppler exam. Alternative sites include the brachial, axillary [1], and posterior tibial arteries. The importance of careful site selection cannot be overemphasized; frequently, patients will require long-term monitoring, and the possibility of complications increases with the length of monitoring.

INSERTION. The area to be used is first prepared with povidone-iodine (Betadine), and, using sterile technique (i.e., gloves and sterile tray), the area is infiltrated with 1% lidocaine. A suitable 18- or 20-gauge polyethylene catheter, as used in intravenous therapy, should be inserted. In general, it is preferable to avoid using an obturator with these lines, since repeated withdrawal of the obturator and its replacement will increase incidence of infection. Utilizing the percutaneous technique, the catheter is inserted until a flow of blood is obtained. Then the catheter is advanced to the hub, and the internal stylet removed.

It is our practice to allow three attempts at percutaneous placement. If insertion is unsuccessful, a small cutdown is done over the artery, and the catheter is then placed under direct vision [2]. This avoids repeated trauma to the artery and possible impairment of circulation owing to hemorrhage within the arterial wall. Once the line is in place, the site is dressed with Betadine ointment and a sterile dressing; the arm (if the radial or brachial artery is used) can then be placed on an arm board. An arm board is essential if the line is in the brachial artery because of the movement at the antecubital fossa.

LINE MAINTENANCE. The hub of the catheter is connected to pressure-resistant tubing (e.g., Sorenson PT-30 arterial pressure tubing[1]), an essential in preventing transmission of the pressure through the walls of the tubing. In addition, the length of tubing between the cannula and transducer should not be excessive. Hughes and Prys-Roberts [14] have recommended that the tubing between transducer and patient be limited to 60 cm (23.6 in.). However, in practice, we have found this limit too restrictive for patient movement, and we have therefore increased it to 152 cm (60 in.). A continuous flush device (Sorenson Intraflo-CFS-03F[1]) is also connected between the transducer and cannual. This allows a constant flow through the line of 3 to 5 ml/hr [8, 11, 15, 19]. The flush device is connected to a 500-ml bag of fluid that has a blood infusion pump (Fenwall BD-1[2]) inflated around it to a pressure of 300 mm Hg, which overcomes the pressure in the arterial system. To the bag of fluid we add 10 to 20 mg of heparin. At the flow rate of the device, the heparin and fluid administration is minimal. Furthermore,

---

[1] Sorenson Research Company, Salt Lake City, Utah.
[2] Fenwal Laboratories, Inc., Morton Grove, Ill.

it has been reported that the use of this system has reduced the incidence of thromboembolic events that result with this technique [8].

Alternatively, if a transducer is not available, the patient's arterial line can be connected to a disposable continuous blood pressure monitor.[3] When this is used, a device with a low rate of 30 ml/hr (Sorenson Intraflo-CFS-30) is recommended if continuous monitoring is desired; or if intermittent monitoring is to be employed, the 3- to 5-ml flow device is adequate.

The dressing and tubing should be changed every 48 hours, but if any leakage should occur, the site must be immediately inspected. In our institution, all arterial lines are sutured in place to prevent accidental loss of the line. In addition, we do not use an antibiotic ointment at the catheter-skin interface, since this seems only to select the organisms that will grow at this site. Instead, we use an antibacterial ointment (Betadine).

DISPLAY. Continuous monitoring of the arterial pressure waveform is desirable. It not only allows one to detect mechanical problems (e.g., damping due to air bubbles in the line), but also allows observation of the contour and upstroke of the arterial pulse. The use of digital rather than analog pressure meters has become popular, allowing the pressure to be seen more easily from a distance and avoiding misinterpretation of exactly where the analog needle is when pressure is measured. Most systems allow the operator to select systolic, diastolic, or mean pressure for numerical display on the meter.

SAMPLING. Arterial lines can also be used for blood sampling. In patients requiring frequent arterial blood gases, the placement of an indwelling line for this purpose alone is justified to avoid the discomfort and possible complications of repeated arterial puncture. Before taking the sample, withdraw enough blood from the line to ensure that the sample is not contaminated by the fluid running in the arterial line. It is important to keep track of the amount of blood withdrawn for samples, as well as any that may have been discarded. Critically ill patients often have frequent enough blood samples withdrawn to amount to 250 ml in a 24-hour period. If this blood loss is not recorded, the unexplained drop in hematocrit may prompt unnecessary diagnostic procedures for occult blood loss.

In addition, it is important never to draw blood for coagulation studies (e.g., for prothrombin time, partial thromboplastin time) from an arterial line, since even a small amount of heparin can lead to erroneous results. Aside from coagulation parameters, blood for other tests (e.g., chemistries, white cell count, hematocrit) can be drawn from the line.

CENTRAL VENOUS PRESSURE
The measurement of central venous pressure (CVP) is frequently used by those caring for critically ill patients. When one understands its limitations, CVP measurement can be used effectively as an aid in their management.

[3] RamTech, Inc., Tampa, Fla.

INSERTION

All central venous lines should be inserted under sterile technique. Routes of insertion include internal jugular, subclavian, and antecubital veins. Our preference is the infraclavicular approach to the subclavian vein. The complications of subclavian puncture can be reduced greatly by careful attention to anatomic landmarks and proper technique (outlined in detail in Chapter 17).

MEASUREMENT AND INTERPRETATION

In most institutions, CVP lines are attached to water manometers to allow intermittent measurement of pressure. Civetta [5] has pointed out the value of measuring CVP with a transducer.

The range of normal values for CVP is considerable (e.g., 5–12 cm H_2O). In certain conditions, the patient may actually require an elevated CVP to maintain effective cardiac output (e.g., in chronic lung disease).

The most common misinterpretation of CVP occurs when one inserts the line and then attempts to assess the state of hydration based on a single measurement. The CVP permits one to assess only the ability of the right side of the heart to accommodate the volume being returned to it. The CVP is the function of four measurable, independent forces [15]:

1. The volume and flow of blood in the central veins.
2. The distensibility and contractility of the right chambers of the heart during filling of the heart.
3. Venomotor activity in the central veins.
4. Intrathoracic pressure.

Another misinterpretation of CVP data occurs when one attempts to extrapolate information relative to left ventricular performance from the CVP. As will be emphasized in this chapter, CVP cannot be substituted for the assessment of left ventricular performance.

As with all pressure measurements, the reference level (zero point) is extremely important when measuring CVP. An analysis of this and other subjects relating to the measurement and interpretation of CVP determinations has been published by Guyton and Jones [13].

THE SWAN-GANZ CATHETER

With the introduction of the Swan-Ganz catheter [22], a new era in the monitoring of critically ill patients began. In addition to its uses in monitoring, this catheter has now been modified to allow ventricular pacing as well. Four advantages of the Swan-Ganz catheter over the conventional CVP measuring devices have been pointed out by Thompson [25].

1. It permits measurement of pulmonary arterial diastolic and wedge pressures that estimate left ventricular filling pressures.

2. Continuous monitoring of pulmonary arterial systolic and mean pressures reflects changes in pulmonary vascular resistance (PVR) secondary to hypoxemia, pulmonary edema, pulmonary emboli, and pulmonary insufficiency.
3. It allows sampling of mixed venous blood for measurement of arteriovenous oxygen content difference, Fick cardiac output, and venoarterial admixture ($\dot{Q}s/\dot{Q}T$).
4. It permits the measurement of cardiac output by the thermodilution technique [10].

CATHETER LUMENS

PROXIMAL LUMEN. The proximal lumen lies 30 cm proximal to the distal lumen, and in the person of average size it lies in the superior vena cava at the atrial junction or in the right atrium. When using the catheter for the measurement of cardiac output by thermodilution, it is essential that this lumen (i.e., the injectate port) be properly positioned. Should catheters with modified injectate-port distances be required, they can be obtained by special order from the manufacturer.[4]

The proximal lumen can also be used to monitor CVP and to infuse fluids. Because of the small lumen size, the rate of fluid administration through it is somewhat limited. We routinely add 10 to 20 mg of heparin to each 1,000 ml of fluid to prevent clotting in the line.

DISTAL LUMEN. The distal lumen lies in the pulmonary artery. It should be connected to a transducer for continuous pressure monitoring. A 500-ml bag with a blood infusion pump inflated to 300 mm Hg around the intravenous bag is connected to the distal catheter lumen, and 10 mg of heparin is added to the bag to prevent clotting. A continuous flow device (Sorenson Intraflo-CFS-30) is used to maintain patency while minimizing the amount of fluid infused. Blood withdrawn from this lumen when the catheter is in the pulmonary artery and when the balloon is deflated is mixed venous blood. At least 10 ml of blood should be withdrawn before sampling from the line to avoid contamination of the sample with the intravenous fluid. Again, because of the heparin, no blood for coagulation studies should be withdrawn from this line.

BALLOON LUMEN. The balloon lumen connects to the balloon on the catheter (the balloon capacity is imprinted on the catheter). The balloon should never remain inflated longer than 30 to 60 seconds. If balloon rupture is suspected, the lumen should be covered with adhesive tape to avoid accidental injection of air. When using plastic syringes (3 cc), if the air is injected and the plunger does not come back on its own, balloon rupture should be suspected. Also, when the balloon is broken, blood will sometimes come back through this lumen.

[4] Edwards Laboratories, Santa Ana, Cal.

INSERTION

The Swan-Ganz catheter may be inserted either percutaneously or by cut-down. The introduction of percutaneous introducers[5] has aided in the insertion of the catheter.

Once a central venous line is placed through the internal jugular or subclavian route, a coiled spring guide wire is introduced through it. The central venous catheter is removed, and a dilator-introducer is passed over the wire. The dilator and wire are then removed, leaving the introducer in place. Through this, the Swan Ganz catheter can be inserted with ease. A detailed description of the technique used in passing the catheter, as well as examples of pressure tracings, can be found in Chapter 10. To reduce the chance of infection once the catheter is in place, the following guidelines have been established: (1) the catheter skin interface is cleaned every 48 hours and covered with Betadine ointment; (2) all intravenous and pressure-resistant tubing is changed every 48 hours; and (3) an airtight dressing is placed over the catheter insertion site.

MONITORING

The monitoring of pulmonary artery pressure and pulmonary capillary wedge pressure (PCWP) requires a transducer and an oscilloscope. Because pulmonary artery pressure and PCWP are in the low ranges (i.e., usually less than 30 mm Hg), it is absolutely essential that the tubing between the catheter and transducer be pressure-resistant (noncompliant), thus avoiding any dissipation of pressure into the walls of the tubing.

To monitor PCWP, the balloon is inflated. It is important to observe the pressure waveform during inflation so that as soon as a wedge pattern is observed, no more air will be introduced. This method is superior to those in which a fixed volume of air is injected. (*Note:* When an intracardiac shunt exists, carbon dioxide should be used instead of air. In addition, it must be kept in mind that the use of air entails the possibility of balloon rupture and air embolism.) Also, the catheter can migrate further into the pulmonary artery, and thus a smaller volume of air is required for wedging. Therefore, careful balloon inflation is important in preventing balloon rupture, and in avoiding overinflation and spurious readings (if the balloon is overinflated, it may cover the distal catheter lumen, and a high pressure reading will then be obtained).

PULMONARY ARTERY PRESSURE. Pulmonary artery pressure is continuously monitored through the distal lumen of the Swan-Ganz catheter as long as the balloon is deflated and the catheter is properly positioned. The lumen's patency is maintained using a pressure system, as described for arterial lines.

Mean pulmonary artery pressure ($\overline{PA}$) is normally in the range of 9 to 17 mm Hg. Several factors can lead to an elevation in $\overline{PA}$. These include:

[5] Edwards Laboratories, Santa Ana, Calif.

1. Pulmonary vascular disease (e.g., chronic lung disease).
2. Intracardiac shunts (i.e., left-to-right shunts) that cause an increase in pulmonary blood flow.
3. Chronic elevation of pulmonary venocapillary, or left atrial pressures, or both. Acute elevation in $\overline{PA}$ without any substantial elevation of mean PCWP ($\overline{PCWP}$) may be the result of (a) massive pulmonary embolism or multiple small emboli, (b) pulmonary vascular obstruction such as may occur following lobar atelectasis or (c) hypoxia.

These situations usually imply an increase in PVR, which may also be present in patients with pulmonary insufficiency.

In the absence of increased PVR and abnormal left ventricular function, the pulmonary arterial end-diastolic pressure will closely approximate PCWP, mean left atrial pressure, and left ventricular end-diastolic pressure. Therefore, should rupture of the balloon on the Swan-Ganz catheter occur, one may use pulmonary arterial end-diastolic pressure to approximate PCWP, provided, of course, that there is neither acute nor chronic elevation of PVR.

Blood sampled from the pulmonary artery is true mixed venous blood and allows calculation of the arteriovenous oxygen content difference (a-$\overline{v}$ DCO$_2$) when blood is simultaneously drawn for blood gases and hemoglobin. This can then be used in the calculation of cardiac output by the Fick method and the measurement of $\dot{Q}s/\dot{Q}T$ (see calculations later in this chapter).

PULMONARY CAPILLARY WEDGE PRESSURE. The normal range for PCWP is 5 to 12 mm Hg. However, when left ventricular compliance is decreased (e.g., following acute myocardial infarction and in sepsis), the optimal PCWP may range as high as 20 mm Hg. The maximizing of this pressure (preload) will be reflected by the slope of the left ventricular function curve, as will be shown later in this chapter.

Because there are no valves between the left atrium and pulmonary arteries, the inflation of the balloon on the Swan-Ganz catheter occludes proximal flow, and the pressure obtained is a back pressure from the left atrium. The PCWP correlates well with mean left atrial pressure and reflects pulmonary venocapillary hydrostatic pressure. In addition, in the absence of mitral valvular disease, PCWP will closely approximate left ventricular end-diastolic pressure.

The PCWP is also used to assess pulmonary capillary hydrostatic pressure. As PCWP (i.e., hydrostatic pressure in the pulmonary capillaries) increases, the tendency for fluid to transudate into the lung interstitium increases. The balance between hydrostatic and colloid osmotic pressure is the factor that acts to keep the alveolus dry [27]. As the hydrostatic pressure in the pulmonary capillaries increases, pulmonary congestion increases.

Forrester and Swan [9] have found the following relationships between PCWP and the radiologic manifestations of pulmonary congestion:

1. When the PCWP is less than 18 mm Hg, there are no radiologic signs of pulmonary congestion.
2. At a PCWP of 18 to 20 mm Hg, there is onset of pulmonary congestion, with the roentgenogram showing engorgement of the hilar vessels secondary to a redistribution of pulmonary blood flow.
3. When PCWP increases to 20 to 25 mm Hg, the congestion is mild to moderate, with the chest film showing perihilar haze and periacinar rosettes.
4. At PCWP of 25 to 30 mm Hg, the congestion can be classified as moderate to severe, and the roentgenogram will show coalescence of periacinar rosettes.
5. When PCWP is over 30 mm Hg, pulmonary edema is usually present, and the chest x-ray film shows the classic findings of pulmonary edema.

LENGTH OF MONITORING

It is often asked how long Swan-Ganz catheters should be left in place. We have left catheters in as long as 12 days without a complication. In spite of this, catheters should be left in no longer than necessary, and we usually try to remove them within 72 hours after insertion.

CARDIAC OUTPUT

Cardiac output is defined as the quantity of blood pumped by the heart each minute, and it is conventionally expressed in liters per minute. However, one usually indexes cardiac output to compensate for the size difference found among patients. Indexing is accomplished by using a body surface area nomogram (see Appendix 3). The normal cardiac index is 2.8 to 3.2 liter/min/M^2.

MEASUREMENT OF FACTORS CONTROLLING STROKE VOLUME

Cardiac output is the product of heart rate and stroke volume. Stroke volume, in turn, is controlled by three factors: preload, afterload, and contractility.

PRELOAD. Preload is the diastolic volume distending the relaxed ventricular wall. As pointed out, this can be assessed by measuring PCWP—in the absence of mitral valvular disease, PCWP is equivalent to left ventricular end-diastolic pressure. (See Pulmonary Capillary Wedge Pressure for values.)

AFTERLOAD. Afterload is the resistance to ventricular ejection [31]. Clinically, this is determined by measuring systemic vascular resistance also termed *total peripheral resistance*). The normal value for systemic vascular resistance is 900 to 1200 dynes $\times$ sec $\times$ cm^{-5}. In general, there are two indications for afterload reduction in the critically ill patient: (1) an increased PCWP (i.e., 18 mm Hg or greater) with an elevated systemic vascular resistance and a reduced cardiac index, and (2) mitral regurgitation.

When employing afterload reducers, one must pay close attention to the patient's blood pressure. If afterload reduction is employed in patients to reduce myocardial infarct size, the reduction in arterial pressure (i.e., diastolic pressure) may affect coronary perfusion. In some cases, it may be desirable to combine afterload reduction (also termed *systolic unloading*) with external counterpulsation (also termed *diastolic augmentation*). A complete discussion of this subject is beyond the scope of this chapter (see Chapter 13).

CONTRACTILITY. Contractility is the ability of the heart to alter its contractile force and velocity independent of fiber length. Clinically, one can assess myocardial contractile state by determining dp/dt, systolic ejection fraction, or by constructing ventricular function curves.

VENTRICULAR FUNCTION MONITORING

The right and left ventricles operate as pumps connected in series. Because of this relationship, the output of the two ventricles must be equal. However, the functional state of the ventricles and the output pressures they face are usually significantly different. To compensate for these differences, the ventricles must independently respond by changes in contractility and/ or changes in the Frank-Starling mechanism, which relates the energy of contraction to end-diastolic fiber length.

Monitoring of ventricular function by relating ventricular end-diastolic pressure to ventricular stroke work provides valuable information regarding the state of ventricular performance. This is accomplished by calculating ventricular stroke work by the conventional formula and plotting it on the ordinate as a function of ventricular end-diastolic pressure, which is plotted on the abscissa. Central venous pressure measurements are substituted for the direct measurement of right ventricular end-diastolic pressure. This has been shown to be a valid assumption in the absence of tricuspid valvular disease. The left ventricular end-diastolic pressure is obtained by measuring PCWP.

The analysis of ventricular function measurements has shown four major uses of these determinations in critically ill patients: (1) to assess the state of biventricular performance; (2) to aid in the recognition of early ventricular impairment; (3) to assess the effect of a given pathologic process (e.g., sepsis, myocardial infarction, or pulmonary insufficiency) on ventricular performance; and (4) to aid in evaluating and directing therapy in critically ill patients.

As shown in Figure 5-1, the slope, shape, and scales of the right and left ventricular function curves are different. Thus, it can readily be seen that assumptions made by relating right ventricular end-diastolic pressure to left ventricular stroke work are subject to substantial error. This is, in fact, what occurs frequently when one attempts to use CVP as the sole indicator of left ventricular function.

Under normal conditions, as ventricular end-diastolic pressure increases,

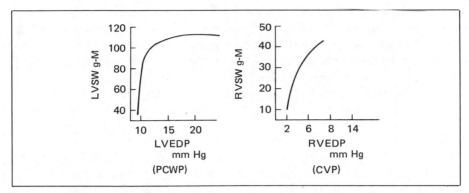

FIGURE 5-1. Examples of right (RV) and left (LV) ventricular function curves. It is important to note that stroke-work scales, as well as shape and flow of curves, are significantly different. This illustrates the inadequacy of utilizing CVP measurements as a reflection of left ventricular function. LVEDP and RVEDP = left and right end-diastolic pressure respectively; SW = stroke work.

a rapid rise in ventricular stroke work is observed, with this rise reaching a plateau at higher filling pressures. Thus, controlled volume infusions are given to elevate end-diastolic pressure and to obtain maximal ventricular stroke work [18]. An evaluation of these curves is then possible, observing whether a favorable effect (i.e., a left and upward shift in the curve) or an unfavorable effect (i.e., a right and downward shift in the curve) has occurred. We have used the finding of a right and downward shift in the curve as evidence of a failing heart.

There are certain limitations to the use of ventricular function monitoring. These are as follows:

1. The Frank-Starling mechanism relates end-diastolic fiber length to the energy of contraction. In clinical monitoring of ventricular function, end-diastolic pressure is substituted for the measurement of end-diastolic fiber length. End-diastolic pressure is not a linear function of end-diastolic fiber length, but it is a useful clinical approximation.
2. Changes in ventricular distensibility may render end-diastolic pressure an unreliable indicator of acute changes in chamber size or fiber length.
3. Substantial evidence indicates that a considerable dilatation of the left ventricle may occur as a structural change in the absence of a change in fiber length.
4. Because of the geometric relationship of the right to the left ventricle in the closed pericardial sac, the Frank-Starling curve may falsely reflect left ventricular function [16].

Despite these limitations, the use of serial measurements of ventricular end-diastolic pressure and ventricular stroke work and the subsequent construction of ventricular function curves will provide valuable information on the state of ventricular performance.

Additional hemodynamic parameters can be calculated from existing for-mulas to supplement the directly measured values—e.g., pulmonary vascu-lar resistance, oxygen consumption, arteriovenous oxygen content differ-ence, and oxygen availability (see Appendix 2). Only together can these hemodynamic parameters be used to construct a physiologic profile from which a scientific therapeutic approach to the critically ill patient can be derived. (See Appendix 4 for a list of commonly used vasoactive drugs.)

RESPIRATORY MONITORING
Respiratory function monitoring serves as the basis for the establishment of guidelines to be used as the criteria for the initiation of oxygen therapy, the use of mechanical ventilatory support, and the discontinuation of these respiratory support techniques.

Perhaps one of the most important roles for respiratory function moni-toring is in those patients admitted to the intensive care unit (ICU) for a problem other than pulmonary insufficiency. In these patients, careful sur-veillance of respiratory function status can often allow early recognition of respiratory impairment and thereby often avoid the morbidity and mortality associated with pulmonary insufficiency.

BLOOD GASES
PO_2, PCO_2, pH, HCO_3^- and percent saturation provide the initial parameters for assessing pulmonary status in the critically ill patient.

Blood gas measurements can provide information regarding oxygen trans-port, the efficiency of gas exchange, acid-base status, and the adequacy of alveolar ventilation. They can also be used in the calculation of param-eters that aid in the determination of shunting in the lung and cardiac output (by the Fick method). The importance of blood gases cannot be overemphasized. However, one must not rely solely on them, or on any other measurement, in the care of the critically ill.

Before discussing the interpretation of blood gas measurements, it is helpful to review certain basic chemical principles as well as the basics of blood gas analysis itself. In this way, one is in a better position to interpret these physiologic data.

THEORETICAL CONSIDERATIONS
BAROMETRIC PRESSURE
The molecules that are present in the earth's atmosphere have weight and exert a force on the earth that is great enough to support a column of mer-cury 760 mm high at sea level. This is termed the *atmospheric* (*barometric*) *pressure.*

DALTON'S LAW
The earth's atmosphere is composed of several gases, the major ones being nitrogen and oxygen. Dalton's law states that the total atmospheric pres-

sure is the sum of the individual gas pressures and that each of these partial pressures is as though that gas alone occupied the space. Dry air is composed of 79.03 percent nitrogen, 20.93 percent oxygen, and 0.04 percent carbon dioxide.

To determine the partial pressure of any gas, one needs to know both the barometric pressure (PB) and the fractional concentration of the gas that is under consideration. To calculate the partial pressure of a given gas, one multiplies the fractional concentration of the gas by the barometric pressure.

Example

To determine the partial pressure of oxygen in room air:

Barometric pressure = 760 mm Hg

Fractional concentration of O_2 (FiO_2) = 20.93%

$$PO_2 = 760 \times 0.2093$$

The PO_2 is then calculated as 159 mm Hg.

HENRY'S LAW

The amount of gas that will dissolve in a liquid at a given temperature is directly proportional to the partial pressure of that gas in the gas phase. However, this law applies only to that fraction of the gas physically dissolved in the liquid and not to the fraction of gas that is combined chemically with either the liquid or a solute within the liquid. Both carbon dioxide and oxygen dissolve physically in plasma. Carbon dioxide, however, also reacts chemically with water, and both carbon dioxide and oxygen react chemically with hemoglobin. Henry's law applies only to the physically dissolved fractions of these two gases. Therefore, it is only the physically dissolved gas that exerts a partial pressure in the plasma and not the gas that is chemically combined.

When the partial pressure in the liquid is equal to the partial pressure of the gas that is chemically combined, the two phases are in equilibrium. A change in either will disrupt this equilibrium and cause a corresponding change in the opposite phase until equilibrium is reestablished.

The amount of carbon dioxide and oxygen that is physically dissolved in plasma is dependent on the solubility coefficient for the gas, the temperature, and the partial pressure of the gas. At 37° C, the solubility coefficient of oxygen is 0.0031 vol%/mm Hg and of carbon dioxide, 0.063 vol%/mm Hg. For example, to determine the partial pressure of oxygen dissolved in plasma when the arterial PO_2 is 215 mm Hg, one multiplies 215 mm Hg by 0.0031 vol%/mm Hg, which equals 0.6665 vol%. As one can see, the amount of gas physically dissolved will be relatively small except at extremely high partial pressures of a given gas (i.e., inhalation of 100% oxygen, and especially hyperbaric oxygen).

In review:

1. The total volume of gas in a solution is equal to the sum of the volume of physically dissolved gas plus that volume of gas chemically combined with other solutes (i.e., hemoglobin).
2. The total concentration of oxygen and carbon dioxide in blood is much greater than the concentration of physically dissolved oxygen and carbon dioxide.
3. The partial pressure of a gas in solution is proportional *only* to the amount of gas that is physically dissolved and not to the total concentration of the gas.
4. The chemical reactions as well as the physiologic properties of gases depend on the partial pressure of those gases rather than on their total concentration in solution.
   Example: The concentration of physically dissolved oxygen, which is proportional to PO_2, affects the rate of diffusion of oxygen into and out of capillaries and red cells. Furthermore, the PO_2 is one of the factors that determines the amount and rate at which oxygen combines with hemoglobin.

WATER VAPOR PRESSURE

Water vapor pressure (P_{H_2O}) increases and decreases in direct relation to temperature (Table 5-1). The importance of water vapor pressure is primarily in its effect on diluting the gases in dry air. Therefore, dry air, when inspired, is free of P_{H_2O}. However, by the time this air reaches the bronchioles, its effect on oxygen is to have lowered its partial pressure by approximately 10 mm Hg.

The PaO_2 of alveolar air is therefore equal to barometric pressure minus water vapor pressure times the fractional oxygen concentration (FiO_2). Mathematically, this can be expressed as:

$$PaO_2 = (PB - P_{H_2O}) FiO_2$$

In the case of room air at 37° C, this makes $PaO_2 = 149$ mm Hg.

TECHNICAL ASPECTS OF BLOOD GAS ANALYSIS

The actual measurement of blood gases is extremely important, since the results often serve as a guide to therapy. Therefore, a brief explanation of how the determinations are made follows.

pH

The glass pH electrode contains an inner chamber in which a solution of a "known" pH is sealed. The electrical potential generated between the outside of the electrode and the inner "known" solution is then read directly as the pH of the blood by the blood gas machine.

In practice, the inner reference is a calomel reference electrode that is surrounded by a solution of a "known" pH. A difference in electrical potential between the inside and the outside is generated when the blood is introduced, using saturated potassium chloride (KCl) as the conductor. This difference in electrical potential is the pH of the blood and is read as such by the blood gas machine.

TABLE 5-1. Water Vapor Pressure in Relation to Temperature

Temperature		P_{H_2O}
°C	°F	(mm Hg)
35	95	42.18
36	96.8	44.56
37	98.6	47.07
38	100.4	49.69
39	102.2	52.44
40	104.0	55.32

PCO_2

The electrode that measures PCO_2 is called the Severinghaus electrode and was originally designed by Stow and Severinghaus. PCO_2 is measured by dissolving carbon dioxide in the blood in an aqueous medium. Acid is then formed, and this changes the pH of the electrolyte contained within the electrode. The Severinghaus electrode measures the change in pH of the electrolyte due to the flow of carbon dioxide through a gas-permeable membrane that covers the electrode. This pH value is then converted electronically to the corresponding PCO_2 value by the blood gas machine.

PO_2

The Clark electrode is used to measure PO_2 and is referred to as an oxygen electrode. Inside the electrode is a platinum wire. Oxygen molecules are broken down rapidly on this surface, causing a change in ionic current that is then measurable as a change in current flow between the silver cathode and the platinum anode. Thus, the oxygen molecule is broken down in the oxygen electrode, electrons are generated, and these electrons in the form of electrical current are read by the blood gas machine and converted into a corresponding PO_2 value.

BICARBONATE

In most institutions, the bicarbonate that is reported with the blood gas results is a standard bicarbonate, as opposed to an actual bicarbonate. Unless otherwise specified, one should assume that the bicarbonate reported with the blood gases is a standard bicarbonate, which is based on pH and PCO_2 and is calculated by the Henderson-Hasselbalch equation.

It is important to remember that *bicarbonate represents the major blood base*.

PERCENT SATURATION

Percent saturation (SO_2) is obtained in one of two ways: by calculation, using a special slide rule based on PO_2 and pH, or by a reading on an oximeter (i.e., spectrophotometrically). The latter method is more accurate, since it involves direct reading of the percent oxyhemoglobin saturation. There are many instances in which the spectrophotometric method has distinct advantages over the calculator—for example, in the patient in whom the oxyhemoglobin dissociation curve is shifted, as is frequently encountered in the critically ill patient, and in the patient who has a high percentage of carboxyhemoglobin in his blood. In the latter case, the calculator does not know what percentage of the oxygen that is analyzed is present as carboxyhemoglobin and has no way to compensate for this factor.

The commercial oximeter available in many institutions is equipped so that it will also give readings for hemoglobin and percent carboxyhemoglobin saturation.

THE CONCEPT OF IN VITRO

One factor often overlooked when interpreting blood gas results is that these measurements have been made in vitro and not in vivo. Probably one of the most significant variables in in vitro measurement of blood gases is the effect of temperature. All blood gas machines are so equipped that the specimen is brought to a given temperature (i.e., usually 37° C) either before or during the analysis. PO_2 and PCO_2 vary directly with temperature at the following rates: 4 percent per degree centigrade for PCO_2 and 7 percent per degree centigrade for PO_2.

Although in most cases the fact that blood gases are measured at 37° C in the laboratory is not significant, there are situations in which this fact could assume real importance (e.g., in operations performed while the patient is on controlled hypothermia). Any corrections for these temperature factors must be made by the physician, since most laboratories do not correct blood gases for temperature. It should also be pointed out that other factors can be corrected for in blood gases (in particular, the effect of pH on percent saturation). Again, this is not done by the laboratory, but various nomograms are available for use in these situations (see Appendix 3).

THE RELIABILITY OF RESULTS

The key question about any laboratory report is whether or not the results are correct. Often, physicians may take the attitude that if the result is what they expected, it is correct. This is a dangerous assumption. Others may take the attitude that results that come from their laboratory must be correct. This, too, is fallacious. One must scrutinize all laboratory results with a critical eye, and when a significant question of accuracy arises, the test must be repeated.

One way to minimize some uncertainties is to investigate the laboratory's quality control program. In the case of blood gas measurements, various methods of quality control are available to a laboratory. These methods all involve the use of a known value solution for comparison with the value

TABLE 5-2. Normal Blood Gas Values

Blood Gas	Arterial	Mixed Venous
pH	7.40 (7.35–7.45)	7.36 (7.31–7.41)
PCO_2	35–45 mm Hg	41–51 mm Hg
PO_2	80–100 mm Hg	35–40 mm Hg
HCO_3^-	22–26 mEq/L	22–26 mEq/L
SO_2 (% saturation)	95 or greater	75 (70–75)
Base excess	−2 to +2	−2 to +2

generated by the machine. Quality control of the PO_2 is the most difficult, but it can be accomplished with a tonometer. A tonometer allows equilibration of a blood specimen with a gas of a known oxygen concentration, thus establishing the PO_2 the machine should get for the equilibrated sample.

CLINICAL INTERPRETATION OF BLOOD GASES

The increased clinical use of blood gas determinations has led to the proliferation of books and articles dealing with the measurement and interpretation. The material to be presented in this section is not intended to replace other available references and will not add significantly to what has already been contributed. Rather, our goal is to provide a review for quick reference.

As with most tests, there are "normal" values for blood gases. However, these should not be overemphasized, since the patient's previous pulmonary status often has not been normal. Whenever possible, baseline or preoperative blood gas values should be obtained, especially when the patient is having major surgery. Also, when indicated, a complete pulmonary function work-up can be invaluable for preoperative preparation, anesthesia evaluation, and postoperative management.

Representative blood gas values for arterial and mixed venous blood are listed in Table 5-2. In any comparisons with these values, however, both the patient's age and previous pulmonary status must be taken into account, and it must be kept in mind that normal values for mixed venous blood gases are more variable than are those for arterial blood gases.

pH

The pH determines the patient's acid-base status (see Chapter 16). An arterial pH less than 7.35 indicates acidemia; an arterial pH greater than 7.45 indicates alkalemia.

The following terms relate to pH:

1. *Acidemia:* an arterial pH of less than 7.35
2. *Acidosis:* the process that gives rise to acidemia
3. *Acidotic:* pertaining to acidosis

4. *Alkalemia:* an arterial pH greater than 7.45
5. *Alkalosis:* the process that gives rise to alkalemia
6. *Alkalotic:* pertaining to alkalosis

The pH allows one to determine whether or not acidemia or alkalemia exists or, if both are present, which one is predominating. The pH is defined as the negative log of the hydrogen ion concentration. The Henderson-Hasselbalch equation is the mathematical statement of pH and is written as follows:

$$pH = pK + \log (base/acid)$$

The pK is defined as the pH at which a substance is half dissociated and half undissociated. The pK of blood under physiologic conditions is 6.1. In the Henderson-Hasselbalch equation, the base is bicarbonate (HCO_3^-), and the acid is carbonic acid. The normal ratio between bicarbonate and carbonic acid is 20 : 1. This is an important relationship to keep in mind. One may determine the value for carbonic acid by multiplying the PCO_2 by 0.03.

$PaCO_2$

The partial pressure of arterial carbon dioxide ($PaCO_2$) is the "respiratory parameter," and, as such, it allows one to assess the adequacy of alveolar ventilation. In addition, the arteriovenous carbon dioxide difference is primarily determined by the metabolic rate (the venous blood must be mixed venous blood for this determination). Therefore, the $PaCO_2$ is a reflection of the adequacy of the alveolar ventilation in relation to the metabolic rate.

$PaCO_2$ may be normal, increased (hypercapnia), or decreased (hypocapnia). A normal $PaCO_2$ means normal alveolar ventilation; an increased $PaCO_2$, hypoventilation; and a decreased $PaCO_2$, hyperventilation. Of course, this is an oversimplification, and one must remember that changes in $PaCO_2$ can occur as compensation for metabolic disturbances, as well as primarily on a respiratory basis.

$PaCO_2$ also has an effect on pH. As previously stated, the pH is the result of the ratio of plasma bicarbonate to plasma carbonic acid, normally 20 : 1. Assuming that HCO_3^- remains within the normal range, a relationship between pH and H_2CO_3 results. This represents the pH change that is secondary to changes in alveolar ventilation (i.e., changes in acid-base status due to respiration). The relationship is inverse and is nearly linear. Because of this, the following guideline can be put forth: for every increase of 20 mm Hg in $PaCO_2$ the pH will decrease by 0.10 units, and for every decrease of 10 mm Hg in $PaCO_2$ the pH will increase by 0.10 units.

PaO_2

The arterial oxygen tension (PaO_2) by itself provides little physiologic information beyond indicating the adequacy of arterial oxygenation. The true value of arterial oxygen tension is that PaO_2 and FiO_2 considered together provide information relative to the efficiency of oxygen exchange.

It is important to remember that PaO_2 will be affected by the presence of preexisting lung disease as well as by age, and both must be taken into account in interpreting a patient's PaO_2.

Since oxygen is essential for cellular function, it is not only valuable to assess the adequacy of supply (i.e., the PaO_2) but equally important to assess delivery of oxygen. Oxygen transport is considered in detail in Chapter 24, but a brief mention of *mixed venous oxygen tension* and/or saturation measurements is useful at this point.

The partial pressure of oxygen in mixed venous blood ($P\bar{v}O_2$), or the oxyhemoglobin saturation of mixed venous blood ($S\bar{v}O_2$), reflects the amount of oxygen that has been removed during passage through the body. Assuming normal conditions, if the arterial oxygen saturation (SaO_2) is 100 percent, one can expect 25 percent of the oxygen to be utilized during passage through the body (i.e., from the aortic root to the right ventricle). This means that the normal $P\bar{v}O_2$ should be about 40 mm Hg, which corresponds to a $S\bar{v}O_2$ of 75 percent (i.e., assuming a normal pH and oxygen dissociation curve). With this knowledge, one can see that a $P\bar{v}O_2$ less than 40 mm Hg reflects increased oxygen extraction by the tissues; a $P\bar{v}O_2$ greater than 40 mm Hg indicates decreased oxygen extraction by the tissues. Additionally, if the $P\bar{v}O_2$ drops below 25 to 30 mm Hg, there is reason to believe that tissue oxygenation may be impaired.

BICARBONATE

The normal value for HCO_3^- is 22 to 26 mEq/liter (with a mean value of 24 mEq/liter). As the $PaCO_2$ is referred to as the respiratory parameter, the HCO_3^- can be called the metabolic parameter. As such, HCO_3^- is primarily a function of the kidneys (this, of course, is somewhat of an oversimplification).

As the kidneys are the prime regulators of HCO_3^-, changes in this parameter are slow (24–36 hr) as compared with changes in $PaCO_2$, which can occur within minutes. Plasma HCO_3^- can, however, be manipulated artificially (e.g., by administration of sodium bicarbonate or ammonium chloride) and thereby quickly changed.

Bicarbonate represents the primary blood base. Analysis of bicarbonate may reveal a normal HCO_3^-, an increased HCO_3^-, or a decreased HCO_3^-. Strictly speaking, an increase in bicarbonate will cause a metabolic alkalosis, while a decrease in bicarbonate or an accumulation of acid (e.g., lactic or β-hydroxybutyric acid) will cause a metabolic acidosis. However, whether or not an alkalosis or acidosis can be determined to be present by analysis of pH alone will depend on the respiratory compensation for the underlying process. This will be dealt with further in the discussion of acid-base imbalances in Chapter 16.

To determine whether the metabolic acidosis is due to an increase in measurable or unmeasurable anions the following formula can be used:

Anion "gap" = serum sodium − (bicarbonate + chloride)

NOTE. Bicarbonate may be interchanged with the serum carbon dioxide measurement. If the difference is greater than 15 mEq/liter, there is an increase in unmeasurable anions.

Some of the causes of an increase in measurable anions are renal tubular acidosis, treatment with acetazolamide (Diamox) or ammonium chloride, ureterosigmoidostomy with chloride reabsorption and hyperchloremia, diarrhea, and drainage of pancreatic juice. Some of the causes of an increase in unmeasurable anions are lactic acidosis, renal failure, diabetic ketoacidosis, and poisoning (with salicylate, ethylene glycol, methyl alcohol, paraldehyde).

PERCENT OXYGEN SATURATION

Oxygen saturation is equal to the oxygen content (minus the physically dissolved oxygen) divided by the oxygen capacity (minus the physically dissolved oxygen). In general, an arterial oxygen saturation equal to 90 percent or greater is considered acceptable. This saturation roughly corresponds to a PaO_2 of 60 mm Hg. When dealing with venous blood, an acceptable value for mixed venous oxygen saturation is 75 percent, which corresponds approximately to a PO_2 of 40 mm Hg.

It is important to emphasize that percent saturation is a ratio of concentrations and therefore cannot be a measure of concentration itself. In other words, a low saturation need not mean that the oxygen concentration in blood is low. On the other hand, a normal saturation may be associated with a low oxygen content. For example, a polycythemic sample (hemoglobin equals 22 gm/100 ml) has an oxygen capacity of 300 ml/liter. This may be only 60 percent saturated and contain as much oxygen (i.e., 180 ml/liter) as a normal sample (hemoglobin equals 15 gm/100 ml) with an oxygen capacity of 200 ml/liter that is 90 percent saturated. On the other hand, in anemia, the percent saturation may be normal, but the quantity of oxygen per unit volume of blood is low.

COLLECTION AND TRANSPORTATION OF BLOOD GAS SPECIMENS

HEPARIN. When drawing blood for blood gas analysis, it is essential to en sure that the specimen is adequately anticoagulated. Adequate anticoagulation can be easily achieved utilizing sodium heparin; neither ammonium heparin nor edetate (EDTA) should be used, since both significantly affect pH readings. However, too much sodium heparin can change pH to the acidotic side. A general rule that can be followed is not to use more than 0.05 ml of sodium heparin for each milliliter of blood sample drawn. If the

TABLE 5-3. Effect of Time and Temperature on Blood Gas Parameters

Parameter	37° C	20° C
pH	0.01/10 min	0.001/10 min
$PaCO_2$	1 mm Hg/10 min	0.1 mm Hg/10 min
PaO_2	0.5 vol%/10 min	0.05 vol%/10 min

small amount of heparin is introduced into the syringe, and the syringe is then coated with the heparin, and all but a very small amount of the heparin is expelled, leaving enough to fill the dead space of the syringe, adequate anticoagulation of the specimen can be achieved, with minimal risk of introducing air into the sample.

AIR CONTAMINATION OF THE BLOOD GAS. Frequently, when a blood gas specimen is being drawn, air enters the syringe. It is important to remember that these air bubbles should be removed before the specimen is analyzed. The most dangerous air bubbles are the small ones; because of their increased surface area, they have the greatest effect upon the reading.

PLASTIC SYRINGES. Several studies have disclosed that plastic absorbs oxygen. This process appears to be insignificant in blood gas analysis when the PaO_2 is in the normal range. However, when dealing with a high PaO_2 (i.e., greater than 160 mm Hg) diffusion of oxygen from the syringe into the atmosphere may be hastened by using a plastic syringe.

TRANSPORTATION OF BLOOD GAS SPECIMENS. Blood is living tissue that continues to consume oxygen and produce carbon dioxide even after it is placed in a syringe. Table 5-3 shows the effect of time on blood gas values when the syringe is kept at body temperature. In view of this effect, the sample should immediately be iced completely so that the temperature will not rise above 20° C. When this is accomplished, the changes in $PaCO_2$ and pH will be insignificant even over several hours.

RESPIRATORY FUNCTION MONITORING
Respiratory monitoring can be divided into four major categories: methods of evaluating (1) the adequacy and efficiency of oxygen exchange, (2) the adequacy of ventilation, (3) respiratory mechanics and ventilatory reserve, and (4) ancillary diagnostic techniques.

In addition, recent advances in respiratory monitoring techniques have been made. These include inert gas measurements for assessing ventilation, perfusion inequalities in the lung, measurement of functional residual capacity (FRC), two-compartmental analysis of ventilation, and breathing loop analysis. However, to avoid overcomplicating the discussion, only conventionally used methods will be discussed.

EVALUATING THE EFFICIENCY AND ADEQUACY OF OXYGENATION
ARTERIAL OXYGEN TENSION

Because many patients in the early stage of acute respiratory failure will be able to maintain adequate oxygenation (PaO_2), it is important to evaluate the efficiency of oxygen exchange in the lungs, since this often shows a change before the patient has lost the ability to maintain adequate oxygenation. One of the most sensitive indicators of early respiratory impairment is the alveolar-arterial oxygen gradient [$P(A-a)O_2$].

ALVEOLAR-ARTERIAL OXYGEN GRADIENT

The $P(A-a)O_2$ may be measured at any given FIO_2; however, it is most commonly determined with the patient inhaling 100% oxygen ($FIO_2 = 1.0$).

When the patient is on an FIO_2 of 1.0, the oxygen tension is the same in all ventilated alveoli (i.e., the partial pressure of oxygen in all ventilated alveoli is the same; the PO_2 in the alveolus is abbreviated as PAO_2). Under these circumstances (i.e., $FIO_2 = 1.0$), the $P(A-a)O_2$ is a reflection of physiologic shunting in the lung, i.e., of alveoli that are perfused but not ventilated. It must be noted that the calculation of the $P(A-a)O_2$ at $FIO_2 = 1.0$ has recently been the center of attention in the literature. The concern is the result of the finding that inhalation of 100% oxygen, even for short periods of time, causes absorption atelectasis with resultant increase in shunt. Briefly, this occurs when the airway becomes obstructed (e.g., secondary to a mucous plug or airway closure). In this situation, the flow of oxygen out of the alveolus occurs rapidly because of the large diffusion gradient between PAO_2 and $P\bar{v}O_2$. After the oxygen has left the alveolus only the pressure due to PCO_2 and PH_2O remains because the nitrogen normally present has been washed out. With the nitrogen "splint" gone, there may be insufficient pressure to maintain the alveolus in an open state. When absorption atelectasis occurs, it may be difficult to reopen the alveolus because of the surface tension of such small units. Clinically, it may require high inspiratory pressures to open these atelectatic units [17, 26, 28].

CALCULATION OF THE $P(A-a)O_2$ AT FIO_2 OF 1.0. The patient should be placed on 100% oxygen for 10 to 20 minutes. (In the nonemphysematous patient, the period required is usually less than 10 min, but because it is often difficult to assess pulmonary function status in these patients, a period of 20–30 min is used.) During this period of time the patient must not be disconnected from the ventilator, and physical activity should be held to a minimum. Arterial blood gases are drawn and the corrected barometric pressure (PB) obtained. The following example is provided to illustrate the calculation of the $P(A-a)O_2$ ($FIO_2 = 1.0$).

Example
Following the inhalation of an FIO_2 of 1.0 for 20 minutes, the following values for arterial blood were obtained: pH, 7.48; $PaCO_2$ 39 mm Hg; PaO_2, 325 mm Hg;

HCO_3^-, 28 mEq/liter; SaO_2, 99.7%. The barometric pressure reading was 752 mm Hg. Taking these values, the calculation is made as follows:[6,7]

P_B	752 mm Hg
P_{H_2O}	−47
Corrected P_B	705
P_ACO_2	−39
P_AO_2	666
PaO_2	−325
$P(A-a)O_2$	341 mm Hg

CALCULATION OF THE $P(A-a)O_2$ AT AN FIO_2 LESS THAN 1.0. When the FIO_2 is reduced below 1.0, the calculation of the $P(A-a)O_2$ becomes a more complex task. Two additional formulas can be used. The alveolar air equation [7] is the most accurate. It requires measurement of the respiratory quotient (RQ) (i.e., the ratio of the volume of carbon dioxide produced to the volume of oxygen consumed), although some authors suggest that rather than actually measuring RQ, one should assume it to be normal (i.e., equal to 0.8). However, this is often not true, especially in the critically ill patient. The second formula, proposed by Thal et al. [24], is admittedly less accurate but can prove useful when RQ cannot be measured.

The alveolar air equation. The alveolar air equation is calculated as follows:

$$P_AO_2 = P_IO_2 - P_ACO_2 \left[FIO_2 + \frac{1 - FIO_2}{R} \right]$$

where

P_AO_2 = partial pressure of oxygen in the alveolus

P_IO_2 = moist inspired oxygen tension

FIO_2 = fractional inspired oxygen concentration

P_ACO_2 = partial pressure of carbon dioxide in the alveolus (can be assumed, as before, to be the same as $PaCO_2$)

R = respiratory quotient

FACTORS INFLUENCING THE ALVEOLAR-ARTERIAL OXYGEN GRADIENT. The factors that affect the alveolar-arterial oxygen gradient [20] are as follows:

---

[6] The value for water vapor pressure (P_{H_2O}) is dependent on the patient's temperature. To simplify the calculation the value at 37° C is used.

[7] Variations in P_ACO_2 due to ventilation-perfusion inequalities are small as compared with the P_AO_2 during oxygen breathing. The error made in assuming that P_ACO_2 equals P_ACO_2 is therefore negligible.

1. The magnitude of the right-to-left shunt ($\dot{Q}s/\dot{Q}T$)—i.e., that portion of cardiac output flowing past nonventilated alveoli (see below).
2. The fractional inspired oxygen concentration FIO_2 (i.e., any ventilation-perfusion inequality has a greater role when less than 100% oxygen is inspired).
3. The arteriovenous oxygen content difference (a-$\bar{v}DCO_2$).
4. Oxygen consumption, through its effect on mixed venous oxygen content.
5. Cardiac output:
   a. Secondary to changes in the a-$\bar{v}DCO_2$ when oxygen consumption remains constant.
   b. Secondary to redistribution of pulmonary blood flow.
6. The position of the arterial point on the oxyhemoglobin dissociation curve.
7. The position (i.e., configuration) of the oxyhemoglobin dissociation curve.

THE PERCENT OF PULMONARY SHUNT

The percent of pulmonary shunt ($\dot{Q}s/\dot{Q}T$) (i.e., the right-to-left shunt) is defined as that portion of the cardiac output ($\dot{Q}T$) (pulmonary blood flow) that is perfusing unventilated alveoli ($\dot{Q}s$). Thus, measuring the shunt enables one to quantitate the percentage of cardiac output that returns to the left heart unoxygenated (i.e., with a PO_2 equal to that of the mixed venous blood). This is often also referred to as pulmonary venous admixture. There are four causes of total pulmonary shunting: (1) impaired diffusion, (2) ventilation-perfusion inequalities, (3) anatomic shunts (e.g., in the normal person, this is due to blood returning to the left heart via the bronchial and thebesian veins), and (4) alveolar collapse (i.e., where the $\dot{V}A/\dot{Q} = 0$). In the normal person, $\dot{Q}s/\dot{Q}T$ is in the range of 3 to 5 percent; however, in the critically ill patient, a shunt of 15 percent is not at all uncommon.

The $\dot{Q}s/\dot{Q}T$ can be measured with the patient either on 100% oxygen or on a lesser oxygen concentration. There are, however, certain advantages to measuring the percent of shunt on an FIO_2 of 1.0. When the patient is breathing 100% oxygen, the calculation of the $\dot{Q}s/\dot{Q}T$ is simplified (because the calculation of the $P(A-a)O_2$, which is required in the shunt equation, is simplified). In addition, when the patient is on an FIO_2 of 1.0, the causes of total pulmonary shunting are reduced to only anatomic shunting and alveolar collapse (i.e., alveoli that are perfused but unventilated). However, while placing the patient on an FIO_2 of 1.0 simplifies the calculation of $\dot{Q}s/\dot{Q}T$ and reduces the causes of shunting, one must keep in mind the effect that an FIO_2 of 1.0 alone may have on alveoli (i.e., absorption atelectasis) [29].

CALCULATION OF $\dot{Q}s/\dot{Q}T$. To calculate the percent of pulmonary shunt ($\dot{Q}s/\dot{Q}T$), one must have the following information: (1) the PAO_2 (i.e., the PO_2 in the alveolus), (2) the PaO_2 (i.e., the arterial PO_2), (3) the arteriovenous oxygen content difference (a-$\bar{v}DCO_2$) (the calculation of which also requires that one know the patient's hemoglobin).

The patient is placed on 100% oxygen for 10 to 20 min, and then arterial and mixed venous blood gases are obtained along with the measurement of hemoglobin. Precise calculation of $\dot{Q}s/\dot{Q}T$ requires that mixed venous blood be withdrawn from the pulmonary artery (e.g., by using the Swan-Ganz catheter).

The $\dot{Q}s/\dot{Q}T$ is then calculated from the following formula. The only additional requirement for calculating the shunt is that the PaO_2 must be at least 150 mm Hg (at this level, hemoglobin is fully saturated with oxygen, and any further increases in PaO_2 only affect the amount of dissolved oxygen in plasma). If the PaO_2 is less than 150 mm Hg, another formula must be used.

CALCULATION OF THE $\dot{Q}s/\dot{Q}T$ WHEN THE PaO_2 IS AT LEAST 150 MM HG. When the PaO_2 is at least 150 mm Hg, the $\dot{Q}s/\dot{Q}T$ is calculated as follows:

$$\dot{Q}s/\dot{Q}T = \frac{(P_AO_2 - PaO_2) \times 0.0031}{a\text{-}\bar{v}DCO_2 + (P_AO_2 - PaO_2) \times 0.0031}$$

where

$\dot{Q}s$ = unventilated alveoli
$\dot{Q}T$ = cardiac output
P_AO_2 = partial pressure of oxygen in the alveolus
PaO_2 = partial pressure of oxygen in arterial blood
0.0031 = solubility coefficient (Bunsen) for oxygen dissolved in plasma
a-$\bar{v}$DCO$_2$ = arteriovenous oxygen content difference

The P_AO_2 is calculated in the same way as previously described. The arteriovenous oxygen content difference is calculated as follows:

a-$\bar{v}$DCO$_2$ = CaO$_2$ − C$\bar{v}$O$_2$

where

CaO$_2$ = (Hb × 1.39) SaO$_2$ + (PaO$_2$ × 0.0031)
C$\bar{v}$O$_2$ = (Hb × 1.39) S$\bar{v}$O$_2$ + (P$\bar{v}$O$_2$ × 0.0031)
CaO$_2$ = the oxygen content of arterial blood
C$\bar{v}$O$_2$ = the oxygen content of mixed blood
Hb = hemoglobin concentration in gm/100 ml
1.39 = ml of oxygen capable of being carried by 1 gm of hemoglobin (theoretical)
SaO$_2$ = oxyhemoglobin saturation of arterial blood
S$\bar{v}$O$_2$ = oxyhemoglobin saturation of mixed venous blood
PaO$_2$ = partial pressure of oxygen in arterial blood
P$\bar{v}$O$_2$ = partial pressure of oxygen in mixed venous blood
0.0031 = solubility coefficient for oxygen physically dissolved in solution [22]

Shunts are now being calculated more frequently on an FIO_2 of 1.0. If the PaO_2 is then less than 150 mm Hg, the following equation must be used.

CALCULATION OF THE $\dot{Q}s/\dot{Q}T$ WHEN THE PaO_2 IS LESS THAN 150 MM HG. At a PaO_2 of less than 150 mm Hg, the $\dot{Q}s/\dot{Q}T$ is calculated as follows:[8]

$$\dot{Q}s/\dot{Q}T = \frac{CcO_2 - CaO_2}{CcO_2 - C\bar{v}O_2}$$

where

$\dot{Q}$ = total pulmonary blood flow
CaO_2 = oxygen content of arterial blood
$C\bar{v}O_2$ = oxygen content of mixed venous blood
CcO_2 = oxygen content of pulmonary capillary blood

In this equation, CaO_2 and $C\bar{v}O_2$ are calculated as described previously. The calculation of CcO_2, however, requires one to assume that this would be the oxygen content that arterial blood would have if fully equilibrated with alveolar air. This is necessary because of the inaccessibility of pulmonary capillary blood for direct measurement. For example, a patient with an FIO_2 of 0.5 has the following values: Hb = 15 gm/100 ml, PaO_2 = 105 mm Hg, SaO_2 = 99.2%. The values for mixed venous blood are as follows: $P\bar{v}O_2$ = 40 mm Hg, and $S\bar{v}O_2$ = 75%. Before calculating the $\dot{Q}s/\dot{Q}T$, it is necessary to determine the PAO_2 (the calculation is explained on p. 87). In this case, the PAO_2 was calculated to be 650 mm Hg. Now that all the necessary information for the calculation of $\dot{Q}s/\dot{Q}T$ has been obtained, one can proceed with the calculation of CcO_2, CaO_2, and $C\bar{v}O_2$.

CcO_2 = (Hb × 1.39) SaO_2 + (PAO_2 × 0.0031)

Note
Because the PO_2 of alveolar air on 100% oxygen will always exceed 150 mm Hg, one can assume that the saturation of blood exposed to alveolar air (i.e., pulmonary capillary blood) will be 100%.

CcO_2 = (15 × 1.39) + (650 × 0.0031)
CcO_2 = 22.86 vol%
CaO_2 = (15 × 1.39) .992 + (105 × 0.0031)
CaO_2 = 21.00 vol%
$C\bar{v}O_2$ = (15 × 1.39) .75 + (40 × 0.0031)
$C\bar{v}O_2$ = 15.76 vol%

The calculation of $\dot{Q}s/\dot{Q}T$ is now completed as follows:

[8] The formula described above can also be used when the PaO_2 is 150 mm Hg or greater. However, when this condition is met, it is easier to use the formula given on page 89.

$$\dot{Q}s/\dot{Q}\textsc{t} = \frac{22.86 - 21.00}{22.86 - 15.76}$$

$$\dot{Q}s/\dot{Q}\textsc{t} = 0.26$$

Note
This value is then converted to a percentage by multiplying it by 100.

$$\dot{Q}s/\dot{Q}\textsc{t} = 26\%$$

EVALUATING THE ADEQUACY OF VENTILATION
The $PaCO_2$ is a reliable indicator of the adequacy of alveolar ventilation.

TIDAL VOLUME
Tidal volume ($V\textsc{t}$) is defined as the volume of air moved in or out of the lungs in any single breath. If the tidal volume is depressed, the patient may have difficulty in both oxygenation and ventilation.

$V\textsc{d}/V\textsc{t}$ (PHYSIOLOGIC DEAD SPACE)
Frequently, the critically ill patient will hyperventilate, yet his $PaCO_2$ will be normal. This is because of increased physiologic dead space, that portion of the tidal volume that does not exchange with pulmonary blood. While this may be obvious in some patients, there are others in whom this observation is not so easily made. In these situations, the measurement of $V\textsc{d}/V\textsc{t}$ may prove useful. The normal value for $V\textsc{d}/V\textsc{t}$ is from 0.2 to 0.4. The derivation of this formula [3] will not be presented here. The formula that is used clinically is derived from Bohr's equation and is as follows:

$$V\textsc{d}/V\textsc{t} = \frac{PaCO_2 - P\bar{E}CO_2}{PaCO_2}$$

where

$V\textsc{d}$ = dead space
$V\textsc{t}$ = tidal volume
$PaCO_2$ = arterial carbon dioxide tension
$P\bar{E}CO_2$ = mean expired carbon dioxide tension

The classic case in which one finds an increased $V\textsc{d}/V\textsc{t}$ is pulmonary embolism. In this situation, there are areas of lung that are ventilated but unperfused. While pulmonary embolism is the classic case, changes in $V\textsc{d}/V\textsc{t}$ also occur following shock and in pulmonary insufficiency. The $V\textsc{d}/V\textsc{t}$ will vary with changes in either anatomic or alveolar dead space or tidal volume. However, $V\textsc{d}/V\textsc{t}$ does not differentiate anatomic from alveolar dead space, nor does it differentiate dead space change from ventilation-perfusion inequalities.

The clinical measurement of V_D/V_T is primarily of value when the tidal volume is greater than normal and when the increased tidal volume is relatively consistent. These conditions are met by most patients who are on mechanical ventilatory assistance.

The following are some situations in which one can observe an increased V_D/V_T:

1. In nonperfusion of a ventilated alveolus (e.g., a pulmonary embolus).
2. In hypotension, in which gravity and a low pulmonary artery pressure promote a redistribution of blood volume and flow, favoring the dependent portion of the lung, so that many alveoli are ventilated but unperfused.
3. When there is an increase in mean airway pressure, occurring in some alveoli to the extent that the capillary perfusion during the respiratory cycle causes a redistribution of blood flow to the remainder of the lung. In the presence of refractory atelectasis, a portion of this redistributed blood flow will go to atelectatic areas. As a result, both V_D/V_T and $\dot{Q}_S/\dot{Q}_T$ are increased.

EVALUATING RESPIRATORY MECHANICS AND VENTILATORY RESERVE

In addition to the evaluation of oxygenation and ventilation, it is necessary to consider the mechanics and work of breathing. The respiratory rate as a function of labored breathing, vital capacity, inspiratory force, functional residual capacity (FRC), and compliance are parameters that can be used.

VITAL CAPACITY

Vital capacity is defined as a maximal expiration following a maximal inspiration. Normally, vital capacity should be in the range of 60 to 70 ml/kg. In the critically ill patient, a vital capacity of less than 15 ml/kg is an indication for mechanical ventilatory assistance. Conversely, patients on ventilatory assistance can be considered ready for weaning when their vital capacity is at least 10 ml/kg. When the vital capacity reaches 15 ml/kg, the patient will probably be able to tolerate being off the ventilator permanently.

INSPIRATORY FORCE

This measurement is based on experience that has shown that the muscular power needed to generate a vital capacity of 15 ml/kg produces a negative inspiratory force of more than -25 cm H_2O within 20 seconds.

Inspiratory force is measured as the maximal pressure below atmospheric pressure that a patient can exert during a period of 10 to 20 seconds against a completely occluded airway. This measurement is not dependent on the cooperation of the patient and is particularly useful with unconscious or anesthetized patients. The normal value for inspiratory force is -75 to -100 cm H_2O. The measurement of inspiratory force requires only the following: a face mask or a connector to an endotracheal or tracheostomy tube and a manometer capable of registering pressure below atmospheric pressure.

FUNCTIONAL RESIDUAL CAPACITY

Functional residual capacity (FRC) is defined as the gas remaining in the lung following a normal expiration. Its measurement [6, 29] has been receiving increased attention in the literature. This is because of the observation that patients with pulmonary insufficiency have decreased FRC. It has also been observed that positive end-expiratory pressure (PEEP) increases FRC. Although methods to measure FRC are not routinely available, there are several methods that can be clinically applied at the bedside.

COMPLIANCE

Compliance is defined as the forces resisting expansion of the lung. There are a variety of methods available to measure compliance, but the discussion here will be confined to the measurement of so-called effective dynamic compliance (EDC).

Compliance is measured as volume change per pressure change (ml/cm H_2O). Effective dynamic compliance measurements should not be confused with static compliance measurements (i.e., when no air is moving); rather, they indicate changes in lung compliance (i.e., the stiffness of the lungs).

The interpretation of EDC is not without problems, since it is affected by high airway pressures and the distensibility of the tubing used on the respirator. Despite these problems, we have used it to indicate a trend. As EDC increases, the lung is becoming less stiff; conversely, as EDC decreases, the lung is becoming stiffer. That is to say, as EDC increases, it takes less pressure to produce a given tidal volume. A sudden decrease in EDC may be an indicator of a blocked airway, and this cause should be ruled out before assuming that the lung has become stiffer.

To measure EDC, one divides the tidal volume by the peak airway pressure.

EDC = tidal volume (ml)/peak airway pressure (cm H_2O)

ANCILLARY TECHNIQUES

CHEST ROENTGENOGRAMS

Chest roentgenograms are routinely taken in patients with pulmonary insufficiency. However, roentgenographic changes are late in such patients.

AUSCULTATION

A physician would not be a physician without a stethoscope, and even though auscultatory changes come very late in pulmonary insufficiency, the physician must frequently auscultate the patient's chest to detect gross changes. For example, a pneumothorax may develop in a patient on PEEP,

TABLE 5-4. Guidelines for the Institution and Discontinuation of Mechanical Ventilatory Support in Patients with Pulmonary Insufficiency

Parameter	Normal Range	Indication for Ventilatory Assistance	Indication for Weaning
Mechanics			
Respiratory rate	12–20	>35	<30
Vital capacity (ml/kg of body weight)[a]	65–75	<15	12–15
FEV_1 (ml/kg of body weight)[a]	50–60	<10	>10
Inspiratory force (cm H_2O)	75–100	<25	>25
Oxygenation			
PaO_2 (mm Hg)	100–75 (room air)	<70 (on mask O_2)	. . .[b]
$P(A-a)O_2$ ($FIO_2 = 1.0$) (mm Hg)[c]	25–65	450	<400
Ventilation			
$PaCO_2$ (mm Hg)	35–45	>55[d]	. . .[e]
VD/VT	0.25–0.40	>0.60	<0.58

[a] Patient's ideal weight is used if weight appears grossly abnormal.
[b] When the physician is deciding to wean the patient, the $P(A-a)O_2$ ($FIO_2 = 0.50$ or 1.0) serves as a better criterion than any given PaO_2.
[c] The $P(A-a)O_2$ is measured after the patient has been on an $FIO_2 = 1.0$ for 10–20 min (in the nonemphysematous patient 10 min is adequate). *Note:* It was mentioned earlier that there are certain problems associated with measuring the $P(A-a)O_2$ at an FIO_2 of 1.0. If, however, it must be measured at 1.0, the patient should be sighed (i.e., the lungs hyperinflated) with nitrogen-containing mixtures following the discontinuation of the the 100% oxygen.
[d] Except in patients with chronic hypercapnia.
[e] Since $PaCO_2$, while the patient is on the ventilator, is a function of the respirator settings as well as the patient's lungs, it is not a useful measurement for assessing readiness for weaning.

Note: The temptation to rely on a list of objective criteria as the definitive ruling on intubation and weaning is great. However, it should be kept in mind that the trend of values is more important than any given value alone.

Source: Modified from R. S. Wilson and H. Pontoppidan. Acute respiratory failure. *Crit. Care Med.* 2:293, 1974.

and in this instance the stethoscope and chest roentgenogram will prove useful. In this situation, blood gases would probably also reveal a deterioration in PaO_2 secondary to pneumothorax.

GUIDELINES FOR THE INSTITUTION AND DISCONTINUATION OF MECHANICAL VENTILATORY ASSISTANCE

In summary, respiratory monitoring is now the established method by which data are obtained for the initiation and cessation of mechanical ventilatory assistance (see Table 5-4). Several excellent reviews and articles have been published on this subject [20, 30], which is dealt with in more detail in Chapters 6 and 8.

Subjective decisions no longer have a place in the determination of the need for mechanical ventilatory assistance.

REFERENCES

1. Adler, D. C., and Bryan-Brown, C. W. Use of the axillary artery for intravascular monitoring. *Crit. Care Med.* 1:148, 1973.
2. Bartlett, R. H., and Munster, A. M. An improved technique for prolonged arterial cannulation. *N. Engl. J. Med.* 279:92, 1968.
3. Bendixen, H. H., et al. *Respiratory Care.* St. Louis: Mosby, 1965. Pp. 17–20.
4. Berne, R. M., and Levy, M. N. The Arterial System. In *Cardiovascular Physiology* (4th ed.). St. Louis: Mosby, 1977.
5. Civetta, J. M. The daily problems in the intensive care unit. *Adv. Surg.* 8:243, 1974.
6. Comroe, J. H., et al. *The Lung: Clinical Physiology and Pulmonary Function Tests* (2nd ed.). Chicago: Year Book, 1962. Pp. 15–19.
7. Comroe, J. H., et al. *The Lung: Clinical Physiology and Pulmonary Function Tests* (2nd ed.). Chicago: Year Book, 1962. Pp. 339–341.
8. Downs, J. B., et al. Prolonged radial-artery catheterization: An evaluation of heparinized catheters and continuous irrigation. *Arch. Surg.* 108:671, 1974.
9. Forrester, J. S., and Swan, H. J. C. Acute myocardial infarction: A physiological basis for therapy. *Crit. Care Med.* 2:283, 1974.
10. Ganz, W., and Swan, H. J. C. Measurement of blood flow in thermodilution. *Am. J. Cardiol.* 29:241, 1974.
11. Gardner, R. M., et al. Percutaneous indwelling radial-artery catheters for monitoring cardiovascular function: Prospective study of the risk of thrombosis and infection. *N. Engl. J. Med.* 290:1227, 1974.
12. Geddes, L. A. *The Direct and Indirect Measurement of Blood Pressure.* Chicago: Year Book, 1970.
13. Guyton, A. C., and Jones, C. E. Central venous pressure: Physiological significance and clinical implications. *Am. Heart J.* 86:431, 1973.
14. Hughes, V. G., and Prys-Roberts, C. Intra-arterial pressure measurements: A review and analysis of methods relevant to anaesthesia and intensive care. *Anaesthesia* 26:511, 1971.
15. Jacobson, E. D. A physiologic approach to shock. *N. Engl. J. Med.* 278:834, 1968.

16. Laver, M. B., et al.   Right and left ventricular geometry: Adjustments during acute respiratory failure. *Crit. Care Med.* 7:509, 1979.
17. McAslan, T. C., et al.   Influence of 100% oxygen in intrapulmonary shunt in severely traumatized patients. *J. Trauma* 13:811, 1973.
18. Manny, Jonah, et al.   Myocardial performance curves as a guide to volume therapy. *Surgery, Gynecology & Obstetrics* 149:863, 1979.
19. Massachusetts General Hospital.   *Concepts of Intra-Aortic Balloon Pumping: An Interdisciplinary Approach.* Section III. Boston: Avco Everett Medical Products, 1974.
20. Pontoppidan, H., et al.   Acute respiratory failure in the adult. *N. Engl. J. Med.* 287:745, 1972.
21. Rushmer, R. R.   Systemic Arterial Pressure. In *Structure and Function of the Cardiovascular System* (2nd ed.). Philadelphia: Saunders, 1976.
22. Swan, H. J. C., et al.   Catheterization of the heart in man with use of a flow-directed balloon-tipped catheter. *N. Engl. J. Med.* 283:447, 1970.
23. Tarazi, R. C., and Gifford, R. W.   Systemic Arterial Pressure. In W. A. Sodeman and W. A. Sodeman, Jr. (Eds.), *Pathologic Physiology: Mechanisms of Disease* (6th ed.). Philadelphia: Saunders, 1979.
24. Thal, A. P., et al.   *Shock: A Physiologic Basis for Treatment.* Chicago: Year Book, 1971. Pp. 201–203.
25. Thompson, W. L.   Introduction: A Perspective. In *The Cell in Shock.* Kalamazoo, Mich.: Upjohn, 1974.
26. Wagner, P. O., et al.   Distributions of ventilation-perfusion ratios in acute respiratory failure. *Chest* (Suppl.) 65:325, 1974.
27. Weil, M. H., et al.   Routine plasma colloid osmotic pressure measurements. *Crit. Care Med.* 2:229, 1974.
28. West, J. B.   Pulmonary gas exchange in the critically ill patient. *Crit. Care Med.* 2:171, 1974.
29. West, J. B.   *Respiratory Physiology: The Essentials* (2nd ed.). Baltimore: Williams & Wilkins, 1979.
30. Wilson, R. S., and Pontoppidan, H.   Acute respiratory failure. *Crit. Care Med.* 2:293, 1974.
31. Zorab, J. S.   Continuous display of arterial pressure. *Anaesthesia* 24:3, 1969.

SELECTED READINGS

HEMODYNAMIC MONITORING

Bland, R., et al.   Physiologic monitoring goals for the critically ill patient. *S.G. & O.* 147:833, 1978.
Ellertson, D. G., et al.   Pulmonary artery monitoring in critically ill surgical patients. *Am. J. Surg.* 128:791, 1974.
Lozman, J., et al.   Correlation of pulmonary wedge and left atrial pressures. *Arch. Surg.* 109:270, 1974.
Shapiro, A. R., et al.   Interpretation of alveolar-arterial oxygen tension difference. *S.G. & O.* 144:547, 1977.
Stürm, J. A., et al.   Cardiopulmonary parameters and prognosis after severe multiple trauma. *J. Trauma* 19:305, 1979.

RESPIRATORY MONITORING

Avery, M. E., and Fletcher, B. D. *The Lung and Its Disorders in the Newborn Infant* (3rd ed.). Philadelphia: Saunders, 1974.

Ayres, S. M., et al. *Care of the Critically Ill* (2nd ed.). New York: Appleton, 1974.

Bates, D. V., et al. *Respiratory Function in Disease: An Introduction to the Integrated Study of the Lung* (2nd ed.). Philadelphia: Saunders, 1971.

Berk, J. L. (Ed.). A physiologic approach to critical care. *Surg. Clin. North Am.* 55:3, 1975.

Berk, J. L., et al. Pulmonary insufficiency caused by epinephrine. *Ann. Surg.* 178:423, 1973.

Civetta, J. M. Intensive Care Unit and Practical Pulmonary Function Tests. In M. Lichtiger and F. Moya (Eds.), *Introduction to the Practice of Anesthesia* (2nd ed.). New York: Harper, 1978.

Comroe, J. H. *Physiology of Respiration* (2nd ed.). Chicago: Year Book, 1974.

Filley, G. F. *Acid-Base and Blood-Gas Regulation.* Philadelphia: Lea & Febiger, 1971.

Finch, C. A., and Lenfant, C. Oxygen transport in man. *N. Engl. J. Med.* 286: 407, 1972.

Hills, B. A. *Gas Transfer in the Lung.* London: Cambridge University Press, 1974.

Laver, M. B. Acute respiratory failure: More questions, fewer answers. *Anesthesiology* 43:611, 1975.

Moore, F. D., et al. *Post-Traumatic Pulmonary Insufficiency: Pathophysiology of Respiratory Failure and Principles of Respiratory Care after Surgical Operations, Trauma, Hemorrhage, Burns and Shock.* Philadelphia: Saunders, 1969.

Nunn, J. F. *Applied Respiratory Physiology with Special Reference to Anesthesia.* New York: Appleton, 1969.

Petty, T. L. *Intensive and Rehabilitative Respiratory Care* (2nd ed.). Philadelphia: Lea & Febiger, 1974.

Pontoppidan, H., et al. *Acute Respiratory Failure in the Adult.* Boston: Little, Brown, 1973.

Pontoppidan, H., et al. Respiratory intensive care. *Anesthesiology* 47:96, 1977.

Shapiro, B. A. *Clinical Application of Blood Gases* (2nd ed.). Chicago: Year Book, 1977.

Sladen, A., et al. Pulmonary complications and water retention in prolonged mechanical ventilation. *N. Engl. J. Med.* 279:448, 1968.

Suter, P. M., et al. Shunt, lung volume and perfusion during short periods of ventilation with oxygen. *Anesthesiology* 43:617, 1975.

Webb, W. R. (Ed.). Pulmonary problems in surgery. *Surg. Clin. North Am.* 54:5, 1974.

Wilson, R. F., and Sibbald, W. J. Acute respiratory failure. *Crit. Care Med.* 4:79, 1976.

John H. Siegel / 6. ACUTE
POSTTRAUMATIC
PULMONARY INSUF-
FICIENCY AND THE
ADULT RESPIRATORY
DISTRESS SYNDROME

In the critically ill or injured patient, no other pathologic process poses greater hazard than the development of the acute respiratory insufficiency syndrome. The initiating mechanisms can occur with major thoracic or nonthoracic trauma, burns, hemorrhagic shock with volume replacement, severe sepsis, and with certain nonspecific inflammatory diseases such as pancreatitis or in transplantation rejection crises [24].

FUNDAMENTAL PATHOLOGIC MECHANISMS
There is considerable dispute about the existence of a common set of etiologic factors that are responsible for the initiation of this syndrome. Blaisdell [3] maintains on the basis of his studies that the common initial event is the formation of platelet microaggregation in the pulmonary capillary bed, which produces early microvascular obstruction and is associated with the release of vasoactive substances. The latter by-products of platelet aggregation, which may be fibrinopeptides [2], are believed to cause changes in alveolar capillary permeability that appear to persist long after lysis of the microaggregates occurs and the vasoconstrictor phase of the disease is at an end. While the mechanistic explanation advanced by Blaisdell is not as yet universally accepted, there is no question but that the fundamental pathophysiology is a consequence of injury to the alveolar capillary. Thus, capillary membrane permeability, a major factor in the Starling hypothesis of the absorption of fluids from connective tissue spaces as applied to the lung, is altered in a deleterious manner. The impressive evidence marshalled by Levine et al. [20] and by Staub [43] conclusively supports the fundamental validity of the Starling equation as a means of explaining and understanding the interaction of various factors in initiating and enhancing the pathologic process producing the acute respiratory distress syndrome (RDS).

Stated briefly, this hypothesis indicates that the flow of fluid ($\dot{Q}_f$) from alveolar capillary to pulmonary interstitium is a function of the filtration coefficient of the capillary membranes (K_f) times the intramicrovascular (P_{IV}) to extramicrovascular (P_{EV}) pressure gradient; minus the reflection coefficient (σ) (expressing the relative permeability of the membrane to solute as opposed to water), times the intramicrovascular (Π_{IV}) to extramicrovascular Π_{EV}) osmotic pressure gradient.

$$\dot{Q}_f = K_f \left[(P_{IV} - P_{EV}) - \sigma(\Pi_{IV} - \Pi_{EV})\right] \tag{1}$$

This relationship applies at all points along the alveolar capillary from the arterial inflow end to the venous outflow end. From it one can see how alterations in each of the factors, or a combination of any, can enhance the flow of capillary fluid into the pulmonary alveolar interstitial space at the arterial side and concomitantly retard the flow of pulmonary interstitial fluid back from the interstitium into the venous side of the pulmonary capillary. At a given capillary membrane permeability (K_f), the values for ($P_{IV} - P_{EV}$) and $\Pi_{IV} - \Pi_{EV}$) change continuously along the length of the alveolar capillary surface from inflow to outflow, as a function of the relative difference between pulmonary arterial and left atrial pressures and the extravascular tissue pressures, and the net flow of intravascular protein molecules (primarily albumin) across the alveolar capillary at each point.

Understanding the importance of the transcapillary pressure gradient is not difficult. However, the importance of the net transcapillary flow of large protein molecules that exert the intravascular colloid oncotic pressure may need some further explanation to clarify the pathologic implications of colloid deficits in the genesis of this syndrome. The net flow of plasma proteins across the alveolar capillary membrane is a separate but related factor governing the rate of fluid transport from alveolar capillary to pulmonary interstitial space. This colloid flow ($\dot{Q}_s$) is a function of the permeability of the capillary membrane to the protein molecule in question (ω), times the transcapillary osmotic pressure gradient ($\Pi_{IV} - \Pi_{EV}$), plus 1, minus the reflection coefficient (σ), times the membrane concentration of the same protein ($\overline{C}_s$), times the net transvascular flow of fluid ($\dot{Q}_f$).

$$\dot{Q}_s = \omega \, (\Pi_{IV} - \Pi_{EV}) + (1 - \sigma) \, C_s \dot{Q}_f \tag{2}$$

As a result of these fundamental relationships, it becomes clear why when an increase in pulmonary alveolar permeability occurs, there is an increased net flow of both plasma fluid and protein molecules (mostly albumin) into the pulmonary interstitial space. The absolute rate of this flux and its direction are a function of the pulmonary intravascular hydrostatic pressure, which determines the value for P_{IV} in equation 1. As pulmonary intramicrovascular hydrostatic pressure is increased by a rising left atrial pressure due to cardiac failure or a cardiac hyperdynamic state (both of which institute a volume or flow load on the heart, moving the cardiac intraventricular pressure to a higher point on the end-diastolic pressure-volume relationship), the net transfer of both fluid and plasma proteins from capillary lumen to pulmonary interstitial space will increase at a normal alveolar capillary permeability and will be markedly enhanced if capillary permeability is decreased. Such changes in pulmonary capillary permeability have been described as occurring with shock, sepsis, and after certain toxic drugs such as heroin or alloxan [43].

In a similar fashion, reduction in the colloid oncotic pressure of the plasma, either by nutritional dysfunction (cirrhotic liver disease, malnutrition, cancer), iatrogenic replacement of intravascular losses with noncolloid-containing fluids, inflammatory loss of intravascular colloid with a low oncotic plasma refill (pancreatitis, burn, peritonitis), or any combination of these events, will reduce the Π_{IV} term in equation 1. This will reduce the effectiveness of the intravascular osmotic pressure in modifying the intravascular-extravascular pressure gradient ($P_{IV} - P_{EV}$) in determining the level and direction of fluid flow from pulmonary capillary to interstitial space.

The clinical evidence of increased pulmonary extravascular water in various posttraumatic lung syndromes seen by Gump et al. [11] is consistent with the Starling hypothesis expressed above, as is the relationship between a reduced serum oncotic pressure and the development of pulmonary edema at low intravascular hydrostatic pressures noted experimentally by Guyton and Lindsey [12].

RELATIONSHIP OF PATHOPHYSIOLOGIC MECHANISMS AND PULMONARY DYSFUNCTION

Changes in the permeability characteristics of the alveolar capillary membranes, whether or not enhanced by concomitant alterations in pulmonary microvascular pressure, or plasma oncotic pressure, or both, have been shown to produce an enhanced pulmonary lymph flow. Under ordinary circumstances, the alveolar epithelium is impermeable to fluid exchange. Consequently, when the gradient of fluid and protein movement into the pulmonary interstitial space exceeds the transport capacity of the lung lymphatics, interstitial edema occurs. The earliest result of this fluid exchange–transport imbalance is edema in the loose connective tissue surrounding the respiratory bronchiole and its accompanying arteriole, venule, and lymphatics. Somewhat later, true interstitial alveolar edema occurs, and finally, very late in the process, alveolar flooding occurs when the tissue pressure exceeds the threshold value for fluid flow across the alveolar epithelial membrane, or perhaps when the fluid in the interstitium breaks into the respiratory bronchiole [44].

The mechanical consequences of this microscopic process are (1) a reduced respiratory bronchiolar diameter, owing to peribronchiolar edema, with an increase in small-airway resistance, and (2) an altered modulus of alveolar elasticity, owing to alveolar interstitial edema, producing a reduced lung compliance. As a result, it becomes harder to distend these impaired alveoli with the normal mouth to negative intrapleural driving pressure gradient, since at a reduced compliance a given level of inspiratory pressure produces a reduced lung volume. By virtue of the specific nature of the initiating pathologic mechanisms, superimposed on already existing normal ventilation-perfusion inequalities (related to the gravitational factors that favor perfusion over ventilation in the dependent portions of the lung, and ventilation over perfusion in the nondependent lung), the reduction in alveolar compliance is distributed nonuniformly over the lung. The net result is a reduction in the total alveolar volume, specifically in the alveolar volume at the end of a tidal respiration, or the functional residual capacity (FRC). This nonuniform reduction in FRC is delineated by a curve of nitrogen washout from the lung that is multiexponential and more rapid than normal [9, 32].

As the alveolus becomes more difficult to distend, and as the resistance to airflow in and out increases, two things happen that tend to compromise alveolar volume further. The first is that inspired air tends to be diverted into the more compliant normal alveoli, overdistending them while further reducing the gas volume of the less compliant alveoli. Second, as airflow in and out of an alveolus is compromised, the intra-alveolar gas tends to come more into equilibrium with mixed venous blood, resulting in a lower P_AO_2 and a higher P_ACO_2, reducing the total intra-alveolar gas partial pressure. As long as there is an intra-alveolar component of inert gas such as nitrogen (P_AN_2) representing a major fraction of the total intra-alveolar partial pressure, no major change in alveolar distending pressure occurs, even in compromised alveoli. However, as the oxygen concentration in the inspired air [F_IO_2] is increased, the fraction of structural gas (F_IN_2) contributing to the total partial pressure is reduced; and with continued uptake of oxygen from the partially obstructed but totally perfused alveolus, the intra-alveolar partial pressure falls, thus further accelerating the tendency toward alveolar collapse. This accounts for the progressive falls in FRC seen in patients with posttraumatic lung syndromes who are ventilated on 100% oxygen, even for brief periods, as during quantitative pulmonary shunt determinations.

The reduction of FRC seen in patients with RDS is physiologically correlated with the reduced compliance, increased airway resistance, and increase in the percentage of pulmonary venoarterial admixture (percent shunt) (Fig. 6-1) [13, 28, 32]. This increase in pulmonary shunting is due to perfusion through areas of collapsed alveoli. This occurs even though the loss of alveolar volume results in the diversion of most of the alveolar perfusion to distended alveoli (due to increased vascular resistance in the collapsed segment), since about 30 percent of the blood flow remains to perfuse the collapsed alveolus. In turn, this shunting produces a fall in arterial oxygen

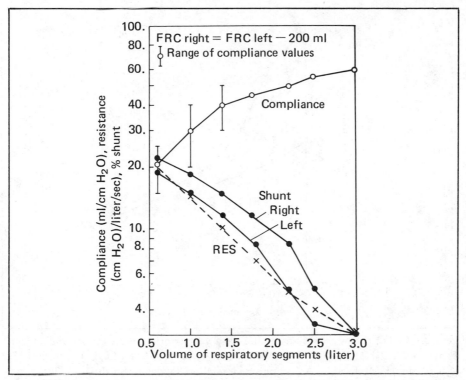

FIGURE 6-1. Physiologic coupling between respiratory segment volumes, total lung compliance and resistance, and pulmonary shunting in each lung. Note that in this simulation example, functional residual capacity (FRC) reduction is nonuniform, being greater on the right than on the left. (From J. H. Siegel and E. J. Farrell, A computer simulation model to study the clinical observability of ventilation and perfusion abnormalities in human shock states. *Surgery* 73:898, 1973.)

tension (PaO_2) and a widening of the alveolar-arterial [$P(A-a)O_2$] gradient at any given FIO_2.

Figure 6-2 shows the relationship between the arterial oxygen tension (PaO_2) with increasing percentage of pulmonary venoarterial admixture on 100% FIO_2, and on room air (20.9% FIO_2). From this figure, it is obvious that an increased FIO_2 will help maintain PaO_2 at the lower-percentage shunts, but when pulmonary shunting is greater than 30 percent, increasing the oxygen concentration in the inspired gas has only minimal beneficial effect.

On the other hand, increasing the volume of perfused alveolar segments available for ventilation (FRC − anatomic dead space) will significantly increase arterial oxygen tension (PaO_2) at any FIO_2 (Fig. 6-3). From this figure it can also be seen that one may avoid a potentially dangerous FIO_2 increase (above 50% FIO_2) by instituting therapeutic measures designed to

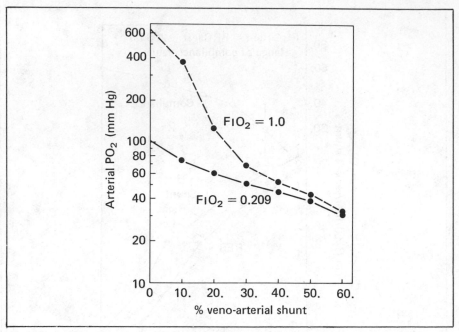

FIGURE 6-2. Effect of increasing pulmonary venoarterial shunt on arterial oxygen tension (PaO$_2$) at FiO$_2$ = 1.0 (100%) and FiO$_2$ = 0.209 (20.9%). (From J. H. Siegel and E. J. Farrell, A computer simulation model to study the clinical observability of ventilation and perfusion abnormalities in human shock states. *Surgery* 73:898, 1973.)

increase effective FRC; for example, increased ventilatory volume and/or the use of continuous end-expiratory pressure to shift the lung with reduced compliance to a more favorable pressure-volume relationship. In addition to the factors previously mentioned, the use of respiratory support techniques that avoid a high FiO$_2$ may also prevent the addition of the specific toxic effects of high oxygen concentrations, which include impairment of respiratory epithelial cell ciliary function, decrease in pulmonary surfactant, and injury to capillary endothelial cells.

RESPIRATORY CONTROL, VENTILATION, AND THE WORK OF BREATHING

It is important to emphasize that the respiratory response of the patient with the posttraumatic lung syndrome represents the interaction of respiratory control mechanisms with the impaired mechanical capabilities of the lung. Under normal circumstances, respiratory regulation is effected through interaction between blood chemoreceptors and the central nervous system respiratory control center. This system mediates the rate and depth of ventilation and functions as a feedback servocontrol mechanism. Under ordi-

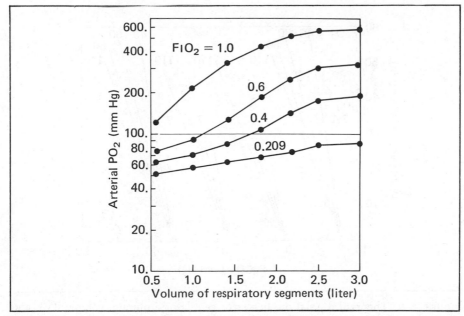

FIGURE 6-3. Effect of increasing volume of respiratory segments (functional residual capacity minus anatomic dead space) on PaO_2 at $FiO_2 = 1.0$ (100%), 0.6 (60%), 0.4 (40%), and 0.209 (20.9%). (From J. H. Siegel and E. J. Farrell, A computer simulation model to study the clinical observability of ventilation and perfusion abnormalities in human shock states. *Surgery* 73:898, 1973.)

nary circumstances, increases in minute volume appear to be a linear function of increases in arterial carbon dioxide ($PaCO_2$), with the exact slope of the relationship dependent on the PaO_2 and the intercept dependent on arterial pH (pHa) (Fig. 6-4) [19]. Consequently, at a given pHa, ventilatory minute volume ($\dot{V}$) will increase in response to arterial hypoxia as long as $PaCO_2$ remains constant. However, the natural response of this control mechanism to arterial hypoxemia is increased $\dot{V}$, with a consequent reduction first in $PACO_2$ and then in $PaCO_2$ and a shift in pHa to a higher level on a respiratory basis. This in turn permits a lower V at a lower $PaCO_2$, and the resultant new equilibrium reduction in alveolar PCO_2 ($PACO_2$) allows a higher PAO_2 and PaO_2 at any given FiO_2 and $P(A-a)O_2$ gradient, thus tending to correct the arterial hypoxemia.

Unfortunately, when the pathologic process producing hypoxemia is associated with a reduction in lung compliance, the normal arterial regulation response is impaired, since it takes a greater mechanical effect to generate the negative intrapleural pressure needed to achieve lung distention by the muscular bellows of the chest wall and diaphragm. Whereas the normal response is to increase ventilation ($\dot{V}$) by increasing the tidal volume, when

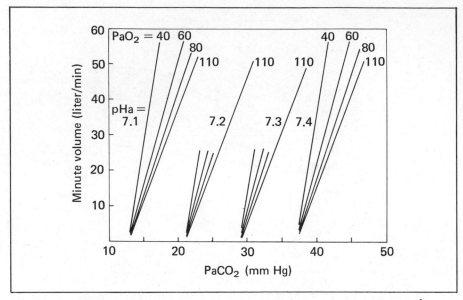

FIGURE 6-4. Theoretical relation between ventilatory minute volume (V̇) and PaCO₂, pHa, and PaO₂. (From R. H. Kellogg. Central Chemical Regulation of respiration. In W. O. Fenn and H. Rahn (eds.). *Handbook of Physiology* (3rd ed.). Baltimore: Williams & Wilkins, 1964. Cited in J. H. Siegel and E. J. Farrell, A computer simulation model to study the clinical observability of ventilation and perfusion abnormalities in human shock states. *Surgery* 73:898, 1973.)

the mechanical capabilities of the thorax are exceeded, a sufficient negative intrapleural pressure cannot be achieved, so that tidal volume cannot be increased. However, the patient still responds to the dictates of his respiratory controller by increasing respiratory rate in an attempt to increase minute ventilation (V̇). This is manifested clinically by the appearance of rapid but shallow respirations in which the patient's tidal volume exchange is only slightly larger than the anatomic dead space of the mouth and tracheobronchial tree. As a result of these large increases in ventilatory rate with only small increases (or even decreases) in V̇, the dead space exchange (V̇D) rises in proportion to the alveolar ventilation (V̇A), and the ventilatory dead space to tidal volume ratio (VD/VT) rises, without the necessity of a concomitant reduction in the distribution of alveolar perfusion. Of course, if there is also an element of decreased or maldistributed alveolar perfusion, those unperfused but ventilated alveoli will become respiratory dead space, further reducing the alveolar exchange and also increasing the VD/VT ratio.

The demands of the respiratory control mechanism drive the patient with hypoxia or hypercapnia to attempt to compensate for the decreased lung compliance by increasing the forceful bellows action of the chest wall and diaphragm. The result is an increased ventilatory work ($\dot{W}$) per liter ventilation. Ordinary exercise or the normal response to carbon dioxide retention by rebreathing or increasing extra pulmonary dead space will increase both $\dot{V}$ and $\dot{W}$, but the normal ratio of respiratory work per liter ventilation remains less than 0.08 kgM/liter. However, when lung compliance falls as a result of the posttraumatic lung syndrome, the work per liter ventilation rises sharply. Peters and Hilberman [25] have shown that early respiratory insufficiency can be delineated by a $\dot{W}/\dot{V}$ ratio of greater than 0.08 kgM/liter and that mechanical ventilation for respiratory support is indicated when the $\dot{W}/\dot{V}$ ratio exceeds 0.18 kgM/liter.

In addition to the mechanical cost to the critically ill patient struggling to breathe against an increased $\dot{W}/\dot{V}$ ratio, there is the increased oxygen cost of breathing. In the critically ill patient, especially one with a low cardiac output, the increased oxygen consumption due to respiration becomes significant and will in itself contribute to arterial hypoxemia by lowering the mixed venous oxygen content ($C\bar{v}O_2$). This in turn will place the patient on a steeper portion of his oxyhemoglobin dissociation curve, thus requiring a greater oxygen uptake on passage through the lung to reach a hemoglobin saturation that is in equilibrium with an acceptable PaO_2. If significant pulmonary venoarterial admixture is already present as a result of atelectasis and reduction in FRC, even a small further reduction in $C\bar{v}O_2$ may have a profound effect on the final arterial oxygen tension.

CARDIORESPIRATORY INTERACTIONS

The limitations imposed on respiratory gas exchange by the pathologic mechanisms previously described appear to be critical factors in the survival of the patient with acute adult RDS. Although many sophisticated measurements of lung function can be made, a simple and practical bedside measure of overall difficulty in oxygen exchange that is useful as a clinical index of the severity of the respiratory difficulty is the oxygen exchange ratio [35]. This is the extent of the alveolar arterial oxygen gradient [$P(A-a)O_2$] normalized by the level of arterial oxygen tension (PaO_2), to adjust for the fact that most patients with severe impairment are breathing gas mixtures with increased oxygen fractions (FiO_2). This $P(A-a)O_2/PaO_2$ ratio is related to the physiologic factors that result in desaturation of arterial blood. If measured at 100 percent FiO_2 to eliminate ventilation inequalities, it will reflect the percentage of physiologic pulmonary venoarterial admixture; at FiO_2 fractions less than 100 percent, it includes the net sum of all factors contributing to poor oxygen exchange between inspired gas and blood. These include: ventilatory exchange inequalities between alveoli; ventilation-perfusion disparities caused by atelectasis, pulmonary alveolar fluid, or exudate; and veolar cell membranes due to interstitial edema or membrane permeability alterations in the diffusion gradient between the alveolar capillary and alchanges.

The oxygen exchange ratio is computed as follows:

Barometric pressure	760 mm Hg
$- P_{H2O}$ at body temperature (e.g., 98.6° F) $-$	47 mm Hg
	713
$\times F_{I}O_2$ (e.g., 40%)	$\times$ 0.40
	285
$- PaCO_2$ (considered $\cong PACO_2$)	$-$ 40 mm Hg
PAO_2 mean (all factors, on $F_{I}O_2$ 40%)	245 mm Hg
$- PaO_2$ (on $F_{I}O_2$ 40%)	$-$ 55 mm Hg
$P(A-a)O_2$ gradient (all factors)	190 mm Hg
$P(A-a)O_2/PaO_2$ ratio (190/55)	3.46

While the oxygen exchange ratio $[P(A-a)O_2/PaO_2]$ is a somewhat imprecise measure, being influenced by all the factors that impair oxygen exchange, it nevertheless appears to be an especially good discriminator and predictor of mortality in critically ill patients with respiratory dysfunction. It also has the advantage that it can be estimated without equilibration on 100 percent $F_{I}O_2$, which has been shown to produce further reductions in FRC in the patient with the adult respiratory distress syndrome. This index of pulmonary capability becomes an especially good parameter when it is considered as a function of myocardial contractile dynamics, as measured by the cardiac mixing time (tm) (Fig. 6-5), which has previously been shown to be a correlate of changes in myocardial contractile function [34]. The cardiac mixing time, measured from the exponential downslope of the indicator dilution curve, is directly related to the changes in the duration of isometric pressure development in the left ventricular myocardium. As myocardial contractility increases, both the time to the peak rate of isometric pressure development (Δt dp/dt) and the cardiac mixing time (tm) shorten proportionately; thus, a higher contractility results in a more dynamic myocardium.

The relationship between oxygen exchange capability $[P(A-a)O_2/PaO_2]$ and myocardial contractile function is shown in Figure 6-5, which contains 751 samples from 95 patients in various forms of shock and from 62 nonshock, preoperative control patients of a similar age, sex, and disease distribution. Those samples obtained within 48 hours of death are shown as boldface **D** letters. In preoperative nonshock patients, a $P(A-a)O_2/PaO_2$ ratio of less than 0.6 and a cardiac mixing time (tm) of less than 6.5 sec have been shown to have a statistically significant favorable prognosis for surgery, and these limits are shown here for comparison. Also shown is the region inhabited by nonshock patients in a control or reference state

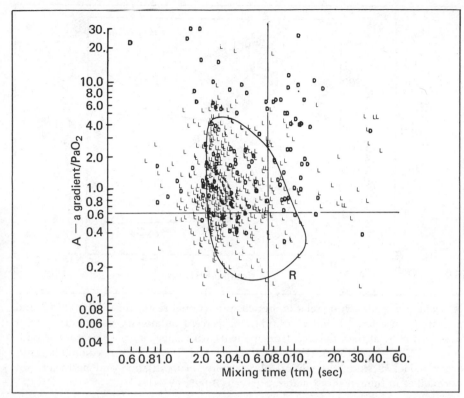

FIGURE 6-5. Cardiorespiratory interactions and their effect on mortality in shock. Boldface **D**s represent samples from patients dying within 48 hr. Lightface *L*s represent patients surviving more than 48 hr. Control group (R) limits are outlined. (From J. H. Siegel et al., Cardiorespiratory interactions as determinants of survival and the need for respiratory support in human shock states. *J. Trauma* 13:602, 1973. Copyright 1973, The Williams & Wilkins Co., Baltimore.)

(R region). As can be easily seen, while deaths within 48 hours can obviously occur in shock patients in all physiologic regions, it is obvious that either an increasingly unfavorable oxygen exchange ratio (reflecting worsening pulmonary function) or a lengthening cardiac mixing time (reflecting deteriorating myocardial function) appears to result in a greater percentage of samples reflecting death within 48 hours.

It can also be seen that while either poor respiratory exchange or poor myocardial contractile function alone has a poor prognosis in shock, the combination of the two is highly lethal unless corrected. This point is even more forcefully made by the exceptions to this rule shown in Figure 6-5—samples from surviving patients in which the cardiac mixing time (tm) was greater than 15 seconds, which is a severe level of myocardial depression.

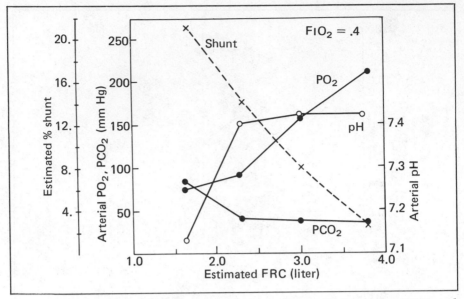

FIGURE 6-6. Simulation of relation between functional residual capacity (FRC) and alterations in arterial blood gases, pH, and percent pulmonary venoarterial shunt based on clinical data derived from patients with shock and respiratory insufficiency. $FIO_2 = 0.4$ (40%). (From J. H. Siegel and E. J. Farrell, A computer simulation model to study the clinical observability of ventilation and perfusion abnormalities in human shock states. *Surgery* 73:898, 1973.)

These all came from patients with acute myocardial infarction shock who were temporarily or successfully resuscitated by intra-aortic balloon counterpulsation [33].

While impairment of oxygen exchange is coupled with minimal reductions in FRC and thus is seen early in the development of acute RDS, when marked reductions in alveolar volume occur, carbon dioxide exchange is also impaired, and hypercapnia results (Fig. 6-6). The importance of respiratory limitations of carbon dioxide exchange in the respiratory distress of shock states caused by sepsis, trauma, hypovolemia, or myocardial infarction is shown in Figure 6-7. This figure shows the relationship among arterial pH, arterial PCO_2, and arterial bicarbonate concentration. The data points are labeled to show samples obtained within 48 hours of death in shock patients. As can be seen in the figure, the region also containing preoperative controls in the reference (R) state is delineated for comparison. As shown, a significant mortality occurs in shock patients who maintain an essentially normal acid-base balance. However, increased metabolic acidosis (metabolic acid > 10 mm/liter) is associated with a higher percentage of samples reflecting imminent death. More important, with relation to the late respiratory distress syndrome, is that lower levels of metabolic acid can be

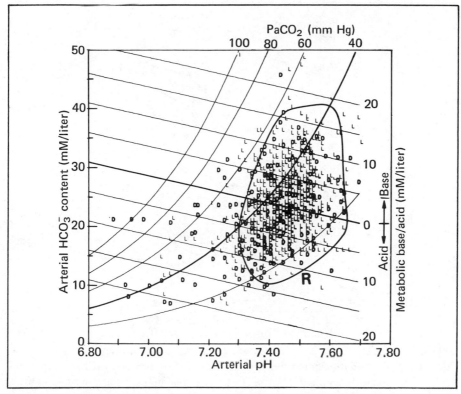

FIGURE 6-7. Acid-base relationships and their effect on mortality in shock. For key, see legend of Figure 6-5. (From J. H. Siegel et al., Cardiorespiratory interactions as determinants of survival and the need for respiratory support in human shock states. *J. Trauma* 13:602, 1973. Copyright 1973, The Williams & Wilkins Co., Baltimore.)

associated with a poor prognosis when respiratory exchange of carbon dioxide is also impaired ($PaCO_2$ > 60 mm Hg), producing a combined respiratory and metabolic acidosis.

ROLE OF THE HYPERDYNAMIC STATE IN THE ADULT RESPIRATORY DISTRESS SYNDROME

The development of adult RDS and its net effect on the maintenance of acceptable levels of arterial blood gases cannot be separated from consideration of the adequacy of cardiac function. A variety of clinical studies have demonstrated the need for an increased cardiac output in peripheral failure states associated with sepsis, decompensated liver disease, and trauma; and it is now becoming clear that a relative hyperdynamic cardiac state is also essential if survival is to be achieved in severe respiratory insufficiency associated with the adult RDS of posttraumatic states.

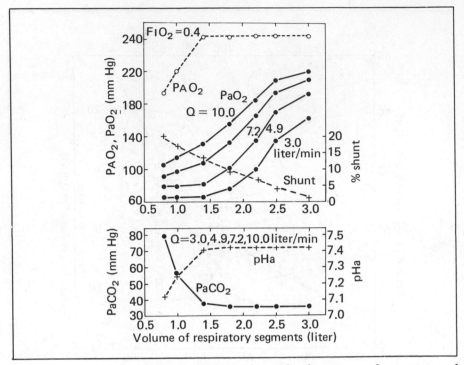

FIGURE 6-8. Systematic simulation of interrelationship between cardiac output and reduced respiratory segment volume (functional residual capacity minus anatomic dead space). Based on clinical data from patient in shock with an acute respiratory distress syndrome. $FiO_2 = 0.4$ (40%). (From J. H. Siegel and E. J. Farrell, A computer simulation model to study the clinical observability of ventilation and perfusion abnormalities in human shock states. *Surgery* 73:898, 1973.)

The reason for this contention is shown in Figure 6-8, which demonstrates the interrelationship between the level of cardiac output and the degree of reduction in FRC due to atelectasis or pulmonary consolidation. It also shows why a patient with a reduced alveolar volume, and coupled shunting, must maintain a hyperdynamic circulation to survive. As noted earlier, the level of $PaCO_2$ and pHa are mainly dependent on the absolute alveolar volume available for respiratory gas exchange but are little influenced by wide changes in cardiac output. This is the result of the high diffusability of carbon dioxide, the much greater carrying capacity of blood for carbon dioxide than for oxygen, and the near linearity of the carbon dioxide dissociation curve. Consequently, once critical minimum levels of alveolar exchange surface and minute volume gas exchange of these alveoli are available, a near-normal $PaCO_2$ can be maintained.

However, in comparison with carbon dioxide exchange, the poorer diffusion characteristics of oxygen, the smaller oxygen-carrying capacity of the blood, and the nonlinear oxyhemoglobin dissociation curve markedly limit the rate of alveolar-capillary oxygen transport. As a result, oxygen exchange is impaired at levels of available alveolar surface that are far greater than that needed for adequate carbon dioxide exchange. This effect is compounded further by the venoarterial shunting that is physiologically coupled to alveolar collapse and occurs in the nonventilated but perfused alveoli. It is this shunting that necessitates a higher blood flow across the functioning alveolar-capillary exchange surfaces if arterial oxygen tension (PaO_2) is to be maintained at normal levels.

THERAPEUTIC IMPLICATIONS
GENERAL PRINCIPLES
The complexity of the pathophysiologic processes involved in the adult respiratory distress, or posttraumatic lung, syndromes mandate that specific therapy be directed at the prevention or amelioration of each aspect of the process. As a useful organizing principle, it is valuable to address the variables in the Starling equation previously discussed.

As a prophylactic measure, it is important to eliminate factors that may induce alterations in membrane permeability in shock or other stress situations. These include strenuous efforts to avoid anoxic injury that may alter membrane permeability and to reduce pathophysiologic factors that may enhance or initiate platelet aggregation and intravascular coagulation. Specifically, there should be an aggressive attempt at prompt treatment of hypotension by volume infusion. In massive blood transfusions, every effort should be made to utilize a micropore filter to avoid infusions of platelet aggregates and other types of microemboli. Nonviable tissues productive of thrombogenic and vasoactive polypeptides should be promptly debrided, and areas of overt infection or sites of potential sepsis must be drained early and effectively to avoid a systemic septic component.

During resuscitation, or in the intraoperative or postoperative period, excessive volumes of noncolloid-containing crystalloid solutions that may lower colloid oncotic pressure should be avoided wherever possible. If massive fluid replacement is necesssary during surgery, endotracheal intubation and volume-controlled ventilation should be continued in the immediate postoperative period until it is clear that RDS is not present and ventilatory support is not needed. In general, the lowest FiO_2 compatible with an acceptable PaO_2 should be used.

PRINCIPLES OF VENTILATORY SUPPORT
Once the posttraumatic syndrome, or adult RDS, has become apparent, as evidenced by a falling PaO_2 in spite of progressive increases in FiO_2, or a widening $P(A-a)O_2$ gradient at a given level of FiO_2, it is imperative that supportive measures be instituted immediately. To wait until the late manifestations of this process occur (significant reduction in pulmonary com-

pliance, increases in respiratory work, a marked fall in PaO_2, and a rising PaCO₂) is to flirt with disaster, since cardiorespiratory arrest is not uncommon under these circumstances.

The first priority in such a patient must be to ensure adequate ventilation of atelectatic or underventilated alveoli and not merely to increase FIO_2 without effective ventilatory support, which will only promote an accelerated alveolar collapse with atelectasis and physiologically coupled pulmonary venoarterial shunting. Ventilatory compensation for the reduction in compliance and FRC requires intubation and mechanical ventilation by a volume-controlled ventilator, with the addition of an intra-alveolar distending force capable of overcoming the factors promoting alveolar collapse. The value of this concept was demonstrated by Ashbaugh et al. [1], who employed continuous positive end-expiratory pressure (PEEP) to reverse the hypoxemia of the posttraumatic lung syndrome. Many careful investigators have confirmed this approach and have shown that the markedly reduced FRC found in this syndrome is increased by this therapeutic maneuver.

PRINCIPLES OF CARDIORESPIRATORY SUPPORT
The previously described interaction between the adequacy of cardiac function and pulmonary dysfunction has a number of important therapeutic implications. Since the intramicrovascular hydrostatic pressure plays a major role in regulating the flow of intravascular fluid and protein into the pulmonary lymph, there is a real value in reducing pulmonary capillary venous pressure by lowering left atrial mean pressure. Furthermore, as shown in Figure 6-8, in the presence of pulmonary dysfunction associated with shunting, pulmonary oxygen exchange in the remaining perfused and ventilated alveoli, and consequently PaO_2, can be improved by increasing cardiac flow. Conversely, any therapeutic maneuver that increases FRC and thus reduces shunting but which also depresses cardiac flow, such as excessive end-expiratory pressure, will result in a reduced oxygen exchange and a lower PaO_2. If the reduction in cardiac output is a result of increased cardiac failure with an increase in left atrial mean pressure, the negative effects on oxygen exchange and PaO_2 may be compounded by an actual increase in pulmonary lymph flow and a progression of the initiating pathogenic process. Similar increases in left atrial mean pressure may follow cardiac decompensation resulting from high output failure in the hyperdynamic state; consequently, the patient with high cardiac flow must also be carefully observed for quantitative evidence of cardiac failure.

For all of these reasons, one may maximize the therapeutic effectiveness of the ventilatory support measures by also effecting cardiac inotropic support. The use of continuous intravenous infusion of isoproterenol in small doses (0.25–1.0 μg/min total dose titrated to heart rate) alone, or in combination with dopamine (3.0–5.0 mg/kg/min) or with glucagon infusion

(3 mg/hr) produces a significant inotropic and flow effect, with little tendency to excessive tachycardia or arrhythmia [39]. Rapid-acting digitalis preparations such as digoxin (75–80% of the estimated full digitalizing dose adjusted to age and level of renal function) are also a valuable therapeutic modality if potassium levels are maintained within normal limits.

PRACTICAL BEDSIDE CONSIDERATIONS IN CARDIORESPIRATORY SUPPORT MEASURES

Once alerted to the possibility of the development of posttraumatic RDS by a falling PaO_2 on a given FiO_2, or a $P(A-a)O_2/PaO_2$ ratio near to or greater than 2.0, it is the surgeon's responsibility to undertake serial quantification of the degree of respiratory difficulty to determine the need for mechanical support. As indicated earlier, perhaps the most useful parameter to measure other than the arterial blood gases and pH is a quantification of FRC, both with regard to absolute volume level and the monoexponential or multiexponential character of the gas washout. However, the measurement devices and trained technicians may not always be available. Therefore, a useful approach is provided by the application (in reverse) of the concept of a respiratory weaning score as suggested by Chodoff and Margand [4], which involves the evaluation of several variables representing different aspects of ventilatory function—namely, oxygen exchange, carbon dioxide exchange, and mechanical efficiency (Table 6-1). By scoring several variables in each group and dividing by the number of variables scored, an overall estimate of respiratory effectiveness can be obtained. Unquestionably, some variables deserve more weight than others in a given patient, but this approach provides a logical basis for considered action. Patients who have a score of 2 or less should be placed on mechanical ventilator support. Those with higher scores may be managed by other means, provided the score continues to improve or remains constant on successive evaluations over the period of observation in the intensive care unit.

When ventilatory support is indicated in RDS, intubation and volume-controlled ventilation are essential. If synchronization of the patient's respiration is not possible during respiratory assistance, total ventilatory control must be obtained, either by depressing the respiratory control mechanism with morphine or by neuromuscular blockade using curare or pancuronium (Pavulon). We prefer the latter agent (Pavulon, 1–4 mg IV every 1–4 hr to obtain control), since morphine tends to depress other visceral functions, and curare may cause hypotension in patients with borderline circulatory compensation.

After mechanical support has been initiated, the surgeon must decide whether or not end-expiratory pressure is indicated. This can only be determined by again quantifying the parameters of gas exchange and FRC (since some of the parameters of mechanical efficiency that require muscular function will be artificially depressed due to the neuromuscular block-

TABLE 6-1. Scoring of Variables for Overall Estimate of Respiratory Effectiveness

	Points		
	1	2	3
OXYGEN EXCHANGE			
PaO_2 on 40% O_2	$\leq$80	$\leq$70	$\leq$75
$P(A\text{-}a)O_2$ on 100% O_2	$\geq$300	$\geq$250	$\leq$200
$P(A\text{-}a)O_2/PaO_2$	$\geq$2.0	>1.0	$\leq$0.8
$\dot{Q}s/\dot{Q}T$	$\geq$20%	>15%	$\leq$10%
CARBON DIOXIDE EXCHANGE			
$PaCO_2$	$\geq$60	>55	$\leq$50
V_D/V_T	$\geq$0.6	$\geq$0.5	$\leq$0.4
pH (on respiratory basis)	$\leq$7.30	<7.35	$\geq$7.40
Base excess	$\pm$7	$\pm$5	$\pm$3
MECHANICAL EFFICIENCY			
Resting tidal volume in ml/kg body weight	$\leq$4	$\leq$5	$\geq$5.5
Maximum effective respiratory volume/resting tidal volume ratio[a]	$\leq$1.5	$\leq$2.0	$\geq$3.0
Effective compliance[b]	$\leq$30	$\leq$40	$\geq$45
VC/PVC $\times$ 100[c]	$\leq$25	$\leq$30	$\geq$35
Inspiratory force	$\geq$ -20	$\leq$ -25	$\leq$ -35
Respiratory rate	>35	$\leq$30	$\leq$25
Bronchospasm	moderate	minimal	absent
Secretions	moderate	minimal	absent

[a] The maximum expired volume that the patient can take at the time; it is similar to vital capacity except that since the patient is usually not capable of doing a true vital capacity, it is usually somewhat less than this value. This ratio is not valid unless resting tidal volume is at least 4 ml/kg body weight.
[b] Effective compliance = tidal volume/peak airway pressure (measured on a ventilator).
[c] Percent of predicted vital capacity.

ade). If there is no improvement in oxygen exchange, shunting, $PaCO_2$, V_D/V_T, effective compliance, or FRC, PEEP should be added in increments of 2 to 5 cm H_2O until an acceptable level of gas exchange is obtained. It is usually not necessary to increase PEEP above 15 cm H_2O.

A preferable mode of therapy is for the intubated patient to be maintained on intermittent mandatory ventilation (IMV). On IMV, the patient's respiratory control is not paralyzed; rather, the patient is allowed to breathe spontaneously, and at a fixed number of times per minute the respirator expands the lung to a present volume, when tripped by a voluntary inspiratory movement. Usable with low levels of PEEP, this IMV technique is a practical and safe way of weaning a ventilator-dependent patient back to spontaneous, unsupported respiration. Since both rate and volume can be adjusted, IMV permits the patient gradually to regain respiratory muscle tone, without risk of hypoxemia or hypercarbia should the lungs' efforts prove insufficient to meet the metabolic demands at a given time in the RDS recovery course.

It is important to monitor the effects of these ventilatory maneuvers on fluid balance, arterial PaO_2, pH, and $PaCO_2$, to check for respiratory complications such as pneumothorax, as well as for decreased cardiac output. The latter may be measured directly by indicator dilution techniques. If this is done, a measure of myocardial contractile function—cardiac mixing time (tm), from which an estimate of the minute cardiac ejection fraction $(EFx = 1 - (3tm/60))$ can be made—may also be used as a guide to the need for inotropic support. However, if facilities for formal cardiac output studies are not available, a crude but reasonable estimate of cardiac output may be made from quantification of the arteriovenous oxygen content difference $[C(a\text{-}\bar{v})O_2]$. This can easily be done at the bedside by inserting a flow-directed low right atrial catheter using the intracardiac ECG obtained through a salt bridge (7% Na_2HCO_3) and monitored via the V lead of a standard ECG for guidance in placement. Alternatively, a Swan-Ganz pulmonary artery catheter can be placed; however, this is not necessary in most cases and is associated with a greater complication rate. The right heart catheter will provide a reasonable mixed venous blood sample to be compared with a simultaneously drawn arterial sample. Since the quantity of oxygen carried in plasma is less than 1 percent under isobaric conditions, a simple estimate of a a-$\bar{v}O_2$ content difference can be made from the hemoglobin concentration and percent saturation of each sample.

The arteriovenous oxygen content difference is calculated as follows:

	Hgb (gm)	×	Saturation (percent as decimal)	×	1.34 =	Est. O_2 content (vol%)
Arterial	10.0	×	.90	×	1.34 =	12.1
Mixed venous	10.0	×	.40	×	1.34 =	5.4
a-$\bar{v}O_2$ difference						6.7

In general, the level of a-$\bar{v}O_2$ difference is inversely proportional to the cardiac output. While there is a relatively wide spread of high cardiac outputs at the narrower a-$\bar{v}O_2$, the relationship between content difference and flow is reasonably linear [35]. As a rule of thumb for guidance in estimating the level of cardiac output, the effect of ventilatory support with end-expiratory pressure, and the need for cardiac inotropic support, one may consider the following relationships:

a-$\bar{v}O_2$ diff. (vol%)		Cardiac index (L/min/M^2)
>6	$\cong$	<2
>5	$\cong$	<3
4	$\cong$	3
>3	$\cong$	<4
<3	$\cong$	>5

By also considering the level of right atrial pressure (or pulmonary wedge pressure), one may also plot a rough Starling-Sarnoff ventricular function curve of flow versus filling pressure as a crude guide to the adequacy of ventricular function.

The following are guidelines for therapeutic intervention with cardiac inotropic support [33]:

Tm	a-$\bar{v}O_2$ diff.	P(A-a)O$_2$	PaCO$_2$	pHa	pH$\bar{v}$
>6.5 sec	>5.3 vol% or <2.6 vol%	>1.8	>48 mm Hg	<7.35	<7.32

It is obvious that the more precise the quantification of cardiorespiratory function can be, the better able the surgeon will be to make valid therapeutic decisions in this difficult clinical context.

PRINCIPLES GERMANE TO ENHANCING THE OXYGEN TRANSPORT CAPACITY OF THE BLOOD

There are other factors that may be of therapeutic significance in the patient with acute postinjury RDS. Certainly, one must pay special attention to the maintenance of an effective red cell mass, both quantitatively and qualitatively. The absolute level of hemoglobin must not be allowed to drop below 10 gm/100 ml. Because of the deleterious effects on oxygen transport of the infusion of ordinary banked blood containing red cells in which the oxygen-hemoglobin dissociation curve is shifted to the left, when transfusion is needed, every effort should be made to administer fresh or fresh frozen reconstituted red cells that have relatively normal dissociation curve characteristics. In patients with respiratory distress developing after a prolonged course complicated by sepsis or inanition in whom serum phosphates may be low, the use of hyperalimentation mixtures containing at least 25 mEq/liter of phosphate (PO$_4$) ion will result in a significant therapeutic shift to the right in the abnormal oxyhemoglobin dissociation curve. While the net effect of such correction is small, it may be critical in the patient in whom all other aspects of respiratory compensation are stretched to the breaking point.

PRINCIPLES OF FLUID MANAGEMENT

It is also important to consider therapeutic approaches to the abnormal pulmonary fluid retention implicated in the genesis of RDS. The observations of Skillman et al. [40] have demonstrated the value of elevating the colloid oncotic pressure in effecting an increase in PaO_2 in postoperative patients in whom acute postinjury RDS has developed after major surgery with massive intraoperative crystalloid replacement. This therapeutic approach to correcting the pathologic increases in lung water is consistent with the theory of pathogenesis based on the Starling hypothesis. Its effect can be enhanced by the simultaneous use of cautious diuretic therapy, using furosemide or ethacrynic acid to remove the excess returning extracellular third-space volume and thus preventing circulatory volume overload.

THE ROLE OF CORTICOSTEROID HORMONES
The role of corticosteroids in ameliorating the pathogenetic factors in acute RDS is controversial. Some experimental studies suggest that very large doses of corticosteroids (methylprednisolone, 30 mg/kg, or dexamethasone 5 mg/kg, IV bolus) may have a protective effect when given before injury. However, at present, no statistically significant data are available that show an unequivocally beneficial role for this class of agents in human posttraumatic pulmonary insufficiency. It would seem likely that if there is a therapeutic role for corticosteroids in this pathophysiologic state, this would be before the syndrome is well established. Any continuing use of corticosteroids must be weighed against the likelihood of enhancing bacterial invasion of the already traumatized lung parenchyma.

BACTERIAL CONTROL
It is essential that all patients with RDS be monitored daily by endotracheal culture, or smears, or both. Specific antibiotics should be used only when indicated by clinical and bacteriologic criteria. Both aerobic and anaerobic organisms should be monitored, since with improved anaerobic culture techniques, infection with anaerobic organisms is becoming increasingly recognized as a pathologically significant cause of pulmonary sepsis. Generally, prophylactic antibiotics are not effective, and their use enhances the risk of replacement of normal flora with resistant pathogenic organisms endemic in the intensive care environment.

SPECIFIC CLINICAL PROBLEMS
The acute posttraumatic respiratory distress syndrome described by Blaisdell [3] as being the result of platelet microaggregation is an important but probably late manifestation of major injury with hemorrhage and soft tissue damage. However, the most common form of acute respiratory insufficiency as an early feature of a life-threatening disease process occurs in sepsis [5, 36, 45]. It has also been noted that the severity and duration of the RDS is more pronounced in major sepsis than after major traumatic or hemorrhagic shock [5, 45]. Patients with acute myocardial infarction [29, 35, 41] or trauma [11, 23, 26, 28] and cardiac surgical patients who manifest myocardial depression after cardiopulmonary bypass [8, 26, 27] have

also been shown to develop an RDS picture. These observations suggest that although all of these clinical conditions may produce increased pulmonary venoarterial admixture as a consequence of pulmonary shunting, a somewhat different mixture of the known pathophysiologic mechanisms may be involved in each type of process.

These different clinical pictures underscore the fact that there are differences between the relative importance of factors producing local pulmonary capillary endothelial injury [3, 43] and interstitial edema [13, 17, 20], and those related to systemic and pulmonary hemodynamic abnormalities that produce pulmonary shunting on the basis of acute ventilation-perfusion disparities [7, 8, 15, 18, 36, 42, 47]. The studies of Clowes [5, 6] and Mac-Lean [21] have shown that the earliest manifestations of arterial hypoxemia accompanied by increased pulmonary venoarterial shunting are frequently associated with a normal chest x-ray. Clowes and associates [5] showed that the late features of the respiratory disease, commonly called shock lung, occur when the microscopic picture of interstitial edema, leukocyte septal invasion, and intravascular congestion (Stage I) progresses to diffuse alveolar collapse and bronchopneumonia (Stage II).

The critical importance of the relationship between the pulmonary and the systemic manifestations of sepsis has been pointed out by Siegel and his colleagues [35, 38], who have shown that the increase in pulmonary shunting seen in sepsis is directly related to the magnitude of the abnormalities in peripheral vascular tone [36, 38]. More recent studies by this group [31, 34, 35] have demonstrated that the severity of the septic process can be quantified by a multivariable physiologic classification technique. By means of this organizational framework, the peripheral and pulmonary hemodynamic relationships can be shown to be a direct manifestation of the fundamental abnormalities in intracellular metabolism and the consequent alterations in organ substrate metabolism and the fuel energy deficit [30, 31].

The basic pattern of cardiovascular abnormalities in sepsis contrasted to those seen in patients with cardiogenic and hypovolemic syndromes is shown in Figure 6-9. In this figure the interrelation among cardiac output (CO), total peripheral resistance (TPR), cardiac ejection fraction (EFx), and cardiac minute work is shown. In contrast to the cardiogenic patients, the septic patients in general have a marked hyperdynamic response. They have higher CO and larger cardiac ejection fractions (EFx) and do a larger amount of cardiac minute work (> 6.28 kgM/min) in spite of a lower TPR than the cardiogenic or hypovolemic patients. When a septic patient develops some degree of myocardial depression (EFx < 60%), he behaves much as does a cardiogenic patient. As a result of the hyperdynamic state, which produces a large amount of flow-related cardiac work in septic patients with evidence of a large cardiac sympathetic response (EFx > 75%), the myocardial fuel requirements and oxygen consumption would be expected

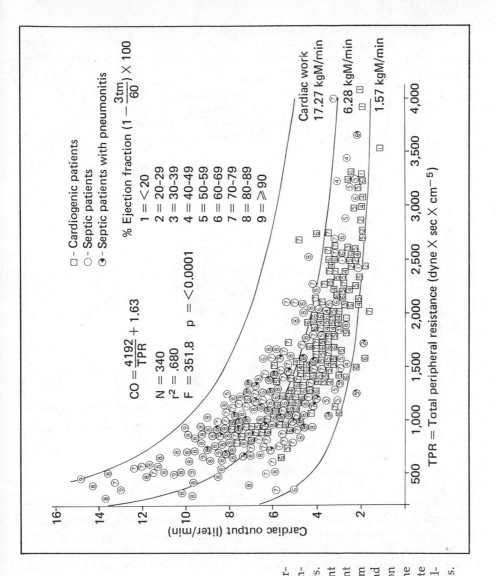

FIGURE 6-9. Relation between cardiac output (CO) and total peripheral resistance (TPR) in 340 studies.
Individual points labeled by percent
ejection fraction. Lines of constant
cardiac work are shown. (From
J. H. Siegel, I. Giovannini, and
B. Coleman, Ventilation: perfusion
maldistribution secondary to the
hyperdynamic cardiovascular state
as the major cause of increased pulmonary shunting in human sepsis.
J. Trauma 19:432, 1979.)

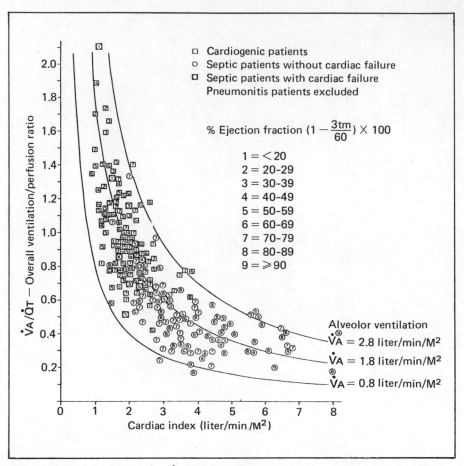

FIGURE 6-10. Relation of $\dot{V}_A/\dot{Q}_T$ to cardiac index. Points labeled by percent ejection fraction. Lines of constant alveolar ventilation are shown. Note that the septic patients have lower $\dot{V}_A/\dot{Q}_T$, higher cardiac index (CI), and larger ejection fractions than cardiogenic patients. (From J. H. Siegel, I. Giovannini, and B. Coleman, Ventilation : perfusion maldistribution secondary to the hyperdynamic cardiovascular state as the major cause of increased pulmonary shunting in human sepsis. J. Trauma 19:432, 1979.)

to be very large. Consequently, the septic patient's myocardial function is likely to be especially vulnerable to any RDS-induced arterial hypoxemia.

The increased cardiac index which occurs in the septic patient is associated with a fall in the overall ventilation : perfusion ratio ($\dot{V}_A/\dot{Q}_T$) compared either to normal patients (normal $\dot{V}_A/\dot{Q}_T = 0.8$ at CI = 3.1 L/min/M²) or to patients with cardiogenic syndromes. This is shown in Figure 6-10, which demonstrates the effect of EFx on the interaction between $\dot{V}_A/\dot{Q}_T$ and pulmonary blood flow (cardiac index). Also shown are lines of constant alveolar minute ventilation ($\dot{V}_A$). It can be seen that the septic patients with the highest blood flow (CI) and the largest cardiac ejection fraction are also the patients with the lowest $\dot{V}_A/\dot{Q}_T$ [36]. In contrast, patients with cardiogenic syndromes have low cardiac outputs, decreased EFx, and a higher than normal $\dot{V}_A/\dot{Q}_T$. The cardiogenic patient may be relatively underventilated due to interstitial edema with alveolar collapse or pulmonary edema, but the septic patient requires a very large minute volume ($\dot{V}_E$) to get even a small $\dot{V}_A$. Because of the extremely low $\dot{V}_A/\dot{Q}_T$, previously normally perfused alveoli are converted into very large volumes of noneffective dead space ventilation, and V_D/V_T rises due to the diversion of perfusion to a more restricted set of pulmonary beds.

The low $\dot{V}_A/\dot{Q}_T$ associated with the occurrence of the hyperdynamic septic syndrome also has as its consequence a marked increase in pulmonary venoarterial admixture ($\dot{Q}_S/\dot{Q}_T$) as the high flow perfuses a larger percentage of poorly ventilated alveolar segments. The relationship between $\dot{V}_A/\dot{Q}_T$, shunt ($\dot{Q}_S/\dot{Q}_T$), and dead space (V_D/V_T) is shown in Figure 6-11. This figure also shows the mean $\pm$ SEM and $\pm$ 95 percent ($\pm$ 2 SD) confidence limits of the $\dot{Q}_S/\dot{Q}_T$ and $\dot{V}_A/\dot{Q}_T$ relationship for all septic and nonseptic patients without clinical pneumonitis. As can be seen, patients with cardiogenic syndromes have higher $\dot{V}_A/\dot{Q}_T$, moderate increases in $\dot{Q}_S/\dot{Q}_T$, and small increases in V_D/V_T compared to normal ($\dot{V}_A/\dot{Q}_T = 0.8$, $\dot{Q}_S/\dot{Q}_T < 10\%$, $V_D/V_T = 0.3$). In contrast, the hyperdynamic septic patients with large CI and EFx (Fig. 6-10) and low TPR (Fig. 6-9) have markedly reduced $\dot{V}_A/\dot{Q}_T$ but large increases in $\dot{Q}_S/\dot{Q}_T$ and V_D/V_T. This suggests that the primary reason for the increased shunt ($\dot{Q}_S/\dot{Q}_T$) seen in the septic patients is due to the disproportionate flow of pulmonary blood flow through *dependent* lung beds where alveolar ventilation is poor. This results in the diversion of blood flow away from the nondependent pulmonary beds with a proportionate conversion of these alveoli to dead space (V_D/V_T). When pulmonary microatelectasis or alveolar consolidation occurs as a secondary phenomenon with the development of septic pneumonitis, an additional factor of pathologic anatomic shunting is added to the functional physiologic shunt induced by the $\dot{V}_A/\dot{Q}_T$ maldistribution. Consequently, the patient with septic pneumonitis has a higher $\dot{Q}_S/\dot{Q}_T$ for a given $\dot{V}_A/\dot{Q}_T$ than does the ordinary hyperdynamic septic patient and falls above the $+95\%$ confidence limits for the $\dot{Q}_S/\dot{Q}_T$ to $\dot{V}_A/\dot{Q}_T$ relationship (Fig. 6-11).

The dependence of $\dot{V}_A/\dot{Q}_T$, $\dot{Q}_S/\dot{Q}_T$, and V_D/V_T in sepsis on flow (CI) and cardiac ejection fraction is consistent with experimental evidence [7, 22] that the distribution of the pulmonary blood flow and thus the ventilation-perfusion and shunt distribution are hemodynamically determined by the gradient between pulmonary arterial inflow and the pulmonary venous outflow pressures relative to the intra-alveolar pressure, and also that this three-way pressure relationship regulates the effective level of pulmonary alveolar perfusion.

The pulmonary venous pressure level is set by the level of left atrial

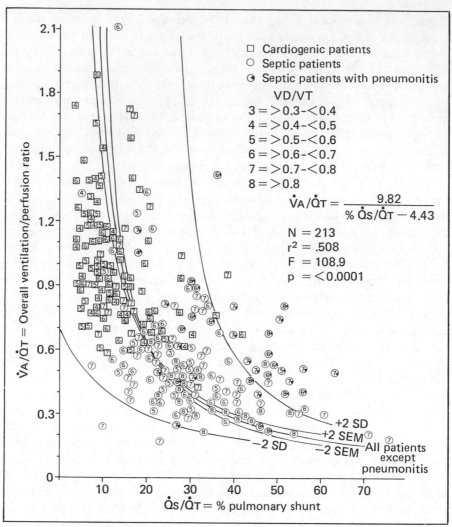

FIGURE 6-11. Relation of the $\dot{V}_A/\dot{Q}_T$ to $\dot{Q}_S/\dot{Q}_T$, with points labeled by V_D/V_T level. Note that the septic patients without pneumonitis tend to have a lower $\dot{V}_A/\dot{Q}_T$ and higher V_D/V_T for a given level of $\dot{Q}_S/\dot{Q}_T$, that the highest $\dot{Q}_S/\dot{Q}_T$ and lowest $\dot{V}_A/\dot{Q}_T$ occur in septic patients, and that septic patients with pneumonitis have a higher shunt for a given $\dot{V}_A/\dot{Q}_T$ and fall outside of the 95 percent confidence limits of the regression for nonpneumonitis patients. (From J. H. Siegel, I. Giovannini, and B. Coleman, Ventilation : perfusion maldistribution secondary to the hyperdynamic cardiovascular state as the major cause of increased pulmonary shunting in human sepsis. *J. Trauma* 19:432, 1979.)

pressure, and it, in turn, is a function of the left ventricular end-diastolic pressure to end-diastolic volume (LVEDV) relationship, left ventricular distensibility. Also, at a given level of myocardial contractility (reflected in the ejection fraction) the forward flow of the heart (CI) is also determined by the LVEDV. Thus, the myocardial function curve is simultaneously the determinant of the rate of pulmonary arterial inflow and the regulator of the pulmonary venous outflow and, as such, is a major factor in determining the distribution of pulmonary perfusion, $\dot{V}_A/\dot{Q}_T$, V_D/V_T, and $\dot{Q}_S/\dot{Q}_T$. This is shown in Figure 6-12, which displays the influence on $\dot{Q}_S/\dot{Q}_T$ of the ventricular function relationship in hyperdynamic septic patients compared to cardiogenic patients and septic patients with myocardial depression producing cardiogenic syndromes. The hyperdynamic septic patients can be seen to fall in a higher range of ventricular function (VF) curves than do the cardiogenic patients. Consequent to this shift to the left in the VF relationship, which produces a lower LVEDV for a higher CI, there is an increase in $\dot{Q}_S/\dot{Q}_T$. The septic patients with the lowest LVEDV and highest pulmonary blood flow (CI) also have the greatest tendency to have $\dot{Q}_S/\dot{Q}_T$ values of greater than 30 percent. Indeed, of nearly all the hyperdynamic septic patients with CI $>$ 4 L/min/M^2 who have shunts, over 30 percent fall at or above the +95 percent confidence limit of the hyperdynamic VF relationship. This suggests that the early $\dot{V}_A/\dot{Q}_T$ maldistribution of sepsis is hemodynamically determined.

The physiologic reasons for this phenomenon are contained in the known dynamic control mechanisms for pulmonary blood flow. As a conceptual description the lung ventilation : perfusion characteristics can be divided into three functional zones on a gravitational basis determined by the "height" of the pulmonary alveolar segment relative to the left atrial pressure [7, 22, 46, 47].

In Zone I, the most superior lung alveolar segments, the pulmonary arterial inflow pressure is greater than the pulmonary venous outflow pressure, but both intravascular pressures are less than the intra-alveolar air pressure, and consequently, no pulmonary blood flow occurs. These alveoli are thus converted to dead space (V_D/V_T).

In Zone II, the functional lung alveoli, the pulmonary arterial inflow pressure is greater than the intra-alveolar pressure, which is, in turn, greater than the pulmonary venous pressure (PVP). In this zone there is pulmonary alveolar perfusion, which is regulated by the intra-alveolar pressure dynamics. Also, since intra-alveolar air pressure is greater than the pulmonary venous capillary pressure, the alveolar capillaries are compressed so that the capillary exchange surface to volume ratio is maximized, and the velocity of capillary blood flow is high for a given level of alveolar blood flow. Most of the pulmonary gas exchange occurs in Zone II lung.

In Zone III, the dependent lung segments, the pulmonary arterial pressure is greater than the intra-alveolar pressure and the pulmonary venous

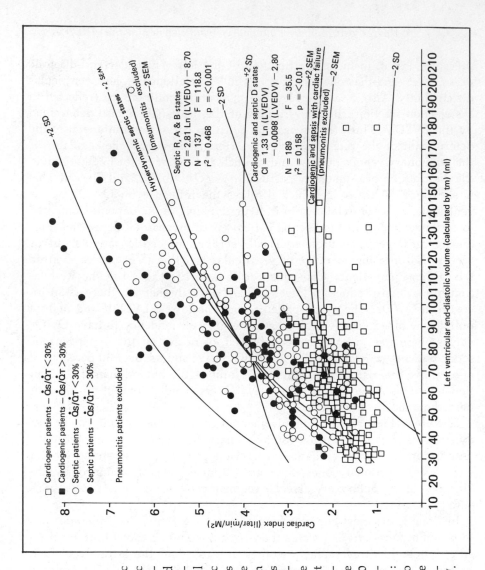

FIGURE 6-12. Relation between cardiac index and left ventricular end-diastolic volume (LVEDV) for septic and cardiogenic patients. The regression and confidence limits for septic R (normodynamic), A (hyperdynamic normal stress response), and B (hyperdynamic metabolic insufficiency) state patients show them to be in a different range of Starling-Sarnoff relationships than the regression and confidence limits for cardiogenic and septic D state patients. The regression slopes of these two groups are significantly different (F ratio, 191.3; $p < 0.0001$). The hyperdynamic septic patients with large CI/LVEDV tend to have $\dot{Q}s/\dot{Q}\tau > 30$ percent. (From J. H. Siegel, I. Giovannini, and B. Coleman, Ventilation: perfusion maldistribution secondary to the hyperdynamic cardiovascular state as the major cause of increased pulmonary shunting in human sepsis. *J. Trauma* 19:432, 1979.)

pressure, but the pulmonary alveolar pressure is less than the pulmonary venous pressure. Consequently, the regulation of blood flow through these alveoli is determined by the PVP. In addition, since intracapillary pressure is greater than intra-alveolar pressure, and this is reflected in the pulmonary interstitial fluid pressure, the alveoli tend to be reduced in air volume compared to Zone I or II. As a result the regional $\dot{V}_A/\dot{Q}$ is low. In those alveoli where the $\dot{V}_A/\dot{Q}$ ratio falls below some critical value, physiologic shunting occurs and a significant $\dot{Q}_S/\dot{Q}_T$ component is present.

An additional feature of the Zone III lung is the tendency for an increased formation of interstitial fluid $\dot{Q}_f$ because of the dynamics of the Starling law of capillary fluid exchange (Equation 1). Since the capillaries in this region are subjected to the highest intracapillary pressure, and have the largest proportion of an already increased pulmonary blood flow by virtue of the high CI and reduced $\dot{V}_A/\dot{Q}_T$, which shifts the blood flow distribution to the more dependent segments, the Starling equation predicts the greatest $\dot{Q}_f$ at a given membrane permeability (K_f) and colloid oncotic pressure gradient σ ($\Pi_{IV} - \Pi_{EV}$). The net result is an increase in pulmonary interstitial fluid volume and pressure and the formation of interstitial and intra-alveolar edema with alveolar microatelectasis and collapse. When this occurs, the previously clear chest x-ray begins to show flocculent exudates distributed to the dependent lung segments. However, since these patients are invariably lying supine in bed, the posterior segments are now the dependent ones, and on routine PA chest x-ray they appear uniformly distributed bilaterally in upper and lower lung fields. When this secondary pulmonary alveolar atelectasis and consolidation occur, the septic patient develops a further increase in pulmonary shunt ($\dot{Q}_S/\dot{Q}_T$), as the pathologic anatomic shunt of alveolar collapse is added to the physiologic shunt produced by the shift to a lower $\dot{V}_A/\dot{Q}_T$ distribution. This is shown in Figure 6-11, in which the septic patients with pneumonitis by x-ray fall above the +95 percent confidence limit of the $\dot{V}_A/\dot{Q}_T$ to $\dot{Q}_S/\dot{Q}_T$ relation for non-pneumonitis patients.

The therapeutic implications of this unbalanced cardiopulmonary relationship seen in hyperdynamic clinical states—as found in sepsis [36], pancreatitis [31], decompensated cirrhotic liver disease [37], and after major traumatic injury [11, 28]—are that a conscious effort must be made to maximize the redistribution of alveolar ventilation by modifying the pattern of breathing and the use of PEEP, and by modifying the distribution of pulmonary blood flow and thus $\dot{V}_A/\dot{Q}_T$ by judicious elevation of the left atrial pressure, using volume loads that will tend to remain in the intravascular compartment (colloid or blood) [36] while at the same time reducing extravascular water by diuresis and crystalloid restriction [40].

Modifying the ventilatory component can be achieved by respiratory intubation or use of a tight-fitting face mask and volume-limited ventilation by either controlled mandatory ventilation (CMV) or intermittent mandatory ventilation (IMV). To this basic respiratory support may be added an inspiratory respiratory hold, which delays the delivery of the major fraction of the inspired volume to the later portion of inspiration to maximize overcoming of the reduced compliance and increased resistance of the small airways. Also, the use of PEEP with either CMV or IMV will tend to prevent expiratory collapse of those alveoli in regions of high pulmonary interstitial fluid pressure and thus drive increased alveolar ventilation down into larger volumes of previously Zone III lung, thereby converting it to effective Zone II lung.

Concomitantly with these respiratory support measures, it is necessary to cautiously increase pulmonary venous pressure by raising LVEDV with colloid or blood volume in the hyperdynamic patient with a very *low* pulmonary wedge or right atrial mean pressure. As shown by Siegel, Giovannini, and Coleman [36], this maneuver will result in an increase in pulmonary blood flow without increasing $\dot{Q}s/\dot{Q}T$ producing an increased $\dot{V}A/\dot{Q}T$ and a fall in VD/VT in the septic hyperdynamic patient who already manifests a large cardiac ejection fraction (EFx). Such cautious volume loading in the hyperdynamic patient is preferable to reducing the cardiac output by negative inotropic measures, since it has been shown that these septic, cirrhotic, or posttraumatic hyperdynamic patients require the high-output state to survive, because of the increased peripheral tissue needs for perfusion. Thus, continued positive inotropic support may be necessary. Also, at a given FRC and contractility level, an increase in cardiac output will increase PaO_2 by reducing shunt, because of a better distribution of $\dot{V}A/\dot{Q}T$ to under-perfused alveolar segments (see Fig. 6-8).

Another important maneuver to improve $\dot{V}A/\dot{Q}T$ distribution and to prevent conversion of Zone III lung into areas of interstitial edema and alveolar collapse is frequently to change the position of the chest so that no area of the lung remains constantly dependent. The best way to do this is by achieving the upright chest for the maximum time period in each day. The patient can be ventilated by CMV or IMV, and PEEP, and can either be seated in the erect position or, if not paralyzed, be ambulated at bedside, even on a respirator. This means that the early stabilization of fractures, by operative means if necessary, is a critical feature of optimal respiratory management in the patient with actual or potential RDS.

THERAPEUTIC PROSPECTS FOR REFRACTORY ACUTE RESPIRATORY INSUFFICIENCY

In refractory cases of acute posttraumatic RDS, the initial clinical investigative studies of Hill et al. [16] and others suggested that there may be a place for prolonged partial extracorporeal oxygenation using a membrane oxygenator (ECMO). However, the benefits of this approach have not been clearly supported by statistically controlled, prospective studies under the ECMO project. Although there are occasional cases in which ECMO has been effective, such a desperate and heroic last-ditch effort should be confined to the few institutions prepared to undertake the necessary complex technologic support and evaluation protocols. At present, it cannot be recommended as a therapeutic measure for general use. Indeed, in most instances, an understanding of the mechanisms of pathogenesis, careful monitoring of the parameters of respiratory effectiveness, and early initiation of and adherence to the principles of respiratory support that have been outlined will substantially reduce the incidence and severity of the posttraumatic lung syndrome. With presently understood "ideal" management, the number of patients requiring extracorporeal support is likely to be small and will be confined largely to patients with major primary pulmonary compression or blast injury and some few patients with fulminant viral or bacterial pneumonitis.

REFERENCES

1. Ashbaugh, D. G., et al.   Continuous positive pressure breathing (CPPC) in adult respiratory distress syndrome. *J. Thorac. Cardiovasc. Surg.* 31:57, 1969.
2. Bayley, T., et al.   Pulmonary and circulatory effects of fibrinopeptides. *Circ. Res.* 21:469, 1967.
3. Blaisdell, F. W.   Pathophysiology of the respiratory distress syndrome. *Arch. Surg.* 108:44, 1974.
4. Chodoff, P., and Margand, P. M.   Use of a respiratory weaning score. *Md. State Med. J.* 22:50, 1973.
5. Clowes, G. H. A., Jr., Hirsch, E., Williams, L., Kwasnik, E., O'Connell, T. F., Ceuvas, P., Saini, V. K., Moradi, I., Farizan, M., Saravis, C., Stone, M., and Kuffler, J.   Septic lung and shock lung in man. *Ann. Surg.* 181:681, 1975.
6. Clowes, G. H. A., Jr., Zuschneid, W., Dragacevic, S., and Turner, M.   The nonspecific pulmonary inflammatory reactions leading to respiratory failure after shock, gangrene and sepsis. *J. Trauma* 8:899, 1968.
7. Edelman, N. H., Gorfinkel, H. J., Lluch, S., Gottschalk, A., Hirsch, L. J., and Fishman, A. P.   Experimental cardiogenic shock: Pulmonary performance after acute myocardial infarction. *Am. J. Physiol.* 219:1723, 1970.
8. Farrell, E. J., and Siegel, J. H.   Cardiorespiratory simulation for the evaluation of recovery following coronary artery bypass surgery. *Computers and Biomed. Res.* submitted for publication 1979.
9. Fowler, W., et al.   Lung function studies VIII. Analysis of alveolar ventilation by pulmonary N_2 clearance curves. *J. Clin. Invest.* 31:40, 1952.
10. Gerst, P. H., Rottenborg, C., and Holaday, D. A.   The effects of hemorrhage on the pulmonary circulation and respiratory gas exchange. *J. Clin. Invest.* 38:524, 1958.
11. Gump, F. E., et al.   Simultaneous use of three indicators to evaluate pulmonary capillary damage in man. *Surgery* 70:262, 1971.
12. Guyton, A. C., and Lindsey, A. W.   Effect of elevated left atrial pressure and decreased plasma protein concentration on the development of pulmonary edema. *Circ. Res.* 7:649, 1959.
13. Hecktman, H. B., et al.   The independence of pulmonary shunting and pulmonary edema. *Surgery* 74:300, 1973.
14. Hedley-Whyte, J., Pontoppidan, H., and Jocelin Morris, M.   The response

of patients with respiratory failure and cardiopulmonary disease to different levels of constant volume ventilation. *J. Clin. Invest.* 45:1543, 1966.

15. Higgs, B. E. Factors influencing pulmonary gas exchange during the acute stages of myocardial infarction. *Clin. Sci.* 35:115, 1968.

16. Hill, J. D., et al. Extracorporeal oxygenation for post-traumatic respiratory failure. *N. Engl. J. Med.* 286:629, 1972.

17. Iliff, L. D., Greene, R. E., and Hughes, J. M. B. Effects of interstitial edema on distribution of ventilation and perfusion in isolated lung. *J. Appl. Physiol.* 33:462, 1972.

18. Kazemi, H., Parsons, E. F., Valenca, L. M., and Streider, D. J. Distribution of pulmonary blood flow after myocardial ischemia and infarction. *Circulation* 41:1025, 1970.

19. Kellogg, R. H. Central Chemical Regulation of Respiration. In W. O. Fenn and H. Rahn (eds.). Respiration, Section 3, *Handbook of Physiology.* The American Physiological Society. Baltimore: Williams & Wilkins, 1964.

20. Levine, D. R., et al. The application of Starling's law of capillary exchange to the lungs. *J. Clin. Invest.* 46:934, 1967.

21. MacLean, L. D., Mulligan, W. G., McLean, A. P. H., and Duff, J. M. Patterns of septic shock in man—a detailed study of 56 patients. *Ann. Surg.* 166:543, 1967.

22. Miner, M. E., and Gonzales, M. D. Variations in pulmonary gas exchange due to changes in pulmonary artery pressure and flow. *J. Surg. Res.* 18:431, 1975.

23. Monaco, V., Burdge, R., Newell, J., Sardar, S., Leather, R., and Powers, S. R. Pulmonary venous admixture in injured patients. *J. Trauma* 12:15, 1972.

24. Moore, F. D., et al. *Post Traumatic Pulmonary Insufficiency.* Philadelphia: Saunders, 1969.

25. Peters, R. M., and Hilberman, M. Respiratory insufficiency: Diagnosis and control of therapy. *Surgery* 71:119, 1967.

26. Peters, R. M., Hilberman, M., Hogan, J. S., and Crawford, D. A. Objective indications for respiratory therapy in post-trauma and post-operative patients. *Am. J. Surg.* 124:262, 1972.

27. Philbin, D. M., Sullivan, S. F., Bowman, F. O., Jr., Malm, J. M., and Papper, E. M. Postoperative hypoxemia: Contribution of the cardiac output. *Anesthesiology* 32:136, 1970.

28. Powers, S. R., Jr., et al. Studies of pulmonary insufficiency in nonthoracic trauma. *J. Trauma* 12:1, 1972.

29. Saunders, K. B. Physiological dead space in left ventricular failure. *Clin. Sci.* 31:145, 1966.

30. Siegel, J. H., Cerra, F. B., Coleman, B., Giovannini, I., Shetye, M., Border, J. R., and McMenamy, R. H. Physiologic and metabolic correlations in human sepsis. *Surgery* 86:163, 1979.

31. Siegel, J. H., Cerra, F. B., Peters, D., Moody, E., Brown, D., McMenamy, R. H., and Border, J. R. The physiologic recovery trajectory as the organizing principle for the quantification of hormonometabolic adaptation to surgical stress and severe sepsis. In W. Schumer, J. J. Spitzer, and B. E. Marshall (eds.), *Advances in Shock Research.* New York: Liss, 1979. Pp. 177–203.

32. Siegel, J. H., and Farrell, E. J. A computer simulation model to study the clinical observability of ventilation and perfusion abnormalities in human shock states. *Surgery* 73:898, 1973.
33. Siegel, J. H., Farrell, E. J., Goldwyn, R. M., and Friedman, H. P. The surgical implication of physiologic patterns in myocardial infarction shock. *Surgery* 72:126, 1972.
34. Siegel, J. H., Farrell, E. J., Lewin, I. Quantifying the need for cardiac support in human shock by a functional model of cardiopulmonary vascular dynamics: With special reference to myocardial infarction. *J. Surg. Res.* 13: 166, 1972.
35. Siegel, J. H., Farrell, E. J., Miller, M., Goldwyn, R. M., and Friedman, H. P. Cardiorespiratory interactions as determinants of survival and the need for respiratory support in human shock states. *J. Trauma* 13:602, 1973.
36. Siegel, J. H., Giovannini, I., and Coleman, B. Ventilation : perfusion maldistribution secondary to the hyperdynamic cardiovascular state as the major cause of increased pulmonary shunting in human sepsis. *J. Trauma* 19(6):432, 1979.
37. Siegel, J. H., Goldwyn, R. M., Farrell, E. J., Gallin, P., and Friedman, H. P. Hyperdynamic states and the physiologic determinants of survival in patients with cirrhosis and portal hypertension. *Arch. Surg.* 108:282, 1974.
38. Siegel, J. H., Greenspan, M., and DelGuercio, L. R. M. Abnormal vascular tone, defective oxygen transport and myocardial failure in human septic shock. *Ann. Surg.* 165:504, 1967.
39. Siegel, J. H., Levine, M. J., McConn, R., DelGuercio, L. R. M. The effect of glucagon infusion on cardiovascular function in the critically ill. *Surg. Gynec. Obstet.* 131:505, 1970.
40. Skillman, J. J., Bloom, G. P., Restall, D. S., Bushnell, L. S., and Salzman, E. W. Loss replacement and rationale for use of albumin in shock. In T. I. Malinin et al. (eds.), *Acute Fluid Replacement in the Therapy of Shock*. New York: Intercontinental Medical Book, 1974.
41. Smith, G., Cheney, F. V., Jr., and Winter, P. M. The effects of change in cardiac output on intrapulmonary shunting. *Br. J. Anaesth.* 46:227, 1974.
42. Stanley, T. H., Lynn, J. K., Wen-Shin, L., and Gentry, B. S. Effects of left atrial pressure on pulmonary shunt and the dead space/tidal volume ratio. *Anesthesiology* 49:128, 1974.
43. Staub, N. C. Pathogenesis of pulmonary edema. *Am. Rev. Respir. Dis.* 109: 358, 1974.
44. Staub, N. C., et al. Pulmonary edema in dogs, especially the sequence of fluid accumulation in lungs. *J. Appl. Physiol.* 22:227, 1967.
45. Vito, L., Dennis, R. C., Weisel, R. D., and Hechtman, H. B. Sepsis presenting as acute respiratory insufficiency. *Surg. Gynec. Obstet.* 138:896, 1974.
46. West, J. B. Regional differences in gas exchange in the lung of erect man. *J. Appl. Physiol.* 17:893, 1862.
47. West, J. B., and Dollery, C. T. Distribution of blood flow and the pressure-flow relations of the whole lung. *J. Appl. Physiol.* 20:175, 1965.

Robert L. Smith / # 7. OXYGEN ADMINISTRATION

One of the most important functions of the lungs is to supply oxygen to the mixed venous blood passing through the pulmonary capillary bed. The proper oxygenation of blood in the lungs depends on many factors that may be affected by disorders of the lungs. Whenever the normal matching of ventilation and blood flow in the myriad of peripheral lung units is disturbed by disease, hypoxemia is a regular consequence. Also, hypoxemia results when the barrier for diffusion of oxygen from the alveoli to the capillaries is increased by diseases such as pulmonary fibrosis. Finally, even though ventilation and blood flow are evenly matched and diffusion is normal, a decrease in the overall level of alveolar ventilation can reduce the partial pressure of oxygen in the alveoli and lead to hypoxemia.

Hypoxemia and the resulting alterations in oxygen delivery to the peripheral tissues can have serious effects on the function of vital organs, including the brain and the heart. Even moderate degrees of brain hypoxia may produce muscular discoordination, restlessness, and confusion. Inadequate oxygen delivery to the heart can eventually result in bradycardia and hypotension. However, hypoxemia and its consequences can be relieved even in the presence of severe lung disorders by the administration of supplemental oxygen.

At sea level, atmospheric air contains 20.93 percent oxygen and has a partial pressure (PO_2) of about 159 mm Hg. As inspired air passes over the upper respiratory tract, it is heated and humidified and its water vapor pressure increases. Because of the uptake of oxygen from the alveoli and the transfer of carbon dioxide from the mixed venous blood into the alveoli, the partial pressure of oxygen in the alveolar air (PAO_2) is only about 100 to 110 mm Hg. Normally the arterial PO_2 is about 80 to 90 mm Hg, depending on age, but this value will be reduced by disorders of the lung that result in a mismatching of ventilation and blood flow or produce a diffusion defect. Regardless of impairments in lung functions, the alveolar PO_2 and, consequently, the arterial PO_2 can be altered by increasing the concentration of oxygen in the inspired air.

FLOWMETERS

The flow of oxygen from either wall or cylinder source is indicated by a flowmeter. The flowmeter produces a pressure drop from 50ψ at the gas

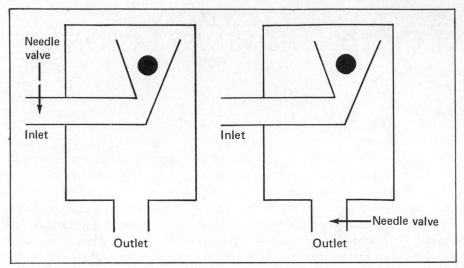

FIGURE 7-1. (A) Nonpressure-compensated flowmeter. (B) Pressure-compensated flowmeter.

inlet to atmospheric pressure at the outlet. A needle valve which controls the flow of oxygen is regulated by an adjusting wheel, and the rate of gas flow is indicated by the level of a ball float suspended in the airstream within the flow tube. The float is suspended in the airstream because of the difference in pressure on either side of the float.

In nonpressure-compensated systems, the needle valve is placed between the gas inlet and the ball float. Normally, the pressure at the gas outlet is at atmospheric levels, but with any narrowing or partial obstruction at the gas outlet, the pressure difference across the float and, consequently, the position of the float will change even though the rate of airflow may be maintained.

The commonly used flowmeters are pressure compensated. The needle valve is located downstream between the ball and the gas outlet so that even with a blockage at the flowmeter outlet, the position of the ball float will accurately reflect the rate of gas flow (Fig. 7-1).

HUMIDIFICATION
Oxygen from both wall and cylinder sources is dry. Even in patients breathing in the usual manner through the nose and mouth, the gas must be humidified or it will produce drying and irritation of the mucous membranes of the upper respiratory tract.

HUMIDIFIERS
Adequate humidification of oxygen delivered at low flow rates to patients breathing by mouth or nose can be achieved with a simple humidifier. The

most commonly used type is the bubble humidifier. From the flowmeter, oxygen passes down a tube and through a porous head submerged under water, forming small bubbles which then return to the surface. As the bubbles rise through the water, the pressure of vaporization forces water vapor into the oxygen. Further vaporization occurs at the water surface when the bubbles break.

The efficiency of the bubble humidifier will depend on a number of factors. Smaller bubbles promote better humidification by increasing the surface area of gas exposed to water. Also, the length of time of contact of gas and water is important in promoting humidification. The humidifier jar must be properly filled to ensure that the bubbles of oxygen pass through as much water as possible.

Oxygen passing through a bubble humidifier is only about 40 percent saturated with water vapor at body temperature; complete humidification is achieved by some water loss from the upper respiratory tract.

METHODS OF OXYGEN ADMINISTRATION

The basic objective of oxygen administration is to increase the concentration of oxygen in the inspired air. This can be accomplished in a variety of ways, depending on the required degree of oxygen enrichment of inspired air and the need for humidification.

Supplemental oxygen is most commonly administered through a nasal cannula, simple face mask, or face mask with reservoir bag using low rates of oxygen flow from a tank or wall source.

In some circumstances, when the concentration of oxygen in the inspired air must be accurately and tightly controlled, a high-airflow system with oxygen enrichment using a jet-mixing or Venturi apparatus is employed.

In patients with endotracheal tubes or tracheostomies, medium- and high-flow systems using a Briggs adaptor or tracheostomy mask are used to ensure not only supplemental oxygen delivery but also proper humidification of inspired air.

NASAL CANNULA

The nasal cannula (Fig. 7-2) consists of two short plastic prongs which fit into the external nares and are connected to the oxygen supply. Because of its comfort and simplicity, the nasal cannula is the preferred method of administration of low to moderate concentrations of supplemental oxygen.

The continuous flow of oxygen through the cannula displaces air in the nasal passages, pharynx, and larynx and creates an oxygen reservoir in this area. When the contents of the pharynx and larynx are added to room air during inspiration, an increase in the concentration of oxygen in the inspired air is achieved.

At a flow rate of 1 liter/min the inspired oxygen concentration increases to approximately 24 percent. At flow rates of 6 to 8 liter/min the reservoir

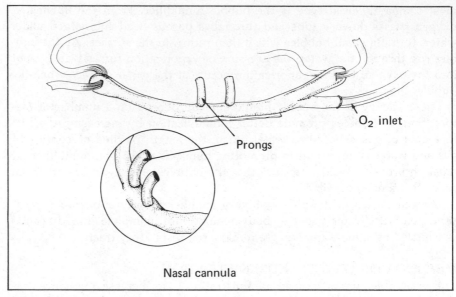

FIGURE 7-2. Nasal cannula.

in the nasopharynx and larynx is generally optimally filled with oxygen and the inspired oxygen concentration rises to about 40 to 45 percent. Further increases in oxygen flow produce little additional increase in the inspired oxygen concentration.

The effect of a given flow of oxygen through the nasal cannula on the overall inspired oxygen concentration will also depend on the size of the tidal volume and the volume of ventilation. If ventilation falls but the oxygen flow is maintained, the inspired oxygen concentration will rise.

Because of variations in the level of ventilation, precise regulation of the inspired oxygen concentration is not possible using a nasal cannula.

In order that oxygen administered by nasal cannula be effective in raising the inspired oxygen concentration, it is clearly important that the nasal passages be patent. However, nasally administered oxygen is as effective in raising the inspired oxygen concentration in mouth breathers as in nose breathers.

The major advantages of the nasal cannula are its simplicity, its comfort, and the fact that oxygen administration does not have to be discontinued during eating or coughing.

FACE MASK

A common alternative method of administering supplemental oxygen is by face mask. Oxygen face masks are shown in Figures 7-3, 7-4, and 7-5. The mask has side ports and may be equipped with a reservoir bag.

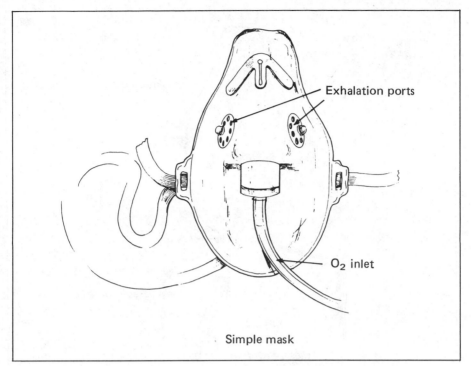

Exhalation ports

O₂ inlet

Simple mask

FIGURE 7-3. Simple mask.

Depending on the presence of a reservoir bag and whether or not the ports are fitted with directional valves, the inspired oxygen concentration can be increased to about 40 to 90 percent using a face mask. The face mask is somewhat less comfortable than the nasal cannula, but the major disadvantage is that the mask must be removed for eating, drinking, coughing, and expectoration.

SIMPLE MASK

Oxygen from a wall or cylinder source passes through the flowmeter and humidifier directly into the mask (Fig. 7-3), displacing air and creating a small oxygen reservoir. During inspiration, the oxygen in the mask is inhaled. In addition, some room air is entrained through the ports and through the spaces between the mask and the face so that the inspired oxygen concentration is considerably less than 100 percent. The extent to which the inspired oxygen concentration can be increased is dependent on the volume of the oxygen reservoir, determined by the size of the mask. Even the simple face mask can provide inspired oxygen concentrations that are higher than can be achieved with the nasal cannula. Generally, oxygen flow rates of 6 to 10 liters/min through a simple face mask raise the inspired oxygen concentration to 35 to 55 percent.

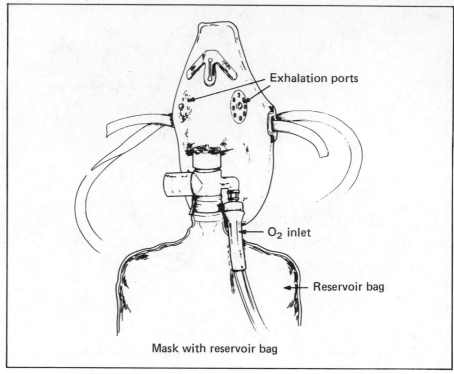

Exhalation ports

O₂ inlet

Reservoir bag

Mask with reservoir bag

FIGURE 7-4. Mask with reservoir bag.

MASK WITH RESERVOIR BAG

Further increases in inspired oxygen concentration can be provided by the addition of a reservoir bag to the face mask (Fig. 7-4), thus enlarging the potential reservoir of oxygen. Inspired gas is made up primarily of the oxygen in the mask and reservoir bag, with smaller amounts of room air passing through the ports of the mask.

During exhalation, most of the expired air passes out through the ports, but some expired air returns to the reservoir bag. This undesirable dead space effect results in a fall in the PO_2 and a rise in the PCO_2 in the bag and must be avoided by ensuring a sufficiently high rate of oxygen flow to keep the bag washed out. Oxygen flow rates of 8 to 10 liter/min are commonly used with the mask and reservoir bag; this provides an inspired oxygen concentration of between 50 and 80 percent. However, the rate of oxygen flow must be adjusted so that inspiration empties the reservoir bag by no more than a half.

MASK WITH RESERVOIR BAG AND DIRECTIONAL VALVES

The flow of room air into the face mask through the side ports during inspiration can be completely prevented by covering the side ports with di-

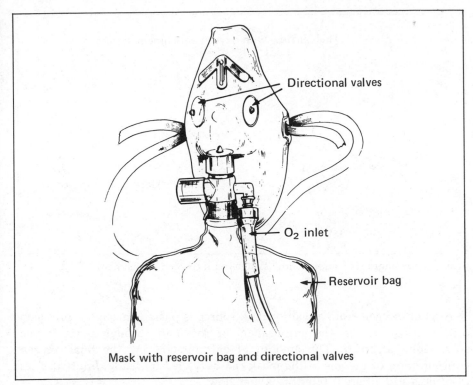

Mask with reservoir bag and directional valves

FIGURE 7-5. Mask with reservoir bag and directional valves.

rectional valves (Fig. 7-5). The entire volume of the breath during inspiration, with the exception of the small amount of air that passes between the mask and face, will then be made up of oxygen from the mask and reservoir bag. When directional valves are employed, it is critical that the rate of oxygen flow be high, in the range of 12 to 15 liter/min. In this manner, the inspired oxygen concentration can be raised to as high as 90 to 95 percent.

Since virtually all of the inspired gas comes from the mask and bag, it is critically important that adequate oxygen flows be maintained. If the reservoir bag is inadvertently allowed to empty, asphyxia may occur, particularly in the debilitated patient.

During exhalation, the port valves open, and expired air passes out of the mask to the atmosphere. The passage of expired air back into the reservoir bag may also be prevented by a directional valve situated between the mask and the bag.

HIGH AIRFLOW SYSTEMS WITH OXYGEN ENRICHMENT

High airflow systems with oxygen enrichment (Fig. 7-6) employ the principle of air entrainment with constant-pressure jet mixing.

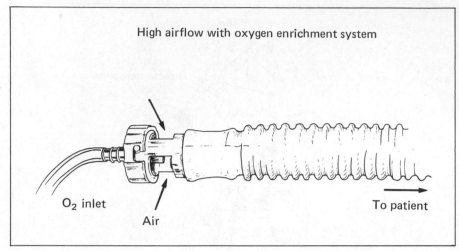

FIGURE 7-6. Diagram of high airflow system with oxygen enrichment.

A jet of oxygen from a wall or tank source is passed through a precision orifice and results in the entrainment of room air through ports in the surrounding cylinder. The amount of entrainment and the final oxygen concentration of the gas in the mask can be varied by using different sizes of orifices and different rates of oxygen flow.

There are commercially available high flow systems designed to deliver oxygen concentrations from 24 to 50 percent.

Data regarding oxygen flow, air/oxygen dilution, and total gas flow are shown in Tables 7-1 and 7-2.

The major advantages of the high airflow systems with oxygen enrichment are that the total gas flow is maintained at high levels and that the concentration of inspired oxygen is kept constant even over a fairly wide

TABLE 7-1. Obtainable Oxygen Concentrations with Low Flow Oxygen Administration Devices

Device	Oxygen flow (l/Min)	Oxygen concentration
Nasal cannula	6–8	40–45%
Simple mask	6–10	35–55%
Mask with reservoir	8–12	50–80%
Mask with reservoir and directional valves	10–15	90–95%

TABLE 7-2. High Airflow Systems with Oxygen Enrichment

Oxygen concentration (%)	Oxygen flow (l/Min)	Air/oxygen ratio	Total gas flow (l/Min)
24	4	25/1	104
28	4–6	10/1	44–66
31	6–8	7/1	48–64
35	8–10	5/1	48–60
40	8–12	3/1	32–48
50	12	1.75/1	33

range of oxygen flow rates and is independent of the size of the tidal volume and the minute volume of ventilation. This is particularly important in patients with chronic obstructive pulmonary disease and alveolar hypoventilation, who tend to hypoventilate progressively as the arterial oxygen tension is increased.

NEBULIZER

Greater humidifying and warming of inspired air are required in patients in whom the normal heating and humidifying mechanisms of the upper respiratory tract are bypassed by a tracheostomy or endotracheal tube.

Large amounts of humidification can be achieved with a nebulizer (Fig. 7-7), a device that produces a suspension of fine water droplets. Basically, a nebulizer is made up of an inlet tube, an attached perpendicular draw tube partly submerged under water, and a baffle. Oxygen passes through the narrow inlet tube at a high flow rate, causing the pressure at the end of the draw tube to fall below atmospheric pressure, according to Venturi's principle. Consequent to the pressure drop within the draw tube, water moves up the tube into the stream of gas and is propelled against the baffle, where the liquid is broken up into a suspension of fine drops, generally ranging in size from 0.5 to 5.0 microns.

The oxygen leaving the nebulizer may be fully saturated at ambient temperature, but the water in the nebulizer must be heated to ensure full humidification at body temperature. By incorporating a heater into the nebulizer, the water can be heated to a level about 10° to 15°C greater than body temperature to compensate for temperature loss as the gas passes along the tubing to the patient (tubing 3–5 ft in length with ¾ in. inside diameter).

When inspired gas is heated and humidified by means of a nebulizer, water loss from the airways can be completely eliminated.

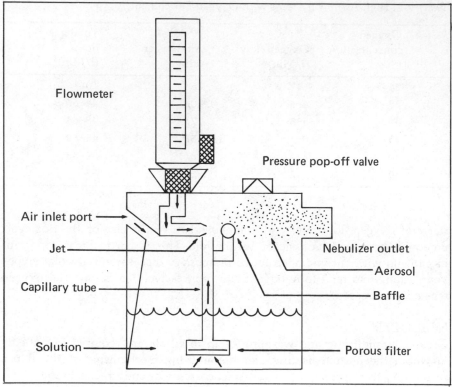

Flowmeter

Pressure pop-off valve

Air inlet port

Jet

Nebulizer outlet

Aerosol

Capillary tube

Baffle

Solution

Porous filter

FIGURE 7-7. Diagram of mechanical nebulizer.

DEVICES FOR THE DELIVERY OF HIGHLY HUMIDIFIED GAS MIXTURES

Warmed and highly humidified gas mixtures must be provided to patients with tracheostomies and endotracheal tubes in order to avoid drying out the tracheal and bronchial mucosa. Humidified gas mixtures may also be administered to patients following extubation and to patients with thick tracheobronchial secretions.

Humidification is provided using a nebulizer. In patients with tracheostomies and endotracheal tubes, the nebulizer is also heated, although in individuals breathing through the mouth and nose, heating of the gas mixture may not be necessary. Some find the heated gas mixtures to be quite uncomfortable.

AEROSOL MASK

This device (Fig. 7-8) consists of a plastic mask with open side ports. The mask is connected to a large-bore delivery tube for the delivery of humidified gas.

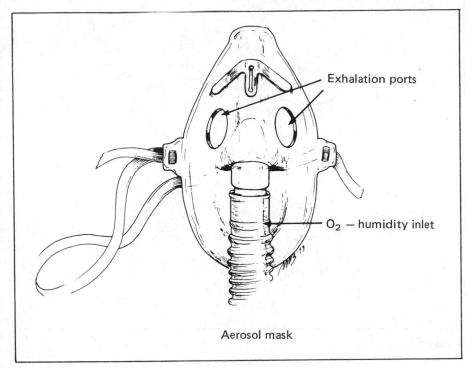

FIGURE 7-8. Aerosol mask.

FACE TENT

The face tent (Fig. 7-9) is a plastic wrap-around, half mask which is positioned around the chin and cheeks. The humidified oxygen mixture is delivered from the bottom of the unit while expired air passes out through the open upper portion.

TRACHEOSTOMY MASK

This consists of a soft, small plastic mask positioned over a tracheostomy tube or stoma (Fig. 7-10). The major disadvantage of this apparatus is that patients are able to breathe unheated and poorly humidified room air around the mask.

BRIGGS ADAPTOR

The use of a Briggs adaptor (Fig. 7-11) or *T* piece in patients with an endotracheal or tracheostomy tube ensures that inspired gas consists only of the prescribed heated oxygen mixture. This large bore *T*-shaped apparatus is fitted directly onto the endotracheal or tracheostomy tube. The heated, nebulized gas mixture is delivered through one limb of the *T*, while expired air leaves by the other. An additional length of tubing fitted to the expira-

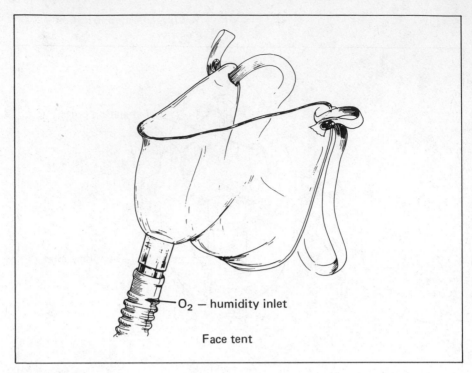

O₂ — humidity inlet

Face tent

FIGURE 7-9. Face tent.

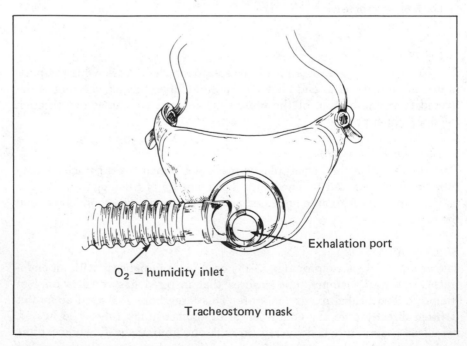

Exhalation port

O₂ — humidity inlet

Tracheostomy mask

FIGURE 7-10. Tracheostomy mask.

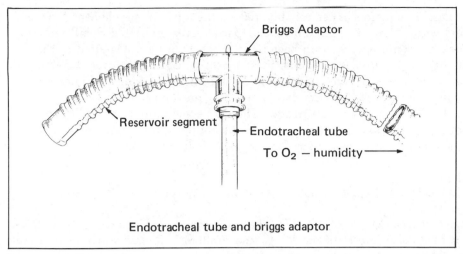

Endotracheal tube and briggs adaptor

FIGURE 7-11. Briggs adaptor.

tory limb of the *T*-piece can serve as a reservoir when the patient's inspiratory flow rate exceeds the rate of flow of the gas mixture from the source.

HAZARDS AND PRECAUTIONS

The administration of supplemental oxygen is clearly important in the management of patients with hypoxemia. However beneficial it may be, oxygen administration is not without risk and potential danger.

Inspired gas must be properly humidified in order to avoid drying of the mucous membranes of the tracheobronchial tree. Improper humidification, particularly with high-airflow systems and in patients with tracheostomies and endotracheal tubes, can interfere with mucociliary clearance mechanisms and result in drying and inspissation of airway secretions.

The prolonged administration of high concentrations of supplemental oxygen can produce toxic effects on the lung. The likelihood of this occurrence can be significantly reduced by ensuring that no more oxygen is given than that required to achieve a normal arterial PO_2.

In patients with chronic obstructive pulmonary disease, alveolar hypoventilation, and chronic arterial hypercapnia, respiratory responses to hypercapnia are blunted, and respiratory stimulation occurs solely as a consequence of hypoxemia. The administration of excessive supplemental oxygen in these patients has a tendency to promote increasing hypoventilation, with a resulting progressive rise in PCO_2. It is particularly important to maintain the inspired oxygen concentration at a fixed, unvarying level by using a high-airflow system with oxygen enrichment and to aim to achieve an arterial PO_2 no greater than 55 to 60 mm Hg.

All parts of any oxygen delivery system must be checked on a regular basis. Flowmeters must reliably reflect the rate of supplemental oxygen delivery. Water in humidifiers and particularly in heated nebulizers may become contaminated with bacteria that can then be transmitted to the patient's respiratory tract. Thus, these pieces of equipment must be changed at least daily. All connections must be tight, and kinking and obstructions due to condensation accumulation in tubing must be avoided.

Finally, oxygen administration should be monitored carefully. The use of arterial blood gases will provide substantial information for evaluating the effectiveness of supplemental oxygen administration.

REFERENCES

1. Egan, D. F. *Fundamentals of Respiratory Therapy* (3d ed.). St. Louis: Mosby, 1977.
2. McPherson, S. P. *Respiratory Therapy Equipment*. St. Louis: Mosby, 1977.
3. Shapiro, B. A., Harrison, R. A., and Walton, J. R. *Clinical Application of Blood Gases* (2d ed.). Chicago: Year Book, 1977.
4. Scacci, R. Air entrainment masks: jet mixing is how they work; the Bernoulli and Venturi principles are how they don't. *Respiratory Care* 24(10), Oct. 1979.

Hillary F. Don / # 8. VENTILATORY MANAGEMENT OF THE CRITICALLY ILL PATIENT

Failure of gas exchange in the lung is common in critically ill patients, regardless of the underlying primary disease. In a majority of patients, it is impossible to identify the exact reason for this failure.

Chief among the predisposing factors is sepsis, where the focus of infection is outside the lung. This is associated with increase in pulmonary vascular resistance, prevention of pulmonary arterial vasoconstriction in response to hypoxia, and pulmonary edema. Other diseases specifically associated with alteration in lung function are heart failure, uremia, hepatic cirrhosis, acute pancreatitis, nonthoracic trauma, central nervous system diseases, and thoracic cage abnormalities.

Instituted treatments may also have associated respiratory complications—for example, immunosuppressive medications predispose to pulmonary infection or may have a direct toxic effect. Finally, major additional factors are the patient's degree of mobility and level of mental obtundation. Inability to move freely or to sit up and decreased cough obviously predispose to the development of atelectasis and pulmonary infections. This is particularly true in the obese patient or the patient with preexisting pulmonary disease.

EARLY DETECTION OF RESPIRATORY DISEASE

The possibility of the development of lung dysfunction dictates the need for close monitoring to detect its onset. In conscious patients, this may be heralded by dyspnea, cough, or chest pain. Auscultation and percussion of the chest, recording of respiratory rate, assessment of intercostal retraction, and tracheal tug are also important.

Analysis of arterial blood for partial pressure of oxygen (PaO_2), carbon dioxide ($PaCO_2$), and pH is an essential guide in the critically ill patient. Arterial oxygen tension must be interpreted with three factors in mind: (1) the inspired oxygen fraction (FiO_2), (2) the alveolar oxygen tension (PAO_2), and (3) the alveolar to arterial oxygen tension gradient [$P(A-a)O_2$].

The FiO_2 is difficult to assess in the patient who is breathing through the normal airway. With a face mask, where delivered oxygen fraction is 1.0,

147

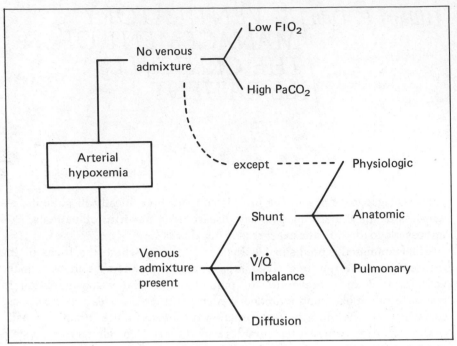

FIGURE 8-1. Causes of arterial hypoxemia. In the figure the dashed line indicates that even in healthy young subjects a small amount of venous admixture is present.

the inspired oxygen fraction may range from 0.3 to 0.6. It can be measured from gas samples taken from the posterior pharynx.

The alveolar oxygen tension is influenced by two major factors: the inspired oxygen tension and alveolar carbon dioxide tension. Alveolar carbon dioxide is approximately equal to $PaCO_2$, and alveolar oxygen tension can be assessed by a simplified form of the alveolar gas equation:

$$PaO_2 = PiO_2 - \frac{PaCO_2}{R}$$

where PiO_2 is inspired oxygen tension in dry gas and R is the respiratory quotient. Elevation of $PaCO_2$, for example, by drug overdose, will necessarily cause a decrease in alveolar, and therefore arterial PO_2, unless inspired oxygen tension is increased.

The alveolar-arterial oxygen tension gradient reflects the presence of venous admixture which is due to shunt, areas of low ventilation-perfusion ratio, or diffusion (Fig. 8-1). The normal or physiologic shunt increases with age, which is an important determinant of PaO_2, such that:

$PaO_2 = 100 - \frac{1}{2}$ (age in years) torr

If $P(A-a)O_2$ is increased due to lung disease, arterial oxygen tension may be normal due to compensatory hyperventilation with lowering of $PaCO_2$ and elevation of PaO_2. Hypocapnia is therefore a frequent early indicator of the development of lung disease.

The chest x-ray is useful but has limited value in the early detection of lung disease. In a reported series, 7 percent of patients with acute respiratory disease had a normal chest x-ray [15]. Equally, a supine portable anteroposterior chest x-ray taken at a small inspiratory lung volume in a normal subject may resemble that of a patient with pulmonary vascular congestion and atelectasis.

In certain disease states, interval measurement of simple pulmonary function may be an appropriate monitor—for example, in a patient with central neurological disease, peripheral neuropathy, myasthenia gravis, or cervical cord injury. The vital capacity measures the resultant difference between the amount of work that can be done, and that needed to be done to inflate and deflate the lungs. A reduction in vital capacity in a patient with myasthenia gravis indicates either a decline in muscle strength or the development of pulmonary parenchymal disease, such as atelectasis. Vital capacity is also impaired by changes in the patient's mental state and level of cooperation.

CAUSES OF RESPIRATORY DISEASE

When lung disease is detected, the cause can be placed in one or more of the following categories:

CENTRAL CONTROL OF RESPIRATION

In the absence of chronic lung disease or other factors such as narcotic administration, elevation of $PaCO_2$ is rarely seen in the early stages of acute lung disease. Hypercapnia therefore necessitates a search for a central or peripheral cause (Table 8-1). In the absence of dyspnea, tachypnea, or marked hypoxemia, central depression of ventilation is commonly found.

A common cause is the use of narcotic analgesia; depression of breathing for up to 6 days following administration of morphine in anuric patients and a similar effect in patients with normal renal and hepatic function after the use of methadone have been shown [32]. Naloxone, a narcotic antagonist with no inherent respiratory effect, can be relatively safely used to test for the presence of narcotics. Nausea, vomiting, and occasionally marked systemic hypertension may, however, follow the administration of naloxone.

Metabolic alkalosis, particularly if produced by nasogastric suctioning, frequently causes hypercapnia. Obesity may be associated with an elevation of $PaCO_2$. The term *Pickwickian* is used to describe the syndrome of obesity, hypercapnia, hypoxemia breathing room air, hypersomnolence, polycythemia, twitching, periodic breathing, and right ventricular hyper-

TABLE 8-1. Causes of Hypercapnia

A. Lung disease present
B. No lung disease present but
  1. Organic disease of the brain
  2. Functional depression
    a. Sleep
    b. Drugs
    c. Oxygen
    d. Metabolic alkalosis
  3. Ventilatory apparatus abnormal
    a. Muscle weakness
    b. Upper or lower airway obstruction
    c. Mechanical deformation of chest wall
  4. Obesity
  5. Ondine's curse
  6. Primary idiopathic hypoventilation

---

trophy or failure. This syndrome may be associated with upper airway obstruction. Different syndromes of sleep apnea have been described, where repeat episodes of apnea lasting more than 10 sec occur during sleep. This is frequently associated with upper airway obstruction, and is relieved by endotracheal intubation or tracheostomy. A central cause is also described.

Ondine's curse was first described in association with bilateral cervical cordotomy, with hypercapnia attributed to deafferentation of the reticular activating mechanism. It has been seen following unilateral cordotomy, cervical laminectomy, and surgery on the bodies of the upper cervical vertebrae, occurring from 1 hour to 1 week after surgery. It usually resolves spontaneously.

MECHANICAL FAILURE OF VENTILATORY PUMP
In the presence of normal central control of breathing, the ventilatory pump may fail owing to a defect of any link of the chain of spinal cord, anterior horn cell, peripheral nerve, neuromuscular junction, respiratory muscles, thoracic cage (including abdomen), and pleural space. The cause may be obvious—for example, trauma to the chest—or subtler, as in hypophosphatemia.

UPPER AIRWAY OBSTRUCTION
Obstruction of the airway is commonly due to collapse of the soft tissues of the upper airway—for example, the tongue or posterior pharynx. Infection of the tonsils, adenoids, or epiglottis may produce supraglottic obstruc-

tion. Acute pharyngotracheitis may cause subglottic obstruction. Spasm or edema of the vocal cords may occur due to reflex stimulation or in association with anaphylactic reaction. A variety of foreign bodies may obstruct the upper airway. The lumen of the airway may also be narrowed by tumor. Extrinsic compression of the airway may occur—for example, with hemorrhage, tumor, or subfascial air.

LOWER AIRWAY OBSTRUCTION
The causes of lower airway obstruction are similar to those that affect the upper airway. Edema, secretions, or spasm of bronchiolar smooth muscle are additional causes of lower airway obstruction.

LUNG DISEASE
Acute disease involving the lung parenchyma predominantly causes hypoxemia rather than hypercapnia; in the early stages, hypocapnia is usual. The following types of lung disease can be identified, although considerable overlap exists.

INFECTION
In the critically ill patient, defense mechanisms are impaired, and uncommon agents may infect the lung. Additionally, the use of immunosuppressive medications may lead to the development of opportunistic infections with unusual bacteria, fungi, viruses, mycoplasma, rickettsiae, and the protozoan *Pneumocystis carinii*. The last organism has been shown to be common [37], but the spectrum of causative organisms is ever-increasing [31]. Examination of the sputum by stain and culture is mandatory, but the diagnosis is frequently elusive. For example, daily acid-fast stain may not uncover mycobacteria, and diagnosis may be established only by biopsy of bone marrow.

Fiberoptic instrumentation has made bronchoscopy relatively easy and safe, even for critically ill patients on mechanical ventilation [35]. Transtracheal aspiration may be helpful [8], but this procedure is associated with cardiac arrhythmias and hypoxemia. Open lung biopsy, with endotracheal intubation and insertion of a chest tube, is perhaps the safest and most fruitful technique for diagnosis of pulmonary infection in the critically ill patient [25, 34].

HIGH PRESSURE PULMONARY EDEMA
In high pressure pulmonary edema, pulmonary extravascular lung water is increased due to an elevation in left atrial pressure. This, in turn, may be due to cardiac arrhythmia, mitral or aortic valvular disease, cardiomyopathy, myocardial ischemia, pericardial tamponade, left atrial myxoma, and expanded intravascular volume.

Suggested by physical examination, the diagnosis is established securely only by measurement of left atrial pressure. Although occasionally directly measured by means of a left atrial catheter inserted during cardiac surgery, left atrial pressure is usually assessed by balloon occlusion of a branch of a pulmonary artery using a flotation catheter. The consequent occlusion, or wedge pressure (PCWP) is elevated if it exceeds 15 torr. Interpretation of the wedge pressure is confused by changes in pleural pressure. During spontaneous breathing PCWP should be measured at the end of exhalation, but may be artificially elevated in the presence of increased expiratory resistance, since pleural pressure remains positive to maintain expiratory gas flow. Positive end-expiratory pressure during mechanical ventilation will also elevate pleural pressure, usually by about one-third to one-quarter of the applied pressure. In these circumstances, an elevated PCWP may be misinterpreted as indicating increased cardiac filling when the reverse may be true [26]. Careful insertion and maintenance of pulmonary artery catheters are essential, since pulmonary complications, such as infarction or pulmonary arterial rupture, have been associated with their use [16].

Low Pressure Pulmonary Edema

Low pressure pulmonary edema is diagnosed if arterial blood gas tensions and chest x-ray film suggest pulmonary edema, but PCWP is normal or low. Newer methods of measurement of extravascular lung water—for example, by double indicators—are becoming helpful in establishing the diagnosis [21].

The causes of this type of edema fall into five categories: (1) circulating toxins (e.g., severe burns, sepsis, acute pancreatitis), (2) hypoproteinemia, (3) damage through the airway (e.g., smoke inhalation, aspiration of gastric contents), (4) neurogenic, and (5) antigen-antibody reaction.

An increase in lung water is a thread running through the pathologic diagnosis in many cases of acute respiratory failure [4]. The title Adult Respiratory Distress Syndrome (ARDS) has been applied to the syndrome of the acute onset of dyspnea, tachypnea, severe hypoxemia, small functional residual capacity, reduced lung compliance, and bilateral infiltrate on chest x-ray. At postmortem, each lung may be increased to 200 to 300 percent of normal lung weight. The syndrome is established only when specific causes of this clinical picture (e.g., infection) are excluded. The causes of ARDS are obscure, but may represent an intravascular microaggregation [5] or central neurogenic [30] etiology.

Pulmonary Embolism by Blood Clot

The accurate diagnosis of pulmonary embolism is important because the treatment results in a significant decrease in mortality; equally, the danger of bleeding from the use of heparin requires that it not be wrongly diagnosed.

Pulmonary embolism can present one of four overlapping clinical pictures [11]: (1) dyspnea with normal chest x-ray; (2) pulmonary infarction with chest pain, dyspnea, and hemoptysis; (3) acute cor pulmonale, with elevation of pulmonary arterial and right atrial pressures when more than 60 percent of the pulmonary vasculature is obstructed (shock may predominate); and (4) unexplained increase in prior left ventricular failure.

The symptoms in one report [3] included chest pain in 88 percent, dyspnea in 84 percent, cough in 53 percent, and hemoptysis in 30 percent of patients with documented pulmonary embolism. The associated clinical signs were a respiratory rate above 16 per minute in 92 percent, rales in 58 percent, pulse rate above 100 per minute in 44 percent, and temperature above 37.8°C in 43 percent of patients. Predisposing factors included current venous disease, immobilization, congestive heart disease, chronic lung disease, a history of a recent surgical procedure, obesity, diabetes mellitus, hypertension, and malignant neoplasm.

Although combined ventilation and perfusion scans are a useful screening test, the definitive diagnosis of pulmonary embolism is made only by pulmonary angiogram.

FAT EMBOLISM

The triad of neurologic dysfunction, respiratory insufficiency, and petechiae which follows trauma, particularly involving long-bone fractures, is imperfectly understood. This syndrome of fat embolism is also found in association with drug overdosage, severe infection, diabetes mellitus, and burns. The diagnosis is supported by the finding of fat globules in the retina and the urine. Stained neutral fat droplets may be identified in rapidly frozen clotted blood [24].

AMNIOTIC-FLUID EMBOLISM

The diagnosis of amniotic-fluid embolism is usually based on presumptive evidence. However, a smear of aspirated right heart blood may reveal lanugo and fetal squamae, confirming the diagnosis of amniotic-fluid embolism.

ASPIRATION OF GASTRIC CONTENTS

There is no discrete clinical picture of aspiration. Acute asphyxia may occur due to obstruction of the larynx or trachea with gastric contents. Obstruction of lobar or segmental airways may result in localized collapse. The syndrome of aspiration of acid gastric secretions (pH < 2.4) is associated with the development of pulmonary edema.

The diagnosis of aspiration is usually based on the clinical history, but may occur silently in the elderly, the sick, or the obtunded patient.

The use of corticosteroids and antibiotics has been advocated, but there is no evidence of a decrease in morbidity when these are employed following aspiration.

PULMONARY HEMORRHAGE

Pulmonary hemorrhage is usually, but not always, accompanied by hemoptysis. The causes include (1) bleeding diathesis, (2) acute infection, (3) tumor, (4) trauma, (5) cardiac disease, (6) thromboembolic disease, (7) idiopathic pulmonary hemosiderosis, (8) pulmonary-renal syndrome (e.g., Goodpasture's syndrome), (9) aspiration of foreign body, and (10) chronic lung disease.

Disseminated intravascular coagulation (DIC) is among the causes of bleeding diathesis. DIC is associated with disseminated cancer, localized ischemia, hypoxia, childbirth, acute infections, burns, trauma, and cardiopulmonary bypass.

DISEASE DUE TO IMMUNOLOGIC
REACTION IN THE LUNG

The acute onset of pulmonary infiltrates on chest x-ray film, dyspnea, fever, and eosinophilia can occur as a hypersensitivity reaction to drugs (Table 8-2) and industrial and animal exposures (Table 8-3). Hypersensitivity reactions may also occur with radiation. Some drugs may cause a dose-related toxicity that is not a hypersensitivity reaction; these include bleomycin and cyclophosphamide. Obviously, it is important to identify the

TABLE 8-2. Drugs Associated with Pulmonary Infiltrates

WITH EOSINOPHILIA

Aminosalicylic acid	Isoniazid
Aspirin	Mephenesin carbamate
Carbamazepine	Nitrofurantoin
Chlorpropamide	Penicillin
Cromolyn sodium	Pituitary snuff
Furazolidone	Sulfonamides
Imipramine	

WITHOUT EOSINOPHILIA

Amitriptyline	Methotrexate
Azathioprine	Narcotics (heroin, methadone)
Cyclophosphamide	Paraquat
Erythromycin	Pentolinium
Hexamethonium	Dextran 40
Hydrochlorothiazide	Blood transfusions
Indomethacin	Ethchlorvynol
Phenylbutazone	Busulfan
Procarbazine	Mecamylamine
Propoxyphene	

TABLE 8-3. Vegetable and Animal Products Associated with Hypersensitivity Pneumonitis

Disease	Source
VEGETABLE PRODUCTS	
Farmer's lung	Moldy hay
Bagassosis	Moldy pressed sugarcane
Sequoiosis	Contaminated wood dust
Humidifier lung	Contaminated home humidifier
Tobacco grower's lung	Tobacco plants
Grain measurer's lung	Cereal grains
Mushroom worker's disease	Moldy compost
Byssinosis	Cotton
ANIMAL PRODUCTS	
Pigeon breeder's disease	Pigeon droppings
Duck fever	Bird feathers

Source: From M. Lopez and J. Salvaggio, Hypersensitivity pneumonitis: Current concepts of etiology and pathogenesis. *Ann. Rev. Med.* 27:453, 1976.

presence of a drug, animal, or vegetable effect on the lung, since withdrawal of the cause will usually resolve the problem.

Other causes of immunologic pulmonary disorders associated with vasculitis include serum sickness, glomerulonephritis, periarteritis nodosa, and systemic lupus erythematosus.

MANAGEMENT OF RESPIRATORY DISEASE

The foregoing discussion indicates a variety of causes for acute respiratory disease, with varying degrees of difficulty in establishing a precise diagnosis. Even when the diagnosis is established, effective therapy may not exist. In a majority of patients, respiratory care is solely supportive—sustaining life while the body itself, or instituted treatment, can repair the damage of the disease process. The manipulation of these supportive modalities to minimize overall toxicity lies at the heart of respiratory care.

OXYGEN ADMINISTRATION

The first indication for increasing inspired oxygen fraction is to maintain a life-supporting PaO_2. The level of PaO_2 below which the function of the body is threatened is approximately 40 torr. In order to provide a safety margin in the event of sudden further deterioration, it is probably safer to maintain a level greater than 60 torr, unless there is a relative contraindication, such as chronic lung disease. Correction of low PaO_2 will also reverse pulmonary vasoconstriction.

The second indication is where a higher than normal PaO_2 is necessary.

In the presence of myocardial ischemia, increased FIO_2 has been shown to reduce infarct size in dogs [29]. It is possible that wound healing is hastened.

Finally, an augmented FIO_2 is indicated as a preventative measure against the development of hypoxemia, for example, in the postoperative period.

HAZARDS OF OXYGEN
The hazards of oxygen are:

1. Combustion.
2. Suppression of respiratory drive, particularly in patients with chronic lung disease, asthma, obesity, kyphoscoliosis, metabolic alkalosis, and central nervous system disease and in the presence of respiratory depressant drugs.
3. Infection owing to a contaminated delivery system.
4. Mechanical failure, providing the patient with either too little or too much oxygen.
5. Drying effect if the gas is not adequately humidified.
6. Retrolental fibroplasia. Although primarily a disease of the premature infant, this entity has been claimed to occur in adults.
7. Lung oxygen toxicity. Scant data are available on the effect of high inspired-oxygen tensions on human diseased lungs, and results from animal experiments require careful interpretation. Oxygen toxicity is modified by species variations, administered drugs, increased resistance of diseased lungs, and attenuation of toxicity by slow increase in FIO_2 up to 1.0. Consequently, the time-dose relationship of oxygen toxicity in the diseased human lung is not known. Life-threatening hypoxemia should not be tolerated because of the fear of oxygen toxicity. In the adult, it is probable that 100 percent oxygen can be tolerated by the sick lung for at least 36 hours. An FIO_2 below 0.6 is probably safe for more prolonged (2–3 wk) periods.
8. Atelectasis owing to the greater solubility of oxygen compared with nitrogen. Studies of this effect have shown conflicting data. Results of the effect of 100 percent inspired oxygen show that the production of trapped gas or loss of functional residual capacity is no greater compared with that at FIO_2 0.3 [13]. Studies on the acute effect of breathing FIO_2 1.0 have demonstrated both an increase and a decrease in venous admixture, depending on the initial shunt [33]. The changes in shunt could be attributed to alterations in the distribution of pulmonary perfusion.

METHODS OF DELIVERY OF OXYGEN

NASAL PRONGS. The advantages of nasal prongs are that they are well tolerated by patients and can be worn while eating. They also provide a low, controlled inspired oxygen fraction, and can be used in addition to a face mask to increase FIO_2 further.

Inspired oxygen fractions from 0.22 to approximately 0.35 can be provided by varying the delivered oxygen flow from 0.25 to 6 liters per minute. Higher flows dry the nasal mucosa, producing discomfort and nasal hemorrhage. Nasal prongs can be used whether the patient breathes through the nose or the mouth.

VENTURI MASK. Venturi masks produce high flow of gas at a known constant oxygen concentration. A flow of 4 to 8 liters per minute enters the device through a narrow orifice. Lateral negative pressure so produced entrains room air. The usual delivered oxygen concentrations are 0.4, 0.35, 0.28, or 0.24. The volumes of air entrained for each liter flow of oxygen are 3, 5, 10, or 20 liters, respectively. Additional humidity can be added by a collar attached around the entrainment ports.

AEROSOL MASK OR FACE TENT. Wide-bore tubing connecting the mask or face tent to a nebulizer allows delivery of humidity and an increased FiO_2. The usual delivered inspired oxygen fraction (FdO_2) is 0.21, 0.4, 0.7, and 1.0. The use of an oxygen-air mixing device to supply the nebulizer gas flow enables any FdO_2 from 0.21 to 1.0 to be delivered.

In the absence of a reservoir of gas, inspired oxygen will be less than FdO_2 whenever the patient's inspiratory flow rate exceeds the flow rate of the delivered gas. An FiO_2 greater than 0.7 is rarely achieved with an aerosol mask delivering an oxygen fraction of 1.0. The difference between FdO_2 and FiO_2 must be taken into account when assessing the severity of defect in gas exchange. If necessary, FiO_2 can be measured by aspirating a gas sample from the oropharynx.

PARTIAL REBREATHING MASK. Narrow-bore tubing connects the partial rebreathing mask to an oxygen flowmeter. The system is designed so that the first portion of the exhaled tidal volume, which is similar to delivered oxygen and carbon dioxide tensions, enters a plastic, collapsible reservoir, to be rebreathed with the next inhalation. It is not designed to rebreathe carbon dioxide. Inspired oxygen fractions of 0.8 may be achieved.

HUMIDITY

In patients breathing through an endotracheal tube, the presence of moist inspired gas is essential to prevent the accumulation of dry secretions, with the danger of airway obstruction. Whether added humidity aids pulmonary toilet by liquefying secretions is disputed. Although few data support its use, it is frequent clinical experience that patients will produce more secretions when given added moisture by the airway. Water can be added either as vapor or as particles. Nebulized water may irritate the airway, provoking bronchospasm. Other hazards are the spread of infection, overheating the inspired gas, and adding excessive water, particularly if an ultrasonic nebulizer is used in children.

PULMONARY PHYSIOTHERAPY

Breathing exercises, postural drainage, percussion, and vibration should be used to provide better expansion of the lungs, improving the mobilization of secretions and creating more effective cough. The effectiveness of physiotherapy in the resolution of pneumonia has been challenged, however [18].

Nasotracheal suctioning may be indicated to stimulate a cough and to aid pulmonary toilet. This mode of therapy is associated with arterial desaturation during the procedure and may provoke cardiac arrhythmia, nasal hemorrhage, or vomiting, with the danger of aspiration.

INTERMITTENT POSITIVE PRESSURE BREATHING (IPPB)

Well established by custom, IPPB is less well documented in its value to prevent or treat lung disease [18]. The objective of the treatment is to increase lung volume during inhalation, opening otherwise closed airways, reexpanding collapsed parts of the lung, and aiding pulmonary toilet. IPPB is helpful if vital capacity is less than 20 ml/kg body weight, when abdominal or thoracic pain limits the willingness of the patient to inhale deeply, or where the patient is fatigued.

An absolute contraindication to the use of IPPB is the presence of pneumothorax without a chest tube in place. Complications of IPPB include insufflation of gas into the gastrointestinal tract, lung disruption, and hyperventilation with hypoxemia when IPPB is stopped.

The procedure of IPPB must be performed with clear objectives and with stated mechanisms for recognizing the achievement of these goals.

INCENTIVE SPIROMETRY

The encouragement of deep inhalation by the use of an incentive spirometer is indicated when vital capacity is greater than 20 ml/kg body weight and the patient's motivation and level of cooperation are judged adequate.

ENDOTRACHEAL INTUBATION

The first indication for endotracheal intubation is to allow positive pressure ventilation. Mechanical ventilation using an iron lung, cuirass or "rain coat" ventilator, or a rocking bed does not require the presence of an endotracheal tube. These types of ventilators are unsatisfactory for acute lung disease, in which positive pressure ventilation is used, necessitating the insertion of an endotracheal tube.

Other indications for endotracheal intubation are to maintain a patent airway, to protect the airway from aspiration, and to facilitate pulmonary toilet. Finally, an endotracheal tube may be used to guarantee an FiO_2 or to apply continuous pressure during exhalation.

DESIRABLE FEATURES OF AN ENDOTRACHEAL TUBE

The tube should be of clear, plastic material, certified for tissue compatibility by animal implantation tests. The material must not irritate mucous membranes and should be smooth and sufficiently flexible to conform to the patient's anatomy. However, the tube should not kink at small radius or flatten due to the pressure of the cuff or the walls of the upper airway.

A radiopaque marker must be present at the distal end of the tube. A side hole (Murphy tip) should also be present.

The cuff should be firmly bonded to the tube and should have a high residual volume with high compliance when inflated.

HAZARDS OF ENDOTRACHEAL INTUBATION

The substitution of an artificial airway for the patient's own is a potentially lethal alteration. The complications of endotracheal intubation include:

1. At the time of insertion, hypoxemia, reflex cardiac arrhythmia, and vomiting with possible aspiration may occur. Trauma to the mucosa or hemorrhage may be caused by the nasal route.
2. The endotracheal tube will introduce infection and break the continuity of the patient's natural lung clearance mechanisms.
3. The tube may be incorrectly placed into the esophagus or a main-stem bronchus. There has been at least one report of a patient swallowing an endotracheal tube. A tracheostomy tube may be accidentally placed in the subcutaneous tissues of the neck.
4. The endotracheal tube may become obstructed by kinking, by an overinflated cuff compressing the tube or evaginating over the end of the tube, or by materials such as blood clot or secretions within the lumen.
5. Erosion of the trachea may occur, with development of a tracheo-mediastinal or -esophageal fistula. Tracheotomy, in particular, may cause erosion of the innominate artery.
6. Following removal of a translaryngeal tube, laryngeal problems such as airway obstruction or hoarseness may occur for a variable length of time. Stenosis of the trachea may also be found

CHOICE OF ROUTE OF TRACHEAL INTUBATION

Three routes are available: nasotracheal, orotracheal, or tracheotomy. The initial route of tracheal intubation in the critically ill patient should be through the nose. The advantages of this technique are that it can usually be inserted during maintained spontaneous breathing without many drugs, it is easy to secure once inserted, and it is more comfortable for the patient than the oral route. The disadvantage of this approach is that the oral route accommodates a shorter tube of wider diameter. A nasal tube can also cause nasal hemorrhage and can be obstructed by pressure from the walls of the nasal passages. Maxillary sinusitis is also more commonly associated with nasotracheal intubation.

Tracheostomy is employed initially only if intubation through the nose or mouth is impossible. The decision to perform tracheostomy in a patient with an existing oral or nasal tube is made to increase the patient's comfort, to allow easier mobilization, to allow short periods of talking if possible, and to permit easier swallowing of food.

The disadvantages of tracheostomy include trauma and hemorrhage at the time of tracheotomy. Pulmonary infection has been shown to be increased, as compared with nasal intubation, in children with burns. Following extubation, tracheal stenosis is much more common following tracheostomy and may approach 30 percent of patients, compared with probably less than 5 percent by the translaryngeal route.

PROCEDURE FOR NASOTRACHEAL INTUBATION

The procedure for nasotracheal intubation must be meticulously planned and prepared. The patient is informed of what is to be done and is connected to a cardiac monitor. The following drugs and equipment must be at the bedside: atropine (0.4 mg); succinylcholine (100 mg); suction apparatus; a hand-ventilating device with appropriate face mask and oxygen supply; endotracheal tubes of the selected size and one size smaller; laryngoscope and blade; Magill forceps; and oral airway.

The nasal mucosa is sprayed with cocaine (4%) to produce topical anesthesia and to shrink the mucosa. The lubricated endotracheal tube is inserted into the nostril and advanced slowly and firmly. Through a feeding tube inserted to the distal end of the endotracheal tube, 1% lidocaine (maximum 10 ml) is injected in front of the tube. The tube is advanced, using audible or visible (by water condensation) guides, through the larynx. The tube is secured, and its position relative to the nares is noted. Auscultation of the chest checks the position of the tube. A chest x-ray is mandatory, however, since auscultation is an unreliable guide.

The equipment and preparation are similar for oral intubation. Topical anesthesia (1% lidocaine) is applied to the tongue, epiglottis, and larynx with direct laryngoscopy before tracheal intubation.

Safeguarding the position and patency of the endotracheal tube is a high priority. The endotracheal tube is anchored by adhesive tape passed around the patient's neck. The distance from the end of the endotracheal tube to the lip or nose is measured and recorded every 2 hours. Warmed humidified gases are always used, to prevent accumulation and drying of secretions within the lumen of the tube.

The endotracheal tube is not changed unless a mechanical defect develops, such as a leak in the cuff.

The cuff is inflated just enough to prevent a leak during positive pressure inflation. The necessary volume is recorded every 8 hours. A hand-ventilating device and an endotracheal tube one size smaller than in use are kept at the bedside.

REMOVAL OF THE ENDOTRACHEAL TUBE

The first criterion for extubation is that the indication for intubation has been corrected. Second, the patient should be conscious and want the tube removed. Coma or an obtunded mental state do not indicate that extubation is impossible, however. In this situation, the ability of the patient to protect the airway can be assessed by whether the patient (1) coughs when a catheter is inserted through the endotracheal tube, (2) gags when the pharynx is stimulated with a tongue depressor, (3) swallows water poured into mouth, and (4) has good tone in the muscles of the jaw.

Extubation of the trachea must be carefully planned, and all the equipment for reintubation must be instantly available. The patient is informed of the plan and should be connected to an electrocardiac monitor. Secretions are aspirated from the trachea and mouth. The patient's lungs are hyperinflated with 100 percent oxygen, and the endotracheal tube cuff is deflated. The tube is withdrawn during exhalation from full inhalation. The patient is provided with humidified oxygen. Laryngeal obstruction is treated with added airway humidity and racemic epinephrine (Vaponefrin) by inhalation. It is our custom to provide the latter drug to all infants and babies immediately following extubation.

MECHANICAL VENTILATION
Mechanical ventilation by intermittent positive pressure (IPPV) will, first, circulate gas in and out of the lungs, increasing minute ventilation (unless dead space increases equally). Hence, impaired minute ventilation can be corrected, and the work normally performed by the patient for spontaneous breathing is taken over by the machine. Second, mechanical ventilation will inflate and deflate the lungs and may increase mean lung volume, improving the distribution of ventilation, decreasing shunt, and allowing clearance of the lung through previously closed airways. Third, mechanical ventilation increases alveolar pressure, which in itself might have an effect on ventilatory and hemodynamic function.

INDICATIONS FOR MECHANICAL VENTILATION

FAILURE TO MAINTAIN ADEQUATE ALVEOLAR VENTILATION. Treatable causes of hypercapnia must first be sought, such as narcotic overdosage or partial neuromuscular block due to the residual effect of relaxant drugs. An elevated $PaCO_2$ is not in itself an absolute indication for IPPV. Some patients with chronic lung disease will tolerate $PaCO_2$ greater than 80 torr, remaining awake, comfortable, and cooperative. An arterial pH below 7.1 is usually considered an indication for mechanical ventilation, however.

RAISED INTRACRANIAL PRESSURE. Deliberate hypocapnia by IPPV may be indicated to lower raised intracranial pressure, in diseases such as Reye's syndrome.

HYPOXEMIA. Perhaps the most frequent indication for mechanical ventilation, a life-threatening PaO_2 will usually be increased by IPPV, probably because the increased tidal volume, provided mechanically, increases mean lung volume. The specific criteria indicating the need for mechanical ventilation are approximately: (1) PaO_2 less than 40 torr on maximal inspired oxygen; (2) the level of obtundation of the patient's mental state, with loss of ability to cooperate with treatments and to communicate changes in symptoms; (3) rapidly progressing respiratory disease; (4) the appearance of intercostal indrawing and tracheal tug during inhalation, indicating increased work of breathing; and (5) elevation of $PaCO_2$.

PROPHYLAXIS. In certain situations, such as in the face of hemodynamic instability, mechanical ventilation may be instituted to maintain ventilatory function.

INCREASED WORK OF BREATHING. Increased work of breathing is disputed as an indication for IPPV, since simply diverting cardiac output from the respiratory muscles to more useful areas of the body is not of great advantage. The increase in the work of breathing might indicate impending respiratory failure.

POSSIBLE THERAPEUTIC BENEFITS. Positive pressure ventilation stabilizes the chest wall of patients with injuries such as flail chest. It may be true that pulmonary collapse and atelectasis benefit physically from IPPV, and normal lung function is more quickly restored.

Choice of Mechanical Ventilator

Since the fundamental purpose of a ventilator is to deliver tidal volume, the cycling from inhalation to exhalation is most effectively achieved by a volume or time mechanism. Pressure-cycled ventilators will fail to deliver the desired tidal volume in the face of changes in airway resistance or lung and chest wall compliance. However, when using uncuffed endotracheal tubes, which will have a variable leak, pressure-cycled ventilators may produce a more constant tidal volume.

The onset of the inspiratory phase should be time-cycled, with the option of the assist mode by pressure. Synchronization of the intermittent mandatory ventilation (IMV) with the patient's spontaneous breath is desirable.

The power source of most ventilators is electricity, but the availability of a ventilator driven by compressed gas allows safer transportation of patients on mechanical ventilation.

The ventilator should be as small and simple as is compatible with its function. It must be reliable and be backed by enthusiastic service. It should have a range of tidal volume suitable for the patient population, from 100 to 2,500 ml. The ventilatory frequency should be from 1 to 60 breaths per minute. The inspiratory flow should be adjustable from 5 to 100 liters/min. An infinitely adjustable range of FiO_2 from 0.21 to 1.0 must be standard. The peak airway pressure must be at least 150 cm H_2O, and the output of the ventilator should vary little at that back pressure.

The patient circuit must be easily sterilizable. Bacterial filters in both the inspiratory and expiratory limbs of the circuit may be advantageous.

A parallel breathing circuit with the same FIO_2 as the ventilator must be available, to allow spontaneous breathing between the mechanical breaths. In the event of failure of the gas supply to the ventilator, a fail-safe device must allow spontaneous breathing of room air. Positive end-expiratory pressure up to 50 cm H_2O should be incorporated.

Alarms for high and low pressure limits, FIO_2, tidal volume, and inspired gas temperature are mandatory.

Hazards of Mechanical Ventilation

MECHANICAL PROBLEMS. Possibly the greatest hazard with the ventilator and its circuitry is mechanical. In one report, mechanical problems occurred in 103 out of 354 separate episodes of acute respiratory failure [47].

DEPRESSION OF CARDIAC OUTPUT. During a spontaneous inhalation, pleural pressure becomes increasingly negative. Positive pressure, on the other hand, creates increasingly less negative pleural pressure and, in fact, may become positive. This increase in pleural pressure increases intrathoracic venous pressure—which, in turn, may reduce venous return, with consequent depression of cardiac output. Pulmonary vascular resistance is also increased.

The rise in venous pressure may increase venous bleeding and elevate the back pressure in the hepatic and renal circulations.

Although cardiac filling may be decreased due to the more positive pleural pressure, it is possible that left ventricular function is aided, since the positive pressure tends to reduce afterload [6].

INTRACRANIAL PRESSURE. Intracranial pressure may increase, but since cerebrospinal fluid pressure rises equally in the closed cranium, the distending pressure across the brain does not increase. The rise in pressure can be minimized in the head-up position. A decrease in cardiac output or systemic mean pressure may cause marked cerebral vasodilatation and an increase in intracranial pressure.

LUNG DISRUPTION. Lung disruption is not infrequent. Air can track from the bronchovascular bundle to the mediastinum, the subcutaneous tissues, and the pleural space. It may track into the retroperitoneum and may appear as free air in the peritoneal space, mimicking the x-ray film of a ruptured abdominal viscus. The incidence of pneumothorax varies from less than 1 to 15 percent [10]. Finally, lung disruption may result in vascular air embolism.

HYPERINFLATION. Hyperinflation, either of both lungs or of discrete areas in the lungs, may occur. This is presumably due to a ball-valve effect aggravated by limited expiratory time.

FLUID RETENTION. Increases in both antidiuretic hormone [23] and aldosterone [9] have been attributed to positive pressure ventilation.

ADJUSTMENT OF TIDAL VOLUME

Tidal volume (VT) is initially set at approximately 15 ml/kg. A high tidal volume is chosen to maintain mean lung volume and to prevent the development of atelectasis. Total compliance has been shown to increase as tidal volume is changed from 5 to 15 ml/kg [42].

Reduction of the size of tidal volume is indicated in patients with chronic lung disease or asthma, where hyperinflation and a markedly positive pleural pressure may develop. An alteration in tidal volume of as little as 100 to 200 ml may lower pleural pressure and increase cardiac output. Gas trapping is detected if initially exhaled volume is less than the volume inhaled. With a time- or volume-cycled ventilator this is seen as an initial stepwise increase in exhaled volume. Prolonged exhalation following disconnection of the ventilator provides further evidence.

A reduction in tidal volume is also indicated in the presence of low chest wall compliance. In this circumstance, the positive pleural pressure on inhalation is accentuated, impeding venous return.

ADJUSTMENT OF INSPIRATORY WAVEFORM

Alterations of inspiratory waveform have been shown to alter the distribution of ventilation and gas exchange [2, 12]. The clinical significance of these findings is not clear. The inspired flow rate should be adjusted to maintain a ratio of inhalation to exhalation of approximately 1 : 1.5.

ADJUSTMENT OF VENTILATOR FREQUENCY

With the tidal volume fixed, the frequency of ventilation is adjusted to maintain $PaCO_2$ at approximately 35 torr. The initial frequency in an adult is between 8 and 14 breaths per minute, and in a child, between 15 and 40 breaths per minute.

Hypocapnia has the hazards of potentiating the effects of digitalis, reducing cerebral blood flow, increasing airway resistance, shifting the oxygen dissociation curve to the left, and causing retention of hydrogen ion by the kidney. If $PaCO_2$ is too low in the presence of satisfactory VT and frequency, mechanical dead space should be inserted in the ventilator circuit.

A modifying factor in the choice of frequency is patient acceptance. Dyspnea can sometimes be relieved by instituting a rapid respiratory rate. A slow rate might be used in the presence of increased airway resistance, promoting more even distribution of inhaled gas. A guide to the appropriate length of exhalation is to ensure that prior to inhalation the exhalation is complete, by watching the spirometer on the ventilator.

Two major modifications of ventilator frequency have been introduced. The first of these is mechanical ventilation at high frequency. At frequencies above 60 per minute, respiration–synchronous variation in blood pressure and flow are eliminated, and spontaneous ventilation usually ceases. This technique appears to simplify the process of mechanical ventilation [38].

The second method is a departure from conventional therapy: the production of high frequency (15 Hz) sine wave oscillation at the airway, with no bulk flow of gas. Elimination of carbon dioxide is normal in human subjects using this technique [7]. The value of this method awaits further clinical trial.

INSPIRED OXYGEN FRACTION
Optimal FIO_2 is that which maintains PaO_2 at approximately 60 torr. Comparative dangers of different levels of FIO_2 are unknown in sick human lungs, but oxygen toxicity is unlikely when FIO_2 is less than 0.6.

SEDATION
Adequate medication should be given to provide sedation or narcosis. Spontaneous ventilation need not be totally suppressed, since the negative pleural pressure may aid venous return.

The choice of drugs is arbitrary. Intravenous morphine sulfate (0.05 mg/kg) or diazepam (0.05 mg/kg) is usually satisfactory. In babies and infants, the use of drugs which block the neuromuscular junction, such as pancuronium (0.05 mg/kg), may be necessary. These drugs have a prolonged effect in patients with impaired hepatic or renal function. The actions of pancuronium and morphine are pharmacologically reversible, however.

DISCONTINUATION OF MECHANICAL VENTILATION
ASSESSMENT OF PATIENT. The criteria for commencing weaning from mechanical ventilation, and its successful accomplishment, have received considerable attention in the literature. No simple factors or combination of factors has been shown to cover all aspects of weaning from mechanical ventilation. The rigid application of criteria based on physiological variables is inappropriate, and probably leads to unnecessarily prolonged periods of mechanical ventilation. Although the management of weaning is tailored to an individual patient, the following represent guidelines.

The initiating indication for mechanical ventilation has been eliminated or modified.

The defect of gas exchange is assessed. In acute lung disease, the usual defect is an increase in venous admixture, $\dot{Q}s/\dot{Q}T$, and in the alveolar to arterial oxygen tension difference, $P(A-a)O_2$. The latter can be assessed by the measurement of PaO_2 following the inhalation of 100 percent oxygen for 30 minutes. A $P(A-a)O_2$ of greater than 300 torr is said to be associated with difficulty in weaning. However, in a series of 80 patients, we found that successful weaning occurred with $P(A-a)O_2$ as large as 580 mm Hg. In fact, improvement in gas exchange may follow tracheal extubation because the patient's own cough may provide a more effective pulmonary toilet.

Assessment of $P(A-a)O_2$ on FiO_2 1.0 is helpful because it presents a wider range of PaO_2 and can be accurately assessed throughout a patient's period of deterioration and recovery. Gas exchange can also be assessed by measuring the $P(A-a)O_2$ on lower inspired oxygen fractions. Data using these values have not been well documented, however. The advantage of using an FiO_2 less than 1.0 is the possibility that 100 percent oxygen itself causes an increase in the shunt [33]. The defect so produced is probably caused by the effect of high FiO_2 on the distribution of pulmonary blood flow.

The use of the alveolar-arterial oxygen tension difference does not take into account the influence of alterations of mixed venous oxygen content on gas exchange. A more accurate assessment is to calculate venous admixture using measured mixed venous oxygen content. This equation takes into account alterations in cardiac output, oxygen consumption, hemoglobin, and the position of the oxygen dissociation curve.

The measurement of $P(A-a)O_2$ or venous admixture on FiO_2 1.0 is normally of limited value in patients with acute exacerbations of chronic lung disease, unless they have superimposed acute pneumonia or pulmonary edema.

The functional state of the lung also can be assessed by measurement of total effective compliance, which should be greater than 20 ml/cm H_2O; by measurement of the fraction of tidal volume (V_T) that is dead space (V_D), which should be less than 0.6; and by measurement of functional residual capacity, which should be greater than 50 percent of predicted.

The mechanical properties of the lung and chest wall are assessed by first temporarily disconnecting the patient from the ventilator and observing a maximum inhalation. There should be no intercostal indrawing or tracheal tug. The presence of either of these motions indicates partial neuromuscular blockade, upper or lower airway obstruction, or decreased lung compliance. Conversely, the movement of the abdomen should be noted. Failure of the abdomen to move outward during the maximum inhalation suggests unilateral or bilateral diaphragmatic paralysis, which may follow surgery in the chest or neck.

Measured vital capacity should exceed 12 ml/kg, but values as low as 5 ml/kg are compatible with successful weaning. Maximum inspiratory pressure generated against a closed glottis should be less negative than −20 cm H_2O.

The control of breathing is assessed first by the mental state of the patient. If the patient is alert and responding appropriately, mechanical ventilation is discontinued and spontaneous breathing of 100 percent oxygen allowed. A lower FiO_2 should be used when indicated—for example, in the presence of chronic lung disease. An obtunded mental state does not contraindicate a trial of spontaneous breathing, but the effect of any depressant drugs such as narcotics previously administered should be reversed, and the trial should be approached more cautiously.

After 30 minutes of spontaneous breathing, $PaCO_2$ should be less than 46 torr. If it is higher, but less than 50 torr, the trial of spontaneous breathing is continued; if $PaCO_2$ remains below 50 torr, extubation can be considered. If it is higher than 50 torr, and pH is below 7.30, further attempts at weaning should be modified (see below) or postponed.

If judged not to need mechanical ventilation, the patient is then assessed for the need for endotracheal intubation, and the endotracheal tube removed if appropriate.

TECHNIQUES OF WEANING. Should the patient be judged as still needing mechanical ventilation, the following options for management are available:

Mechanical ventilation is continued with testing at intervals of 12 to 24 hours to judge possibility of weaning. If the factor influencing the decision is the amount of venous admixture, positive end-expiratory pressure (PEEP) may be added to the exhalation limb of the ventilator.

Alternately, using a parallel breathing circuit, the frequency of mechanical breaths is decreased at appropriate intervals. This technique of intermittent mandatory ventilation (IMV) allows maintenance of safe arterial gas tensions, while providing an increasing amount of spontaneous breathing. The rate of reduction of mechanical breaths is judged from alterations in arterial blood gas tensions, and the symptoms and signs of respiratory distress shown by the patient. This technique is safe, easy to institute, and minimizes mechanical accident and bacterial contamination.

Some patients, particularly those with chronic lung disease, may not tolerate IMV, but accept increasing periods of spontaneous breathing interrupted by short periods of mechanical ventilation.

Spontaneous breathing with continuous positive airway pressure (CPAP) may improve the ability of patients with chronic lung disease to breathe spontaneously, presumably by maintaining airway patency during exhalation. Caution should be exercised, since the resultant increase in functional residual capacity may impede both hemodynamic and ventilatory function.

CONTINUOUS POSITIVE PRESSURE

Although the technique of PEEP breathing dates back more than 40 years, its modern application to the management of acute respiratory disease was described by Ashbaugh et al. in 1969 [1]. The interpretation of the acronyms used to identify different forms of positive pressure breathing varies: for the present description, CPPV (continuous positive pressure ventilation) indicates the maintenance of positive airway pressure throughout the inspiratory and expiratory phases of a mechanical tidal volume; CPPB (continuous positive pressure breathing) refers to spontaneous breathing with positive pressure maintained during both inhalation and exhalation; and EPPB (expiratory positive pressure breathing) indicates spontaneous breathing with positive pressure at the airway only during the expiratory phase.

Positive pressure breathing has its effect presumably by increasing functional residual capacity (FRC), which, in turn, improves the matching of ventilation to perfusion and allows better lung clearance.

Although disputed, the positive pressure itself may improve hemodynamic function through reduction of preload [19] and possibly by reducing left ventricular afterload [6].

INDICATIONS FOR PEEP
There are five basic categories of indications for the use of PEEP:

1. When arterial oxygen tension is sufficiently low to threaten life in the face of maximum inspired oxygen fraction. PaO_2 less than 40 torr, with hemodynamic instability, altered mental state, and the development of metabolic acidosis fulfill this criterion. The addition of PEEP usually increases PaO_2.
2. When life-supporting PaO_2 is maintained only by a potentially life-threatening FIO_2. The use of PEEP will allow reduction of FIO_2, creating an optimal environment for recovery of pulmonary function. However, the relative toxicity of high inspired oxygen fraction compared with PEEP can not be defined. The judgment, for example, that PEEP of 10 cm H_2O plus FIO_2 0.4 is less harmful to the lung than PEEP of 0 cm H_2O plus FIO_2 0.8 is arbitrary.
3. When it is thought that PEEP will actually treat the lung disease. That the actual disease process, and not merely the arterial blood gas, is improved by the use of PEEP is disputed [39]. Although it is probably true that atelectasis or collapse may resolve more quickly when treated with PEEP, it is well established that lung water is not diminished by the addition of PEEP to ventilatory support.
4. Some patients, particularly those with chronic lung disease, may benefit from PEEP during spontaneous breathing. This is presumably the equivalent of breathing with pursed lips. This technique may be assessed in patients who experience difficulty while weaning from mechanical ventilation.
5. Prophylaxis. The newborn, with a chest wall of high compliance, maintains FRC by creating increased laryngeal resistance to flow during exhalation. This is prevented by the presence of an endotracheal tube, and PEEP is indicated in this age group to maintain lung volume and prevent atelectasis. The adult does not usually have a dynamically determined FRC, and the prophylactic use of PEEP is not indicated. The age at which PEEP is no longer advantageous is not identified, but is possibly at approximately 3 years.

HAZARDS OF PEEP
A false sense of security may be the first hazard of PEEP. An improvement in gas exchange following institution of PEEP may not reflect any real change in the amount of lung disease, but might reduce the impetus for a careful and thorough search for the underlying cause of the pulmonary deficit.

An increased risk of lung disruption may be produced. It has been claimed, however, that the risk of pneumothorax even with high levels is no greater than if mechanical ventilation were used without PEEP [22].

Cardiac output may be unchanged or may change in either direction. The determinants of the effect of PEEP on hemodynamics include the blood volume and cardiac status of the patient. In the presence of hypovolemia, cardiac output may fall. If congestive heart failure is present, cardiac output may increase [19]. The benefits of PEEP to hemodynamics in this situation can be through preload or afterload reduction [6]. The presence of decreased lung compliance will attenuate the transmission of positive alveolar pressure to the pleural space [26]. Usually, about one-third of PEEP applied at the airway is seen as changes in pleural pressure. Oxygen transport may decrease, therefore, since an increase in arterial oxygen content may be offset by a decline in cardiac output.

Systemic blood pressure may decrease but is frequently maintained, even in the presence of a fall in cardiac output. Left atrial diastolic pressure, assessed by measurement of pulmonary capillary wedge pressure, is almost invariably elevated when PEEP is added. This does not imply that atrial filling pressure has increased, because pleural pressure may rise equally. In this situation, a decrease in filling pressure may accompany a rise in pulmonary capillary wedge pressure (PCWP). Simultaneous measurements of esophageal pressure allow interpretation of changes in filling pressures [26], but the clinical utility of this technique, in the supine position, has not been established. The changes in right atrial pressures are similar to those in the left atrium.

Pulmonary vascular resistance (PVR) may increase with PEEP, although this is not an universal finding [40]. The change in PVR may cause a decrease in cardiac output. In the presence of an unequal distribution of lung disease, the increase in resistance will be felt primarily by well-ventilated lung, causing a shift of pulmonary blood flow away from well-ventilated areas. In the presence of an intracardiac defect, right to left shunt may be increased. The increase in intrathoracic venous pressure caused by the rise in pleural pressure may increase intracranial pressure, but this is not invariable; an increase in intracranial pressure is most in evidence if mean systemic pressure falls.

The amount of venous admixture is usually diminished by PEEP. The dead space fraction (VD) of tidal volume is usually not altered.

Renal function may be impaired, but probably only as a function of a decrease in cardiac output. Intravenous dopamine will usually correct this alteration in kidney perfusion [20]. An increase in antidiuretic hormone and aldosterone may also occur during therapy with PEEP.

The work of breathing is usually not increased during CPPB, so long as the pressure at the airway does not decrease significantly during spontaneous inhalation. If airway pressure decreases to ambient pressure during inhalation (EPPB), the work of breathing increases linearly to as much as 100 percent with the application of 20 cm H_2O of end-expiratory pressure [17].

Functional residual capacity usually increases with PEEP, although this may not be seen with EPPB [17]. In the adult, the change in FRC is in the order of 100 ml/cm H_2O PEEP. The increase in FRC may be deleterious in a patient with preexisting elevation of FRC or total lung capacity, such as is found in pulmonary emphysema.

CORRECT LEVELS OF PEEP

Although many authors have struggled for the answer, identification of the optimum level of PEEP is not possible at present. It has been stated that the optimum level of PEEP to be applied is that which reduces the amount of venous admixture to near normal [22, 44]. A second published view is that the objective is to maximize oxygen transport [41]. None of these reports, however, has asked the key question, What level of PEEP is associated with the greatest return of pulmonary function in the shortest time and with the least toxicity to the organ systems of the body? The published reports quoted above are concerned with the immediate, short-term effects of PEEP. Looking at the long-term goals of PEEP, one nonrandomized, retrospective study concluded that an improvement in PaO_2 and decrease in shunt fraction following a trial of PEEP portends a favorable outcome, but its continued use appears to prolong life for a few days without affecting hospital mortality [39].

The answer to the question of how PEEP should be optimally used is therefore not apparent at this time. The effect of PEEP must be studied in each individual patient. One system is to apply PEEP when PaO_2 on FiO_2 1.0 has declined to approximately 100 torr. PEEP is added to increase PaO_2 to over 150 torr, allowing FiO_2 to be reduced to 0.8, with PaO_2 at least 60 torr. Acutely deleterious hemodynamic effects of PEEP are sought by measurement of mixed venous oxygen content ($C\bar{v}O_2$), metabolic acidosis, urine output, blood pressure, electrocardiogram, and cardiac output. Central nervous system changes are also assessed. Infusion of fluid or vasopressor agents such as dopamine may be used to offset these harmful effects of PEEP. The trend of the amount of pulmonary disease is then assessed at intervals of 2 to 24 hours, depending on the severity of the defect. If oxygen exchange is further impaired after the initial improvement, PEEP is increased in steps of 3 or 5 cm H_2O to reverse this downward trend. An inspired oxygen of less than 0.6 should be achieved within 24 hours if possible.

TECHNIQUE OF APPLYING PEEP

PEEP should be achieved with a threshold, rather than a flow, resistor. The safest apparatus is probably wide-bore expiratory tubing inserted to the appropriate depth under water. Continuous positive pressure breathing compared to CPPV has a less depressant effect on cardiac output and a lower tendency to produce lung disruption; it has been used successfully in adult patients both with [44] and without endotracheal intubation. We have found the latter technique too difficult and traumatic to the patient's face, for prolonged use.

CPPB is probably preferable to EPPB because the hemodynamic and ventilatory advantages are approximately the same, but the work of breathing is less.

The use of the assist mode for cycling the beginning of a mechanical breath has been shown to have no advantage over controlled ventilation [14].

A continuous negative chest wall pressure has been used in both children and adults as an alternative to PEEP. A sustained improvement in oxygenation has been reported without need for endotracheal intubation [36].

Reducing PEEP
Premature withdrawal of PEEP in the face of an improvement in gas exchange may result in significant deterioration in oxygenation, which may persist even if the previous level of PEEP is restored [28]. It is our practice not to reduce PEEP within 12 hours of establishing a given level. Control measurement of venous admixture or $P(A-a)O_2$ on FiO_2 1.0 are then made before and after reduction in PEEP by 3 to 5 cm H_2O. If a significant increase in $P(A-a)O_2$ (i.e., more than 75 torr) occurs, the initial PEEP is restored.

EXTRACORPOREAL MEMBRANE OXYGENATION
Prolonged extracorporeal membrane oxygenation (ECMO) has been shown to be practical, and survivors are reported [46].

Indications for ECMO
The first indication for ECMO is that a life-supporting PaO_2 cannot be maintained with maximum FiO_2, mechanical ventilation, and PEEP. If a potentially reversible lung condition is suspected, ECMO will usually support life, so that perhaps time, and instituted treatments, will effect recovery.

The second indication is that the alternative support modalities (FiO_2, positive airway pressure) can be reduced to a less toxic range. This supposes that the added burden of ECMO is less harmful than the decreased morbidity of the reduced alternative supports.

The third indication is the conjecture that venoarterial bypass will reduce pulmonary blood flow, and pulmonary capillary and venous pressures, hence improving pulmonary edema and facilitating recovery of normal lung structure. Certainly, ECMO will allow safe therapeutic regimens, such as suctioning or lung lavage, should these not be possible without the support.

METHOD OF ECMO

Three routes are available. The most popular is venoarterial bypass, which may improve oxygenation by three mechanisms: mixing in the aorta of oxygenator's effluent blood with left ventricular output; increased mixed venous oxygen content; and decrease of venous admixture in the lung by vascular decompression. If the improvement in PaO_2 is only by the first of these mechanisms, coronary arterial blood may be significantly desaturated.

The second route is venovenous bypass, which has the disadvantage that the oxygenator may scavenge already oxygenated blood. Additionally, the technique does not provide hemodynamic support, and pulmonary blood flow is not reduced.

The third route is arteriovenous, which has the features of maintaining the load on the left ventricle, and providing limited oxygenator flow.

MANAGEMENT DURING ECMO

The major hazards of ECMO are sepsis and hemorrhage due to the need to heparinize the patient's blood. During bypass, the FiO_2 is reduced to a point compatible with safe oxygenation. An FiO_2 of 0.6 should be achieved. The tidal volume and PEEP should probably be reduced. If, however, PEEP is in fact therapeutic in keeping airways open and allowing lung clearance, the latter move might be detrimental.

FUTURE OF ECMO

The published results of a multi-center randomized study conducted by the NIH showed that mortality of patients supported with or without ECMO was 9.5 and 8.3 percent, respectively [46]. The failure of ECMO to improve survival indicates either that the support was instituted too late, that it is equally as damaging to the lung as FiO_2 and PEEP, or that without more specific treatment, merely buying time with support does not improve salvageability. It was of interest that the incidence of pneumothorax was 45 percent in both groups of patients. There was also no difference in the incidence of septicemia. In the management of the patients described in the report, and with the criteria for selection described, it was concluded that the use of ECMO is not justified until a therapy to produce or accelerate lung healing is available.

LUNG TRANSPLANTATION

Lung transplantation has been attempted, with a maximum survival time of 10 months [43, 45]. The first indication for transplantation is in the presence of permanent destruction of lung tissue to an extent incompatible with a reasonable quality of life. It has also been thought of as providing a temporary, safer, long-term "membrane oxygenator."

OTHER ASPECTS OF MANAGEMENT

BRONCHODILATING AGENTS

Detected increased lower airways resistance should be treated with bronchodilating agents. Initial route of choice is by inhalation, where lower blood levels are associated with similar therapeutic levels in the smooth muscles of the airway. The more specific beta-2 stimulants such as terbutaline (0.75–1.5 mg every 3 hr) should be used. Inhaled atropine (0.05–0.1 mg/kg) can also be used should the beta-2 agents fail to improve airway resistance. Where lung clearance is a problem, inhaled bronchodilators should be used even in the absence of expiratory rhonchi.

Persistent bronchospasm should be treated with the continuous infusion of aminophylline. A bolus of 5 mg/kg is initially given over 20 minutes. A continuous infusion of 0.7 mg/kg/hr is then maintained. Drug dosage is reduced by one-third in the presence of hepatic disease, congestive heart failure, and metabolic acidosis. Dosage is regulated by measuring plasma theophylline levels, which should be between 10 and 20 μg/ml.

CORTICOSTEROIDS

Corticosteroids are of undoubted value in the management of severe asthma. Their use in other forms of acute pulmonary disease is more questionable. Two functions are attributed to the use of steroids: restoring or maintaining capillary wall integrity when this defect is thought to cause pulmonary edema, and aiding regeneration of surfactant production.

NUTRITION

Nutrition is obviously essential in the care of critically ill patients. Nasogastric tube feeding or hyperalimentation should be started as appropriate within 3 days of hospitalization if possible.

MONITORING THE PROGRESS OF PULMONARY DISEASE

The essential question of whether the lung disease is improving, getting worse, or staying the same must be assessed at appropriate intervals. If the answer is that improvement is occurring, it is probably as well to leave the ventilatory support basically unchanged. Should the status be deteriorating, the support or treatment modalities must be reexamined and altered. It is essential, for any particular patient, to examine at intervals the factors that follow changes in pathophysiology most accurately. The more precise the understanding of the abnormalities, the fewer guides are necessary.

The following parameters may be helpful:

1. Simple pulmonary function tests. Measurement of vital capacity (3–5 consecutive measurements) should be made at intervals in cases of muscle weakness (e.g., myasthenia gravis). Forced expiratory volume in 1 sec should also be measured in patients with chronic lung disease or asthma.

2. Alveolar-arterial oxygen tension difference while breathing FiO_2 1.0 for 20 minutes can be measured at intervals. The advantages of this measurement are: it measures the predominant defect in most patients with acute lung disease; it can be used throughout the patient's course and provides easy comparisons of day-to-day alterations; groups of patients can also be easily compared; the range of PaO_2 measured (50–650 torr) allows for accurate interpretation of changes; and the FiO_2 is usually accurate. The disadvantage is that an FiO_2 1.0 may increase the shunt. This is usually immediately reversible on resuming a lower FiO_2 and is probably due to an alteration in pulmonary perfusion distribution [33].

3. Measurement of venous admixture by the application of the equation:

$$\frac{\dot{Q}s}{\dot{Q}t} = \frac{CcO_2 - CaO_2}{CcO_2 - C\bar{v}O_2}$$

where Qs is that portion of total cardiac output ($\dot{Q}t$) which perfuses unventilated alveoli, CcO_2 is capillary oxygen content, CaO_2 is arterial oxygen content, and $C\bar{v}O_2$ is mixed venous oxygen content.

The use of this equation takes account of alterations in $C\bar{v}O_2$, which will increase $P(A\text{-}a)O_2$ in the presence of a constant amount of venous admixture. Mixed venous oxygen content is reduced by a decrease in cardiac output (oxygen consumption being unchanged) or hemoglobin or by a shift of the oxygen dissociation curve to the right.

4. Quantification of the fraction of a tidal breath that is dead space. Measurement of the carbon dioxide tension of mixed expired gas ($P\bar{E}CO_2$) and the tension in arterial blood ($PaCO_2$) allows calculation of dead space ventilation by the Enghoff modification of the Bohr equation:

$$\frac{V_D}{V_T} = \frac{PaCO_2 - P\bar{E}CO_2}{PaCO_2}$$

5. Total effective compliance (tidal volume divided by [peak inspiratory pressure minus positive end-expiratory pressure]) is a guide to improvement of acute lung disease, where either lung compliance is reduced or airway resistance is increased.

6. Functional residual capacity is markedly reduced to less than 50 percent of predicted in many forms of acute lung disease.

7. Pulmonary artery pressure and calculated pulmonary vascular resistance are usually increased in the presence of acute parenchymal lung disease. The increase in PVR may become a primary cause of the development of systemic hypoperfusion as the pulmonary disease progresses. The use of vasodilating agents (e.g., sodium nitroprusside) to increase pulmonary blood flow is monitored by measurement of pulmonary artery pressure and cardiac output.

8. Measurement of PCWP is an essential guide to the management of high-pressure pulmonary edema. It is also of value in the management of fluid balance in acute lung disease where maintenance of low PCWP (< 10 torr) may minimize low pressure edema.

REFERENCES

1. Ashbaugh, D. G., et al. Continuous positive-pressure breathing (CPPB) in adult respiratory distress syndrome. *J. Thorac. Cardiovasc. Surg.* 57:31, 1969.

2. Baker, A. B., et al. Effects of varying inspiratory flow waveform and time in intermittent positive pressure ventilation. II. Various physiological variables. *Br. J. Anaesth.* 49:1221, 1977.

3. Bell, W. R., et al. The clinical features of submassive and massive pulmonary emboli. *Am. J. Med.* 62:355, 1977.

4. Bergofsky, E. H. Pulmonary insufficiency after non-thoracic trauma: Shock lung. *Am. J. Med. Sci.* 264:93, 1972.

5. Berman, I. R. Intravascular microaggregation and the respiratory distress syndromes. *Pediatr. Clin. North Am.* 22:275, 1975.

6. Buda, A. J., et al. Effect of intrathoracic pressure on left ventricular performance. *N. Engl. J. Med.* 301:453, 1979.

7. Butler, W. J., et al. Ventilation of humans by high frequency oscillation. *Anesthesiology* (Suppl.) 51:S368, 1979.

8. Chamarro, H., et al. Tracheobronchial studies via transcricothyroid approach. *J.A.M.A.* 227:631, 1974.

9. Cox, J. R., et al. The effect of positive pressure respiration on urinary aldosterone excretion. *Clin. Sci.* 24:1, 1963.

10. Cullen, D. J., and Caldera, D. L. The incidence of ventilator-induced pulmonary barotrauma in critically ill patients. *Anesthesiology* 50:185, 1979.

11. Dalen, J. E. (ed.). *Pulmonary Embolism.* New York: Medcom, 1972.

12. Dammann, J. F., et al. Optimal flow pattern for mechanical ventilation of the lungs. 2. The effect of a sine versus square wave flow pattern with and without an end-expiratory pause on patients. *Crit. Care Med.* 6:293, 1978.

13. Don, H. F., et al. The effect of anesthesia and 100% oxygen on the functional residual capacity of the lungs. *Anesthesiology* 32:521, 1970.

14. Downs, J. B., et al. Comparison of assisted and controlled mechanical ventilation in anesthetized swine. *Crit. Care Med.* 7:5, 1979.

15. Dyck, D. R., et al. Acute respiratory distress in adults. *Radiology* 106:497, 1973.

16. Foote, G. A., et al. Pulmonary complications of the flow-directed balloon-tipped catheter. *N. Engl. J. Med.* 290:927, 1974.

17. Gherini, S., et al. Mechanical work on the lungs and work of breathing with positive end-expiratory pressure and continuous positive airway pressure. *Chest* 76:251, 1979.

18. Graham, W. G. B., and Bradley, D. A. Efficacy of chest physiotherapy and intermittent positive-pressure breathing in the resolution of pneumonia. *N. Engl. J. Med.* 299:624, 1978.

19. Greenbaum, D. M. Positive end-expiratory pressure, constant positive airway pressure, and cardiac performance. *Chest* 76:248, 1979.

20. Hemmer, M., and Suter, P. M. Treatment of cardiac and renal effects of PEEP with dopamine in patients with acute respiratory failure. *Anesthesiology* 50:399, 1979.

21. Hill, S. L., et al. Changes in lung water and capillary permeability following sepsis and fluid overload. *Crit. Care Med.* 7:137, 1979. (Abstract)

22. Kirby, R. R., et al. High level positive end expiratory pressure (PEEP) in acute respiratory insufficiency. *Chest* 67:156, 1975.

23. Kumar, A., et al. Inappropriate response to increased plasma ADH during mechanical ventilation in acute respiratory failure. *Anesthesiology* 40:215, 1974.

24. Lahiri, B., and ZuWallack, R. The early diagnosis and treatment of fat embolism syndrome: A preliminary report. *J. Trauma* 17:956, 1977.
25. Leight, G. S., Jr., et al. Open lung biopsy for the diagnosis of acute, diffuse pulmonary infiltrates in the immunosuppressed patient. *Chest* 73:477, 1978.
26. Loeber, N. V., and Don, H. F. Effect of lung, chest wall, and total static compliance on pleural pressure changes during mechanical ventilation with PEEP. In Abstracts of Scientific Papers, for the Annual Meeting of the American Society of Anesthesiologists, 1978. P. 449.
27. Lopez, M., and Salvaggio, J. Hypersensitivity pneumonitis: Current concepts of etiology and pathogenesis. *Ann. Rev. Med.* 27:453, 1976.
28. Luterman, A., et al. Withdrawal from positive end-expiratory pressure. *Surgery* 83:328, 1978.
29. Maroko, P. R., et al. Reduction of infarct size by oxygen inhalation following acute coronary occlusion. *Circulation* 52:360, 1975.
30. Moss, G., et al. The centrineurogenic etiology of the acute respiratory distress syndrome. *Am. J. Surg.* 126:37, 1973.
31. Myerowitz, R. L., et al. Opportunistic lung infection due to "Pittsburgh pneumonia agent." *N. Engl. J. Med.* 301:953, 1979.
32. Norris, J. V., and Don, H. F. Prolonged depression of respiratory rate following methadone analgesia. *Anesthesiology* 45:361, 1976.
33. Quan, S. F., et al. The effect of varying inspired oxygen concentrations on calculated intrapulmonary shunt. Abstracts of Scientific Papers for the Annual Meeting of the American Society of Anesthesiologists, 1978. P. 453.
34. Rossiter, S. J., et al. Open lung biopsy in the immunosuppressed patient. Is it really beneficial? *J. Thorac. Cardiovasc. Surg.* 77:338, 1979.
35. Sackner, M. A., et al. Applications of bronchofiberoscopy. *Chest* (Suppl.) 62:70S, 1972.
36. Sanyal, S. K., et al. Continuous negative chest-wall pressure therapy in management of severe hypoxemia due to aspiration pneumonitis: A case report. *Respir. Care* 24:1022, 1979.
37. Singer, C., et al. Diffuse pulmonary infiltrates in immunosuppressed patients. Prospective study of 80 cases. *Am. J. Med.* 66:110, 1979.
38. Sjöstrand, U. Pneumatic systems facilitating treatment of respiratory insufficiency with alternative use of IPPV/PEEP, HFPPV/PEEP, CPPB or CPAP. *Acta Anaesth. Scand.* (Suppl.) 64:123, 1977.
39. Springer, R. R., and Stevens, P. M. The influence of PEEP on survival of patients in respiratory failure. A retrospective analysis. *Am. J. Med.* 66:196, 1979.
40. Sturgeon, C. L., et al. PEEP and CPAP: Cardiopulmonary effects during spontaneous ventilation. *Anesth. Analg.* 56:633, 1977.
41. Suter, P. M., et al. Optimum end-expiratory airway pressure in patients with acute pulmonary failure. *N. Engl. J. Med.* 292:284, 1975.
42. Suter, P. M., et al. Effect of tidal volume and positive end-expiratory pressure on compliance during mechanical ventilation. *Chest* 73:158, 1978.
43. Veith, F. J., et al. Experience in clinical lung transplantation. *J.A.M.A.* 222:779, 1972.
44. Venus, B., et al. Treatment of the adult respiratory distress syndrome with continuous positive airway pressure. *Chest* 76:257, 1979.

45. Vermeire, P., et al. Respiratory function after lung homotransplantation with a ten-month survival in man. *Am. Rev. Respir. Dis.* 106:515, 1972.
46. Zapol, W. M., et al. Extracorporeal membrane oxygenation in severe acute respiratory failure. *J.A.M.A.* 242:2193, 1979.
47. Zwillich, C. W., et al. Complications of assisted ventilation. *Am. J. Med.* 57:161, 1974.

William J. Mandel / # 9. CARDIAC ARRHYTHMIAS

The management of arrhythmias plays a major role in the care of the critically ill patient, since the presence of even minor arrhythmias in this clinical setting may have profound negative hemodynamic effects. It is therefore essential to have accurate electrocardiogram (ECG) evaluation of all patients who are critically ill, preferably by continuous monitoring techniques. Adequate therapy for the arrhythmias encountered can be accomplished only by careful analysis of the ECG waveform. In many instances atrial activity cannot readily be recognized, necessitating the use of special surface lead positions (i.e., Lewis lead), esophageal leads, and/or intracardiac electrogram recordings.

A key part of the management of patients with arrhythmias is to recognize that extracardiac problems may be largely responsible for the basic arrhythmia encountered. Therefore, it is essential to recognize and correct alterations in acid-base balance, gas exchange, electrolyte disorders, hypotension, catecholamine excess, and hypermetabolic states such as hyperthyroidism.

ANTIARRHYTHMIC DRUG THERAPY

QUINIDINE

ELECTROPHYSIOLOGIC EFFECTS

Quinidine has a variety of electrophysiologic effects that are dependent on the particular cardiac tissue studied. Quinidine prolongs atrial refractoriness and depresses intraventricular conduction. In general, it shortens atrioventricular (AV) nodal conduction; the latter effect may be due to a direct or a vagolytic action of the drug.

HEMODYNAMIC EFFECTS

Quinidine is a negative inotropic agent and also causes peripheral vasodilation, possibly by adrenergic blocking action.

ABSORPTION AND METABOLIC FATE

Quinidine, the dextro-isomen of quinine, is almost completely absorbed by the gastrointestinal tract; the extent and rate are dependent on gastric acidity, gastrointestinal tract motility, and the amount of food in the gastrointestinal tract. The molecule is unchanged during absorption. Quinidine is highly protein-bound (approximately 80%), with a peak serum concentration being achieved between 1 and 2 hours. The heart has a high affinity for quinidine, and rapid binding occurs (less than 1 min). Skeletal muscle concentration appears to be only one-tenth that of ventricular muscle concentration, and the concentration in the ventricle is greater than that in the atrium. Quinidine's half-life is between 2 and 3 hours; 95 percent of the administered dose can be recovered in the urine as either quinidine or one of its metabolites. As yet, no significant data are available concerning the antiarrhythmic properties of the metabolites of quinidine.

Dosage, Route, and Serum Levels

In general, quinidine is administered by the oral route every 6 hours. However, occasional patients may require administration every 3 or 4 hours. The total daily dose required is 1.2 to 3.4 gm with a therapeutic serum level range of 2 to 6 mg/liter. The method of quinidine serum level determination may be important in evaluating the dosage. The protein precipitate method measures quinidine plus all metabolites, including water-soluble metabolites. The double-extraction technique measures only quinidine and its dihydroxyquinidine derivative. Stable serum levels during oral quinidine therapy are not observed for 2 to 3 days.

Toxicity

The most common side effect of quinidine therapy is gastrointestinal tract toxicity, usually manifested by nausea, vomiting, and diarrhea. These symptoms are rarely severe enough to warrant discontinuance of the drug. Another significant side effect is the development of cinchonism, which is characterized by tinnitus, visual difficulty, vertigo, and headache. Rarely, one may see thrombocytopenic purpura, exfoliative dermatitis, fever, and respiratory paralysis. In addition, quinidine syncope has been described, which appears to be related to the development of ventricular arrhythmias, presumably due to excessive dosage. Hypotension and diminished cardiac output may also occur because of quinidine's negative inotropic effects and may prove a significant problem in patients with borderline hemodynamic function. Finally, acceleration of the ventricular rate during atrial fibrillation or atrial flutter may occur because of potential vagolytic effects on AV nodal transmission. Quinidine administration in digitalized patients may result in significant elevation of the serum digitalis level and possible precipitation of digitalis intoxication.

Specific Indications

Oral quinidine therapy is useful for the treatment of both atrial and ventricular arrhythmias of all types. Furthermore, it may be used prophylactically following conversion to sinus rhythm from atrial fibrillation, as well as in the early stages of myocardial infarction. Also, it has been shown to have prophylactic benefits in the long-term management of patients with paroxysmal atrial tachycardia with or without Wolff-Parkinson-White syndrome.

AVAILABLE PREPARATIONS
Quinidine for oral administration is available as the sulfate in tablets of 200 or 300 mg, as the polygalacturonate (Cardioquin) in 275-mg tablets, as sustained-release quinidine gluconate (Quinaglute) in 330-mg tablets, or as sustained-release quinidine sulfate (Quinidex) in 300-mg tablets. The sustained-release or long-acting quinidine preparations have been stated to be effective over periods of 8 to 12 hours. However, relatively limited amounts of critical data analysis are available to substantiate these claims. The usual dose for quinidine gluconate in an average-sized patient with normal renal function is 660 mg every 8 hours. Quinidine gluconate is also available for parenteral use in 10-ml vials with 80 mg of quinidine per milliliter.

PROCAINAMIDE
ELECTROPHYSIOLOGIC EFFECTS
The electrophysiologic effects of procainamide are essentially identical with those of quinidine. Specifically, this drug prolongs the effective refractory period of the atrium and His-Purkinje system and abbreviates the effective refractory period of the AV node.

HEMODYNAMIC EFFECTS
Procainamide may significantly lower cardiac output and peripheral vascular resistance. Intravenous administration may also significantly depress glomerular filtration rate and effective renal plasma flow.

ABSORPTION AND METABOLIC FATE
The absorption of procainamide from the gastrointestinal tract is rapid, with the peak effect being seen in 1 to 1½ hours. This drug is sparingly protein-bound and is highly concentrated in cardiac muscle. Approximately 90 percent of the unchanged drug or its metabolites is excreted via the renal route. The half-life for procainamide is approximately 2 to 3 hours.

DOSAGE, ROUTE, AND SERUM LEVELS
Therapy with oral procainamide usually requires a total daily dose of 50 mg/kg given in divided doses every 3 hours. For a more rapid onset of action with oral therapy, it is suggested that a loading dose of 1 gm be given intramuscularly, eliminating the long equilibration that may be necessary by the oral route. Procainamide requires 1 to 2 days to establish a stable serum level when administered orally.

In contrast with quinidine, procainamide is frequently administered by intravenous injection and by chronic infusion. Intravenous administration may be carried out using a dose of 100 mg every 3 to 5 minutes until a total dose of at least 1 gm is given or the arrhythmia is terminated. The dose necessary for satisfactory results with constant infusion is 20 to 80 μg/kg/min with an expected plateau time of approximately 12 hours. Therapeutic serum levels are 4 to 8 mg/liter.

Toxicity

Procainamide may produce clinically significant ventricular arrhythmias that apparently are the result of excessive blood levels. Syncopal episodes, as reported with quinidine, may occur, presumably due to ventricular arrhythmias. In addition, significant depression of blood pressure and cardiac output may be seen. Agranulocytosis and transient psychoses may develop. Other side effects include anorexia, fever, drug rash, nausea, and vomiting. A lupuslike syndrome occurs in a relatively small percentage of patients, usually after at least 2 weeks of oral therapy. However, elevated antinuclear antibody titers will develop in 100 percent of patients after 12 months of oral therapy.

Specific Indications

Indications for procainamide are identical with those for quinidine therapy; these drugs have been found to be effective in a variety of atrial and ventricular arrhythmias.

Available Preparations

Procainamide is available in capsules of 250, 375, and 500 mg for oral administration. It is available as the hydrochloride for parenteral administration in 10-ml ampules containing 100 mg/ml. Procan SR is a new oral preparation of procainamide which enables the clinician to administer the drug every six hours. This preparation is available in 250 and 500 mg tablets.

LIDOCAINE

Electrophysiologic Effects

Lidocaine's electrophysiologic effects differ significantly from those of procainamide and quinidine. The drug has little effect on the sinus node, atrial muscle, or AV node but has a profound effect on the ventricular conduction system and ventricular muscle. It has been shown to shorten markedly the refractory period and action potential duration of both Purkinje fibers and ventricular muscle.

Hemodynamic Effects

No significant changes in cardiac output, left ventricular end-diastolic pressure, dp/dt, or stroke work are observed. Peripheral vascular resistance is variably affected.

ABSORPTION AND METABOLIC FATE

At present, lidocaine is available only for parenteral administration. Its half-life is short (108 min), requiring repeated administration of intravenous boluses or chronic constant infusion. Nevertheless, 6 to 10 hours are required before stable plateau levels are achieved with chronic infusion. The serum blood levels of lidocaine are influenced substantially by decrease in hepatic blood flow with resultant increases in expected serum levels; this is a particular problem in the setting of congestive heart failure or liver insufficiency. If it is deemed essential to increase the infusion rate of lidocaine in response to increasing ventricular arrhythmias, it would appear most prudent to administer sequential small (i.e., 25-mg) boluses at repeated 15-min intervals, in addition to increasing the infusion rate, until a new stable state is achieved. Lidocaine is effectively metabolized only by the liver, without any significant renal excretion; it is less than 10 percent bound to plasma proteins.

DOSAGE, ROUTE, AND SERUM LEVELS

In general, the drug is administered by an intravenous bolus of 1 mg/kg followed by continuous infusion. Lidocaine's effective plasma levels are 2 to 6 mg/liter, necessitating an infusion rate of 20 to 50 μg/kg/min. Lidocaine may also be given by intramuscular (deltoid) injection. Doses of 300 mg will maintain therapeutic serum levels for more than 1 hour.

TOXICITY

The toxic effects of lidocaine are usually restricted to central nervous system dysfunction. These effects in turn are directly related to the serum level of the drug, with toxic manifestations being seen only at serum levels above 7.5 mg/liter. These toxic manifestations range from drowsiness and confusion to respiratory arrest and convulsions.

SPECIFIC INDICATIONS

Lidocaine has been found most useful for the treatment of serious ventricular arrhythmias, usually in the setting of acute myocardial infarction. The drug appears to have no significant effectiveness in the treatment of atrial arrhythmias or AV block. However, in the setting of digitalis intoxication with prolonged AV conduction and ventricular arrhythmias, lidocaine appears to be of great clinical utility.

AVAILABLE PREPARATIONS

Lidocaine as the hydrochloride (without epinephrine) comes in single-dose and multidose ampules in concentrations of 1%, 4%, and 10% (10, 20, 40, and 100 mg/ml).

DIPHENYLHYDANTOIN SODIUM

ELECTROPHYSIOLOGIC EFFECTS

Diphenylhydantoin appears to be identical with lidocaine in its electrophysiologic effects. Specifically, it has limited effect on the sinus node or atrial musculature, abbreviates AV conduction, and markedly shortens the effective refractory period and action potential duration in Purkinje fibers and ventricular muscle.

HEMODYNAMIC EFFECTS

Diphenylhydantoin decreases myocardial contractility, increases coronary flow, increases coronary vascular resistance, and has a variable effect on peripheral resistance and left ventricular end-diastolic pressure.

ABSORPTION AND METABOLIC FATE

Diphenylhydantoin is absorbed slowly from the gastrointestinal tract and has a long half-life. The peak plasma level is achieved 6 to 12 hours after oral administration. Oral administration requires 6 to 7 days before a plateau is reached. The drug is approximately 50 percent bound by plasma protein and is excreted to a very limited extent by the renal route; its main metabolic pathway is that of the liver. Therefore, in patients with decreased hepatic perfusion, liver insufficiency, or both, elevated blood levels of this agent may be anticipated.

DOSAGE, ROUTE, AND SERUM LEVELS

Diphenylhydantoin may be administered orally, intramuscularly, or intravenously. Oral administration requires 300 to 600 mg/day administered in divided doses every 6 or 8 hours. A decreasing loading dose over the first 3 days of therapy may be clinically useful. Intravenous administration can be carried out by giving 100 mg every 3 to 5 minutes until a total dose of 600 mg is achieved or the arrhythmia is terminated. Effective serum levels are 10 to 18 mg/liter.

TOXICITY

Diphenylhydantoin produces central nervous system toxic manifestations, generally in direct relation to the amount of drug administered. These symptoms include tremors, ataxia, nystagmus, drowsiness, and confusion. In addition, with parenteral administration, asystole has been observed, but rarely. Further toxic manifestations include gum hypertrophy, megaloblastic anemia, pseudolymphoma, and drug interaction.

SPECIFIC INDICATIONS

Diphenylhydantoin appears to be useful in the treatment of ventricular arrhythmias with or without AV block in the setting of digitalis intoxication. Furthermore, it appears to be effective in the treatment of other types of ventricular arrhythmias. Parenteral administration is more successful than oral administration.

AVAILABLE PREPARATIONS
Capsules are available in 30- and 100-mg sizes. A suspension of 30 or 125 mg per 5 ml is also available. Parenteral preparations consist of 2- or 5-ml ampules (50 mg/ml) to be mixed just before use.

β-BLOCKING AGENTS
The only β-blocking agent presently available for use as an antiarrhythmic drug in the United States is propranolol. This drug is a competitive β-adrenergic blocking agent, which will inhibit myocardial response to catecholamines. Recently, metoprolol and nadolol cardioselective β-blocking agents have been released for use as an antihypertensive agent. These drugs may have special use in patients with asthma who have need for a β-blocker.

ELECTROPHYSIOLOGIC EFFECTS
Propranolol, in Purkinje fibers, decreases the rate of rise of the action potential upstroke and prolongs the refractory period and conduction time. It also shortens action potential duration. Studies in both experimental animals and man have determined that propranolol significantly prolongs the AV nodal conduction time without altering intraventricular conduction times.

A pronounced electrophysiologic alteration seen following propranolol administration is the decrease in spontaneous sinus node activity.

HEMODYNAMIC EFFECTS
Propranolol is a potent negative inotropic agent and so decreases the force of contraction. In addition, there is a decrease in both the velocity and the extent of fiber shortening following propranolol administration, as well as a drop in dp/dt and an elevation of left ventricular end-diastolic pressure. It also may decrease coronary flow and cause arteriolar constriction and venodilatation. Propranolol produces a decrease in adenyl cyclase activity in the myocardium.

In spite of its effect on the peripheral arterial system, propranolol, especially in hypertensive patients, may produce a significant hypotensive effect.

ABSORPTION AND METABOLIC FATE
Highly variable plasma levels of propranolol are obtained from different patients, suggesting marked variation in the rate of absorption from the gastrointestinal tract from patient to patient, or alterations in metabolism, or both. Peak absorption is 1½ to 2 hours after the oral dose in the fasting state and 2 to 4 hours if taken with a meal. The plasma half-life is 3.2 hours after oral administration; up to 90 percent of the drug is protein-

bound. The drug is extensively metabolized, with only minimal amounts excreted unchanged by the kidneys. The major site of metabolism appears to be the liver.

Dosage, Route, and Serum Levels

For the treatment of recurrent arrhythmias, oral administration of propranolol is usually begun with 5 to 10 mg every 6 hours. The dosage can be increased in a stepwise fashion to as much as 480 mg/day in extremely recalcitrant cases. During oral administration, a stable serum level is achieved in 1 to 2 days.

Propranolol can also be administered intravenously for the urgent treatment of arrhythmias. A dosage schedule should be at the rate of 1 mg intravenously every 1 to 3 minutes, for a total dose of up to 15 mg in recalcitrant cases.

Toxicity

The major toxic effect of propranolol is the development of sinus arrest or marked sinus bradycardia. Complete AV block may also be observed. These findings have generally been seen during intravenous administration at too rapid a rate and in too large a dose.

Hemodynamic side effects include a significant decrease in cardiac output and peripheral blood pressure. In addition, patients may manifest bronchospasm, gastrointestinal distress, or masked hypoglycemia.

Specific Indications

Propranolol's most potent clinical effect is the production of delay in AV nodal conduction. It is very effective for the rapid induction of partial AV nodal delay. It is most appropriately used clinically to slow the ventricular rate in atrial tachyarrhythmias, such as atrial fibrillation and atrial flutter and/or atrial tachycardia. Furthermore, it has been suggested to be of significant benefit for the elimination of arrhythmias due to reentry involving the AV nodal conducting system, such as those seen during episodes of paroxysmal atrial tachycardia. Oral administration has been helpful in the treatment of significant ventricular arrhythmias, especially those that are related to catecholamines, digitalis intoxication, or both.

Available Preparations

Propranolol is supplied in 10-, 20-, 40-, and 80-mg tablets and 1-mg vials for intravenous administration.

Additional β-Blocking Agents

At the present time, outside the continental United States, there are a variety of β-blocking agents available, having slightly different effects in terms of cardiac and extracardiac manifestations of β blockade as compared with propranolol. Clinical use of these drugs in this country awaits the results of further studies.

BRETYLIUM
Bretylium was recognized as a potent antiarrhythmic drug in 1965. Previously, the drug was used as an antihypertensive agent with modest clinical success.

ELECTROPHYSIOLOGIC EFFECTS
Bretylium has complex electrophysiologic effects based on its ability to cause, initially, catecholamine release. In Purkinje fibers, the drug prolongs action potential duration and refractory period, but it does not do this in atrial muscle. It also has been shown to have differential effects in infarcted myocardium. On rare occasions, this agent has been found to convert ventricular fibrillation. More commonly, it has been effective in preventing ventricular fibrillation.

HEMODYNAMIC EFFECTS
The hemodynamic effects of Bretylium are, in part, related to initial release and subsequent blockade of norepinephrine from adrenergic nerve endings.

In clinical use, Bretylium produces an initial mild increase and subsequent modest decrease in systemic pressure. No significant effects have been noted with regard to other parameters of ventricular function, i.e., wedge pressure, cardiac index, and stroke work index.

ABSORPTION AND METABOLIC FATE
Pharmacologic data are limited but in studies with intramuscular dosage the plasma half-life was between 3 and 10 hours. Approximately 80 percent of the drug was excreted in the urine. Suppression of the arrhythmia was not related to the plasma levels of the drug.

DOSAGE, ROUTE, AND SERUM LEVELS
Acute intravenous administration with Bretylium is in a 5- to 10-mg/kg dose given over at least 10 minutes. Maintenance dosage may be given by constant infusion at a dosage of 1–7 mg/min, with mandatory monitoring of blood pressure.

Intramuscular administration may also be utilized with a dosage of 5–10 mg/kg given every 6 hours. It has been recommended that the total 24-hour dosage not exceed 30 mg/kg.

Blood level determinations are not clinically available at this time. However, dosage should be reduced in significant renal insufficiency.

TOXICITY

Hypotension is a frequently observed effect. Nausea and vomiting are also commonly observed, especially if the dose is administered too rapidly. Ventricular arrhythmias may be enhanced in the early stages of administration. Bradycardia has been noted. Rarely, episodes of parotitis have been clinically recognized.

SPECIFIC INDICATIONS

Bretylium is specifically indicated for the treatment of intractable ventricular arrhythmias, especially recurrent ventricular fibrillation. Clinically, the drug has been used only in patients refractory to routine antiarrhythmic agents.

AVAILABLE PREPARATIONS

The drug is available presently only for parenteral use. A 10-ml ampule containing 500 mg is available. The drug should be diluted to a minimum of 50 ml of 5% D/W or saline.

DISOPYRAMIDE

This agent (Norpace) was introduced in the United States in 1977. Clinical experience with this agent is limited but significant data are available concerning its spectrum of activity and toxicity.

ELECTROPHYSIOLOGIC EFFECTS

Disopyramide is similar but not identical with quinidine with regard to electrophysiologic effects. It decreases action potential amplitude and upstroke velocity, resulting in decreased conduction and prolongation of refractoriness in the intraventricular conduction system.

This drug has potent anticholinergic properties that balance the direct depressant effects on the sinus node.

HEMODYNAMIC EFFECTS

Disopyramide has been found to have minor negative inotropic effect. However, in the setting of acute myocardial infarction, the negative inotropic effects seem to be accentuated.

ABSORPTION AND METABOLIC FATE

The drug is well (83%) absorbed from the gastrointestinal tract. The reported half-life has been variable, ranging from 8 to 18 hours.

A significant portion of the unchanged drug and its major metabolite is excreted by the kidneys. The protein binding is concentration dependent, and the free form increases as the total drug concentration increases—i.e., nonlinear pharmacokinetics. The major metabolite is formed in the liver.

Renal insufficiency necessitates significant reduction in the frequency of administration and the total dose administered per day.

DOSAGE, ROUTE, SERUM LEVELS
Disopyramide is clinically available only as an oral agent. Doses range from 300 to 1,600 mg/day administered in divided doses every 6 hours. The therapeutic serum levels are 2 to 5 μg/ml.

TOXICITY
Side-effects are generally related to the drug's potent anticholinergic effects, i.e., dry mouth, blurred vision, constipation, urinary retention, and psychosis. Intraventricular conduction disturbances may occur, especially in patients with preexisting conduction abnormalities.

SPECIFIC INDICATIONS
Disopyramide is particularly useful in the treatment of ventricular arrhythmias. Its usefulness in the treatment of supraventricular arrhythmias has yet to be clarified.

AVAILABLE PREPARATIONS
Capsules are available in 100- and 150-mg sizes.

MISCELLANEOUS ANTIARRHYTHMIC DRUGS
A variety of additional agents have been found helpful for the treatment of arrhythmias in man. Of particular interest is ancillary therapy, such as the use of tranquilizing agents in the setting of recurrent tachyarrhythmias. It has been suggested that central nervous system alterations may be partly responsible for the development or perpetuation of arrhythmias seen in man. In this regard, drugs such as hydroxyzine, chlordiazepoxide, and pentazocine have been found to have some antiarrhythmic effects.

In addition, there are agents available outside the continental United States or only for experimental trial in the United States that are reported to have significant antiarrhythmic action, such as ajmaline, verapamil amiodarone, and aprindine. To date, only limited data are available concerning the clinical efficacy of these drugs.

ARRHYTHMIAS IN DIGITALIS INTOXICATION
A significant percentage of arrhythmias seen in the clinical setting are due to digitalis overdosage. The gamut of arrhythmias produced by digitalis intoxication covers such arrhythmias as paroxysmal atrial tachycardia with block, multiform ventricular extrasystoles, and second- and higher-degree AV block. The treatment of these arrhythmias is dependent on the type observed clinically. For the treatment of significant ventricular arrhythmias,

diphenylhydantoin, lidocaine, and procainamide appear to be highly efficacious. For various types of AV block, diphenylhydantoin appears to be particularly efficacious because it shortens AV nodal conduction time. In addition, a potassium administration is usually of value in all these patients,
including those with various forms of AV block. The use of oral or intravenous potassium in the setting of digitalis-induced AV block can be
considered appropriate if the serum potassium level is less than 4.5 mEq/
liter.

CARDIOVERSION

The use of electrical conversion of tachyarrhythmias has become commonplace since the introduction of the first capacitor-discharged defibrillator
by Lown and his co-workers. Cardioversion requires the use of a synchro-
nizer circuit that will result in discharge of the waveform at the time of the
QRS. This timed discharge will therefore eliminate the possibility of induction of ventricular fibrillation by delivering the electrical discharge outside
the vulnerable period of ventricular repolarization.

INDICATIONS FOR USE

Cardioversion is considered appropriate for attempted conversion of atrial
fibrillation to sinus rhythm, especially if the atrial fibrillation is of short
duration. Anticoagulation should be considered if the patient has a history
of mitral valve disease, systemic embolization, or both. Cardioversion is
also of great value for the treatment of ventricular tachyarrhythmias and
supraventricular tachyarrhythmias that are recalcitrant to medical management. Cardioversion would not be considered beneficial for the treatment
of paroxysmal arrhythmias that are self-terminating, short-lived, or both.

Cardioversion can be performed in patients who have been receiving
digitalis if initial power settings are of very low magnitude. Initial cardioversion in these instances should be attempted with a power setting of 5 to
10 watt-seconds, then increased in a graded fashion with constant ECG
monitoring; if ventricular extrasystoles are seen, cardioversion should be
discontinued. However, if no ventricular extrasystoles are observed, increasing power settings should be used until cardioversion is successful.

ADVERSE EFFECTS

The complications resulting from cardioversion vary. The development of
pulmonary edema following successful cardioversion of atrial fibrillation
has been reported; the mechanism responsible appears to be possible elec-
tromechanical dissociation with mechanical paralysis of the left atrium. In
addition, ventricular tachyarrhythmias may be precipitated in the digitalized patient. Other problems include the development of asystole following cardioversion in patients with sinoatrial node disease or in patients

treated with β-blocking agents. Cerebrovascular accidents presumed secondary to embolism are also a potential, serious problem. A variety of enzymes will be released from skeletal muscle following closed chest cardioversion, resulting in elevation of serum enzymes. Finally, chest burns may occur if electrode solution or paste is not appropriately applied to the chest.

ANCILLARY CARDIOVERSION PROCEDURES

Various analgesic agents have been used to medicate patients before the use of cardioversion, but the most popular agent at present appears to be diazepam in doses from 2.5 to 30 mg given by slow intravenous infusion. This drug should not be administered into intravenous tubing, but directly into the vein. It appears most prudent to consider the ancillary use of premedication such as intravenous meperidine before the use of diazepam so that lower doses of the latter drug may be given and more rapid "anesthesia" induced.

Oxygen should be available for inhalation at the time of cardioversion. Atropine (0.5–1.0 mg) and lidocaine (50–100 mg) should also be at the bedside for intravenous administration if needed. Intubation equipment is also essential.

VASOPRESSOR THERAPY

Many of the serious tachyarrhythmias are associated with significant peripheral hypotension. Nevertheless, restoration of systemic pressure with the use of vasopressors does not usually convert ventricular tachyarrhythmias to normal sinus rhythm; sympathetic stimulation in these patients may in fact enhance the frequency or result in further rhythm deterioration. Therefore, in the setting of serious ventricular arrhythmias with hypotension, immediate attention should be given to restoration of normal sinus rhythm by other means.

However, in the setting of paroxysmal atrial tachycardia, elevation of the peripheral arterial pressure frequently activates parasympathetic input to the heart through carotid sinus and arch reflexes. This intense parasympathetic stimulation frequently converts these arrhythmias if they are due to reentrant activity. It is essential to recognize that relatively modest elevations in blood pressure usually are satisfactory in conversion of these tachycardias, i.e., a systolic pressure rise to 160 mm Hg maximum. Extreme care must be used in monitoring the peripheral arterial pressure during the vasopressor administration to prevent an overshoot of systemic pressure; marked elevations in systemic pressure might result in cerebrovascular accidents due to intracranial hemorrhage. Phenylephrine hydrochloride (Neo-Synephrine) and metaraminol (Aramine) are the drugs generally used, but any vasoconstrictor with α-stimulating characteristics would be appropriate.

ADDITIONAL MEASURES USEFUL FOR THE TREATMENT OF ARRHYTHMIAS

CAROTID SINUS MASSAGE

Carotid sinus massage is extremely useful for the diagnosis and treatment of certain paroxysmal arrhythmias. It is especially useful for the production of AV nodal conduction delay to enable full identification of underlying atrial arrhythmias. Furthermore, certain paroxysmal arrhythmias, such as paroxysmal atrial tachycardia, can be converted with the use of carotid sinus massage. It is interesting to note that the right carotid sinus has been suggested to have dominant innervation of the sinus node area, whereas the left carotid sinus appears to innervate predominantly the AV nodal area.

It is essential to recognize that carotid sinus massage in the elderly patient may produce cardiac asystole, significant cerebrovascular insufficiency, or even central blindness from emboli from the carotid artery. One should not consider the use of carotid sinus massage in patients with bruits in the neck.

EDROPHONIUM ADMINISTRATION

Edrophonium administration has been found useful for the treatment of paroxysmal supraventricular tachyarrhythmias because of its anticholinesterase activity, which resembles that of acetylcholine and therefore results in intense parasympathetic stimulation. This drug may be administered either in an acute intravenous dose (10 mg) or by continuous infusion at a rate of 0.25 to 2.0 mg/min.

ATROPINE ADMINISTRATION

Frequently, clinical situations are encountered of moderate bradycardia or second-degree AV block that appears to be due to enhancement of parasympathetic tone. In these cases, intravenous administration of atropine in doses from 0.5 to 2.0 mg as a bolus will restore normal sinus rate and AV conduction. Under other circumstances, bradycardia may result in more serious arrhythmias, such as those observed during myocardial infarction with the development of idioventricular tachycardia. The latter rhythm can frequently be treated by increasing the sinus rate with atropine administration. However, the resultant sinus rate cannot be predicted from the dose of atropine administered; therefore, episodes of sinus tachycardia may result in patients who are highly responsive to atropine. This overshoot in cardiac rate may be a potential problem because of diminished coronary flow.

TREATMENT OF SPECIFIC ARRHYTHMIAS

ATRIAL PREMATURE COMPLEXES

Atrial premature complexes are usually considered to be benign. However, frequent premature atrial complexes with very short coupling intervals (less than 450 msec) may be precursors of atrial fibrillation. Therefore, in the latter case, antiarrhythmic drug therapy should be considered, with the major drug being quinidine, digitalis, or procainamide. On rare occasions, atrial premature contractions may initiate ventricular tachycardia.

Occasional instances occur when frequent, blocked premature atrial complexes will impair the functional ventricular rate. Antiarrhythmic drug therapy will be required to reestablish an effective ventricular rate.

PREMATURE VENTRICULAR COMPLEXES

Premature ventricular complexes may be observed in patients without evidence of cardiovascular disease. In general, these patients should not be treated unless they are symptomatic or have frequent ventricular premature contractions. On occasion, patients respond to the withdrawal of stimulants, caffeine, tobacco, and/or alcohol. If encountered in the setting of organic heart disease, ventricular premature systoles should be treated if any of the following criteria are met: (1) there are more than 6 ventricular complexes per minute; (2) the ventricular prematures interrupt the T wave; and (3) the ventricular prematures occur in salvos.

The antiarrhythmic drugs that have been found to be successful in the treatment of ventricular premature complexes include quinidine, procainamide, lidocaine, diphenylhydantoin, propranolol, and disopyramide. If significant congestive heart failure is associated with ventricular premature systoles, the extrasystoles may respond to digitalis therapy.

PAROXYSMAL SUPRAVENTRICULAR TACHYCARDIA

Paroxysmal supraventricular tachycardia is characterized by its paroxysmal nature, with ventricular rates between 150 and 250 per minute. It is usually seen in a young patient without obvious organic heart disease. Atrial activity is only occasionally discernible. The rhythm is generally perfectly regular, and the QRS duration is usually normal. However, during these episodes, occasional patients manifest rate-related bundle branch block that may simulate ventricular tachyarrhythmias.

Treatment of an acute episode should be initiated with unilateral carotid sinus massage, edrophonium administration, or both. If this proves unsuccessful, vasopressor therapy directed at increasing the systemic pressure to 130 to 160 mm Hg should be instituted under careful arterial pressure monitoring. If this does not terminate the arrhythmia, repeat carotid sinus massage should be performed, edrophonium readministered, or both. If the latter maneuvers are not successful, rapid intravenous digitalization should be considered for a patient who is hemodynamically stable, or cardioversion should be performed if dictated by the clinical circumstances.

The patient with recurrent episodes of paroxysmal tachycardia should be treated with a combination of digitalis and propranolol. Occasional patients respond to quinidine therapy alone or in combination with digitalis and propranolol. However, in patients with recurrent episodes of atrial tachycardia, underlying accelerated AV conduction may be the physiologic mechanism, and such patients should therefore be evaluated in detail by more sophisticated physiologic studies.

PAROXYSMAL ATRIAL TACHYCARDIA WITH BLOCK

Paroxysmal atrial tachycardia with block, a dysrhythmia characterized by an atrial rate of 150 to 250 per minute and a variable ventricular rate, is considered to be due to digitalis toxicity in approximately two-thirds of cases. In general, the P wave configuration resembles sinus rhythm; in contrast, the atrial rate in atrial flutter is 250 to 350 per minute and has a sawtooth configuration to the P waves.

When this rhythm is related exclusively to digitalis intoxication, digitalis administration should be discontinued immediately. If the clinical situation is stable, observation of the rhythm disturbance may be all that is needed. However, if the serum potassium is in the lower range of normal, potassium may be administered by mouth or intravenously to elevate the serum potassium to the upper range of normal. In addition, propranolol may be used to increase the degree of AV block if clinically indicated.

ATRIAL FIBRILLATION

Atrial fibrillation is a common arrhythmia characterized in the untreated state by chaotic atrial activity and a rapid ventricular response, usually 140 to 200 per minute. P waves are not discernible on the ECG; atrial fibrillation characterized by coarse electrical activity may be observed with a bizarre baseline or with a fine baseline not demonstrating any significant fibrillatory waves. On occasion, with rapid ventricular rates, bizarre QRS configurations may be identified, which may be due to abberrant conduction within the ventricular conducting system.

Extremely rapid ventricular rates due to atrial fibrillation may be seen on rare occasions. Patients with ventricular rates in excess of 250 per minute should be presumed to have Wolff-Parkinson-White syndrome.

In general, this rhythm disturbance is due most frequently to atrial fibrosis and occurs secondary to mitral valve disease or to atherosclerotic or hypertensive cardiovascular disease. Furthermore, atrial fibrillation can develop in patients with significant hyperthyroidism and is usually accompanied by a rapid ventricular rate in such patients. Finally, occasional patients are observed who have paroxysmal atrial fibrillation without a discernible cause ("lone" fibrillators). Rarely, atrial fibrillation may be due to pericarditis, and in older patients, carcinomatous pericardial implantation may be responsible.

Hemodynamically, the loss of the atrial contribution to ventricular filling may result in a diminished cardiac output, with decreases of up to 25 percent. An additional complication is the presence of systemic embolization in patients who have paroxysmal episodes of atrial fibrillation.

The hemodynamic advantage of restoration of sinus rhythm varies from patient to patient. In a younger patient without evidence of atrial disease, restoration of sinus rhythm may result in an increase in cardiac output of up to 25 percent. However, in the older patients with advanced atrial disease, restoration of sinus rhythm may produce little or no increase in cardiac output.

MEDICAL TREATMENT

The method of choice for the control of the ventricular rate in the untreated patient is the administration of digitalis, usually intravenously in a fast-acting preparation. The end point for digitalization would be the presence of a resting heart rate of 60 to 90 per minute, with only a minimal increase observed during mild exercise. Maintenance digitalis should be administered according to the patient's weight and renal function status.

In an occasional patient in whom immediate control of rapid ventricular rates is necessary, the intravenous use of propranolol may be considered appropriate in doses of up to 15 mg given at a rate of 1 mg every 3 minutes.

On occasion, patients will present with atrial fibrillation with a controlled rate (i.e., 60–80/min). In these circumstances no therapeutic intervention should be considered unless the patients require the use of inotropic drugs as part of their medical management.

METHODS OF CONVERSION TO SINUS RHYTHM

In all patients, an attempt should be made to convert atrial fibrillation to sinus rhythm when the patient first presents with arrhythmia. The success rate for conversion to sinus rhythm is dependent largely on the duration of the atrial fibrillation. The success rate diminishes significantly when the duration exceeds 1 month. Furthermore, maintenance of sinus rhythm following successful conversion is highly variable and appears to be related to the underlying pathologic condition.

Anticoagulation should be considered mandatory in all patients who have a history of systemic embolization and in patients who have mitral valve disease. Anticoagulation should be administered for a total of 3 weeks before attempting conversion.

CARDIOVERSION. Patients who are on maintenance digitalis can be electively cardioverted using the graded cardioversion technique. It is generally suggested that the morning dose of digitalis be deleted on the day of cardioversion.

PHARMACOLOGIC CONVERSION. All patients should be adequately digitalized to obtain controlled ventricular rates prior to the attempt at pharmacologic conversion. In general, the most effective agent for the conversion to sinus rhythm is quinidine sulfate. A variety of regimens have been developed for the administration of quinidine for the conversion of atrial fibrillation to sinus rhythm, including the Sokolow method and the Levine method. The Sokolow regimen consists of 5 doses of quinidine sulfate administered at 2-hour intervals, the initial dose being 200 mg. If conversion does not occur, the dose is increased the next day by 100 mg and repeated over the 5 daily doses. The end point is either conversion to sinus rhythm or a daily dosage of up to 4 gm. In contrast, the Levine regimen consists of three daily doses at 4-hour intervals. Each dose is increased by 200 mg until a total daily dose of 3 gm is given.

Utilizing present pharmacologic concepts, one may devise any number of different regimens for quinidine administration, but the Sokolow method has proved to be the most successful for clinical use.

It is essential that the electrocardiogram be continuously recorded during these medical cardioversion procedures, so that early signs of toxicity may be detected.

POSTCONVERSION AND MAINTENANCE THERAPY. *At the time of cardioversion.* No definitive information is available to date on the efficacy of prophylactic antiarrhythmic therapy prior to electrical cardioversion. Nevertheless, it appears prudent to consider the use of intramuscular quinidine a half hour prior to the attempted cardioversion in doses of 200 mg for a 70-kg patient.

Maintenance antiarrhythmic drug therapy. The long-term prognosis for maintenance of sinus rhythm is dependent on the nature of the underlying disease. Nevertheless, it appears prudent to consider long-term antiarrhythmic therapy for most patients, usually quinidine. Doses should be administered so that effective blood levels will be obtained around the clock (2–6 mg/liter). The dosage regimen should be tailored to the patient's body weight and renal function.

Several investigators have commented on the efficacy of propranolol and also of digitalis therapy. To date, however, no definitive studies are available on the long-term effects of antiarrhythmic prophylactic drug therapy in these patients.

ATRIAL FLUTTER
Atrial flutter is characterized by regular atrial rates between 250 and 350 beats per minute. The etiology of this rhythm disturbance is generally considered to be identical with that of atrial fibrillation, except that it is frequently seen in patients with pulmonary disease. Morphologically, the P

wave has a biphasic or sawtooth configuration, which is most clearly seen in leads II, III, and aVF. In the untreated patient there is usually 2 : 1 conduction to the ventricles, with a general ventricular rate of 150 per minute. On occasion, it may be difficult to identify atrial flutter waves clearly. In the latter instance, gentle coronary sinus massage may be utilized to increase the degree of AV block and further delineate flutter waves. Furthermore, prominent a waves may be noted in cervical veins.

This rhythm is usually treated by digitalis administration. In patients with rapid ventricular rates, intravenous digitalis administration should be considered. However, patients with atrial flutter generally need much more digitalis than usual to produce significant AV block. Digitalis administration may result in either increased degrees of AV block, conversion to atrial fibrillation, or conversion to sinus rhythm. In addition, for immediate control of a rapid ventricular rate, the use of intravenous propranolol (see Atrial Fibrillation) may be considered. However, atrial flutter, in contrast with atrial fibrillation, is very sensitive to electrical conversion, and cardioversion is therefore the therapy of choice. Power settings of less than 100 watt-seconds are frequently successful for the conversion of this rhythm disturbance.

VENTRICULAR TACHYCARDIA

Ventricular tachycardia is characterized by ventricular rates of 100 to 250 per minute. Independent atrial activity can generally be observed on the ECG. The QRS configuration is extremely bizarre, but the ventricular rate is generally regular. Patients who have ventricular tachycardia usually have significant hemodynamic depression, with dizziness, syncope, and evidence of acute left-sided failure or angina pectoris, or both. The treatment of sustained ventricular tachycardia should be immediate cardioversion if the patient is hemodynamically compromised. Otherwise, medical management may be considered. In the setting of recurrent bouts of ventricular tachycardia, medical management is essential. Medical therapy includes: (1) lidocaine, (2) oral or intravenous procainamide, (3) quinidine sulfate or gluconate, (4) propranolol, or (5) a combination of these drugs.

Surgical therapy may be considered in the patient whose arrhythmia is recalcitrant to medical therapy and in whom there is evidence suggestive of ischemic heart disease with or without ventricular aneurysm formation. Such a patient may be found to be a suitable candidate for revascularization procedures, ventricular aneurysm resection, or both.

An additional form of ventricular tachycardia has been observed that can be characterized as an escape ventricular rhythm, generally with rates of 50 to 120 per minute. This is seen most frequently in patients with acute myocardial infarction, usually with an inferior infarct. The patients do not appear to have significant hemodynamic abnormalities during this rhythm disturbance. At present, the prognosis of the rhythm disturbance has not been fully delineated, and the need for antiarrhythmic drug therapy is thus uncertain. Attempted medical management should consist of agents that would elevate the basic sinus rate, such as atropine or its derivatives, and possibly the use of antiarrhythmic agents, such as lidocaine.

WOLFF-PARKINSON-WHITE SYNDROME

The Wolff-Parkinson-White syndrome is characterized by alterations in electrical activity secondary to ventricular preexcitation and is frequently associated with a history of paroxysmal arrhythmias. In the majority of patients who have a history of such arrhythmias, paroxysmal supraventricular tachycardia without a Δ wave is observed during this tachyarrhythmia. Medical management for these patients is highly dependent on the electrophysiologic characteristics of the bypass tracts and AV conducting system. Therapy should be tailored to the individual patient and should be based on studies directed at defining the electrical characteristics of these conducting networks.

Atrial fibrillation develops in a small percentage of patients with the Wolff-Parkinson-White syndrome. This group appears to be in jeopardy because of the development of extremely rapid ventricular rates due to anterograde conduction through the bypass tract or tracts. This bypass conduction leads to ventricular rates that on occasion may exceed 300 per minute. These rapid ventricular rates may result in syncopal episodes or in the development of ventricular fibrillation.

In the setting of atrial fibrillation with the Wolff-Parkinson-White syndrome, digitalis administration should be considered contraindicated because digitalis can shorten refractoriness in the bypass tract or tracts and may result in a more rapid ventricular rate. The therapy of choice would be immediate cardioversion or the intravenous administration of drugs that preferentially block the bypass tract, such as lidocaine and procainamide.

CARDIAC ARREST

Cardiac arrest may be due to the development of either ventricular fibrillation or cardiac asystole. In the setting of a witnessed cardiac arrest, it is suggested that a sharp blow with a clenched fist be administered to the midsternum. However, in an unwitnessed arrest, immediate cardiopulmonary resuscitation should be instituted.

RESUSCITATION

SINGLE-PERSON RESUSCITATION TECHNIQUE

In the single-person resuscitation technique, the airway should be checked, foreign bodies removed, and mouth-to-mouth resuscitation begun with four superimposed respirations to hyperinflate the lungs. The carotids should then be immediately checked for restoration of cardiac activity, and if no pulse is discernible, closed-chest massage should be instituted immediately at a cadence of 80 compressions per minute. After 15 chest compressions, the resuscitator should ventilate the patient twice and then resume closed-chest compression for an additional 15 compressions. This should be continued, alternating 15 compressions and 2 respirations, until cardiac action is restored. Every attempt should be made to obtain additional help.

TWO-PERSON CARDIOPULMONARY RESUSCITATION

In the two-person technique, chest compression is performed by one member at a rate of 60 compressions per minute, and the other member performs one respiration after every fifth chest compression; the team alternates when necessary.

MEDICAL MANAGEMENT AT THE TIME OF CARDIOPULMONARY ARREST

If ancillary help is available and an arrest cart is nearby, an intravenous line must be inserted immediately and the patient defibrillated at once. If monitoring is available and the patient was noted to be asystolic, intracardiac administration of epinephrine, 1 ml of 1 : 1000, is required. If fibrillation ensues, the patient should then be defibrillated.

If the patient is found on the floor, resuscitative procedures should continue in this position. If the patient is in bed, a board must be slid under the patient's back to allow for adequate chest compression.

Under no circumstances should any significant delay be allowed to occur before the institution of closed-chest massage. Furthermore, no significant interruptions should be allowed in the sequence of closed-chest massage and ventilation.

In the setting of poor myocardial contractility, consideration should be given to the administration of 10 ml of intracardiac calcium chloride.

If possible, arterial blood gases and serum potassium should be obtained for analysis. All attempts should be made to correct acid-base balance through the use of intravenous bicarbonate. In addition, at the earliest possible point, the patient should be intubated either by the nasotracheal or orotracheal route, so that artificially assisted ventilation may be instituted.

If the patient's arrest occurs outside the hospital, every attempt should be made to ensure rapid transport to the nearest hospital facility that has adequate resources to handle the patient's emergency care.

ATRIOVENTRICULAR BLOCK

In the past several years, the use of intracardiac recording techniques has substantially increased the information available to the clinician relative to the etiology of heart block in man. Utilizing these techniques, investigators have observed that first- and second-degree AV block may occur because of abnormalities throughout the entire AV conduction system, i.e., within the atrium, the AV node, the bundle of His, and the bundle branches. Therefore, therapy should be guided by knowledge of the underlying site of AV block.

In general, it has been observed that the width of the QRS on the standard ECG may serve as an indicator of the area of block that will be encountered by electrophysiologic studies: a narrow QRS generally identifies a supraventricular site of AV block, and a wide QRS identifies a distal conducting system site. Although this relation usually holds regardless of the degree of AV block encountered, there are significant exceptions. Thus, the decision to insert a permanent pacemaker should not be made unless electrophysiologic studies are performed to define clearly the site of block within the AV conducting system.

First-Degree Atrioventricular Block

First-degree AV block is characterized by the presence of a P–R interval in excess of 210 milliseconds. In the majority of patients with first-degree AV block, the delay is due to an abnormality of conduction in the AV node. Nevertheless, block may occur because of delay within the atrium, bundle of His, or bundle branches. In the latter circumstance, first-degree AV block due to delay in the distal conducting system may be of grave prognostic significance if the patient has any evidence suggestive of additional intraventricular conduction delay, i.e., bundle branch block, fascicular block, or both.

Second-Degree Atrioventricular Block

Second-degree AV block is usually divided into two subgroups.

TYPE I. Type I second-degree AV block is characterized by the presence of gradual prolongation of the P–R interval with associated gradual shortening of the R–R interval, until a P wave is not conducted to the ventricles. As observed with first-degree AV block, this rhythm disturbance may be due to delay in conduction within the atrium, the AV node, or the bundle of His. In general, this rhythm disturbance is considered benign and should not warrant medical or pacemaker therapy if the ventricular rate is adequate and the patient suffers no adverse hemodynamic consequences. Nevertheless, in patients who have distal conduction delay accounting for Wenckebach periods, a less optimistic prognosis has been suggested, and these patients should be followed extremely carefully.

TYPE II. Type II second-degree AV block is characterized by stable P–R and stable R–R intervals until suddenly a P wave or waves are found not to conduct to the ventricle. This rhythm disturbance is generally considered to have a poor prognosis, in that more advanced degrees of AV block, syncope, or both frequently develop. Therefore, in a large percentage of patients, permanent pacemaker therapy should be considered. A peculiar situation exists for patients who have second-degree AV block with 2 : 1 conduction to the ventricles. Regardless of the site of AV block, these patients may have significant alterations in hemodynamics because of the extremely slow ventricular rate sometimes observed. Furthermore, these patients may not respond appropriately to exercise in that it may increase the degree of AV block. Therefore, regardless of the site of AV block, many of these patients require pacemaker therapy.

CHRONIC ADVANCED AV BLOCK

CONGENITAL TYPE. Congenital AV block is characterized generally by the presence of a narrow escape pacemaker configuration with ventricular rates of 35 to 60. In addition, the ventricular rate in these patients frequently increases slightly with exercise. The site of block in these patients is generally within the AV node. Their long-term prognosis appears to be reasonably good, although there is evidence to suggest that Adams-Stokes syndrome develops in such patients on occasion. Pacemaker therapy is not indicated in the majority of these patients, but careful long-term follow-up is essential.

ACQUIRED TYPE. The majority of the patients with acquired AV block appear to have distal conducting system disease with escape ventricular pacemakers with rates of 15 to 50 per minute and a wide QRS duration. Some patients manifest this rhythm disturbance on a chronic basis and appear to have a reasonably good hemodynamic function. However, in the majority this rhythm disturbance is acute and there are associated seizure episodes (Adams-Stokes syndrome). The latter group is universally treated by permanent pacing. If chronic advanced AV block is seen in the adult patient without symptoms, permanent pacemaker insertion is not mandatory, but extremely careful follow-up should be instituted.

MANAGEMENT OF ADAMS-STOKES SYNDROME. The immediate management of Adams-Stokes syndrome should be the insertion of a transvenous pacemaker on an emergency basis. If this cannot be done, pharmacologic measures should be taken immediately to enhance the ventricular rate until a pacemaker may be inserted. Isoproterenol appears to be the drug of choice, given by the intravenous route. Immediate intravenous infusion should be begun at a rate of at least 3 μg/min. The patient's ECG should be followed continuously and the dose of isoproterenol altered in response to the rate of the ventricular escape pacemaker. If medical management is not successful, cardiopulmonary resuscitation should be instituted at once until it is possible to insert an emergency transvenous pacemaker.

SELECTED READINGS

Bigger, J. T., et al. Arrhythmias and antiarrhythmic drugs. *Adv. Intern. Med.* 18:251, 1972.

Cranefield, P. F., et al. Genesis of cardiac arrhythmias. *Circulation* 47:190, 1973.

Goldreyer, B. N. Intracardiac electrocardiography in the analysis and understanding of cardiac arrhythmias. *Ann. Intern. Med.* 77:117, 1972.

Harrison, D. C., Meffin, P. J., and Winkle, R. A. Clinical pharmacokinetics of antiarrhythmic drugs. *Prog. in Cardiovasc. Dis.* 20:217, 1977.

Mandel, W. J. *Cardiac Arrhythmias: Their Mechanisms, Diagnosis, and Management.* Philadelphia: Lippincott, 1980.

National Conference Steering Committee, A. S. Gordon, Chairman. Standards for cardiopulmonary resuscitation (CPR) and emergency cardiac care (ECC). *J.A.M.A.* (Suppl.) 227:837, 1974.

Singh, B. N., Collett, J. T., and Chew, C. Y. C. New perspectives in the pharmacologic therapy of cardiac arrhythmias. *Prog. in Cardiovasc. Dis.* 22:243, 1980.

Kanu Chatterjee / 10. ACUTE HEART FAILURE

Cardiac failure may be broadly defined as a condition in which cardiac output is inadequate in relation to the organism's demand. Acute heart failure is difficult to define, but in clinical practice it may be said to be present when the consequences of heart failure are manifested rapidly.

Cardiac output is the product of stroke volume and heart rate. Stroke volume in turn is influenced by the initial muscle fiber length, the preload, the resistance to ventricular ejection, the afterload, and the myocardial contractile state. Inability to maintain cardiac output may therefore be precipitated by decreased end-diastolic volume (preload), increased resistance to left ventricular ejection, a decreased contractile state, and disturbances of heart rate. These mechanisms may be operative either in isolation or in combination.

Acute myocardial infarction is by far the most common and important cause of acute heart failure. Despite the better understanding of the pathophysiology of acute infarction acquired in recent years, treatment of heart failure complicating myocardial infarction still remains one of the most difficult problems in clinical practice. It is becoming increasingly apparent that the conventional therapy of heart failure more often than not is unsuccessful, and a more aggressive therapeutic approach is necessary.

One of the problems in instituting effective treatment is that clinical recognition of the unstable and changing levels of cardiac function that may occur in these patients is often difficult if not impossible. Although abnormal physical signs, such as tachycardia, gallop rhythm, and reversed splitting of the first heart sound, provide information regarding the presence of abnormal cardiac function, they lack useful precision. Hemodynamic monitoring allows more precise diagnosis of the mechanism and degree of depression of cardiac function and is now more often used for the management of cardiac failure following acute myocardial infarction.

HEMODYNAMIC MONITORING

The hemodynamic parameter that provides the most useful information concerning cardiac function is left ventricular filling pressure. Monitoring of central venous pressure (CVP) is not only less useful but also may be misleading when monitoring of left ventricular function is intended. Central venous pressure is right ventricular filling pressure, and although there is normally a good correlation between right and left ventricular filling pressures (LVFP) when both ventricular functions are parallel, gross disparity may occur between CVP and LVFP when one ventricular function is affected in isolation or more than the other. In patients with acute myocardial infarction, the left ventricle is most commonly and predominantly affected. Therefore, monitoring of LVFP is preferable to monitoring CVP.

MONITORING OF LEFT VENTRICULAR FILLING PRESSURE

DIRECT LEFT VENTRICULAR CATHETERIZATION

Left ventricular filling pressure can be most accurately determined by recording left ventricular pressure by placing a catheter inside the left ventricular cavity. However, because of the risks of inducing arrhythmias and thromboembolism, this method is not suitable for the continuous and prolonged monitoring of LVFP that is often required for the proper management of cardiac failure following acute myocardial infarction.

INDIRECT MEASUREMENT OF LEFT VENTRICULAR FILLING PRESSURE

In the absence of mitral valve obstruction, mean left atrial pressure reflects LVFP. Direct determination of left atrial pressure is possible by either retrograde or transseptal catheterization of the left atrium. However, such procedures need a high degree of skill, are associated with significant complications similar to those of direct left ventricular catheterization, and cannot be recommended for routine hemodynamic monitoring of critically ill patients. Because of the absence of valves between the left atrium and pulmonary veins, pulmonary venous pressure is the same as the left atrial pressure. Pulmonary venous pressure can be recorded indirectly by recording "pulmonary artery occluded pressure," which can be obtained by right-sided heart catheterization. This is done either by wedging the tip of a catheter in a very small pulmonary artery branch or by inflating the balloon of a Swan-Ganz balloon flotation catheter placed in a medium or large pulmonary artery branch. In both circumstances, forward transmission of pressure is prevented, and the tip of the catheter records reflected pulmonary venous pressure. Although LVFP can be determined by wedging any catheter used during routine right heart catheterization, this method cannot be recommended for monitoring LVFP in critically ill patients because of several disadvantages, as follows:

1. The use of fluoroscopy is necessary for insertion of such catheters.
2. Each time wedge pressure is to be determined, the catheter must be manipulated.
3. It requires a great deal of skill.
4. Most important of all, serious cardiac arrhythmias may be induced during passage of these catheters through the right ventricle.

These disadvantages were virtually eliminated with the advent of balloon flotation Swan-Ganz catheters, and continuous, safe, and reliable hemody-

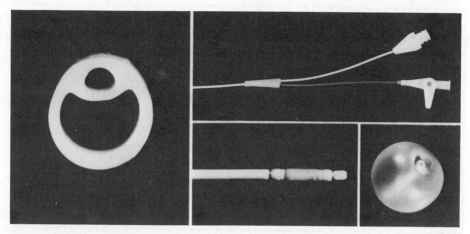

FIGURE 10-1. Cross section of flow-directed balloon catheter (*left*); proximal end of catheter (*top right*); distal end of catheter and inflated balloon (*lower right*). (From H. J. C. Swan et al., Catheterization of the heart in man with use of a flow-directed balloon-tipped catheter. Reprinted by permission of the *N. Engl. J. Med.* 283:447, 1970.)

namic monitoring is now possible even in the most critically ill patients without adding any significant risk to the patient.

MONITORING WITH THE BALLOON FLOTATION CATHETER
IMPORTANT CHARACTERISTICS OF BALLOON FLOTATION CATHETERS
All types of balloon flotation Swan-Ganz catheters have one lumen connected to a latex balloon close to the tip of the catheter. When the balloon is inflated, the surface protrudes above the tip of the catheter. The inflated balloon thus prevents irritation of the endocardium by the tip of the catheter and virtually no arrhythmias are induced during the passage of the catheter (Figs. 10-1 and 10-2). With the balloon inflated, the catheter floats along the bloodstream through the right side of the heart, and it can therefore be passed at the bedside without the use of fluoroscopy. Thus, movement of a critically ill patient to the fluoroscopy unit or the use of portable fluoroscopy is not necessary.

The double lumen Swan-Ganz catheter has, in addition to the lumen connected to the balloon, another lumen that opens at the tip of the catheter (Fig. 10-1). This lumen is of a sufficiently large size to record phasic pressures in the central circulation with an adequate dynamic response and to permit sampling of blood from locations in the right heart and pulmonary arteries. With the catheter in position (i.e., when the catheter tip is in the pulmonary artery branches) and with the balloon inflated, pulmonary capillary wedge pressure (PCWP) is recorded; and with the balloon

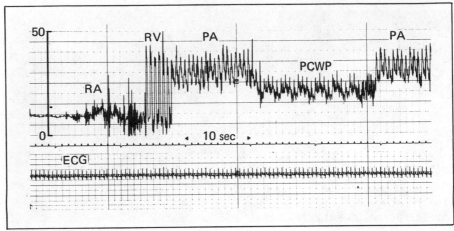

FIGURE 10-2. Pressure recorded during insertion of flow-directed balloon catheter. RA = right atrial pressure; RV = right ventricular pressure; PA = pulmonary artery pressure; PCWP = pulmonary capillary wedge pressure. Pressure scale: 50 mm Hg.

deflated, pulmonary artery pressure is recorded (Fig. 10-2). Pulmonary artery end-diastolic pressure (PADP) is similar to mean PCWP in the absence of significantly increased pulmonary vascular resistance, as in primary lung disease or pulmonary embolism. Therefore, in patients without primary lung disease, PADP can also be used as representative of LVFP.

With the use of the triple lumen Swan-Ganz catheter (Fig. 10-3), cardiac output can be determined by thermodilution technique. The catheter is also passed at the bedside without the use of fluoroscopy. A small thermistor is located close to the tip of the catheter, so that it lies in the main pulmonary artery or its major branches. In addition to the main lumen to record pulmonary artery pressure or PCWP, there is another lumen that opens 28 or 30 cm from the tip, in the high right atrium or right atrial–superior vena cava junction. This orifice is used for the delivery of cold (0–5°C) dextrose solution. The resultant changes in the temperature of the flowing blood are recorded by the thermistor in the pulmonary artery. The degree of cooling of the blood is inversely proportional to the volume flow of blood; the cooler the blood, the less is the volume flow, i.e., the less is the cardiac output, and vice versa.

The advantages of this technique of cardiac output determination in an intensive care area are as follows: (1) it does not require withdrawal of blood; (2) an inert and inexpensive indicator can be utilized; (3) calibration is simple and reproducible; and (4) there is no recirculation peak to complicate the calculation of cardiac output. In the presence of tricuspid regur-

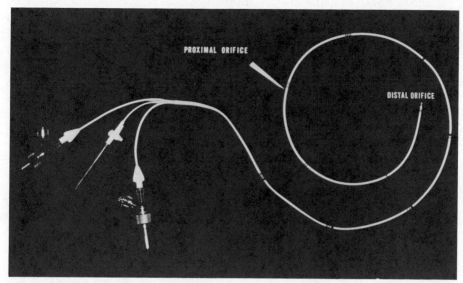

FIGURE 10-3. Flow-directed triple-lumen balloon catheter for measurement of cardiac output by thermodilution. Distance from tip is marked in 10-cm intervals. Position of thermistor proximal to inflated balloon is indicated by arrow. Proximal end of catheter contains two thermistor leads, lumen for inflation of balloon (small syringe), lumen for injection of the cold liquid (large syringe), and distal lumen, connected to a pressure transducer. (From J. S. Forrester et al., Thermodilution cardiac output determination with a single flow-directed catheter. *Am. Heart J.* 83:306, 1972.)

gitation or left-to-right shunt, however, cardiac output cannot be accurately determined by this technique.

In the latest type of Swan-Ganz catheters, right ventricular and right atrial electrodes have been incorporated. This catheter can be used to record right ventricular and right atrial electrograms for the diagnosis of complex arrhythmias, as well as for determination of intracardiac pressures and cardiac output. Furthermore, right ventricular or right atrial electrodes can be used for temporary ventricular, atrial, or atrioventricular sequential pacing.

INSERTION

Before insertion of the catheter, possible balloon leakage should be tested by inflating the balloon under sterile water; the other lumens of the catheter should be flushed with sterile, heparinized saline solution. The outer surface of the catheter should be cleansed thoroughly with water. Rough handling of the tip of the catheter should be avoided to prevent trauma to the balloon.

Balloon flotation catheters are inserted into a vein by a cutdown or by percutaneous technique and advanced to a central venous position with pressure monitoring. The intrathoracic position is recognized by the wide swing in venous pressures that occurs with deep inspiration, which causes marked changes in negative intrathoracic pressure. The central venous position is usually reached when the catheter has been advanced 35 to 40 cm when a right arm vein is used, or 45 to 50 cm when a left arm vein is used (the distance from the tip is marked in 10-cm intervals).

Once the central venous position is reached, the balloon is inflated with 0.8 ml of air if the double-lumen catheter is used, or with 1.2 to 1.5 ml of air if the triple-lumen catheter is used. In the presence of intracardiac shunts, carbon dioxide instead of air should be used for inflation of the balloon to avoid systemic air embolization in case of accidental balloon rupture. (The bursting volume of the balloon is 3 ml.) When the catheter is advanced with the balloon inflated, the catheter passes from the right atrium to the right ventricle, to the pulmonary artery, and then to the pulmonary capillary wedge position, usually in a matter of seconds (Fig. 10-2). Characteristic configurations of atrial, ventricular, pulmonary arterial, and pulmonary capillary wedge pressures are shown in Figure 10-4. When the catheter has been advanced 60 to 70 cm and the right ventricular pressure is not recorded, the catheter should be withdrawn and readvanced.

RECOGNITION OF RIGHT ATRIAL, RIGHT VENTRICULAR, PULMONARY ARTERIAL, AND PULMONARY CAPILLARY WEDGE PRESSURE PULSES

Right atrial traces. The right atrial traces (Fig. 10-4) consist of the positive waves, namely, *a, c,* and *v* when patients are in sinus rhythm. The *a* wave occurs between the P and R waves of the electrocardiogram (ECG). The *c* wave runs on the downslope of the *a* wave; the *v* wave coincides with the T wave of the ECG. The height of the *a* wave in the right atrium is usually higher than the height of the *v* wave in the absence of tricuspid regurgitation and is similar to right ventricular end-diastolic pressure.

Right ventricular traces. When the catheter passes across the tricuspid valve into the right ventricular cavity, characteristic ventricular pressure tracings are recorded (Fig. 10-4). Ventricular pressure tracings usually resemble a cone and consist of one peak during systole. The pressure starts rising a few milliseconds after the R wave of the ECG and reaches its nadir just after the T wave. The early diastolic pressure is lower than the end-diastolic pressure, which is similar to the right atrial pressure.

Pulmonary artery pressure. Pulmonary artery pressure approximately resembles a triangle and can be identified by the presence of the dicrotic notch in the downslope coincidental with the pulmonary valve closure (Fig. 10-4). The early diastolic pressure is always higher than the end-

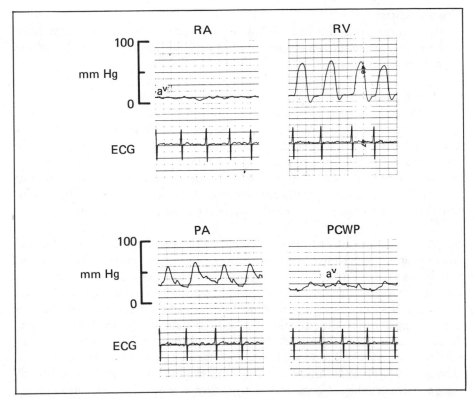

FIGURE 10-4. (*Upper left*) Right atrial (RA) pressure pulse. The *a* wave is between the P and R waves, and the *v* wave coincides with the T wave of the electrocardiogram (ECG). The *c* wave is on the downslope of the *a* wave before the onset of the *v* wave and is not marked. (*Upper right*) Right ventricular (RV) pressure pulse. End-diastolic pressure is the same as mean RA pressure. (*Lower left*) Pulmonary artery (PA) pressure pulse is triangular in shape with dicrotic notch on the downslope; early diastolic pressure is higher than end-diastolic pressure. (*Lower right*) Pulmonary capillary wedge pressure (PCWP) resembles right atrial pressure pulse.

diastolic pressure. It is common to observe artifacts due to catheter movement in pulmonary artery pressure tracings.

Pulmonary capillary wedge pressure pulse. The PCWP pulse (Fig. 10-4) resembles right atrial pressure tracings in configuration. The mean height of the pressure is always lower than the mean of the pulmonary artery pressure. With the balloon deflated, the tracing should show a clear-cut increase in the height of the pressure and change to the pulmonary artery pressure pulse contours.

COMPLICATIONS

Complications with the use of balloon flotation catheters for right heart catheterization are extremely uncommon and can be avoided if the proper guidelines are followed.

THROMBOPHLEBITIS, INFECTION, AND CATHETER CLOTTING. Thrombophlebitis, infection, and catheter clotting occur rarely and can usually be prevented. The incidence of thrombophlebitis can be reduced by properly cleaning the catheter before insertion and by avoiding repeated manipulations of the catheter or using the same vein for multiple catheter insertions. Infection can be avoided by maintaining proper aseptic techniques. Catheter clotting is usually avoided by intermittent flushing of the catheter (every half-hour) with heparinized saline or dextrose solution (5,000 units/500 ml).

BALLOON RUPTURE. With the successive use of the same catheter, it is not uncommon to experience balloon rupture. Thus, the same catheter should not be used more than 2 or 3 times. If balloon rupture occurs with the catheter in place, its flotation properties are lost. Balloon rupture is diagnosed by loss of resistance during deflation and inflation of the balloon and occasionally by blood leaks through the balloon lumen. Once the balloon ruptures, PCWPs cannot be monitored. However, pulmonary artery pressure can still be monitored, and PADP can be used to represent LVFP. The injection of small amounts of air into the central circulation in the absence of intracardiac shunts does not produce any adverse consequences.

THROMBOSIS AND PULMONARY EMBOLISM. In patients with shock, hypercoagulable states, or a preexisting thrombotic tendency, if prolonged monitoring is contemplated, anticoagulation with heparin is recommended to prevent thromboembolic complications.

PULMONARY INFARCTION. Pulmonary infarction occurs rarely and only when the catheter is left in the wedge position for a prolonged period. Therefore, the balloon should be deflated as soon as the wedge pressure is recorded, and under no circumstances should the balloon remain inflated more than 2 or 3 minutes. There is a natural tendency of the catheter to migrate into the distal pulmonary artery branches, and this position can be recognized if the pressure recorded when the balloon is deflated resembles PCWP or damped pulmonary artery pressure. In such circumstances the catheter should be withdrawn until undamped pulmonary artery pressure is recorded.

CATHETER KNOTTING. Catheter knotting is an uncommon complication and occurs when there are kinks in the shaft of the catheter. Therefore, before insertion, the catheter should be examined for the presence of any kinks.

Furthermore, once the catheter tip reaches the right atrium, the catheter should not be advanced too fast.

PULMONARY ARTERIAL PERFORATION. Rupture of pulmonary arterial branches is extremely rare. The risk of rupture is higher in patients with severe pulmonary hypertension. Such complications can be avoided if the following steps are taken:

1. During recording of wedge pressure, the balloon should be kept inflated for a minimal period to lessen the stress on the pulmonary artery wall.
2. The balloon should never be inflated with fluid.
3. The balloon lumen should be identified each time balloon inflation is intended.
4. After initial passage of the catheter, when the balloon is reinflated for recording wedge pressure, the inflation should be done very slowly and stopped as soon as the wedge pressure is recorded to avoid overdistention of the pulmonary artery branches.
5. If the inflation volume necessary to obtain wedge pressure is significantly less than that indicated on the shaft of the catheter, it will suggest that the catheter has probably migrated to small pulmonary artery branches. In such circumstances, the catheter should be pulled back to a position in which full or near-full inflation volume is needed to obtain wedge pressure.

OTHER HEMODYNAMIC PARAMETERS
Monitoring of cardiac output is useful in the diagnosis and management of pump failure. In the presence of severe pump failure or cardiogenic shock, direct intra-arterial pressure should be monitored because marked discrepancies between cuff pressure and intra-arterial pressure may exist in such patients.

DRUG THERAPY OF PUMP FAILURE COMPLICATING MYOCARDIAL INFARCTION
The objectives of the therapy of pump failure are to increase cardiac output and to decrease pulmonary venous congestion. In patients with myocardial infarction, it is preferable that these goals be achieved without enhancing myocardial ischemia.

Cardiac output can be increased by the following mechanisms:

1. An increase in end-diastolic volume, i.e., preload by the Frank-Starling mechanism (volume expansion).
2. An increase in contractility by inotropic agents such as digitalis, norepinephrine, isoproterenol, glucagon, dopamine, and dobutamine.
3. A decrease in resistance to ventricular ejection by the use of vasodilator (afterload) agents such as nitroprusside, phentolamine, nitroglycerin, and trimethaphan.
4. The relief of ischemia, thereby recruiting more functioning myocardial segments, by drugs such as propranolol that decrease myocardial oxygen demand

in relation to supply, or possibly by enhancing oxygen supply by direct myocardial revascularization.
5. An increase in heart rate when stroke volume is more or less fixed by using artificial pacemakers or chronotropic agents such as isoproterenol.

Pulmonary venous pressure can be decreased by the following mechanisms:

1. The depletion of total circulating blood volume with phlebotomies or diuretics.
2. The reduction of effective venous return by peripheral venous pooling, using diuretics, vasodilators, or rotating tourniquets.

VOLUME EXPANSION

Volume expansion is indicated when symptoms or signs of low cardiac output are present due to relative or absolute hypovolemia. The clinical diagnosis is often difficult. However, a history of prolonged use of diuretics prior to infarction, and severe vomiting and diaphoresis at the onset of infarction, predispose to hypovolemia. Along with the clinical features of low cardiac output, jugular venous pressure is usually normal clinically. However, diagnosis and assessment of the results of therapy are greatly facilitated if PCWP or PADP can be monitored. If low cardiac output and hypotension are associated with a PCWP of 14 mm Hg or less, hypovolemia is likely to be present, and volume expansion with intravenous fluid administration is indicated. Rapid infusion of 100 to 200 ml of dextran, salt-poor albumin, plasma, or 5% D/W should be instituted while monitoring changes in PCWP or PADP. If PCWP increases rapidly and exceeds 18 mm Hg without significant improvement in cardiac output, fluid administration should be discontinued. A further increase in PCWP carries the risk of precipitating pulmonary congestion. If cardiac output increases without a rapid increase in PCWP, fluid administration should be continued to maintain PCWP between 15 and 18 mm Hg.

Without hemodynamic monitoring, fluid administration should be undertaken with extreme caution. Frequent physical examinations for signs of congestive failure (increased jugular venous pressure, S_3 gallop, pulmonary rales) are mandatory. If signs of heart failure appear, fluid administration should be immediately discontinued. If there is clinical improvement without signs of heart failure, fluid infusion may be continued at a rate of 100 to 200 ml/hr. Besides the risk of precipitating pulmonary congestion, another potential disadvantage of volume expansion is enhancement of myocardial ischemia by increasing left ventricular volume and radius (Laplace relation).

INOTROPIC AGENTS

The inotropic agents digitalis, isoproterenol, norepinephrine, dopamine, and glucagon are potentially capable of increasing cardiac output by increasing contractility. Increased contractility, however, increases myocardial oxygen demand, which may exceed oxygen supply in the presence of severe obstructive coronary artery lesions, thereby enhancing existing myocardial ischemia. Paradoxically, an increase in contractility may cause deterioration of cardiac performance. The chronotropic effect of some of the inotropic drugs (e.g., isoproterenol, norepinephrine) may also contribute to an increase in myocardial oxygen demand by inducing tachycardia. Most inotropic agents are essentially arrhythmogenic.

Furthermore, improvement in cardiac performance in patients with recent myocardial infarction depends on the degree of responsiveness of the noninfarcted myocardium to inotropic stimulation. Recent studies indicate that the level of circulating endogenous catecholamines is already high in these patients, and it is higher in patients with pump failure and cardiogenic shock. It is possible that noninfarcted myocardial segments are already maximally or near maximally inotropically stimulated, and administration of inotropes may therefore not produce adequate and expected responses. Indeed, clinical experience suggests that the value of inotropic agents in the management of pump failure complicating acute myocardial infarction is extremely limited.

DIGITALIS PREPARATIONS

In patients with recent myocardial infarction when pump failure is not precipitated by tachyarrhythmias, digitalis administration usually does not improve cardiac output significantly ($< 10\%$ of output), and the decrease in pulmonary venous pressure is also minimal. There is also experimental evidence that digitalis may cause an increase in infarct size. Furthermore, in the presence of recent infarction, ventricular irritability is enhanced by digitalis. Therefore, digitalis should be avoided for the management of pump failure complicating myocardial infarction, particularly in the absence of significant cardiomegaly. If pump failure is precipitated by tachyarrhythmias such as atrial fibrillation or flutter with rapid ventricular response, and if such arrhythmias are not readily converted by direct current cardioversion, digitalis preparations may be used to control ventricular rate. Digoxin, when given intravenously, should be administered by infusion, not by bolus. With infusion of digoxin (0.5 to 1 mg), given in 15 to 20 minutes, adverse peripheral vascular effects can be minimized. Once ventricular rate is controlled, digoxin should be continued with 0.125 to 0.25 mg, once a day, as a maintenance dose. At this stage, quinidine (200 to 400 mg every six hours) will frequently convert atrial fibrillation or flutter into sinus rhythm.

NOREPINEPHRINE

Like digitalis, norepinephrine is of little use in the management of pump failure complicating recent myocardial infarction. With higher doses of norepinephrine (> 10 μg/min), systemic vascular resistance may actually increase, which might further decrease stroke volume. Left ventricular end-diastolic pressure and therefore pulmonary venous pressure may also concomitantly increase. Furthermore, like any other inotropic agent, it has the disadvantage of enhancing myocardial ischemia.

ISOPROTERENOL

Despite some improvement in cardiac output that might occur in a dose range of 1 to 8 μg/min, isoproterenol increases myocardial ischemia by its marked inotropic and chronotropic effects. It is also a potent arrhythmogenic. Therefore, it is not recommended for the treatment of pump failure complicating myocardial infarction.

GLUCAGON

With an initial intravenous loading dose of 5 mg, followed by a maintenance dose of 1 mg/min, glucagon may improve cardiac performance but only in patients with mild to moderate left ventricular failure. In patients with severe pump failure or cardiogenic shock, it has little beneficial effect. Nausea, vomiting, and marked hyperglycemia may be troublesome side-effects.

DOPAMINE

Dopamine has been shown to have beneficial hemodynamic effects in some patients with acute myocardial infarction complicated by left ventricular failure and cardiogenic shock. With dopamine, cardiac output increases, along with a slight or no decrease in left ventricular filling pressure. Improvement in urinary output has also been claimed with the use of dopamine, owing to its direct renovascular effects. The recommended dose is 5 to 30 μg/kg/min. With higher doses, significant tachycardia and an increase in systemic vascular resistance may occur.

In the presence of severe hypotension (e.g., systolic pressure less than 85 mm Hg and diastolic pressure less than 60 mm Hg) and severe left ventricular failure, dopamine infusion may be useful to increase arterial pressure. Concomitant increase in cardiac output and a decrease in left ventricular filling pressure may also occur in these patients, indicating improved left ventricular function. Since a relatively larger dose is required to obtain the hemodynamic effects, considerable tachycardia is frequently observed. Augmented inotropic state and tachycardia increase myocardial oxygen demand and may enhance myocardial ischemia in patients with acute myocardial infarction.

DOBUTAMINE

Dobutamine is a new synthetic catecholamine which acts directly on β-adrenergic receptors to increase cardiac contractility and heart rate. Compared with isoproterenol, dobutamine produces less tachycardia. At low doses it may cause slight vasoconstriction, and at higher doses a biphasic vasoconstrictor-vasodilator response may be observed. However, its peripheral vascular effects appear to be less marked than those of isoproterenol or dopamine. In patients with heart failure, dobutamine at infusion rates of 2.5 to 15 μg/kg/min may increase cardiac output and decrease left ventricular filling pressure significantly. Some increase in heart rate and arterial pressure usually accompanies an increase in cardiac output. Enhanced contractile state and tachycardia increase myocardial oxygen demand and coronary blood flow.

AMRINONE

Amrinone is a bipyridine derivative and a nonglycosidic, nonadrenergic inotropic agent. In patients with severe left ventricular failure, it increases cardiac output and stroke volume and decreases left ventricular filling pressure, indicating improved cardiac performance. It does not cause any significant change in heart rate or arterial pressure, but decreases systemic vascular resistance. Since its mode of action is different from that of digitalis or catecholamines, it can be combined with the inotropic agents to produce synergistic effects on left ventricular function. Because amrinone does not appear to cause significant tachycardia or hypertension, an excessive increase in myocardial oxygen demand and, therefore, adverse effects on myocardial metabolism are less likely to occur in patients with ischemic heart disease. After a single intravenous dose (0.75–2.5 mg/kg), the onset of action has been noted within 2 minutes, reaching a maximum in 10 minutes with the hemodynamic effects lasting 60 to 90 minutes. With a continuous infusion (6–10 μg/kg/min) sustained hemodynamic effects are expected. The compound is now being investigated and is not yet available for use by the practicing physician.

VASODILATOR (AFTERLOAD REDUCING) AGENTS

Changes in resistance to left ventricular ejection alter left ventricular pump function. Decreased resistance enhances left ventricular stroke volume and cardiac output. Vasodilator agents such as nitroprusside or phentolamine have been shown to reduce peripheral resistance (resistance to left ventricular ejection) and thereby to improve cardiac performance. Furthermore, because of the venous pooling effect, left ventricular end-diastolic volume and pressure (preload) and pulmonary venous pressure usually decrease significantly (Fig. 10-5). There is some decrease in arterial pressure (afterload) without any change in heart rate and contractile state. Overall myocardial oxygen demand tends to decrease.

Vasodilator therapy may improve the immediate prognosis in patients with recent infarction complicated by severe pump failure with or without clinical features of cardiogenic shock. The major disadvantage of vasodilator therapy, however, is the usual decrease in arterial pressure, which, if pronounced, might restrict coronary blood flow and enhance ischemia.

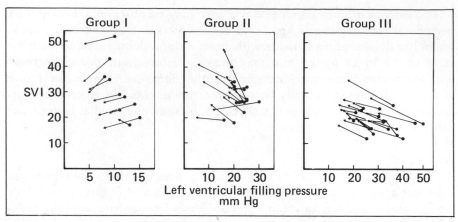

FIGURE 10-5. Individual changes in stroke volume (SVI) and left ventricular filling pressure (LVFP) during vasodilator therapy. Each dot represents baseline measurements; the arrowhead represents measurements during phentolamine or nitroprusside infusion. Group I patients have a baseline LVFP of <15 mm Hg. Group II patients have a baseline LVFP of >15 mm Hg and a SVI of 20 gmM/M². Group III patients have a baseline LVFP of >15 mm Hg and a SVI of ≦20 gmM/M². (From K. Chatterjee et al., Hemodynamic and metabolic responses to vasodilator therapy in acute myocardial infarction. *Circulation* 48:1183, 1973. By permission of The American Heart Association, Inc.)

Arterial pressure, LVFP (PCWP or PADP), and, if possible, cardiac output should therefore be monitored during vasodilator therapy.

For the treatment of pump failure complicating myocardial infarction, vasodilator agents with quickly reversible hemodynamic effects have been advocated. Sodium nitroprusside and phentolamine are examples; the hemodynamic effects are usually reversed within 5 to 10 minutes after discontinuation of these drugs. Both drugs are used intravenously, and the initial dosage should be very low. When sodium nitroprusside is used, the initial dosage should not exceed 16 μg/min. If there is no significant decrease in PCWP and arterial pressure or increase in cardiac output, the dose is increased by 10 to 15 μg every 5 to 10 minutes until the hemodynamic response is adequate. At any dose level, if arterial pressure decreases markedly without significant decrease in PCWP or increase in cardiac output, the therapy should be discontinued. If phentolamine is used (this use of phentolamine is not stated in the manufacturer's official directive), the initial dose should not exceed 0.1 mg/min. Every 5 to 10 minutes, the dose may be increased by 0.1 mg/min up to 2 mg/min.

COMPLICATIONS OF VASODILATOR THERAPY
Several complications may be associated with vasodilator therapy. (1) Unexpected, sudden significant hypotension may occur; in such circumstances,

therapy should be discontinued temporarily, and the legs should be elevated. (2) When nitroprusside is used for more than 2 weeks, hypothyroidism may be induced. (3) Involuntary muscular twitching and even frank convulsions may occur. (4) Hiccups, the mechanism of which remains unexplained, may occur in some patients. (5) Cardiac output may not increase; indeed, it may decrease if there is a marked decrease in LVFP. In such patients, the dose of the vasodilator should be adjusted to maintain the PCWP or PADP between 14 and 18 mm Hg. (6) Cyanide poisoning, thiocyanate toxicity, and methemoglobinuria are rare complications of nitroprusside therapy. During prolonged nitroprusside therapy, particularly in patients with renal failure, serum levels of thiocyanate should be monitored. The toxic concentration of thiocyanate is approximately 12 mg/100 ml.

ROLE OF DIURETICS IN THE MANAGEMENT OF PUMP FAILURE

Potent diuretics such as furosemide are helpful in reducing pulmonary venous congestion. Intravenous furosemide decreases pulmonary venous pressure in 5 to 10 minutes, even before there is any significant increase in urinary output. This early reduction is related to increased peripheral venous capacitance. Potent diuretics should be used cautiously, because they may induce marked and rapid diuresis, with precipitation of hypovolemic shock. Furthermore, associated urinary potassium loss may enhance ventricular irritability. A single intravenous dose of 20 mg of furosemide should be tried initially. Diuretics, although they decrease pulmonary congestion, do not increase cardiac output. Therefore, in the presence of low cardiac output, diuretics alone are not effective.

COMBINATION INOTROPIC AND VASODILATOR THERAPY

Beneficial hemodynamic effects of vasodilators can add to the beneficial effects of inotropic agents. If a vasodilator agent such as sodium nitroprusside or phentolamine does not improve left ventricular failure appreciably, an inotropic agent such as dopamine or dobutamine may be added. This combination therapy may prove particularly beneficial in patients with severe pump failure associated with hypotension. In such patients, dopamine or dobutamine infusion should be started and then a vasodilator drug (nitroprusside or phentolamine) added.

MECHANICAL CIRCULATORY ASSISTANCE AND PUMP FAILURE

The two major objectives of circulatory assistance are (1) to increase arterial pressure during diastole (diastolic augmentation) to maintain or enhance coronary artery perfusion pressure, and (2) to decrease preejection and ejection pressures (systolic unloading) to reduce myocardial work and oxygen demand.

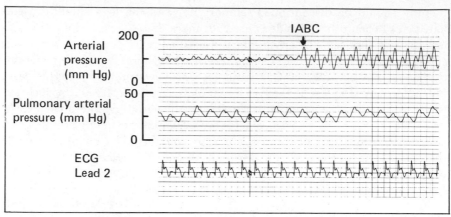

FIGURE 10-6. Intra-aortic balloon counterpulsation (IABC). Balloon is inflated at beginning of diastole to increase diastolic perfusion pressure (diastolic augmentation) and is deflated just before opening of aortic valve (sink, or systolic unloading).

In clinical practice to date, most experience has been gained with the use of intra-aortic balloon devices (Fig. 10-6). Although an improvement in hemodynamics and reversal of shock syndrome have been demonstrated in patients with severe pump failure and cardiogenic shock, the ultimate prognosis has not significantly improved. However, in the presence of severe hypotension (diastolic arterial pressure less than 50 mm Hg) when vasodilator agents cannot be used, circulatory assistance may be the only therapy that can be offered. Circulatory assistance may also be used in conjunction with vasodilator therapy to maintain arterial diastolic pressure. Furthermore, if cardiac catheterization and surgical therapy are indicated, circulatory assistance may be used to stabilize the hemodynamic and clinical states.

The indications for circulatory assistance are as follows: (1) cardiogenic shock secondary to myocardial infarction or myocardial depression following cardiac surgery; (2) acute heart failure refractory to medical therapy; and (3) recurrent life-threatening ventricular arrhythmias unresponsive to pharmacologic agents and artificial pacing.

The contraindications to circulatory assistance are irreversible brain damage, chronic end-stage heart disease, severe associated disease, and incompetent aortic valve.

SURGERY AND PUMP FAILURE
The role of surgical therapy in the management of pump failure and cardiogenic shock is controversial, and such therapy is still in the experimental stage. Aortocoronary artery bypass surgery provides supplementary chan-

nels of blood supply to the ischemic myocardium. Coronary artery bypass surgery with or without infarctectomy has been attempted to revascularize the ischemic myocardium in the peri-infarction zone. It has been hoped that by such revascularization the function of the ischemic myocardium can be significantly restored and pump failure can be reversed. Although some success has been reported, the surgical mortality remains extremely high. Furthermore, if the shock syndrome persists for more than 8 hours, the surgical mortality is virtually 100 percent. The time required for the hemodynamic and angiographic studies that are prerequisites for surgery usually exceeds 8 hours, and therefore the prospect of successful surgery is extremely limited.

CORRECTION OF CONTRIBUTING FACTORS IN PUMP FAILURE

ACID-Base IMBALANCE

Hypoxia, acidosis, and electrolyte imbalance, such as hyperkalemia, not only precipitate but also perpetuate pump failure. Frequent determinations of arterial blood gases and serum electrolytes are mandatory for the proper management of pump failure. Intubation and artificial ventilation should not be delayed if the usual methods of oxygen administration fail to correct hypoxia. Metabolic acidosis should be corrected with intravenous administration of sodium bicarbonate (44–132 mEq, then repeated if required to keep the arterial pH above 7.35).

ARRHYTHMIAS

In some patients, persistent sinus bradycardia and atrioventricular (AV) block or dissociation with relatively slow ventricular response may precipitate or perpetuate severe pump failure. It is desirable in such cases to increase heart rate to an optimal level. Sinus bradycardia can usually be corrected by intravenous atropine sulfate (0.6 mg initial dose; this can be repeated until 1–2 mg have been given), but it should be administered cautiously, because a sudden and rapid ventricular response may enhance ventricular irritability by increasing myocardial oxygen demand. Similarly, isoproterenol may enhance ischemia and ventricular arrhythmias and therefore should be avoided. Atrial pacing in such circumstances may be a safer method of elevation of heart rate. In the presence of AV block, however, ventricular pacing is needed. For management of severe pump failure associated with AV block, ventricular pacing alone may not adequately improve cardiac output. Atrioventricular sequential pacing may in some instances significantly improve cardiac output and should be attempted.

MECHANICAL DEFECTS AND PUMP FAILURE

Severe mitral regurgitation due to papillary muscle infarction and ventricular septal rupture, although uncommon complications of acute myocardial

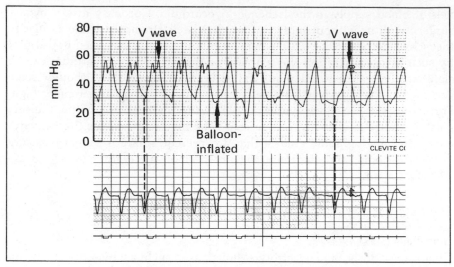

FIGURE 10-7. Diagnosis of mitral regurgitation at the bedside. Note giant v wave in pressure tracing with pulmonary artery occluded and unoccluded.

infarction (occurring in 1–2% of cases), may precipitate severe pump failure and cardiogenic shock despite the presence of a relatively small infarct. Prompt diagnosis and immediate therapeutic intervention are essential. Clinical differentiation between mitral regurgitation and ventricular septal rupture is often difficult. Bedside hemodynamic monitoring with the use of balloon flotation (Swan-Ganz) catheters resolves the difficulty in diagnosis. The presence of giant v waves in the PCWP tracing indicates mitral regurgitation (Fig. 10-7); significantly higher oxygen saturation in the pulmonary artery blood as compared with right atrial blood confirms the diagnosis of ventricular septal rupture (Fig. 10-8).

Pump failure caused by severe acute mitral regurgitation or ventricular septal rupture carries an immediate mortality of 85 to 100 percent. These lesions are potentially surgically correctable, and surgical repair should therefore be considered. In patients with recent myocardial infarction, surgical mortality is extremely high if surgery is performed within 2 weeks of the onset of infarction. The longer surgical therapy can be deferred, the better the expected results.

Unfortunately, it is hardly ever possible to prevent progressive clinical and hemodynamic deterioration with conventional therapy (e.g., digitalis, diuretics). Reduction in systemic vascular resistance by the use of phentolamine or sodium nitroprusside in patients with mitral regurgitation sometimes can improve forward flow and decrease the severity of mitral regurgitation. Similarly, with the use of vasodilators, the magnitude of left-to-right shunt can be decreased by decreasing the ratio of systemic to pul-

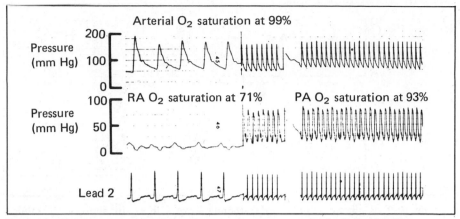

FIGURE 10-8. Diagnosis of ventricular septal rupture at the bedside. Higher oxygen saturation in pulmonary artery (PA) blood as compared with that in right atrial (RA) blood confirms the diagnosis.

monary vascular resistance. Intra-aortic balloon counterpulsation can also improve pump failure in the presence of mechanical defects. Therefore, vasodilator therapy, or circulatory assistance, or both, should be promptly instituted, and surgical therapy should be deferred as long as possible. If, however, hemodynamic and clinical deterioration continues despite vasodilator and circulatory assistance therapy, surgery should be attempted.

RIGHT VENTRICULAR INFARCT
Massive right ventricular infarct as a predominant cause of severe pump failure occurs in less than 7 percent of patients with acute infarction; inferior or posterior myocardial infarction is usually associated with it. The clinical presentation is that of severe right ventricular failure with little or no evidence of left ventricular failure. Hemodynamic monitoring may be useful in the diagnosis, and the hemodynamic picture is characterized by markedly elevated right atrial and right ventricular end-diastolic pressures with normal or reduced right ventricular systolic pressure, reduced or normal pulmonary artery systolic pressure, and normal or only slightly elevated PCWP (Fig. 10-9). Owing to markedly reduced right ventricular output, left ventricular filling pressure becomes inadequate, and left ventricular output therefore decreases.

Volume expansion therapy with administration of intravenous fluids to maintain adequate left ventricular filling pressure and its output despite elevated CVP has been successful in some patients. Vasodilator therapy may improve right ventricular output and therefore left ventricular filling pressure and has also been successful. Appropriate therapy with hemodynamic monitoring improves the prognosis.

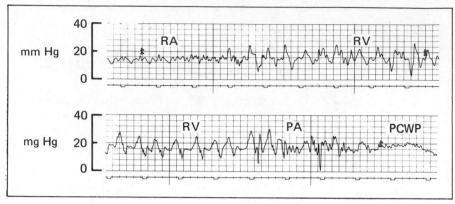

FIGURE 10-9. Right ventricular infarct and pump failure. In appropriate clinical set-up, high right atrial (RA) pressure, markedly elevated right ventricular (RV) end-diastolic pressure with low or normal RV systolic pressure, and normal pulmonary capillary wedge pressure (PCWP) suggest right ventricular infarct.

SUGGESTED APPROACH TO THE TREATMENT OF PUMP FAILURE AND CARDIOGENIC SHOCK AFTER ACUTE MYOCARDIAL INFARCTION

The following guidelines to the therapy of pump failure and cardiogenic shock following acute myocardial infarction are suggested:

1. Monitoring of pulmonary artery diastolic pressure or PCWP and arterial pressure should be instituted; monitoring of cardiac output is desirable whenever possible.
2. Acidosis, hypoxia, and dysrhythmias, if present, should be promptly corrected.
3. Volume expansion with intravenous fluids should be tried if PADP or PCWP is less than 14 mm Hg.
4. Vasodilator therapy, with or without diuretics and with proper hemodynamic monitoring, should be started if the left ventricular filling pressure is high (PADP or PCWP > 18 mm Hg). Normotension and mild to moderate hypotension are not contraindications to the judicious use of vasodilator agents.
5. In the presence of severe hypotension (arterial diastolic pressure < 50 mm Hg), mechanical circulatory assistance with or without vasodilator therapy should be tried.
6. If facilities for mechanical circulatory assistance are not available and if severe hypotension is present, vasopressor agents, including dopamine, may be used, but the results are likely to be unrewarding.
7. When the aforementioned therapeutic measures fail, more heroic measures may be attempted, such as myocardial revascularization with or without infarctectomy.

Other measures that may be used include the administration of morphine, oxygen, and aminophyllin.

Morphine should be used during the acute stage to reduce anxiety and tachypnea. The dose is 10 to 15 mg every 4 to 6 hours. It should be used with great caution in patients with chronic lung disease. A decrease in peripheral and systemic vascular resistance and peripheral venous pooling effect may be the underlying mechanisms of action.

Oxygen (100%) should be given, preferably through positive-pressure breathing apparatus. The value of bubbling oxygen through antifoaming agents (50% ethyl alcohol, propylene glycol, or 2-ethylhexanol) to decrease the respiratory obstruction resulting from the mechanical interference of edema fluid is not yet proved.

If pulmonary edema is associated with severe bronchospasm, intravenous aminophyllin (500 mg) given very slowly (over 15 min) may be tried every 4 hours. However, it should be used cautiously because of its tendency to induce tachyarrhythmias.

CARDIAC TAMPONADE

DIAGNOSIS

Cardiac tamponade is another form of acute heart failure caused by markedly increased intrapericardial pressure. Increased intrapericardial pressure restricts diastolic filling of the heart and causes a marked decrease in cardiac output. Cardiac tamponade may occur with a major or minor pericardial effusion. Rising jugular venous pressure, increasing tachycardia, falling blood pressure with pulsus paradoxus (inspiratory decrease in systolic blood pressure of more than 10 mm Hg) strongly suggest tamponade in a patient with suspected or known pericardial effusion.

Determination of right atrial, right ventricular, pulmonary artery, and pulmonary capillary wedge pressures is sometimes useful for confirmation of the diagnosis; in tamponade, right atrial and ventricular diastolic pressure, PADP, and PCWP are all equal. Hemodynamic monitoring is also useful for assessing the results of therapy.

PERICARDIOCENTESIS

Treatment of cardiac tamponade is specific: removal of the pericardial fluid, or pericardium, or both.

PROCEDURE

For closed pericardiocentesis, the following equipment should be available: 5- and 50-ml syringes; 14-, 18-, and 20-gauge needles (3 in. in length with short bevels); three-way sterile stopcock; rubber connecting tubing; sterile alligator clamps; and an ECG machine and defibrillation equipment. Premedication is usually not required. Pericardiocentesis should be performed with the patient elevated at 60 degrees and with proper aseptic technique.

After administering local anesthesia to the skin and subcutaneous tissue of the selected area, a 20-gauge needle is connected to a 50-ml syringe through a three-way stopcock. The V lead to the ECG machine is then connected to the shank of the needle through the alligator clamp (the ECG machine must be properly grounded). The ECG is monitored continuously. The needle is slowly advanced, without sudden movement and with intermittent gentle suction. Fluid is usually encountered at a depth of 3 to 4 cm with these approaches. Epicardial contact is marked by premature beats or S–T or P–R segment elevation, and the needle is then drawn back. After the presence and depth of fluid has been ascertained, a larger needle may be substituted, and polyethylene catheters may be placed in the pericardial cavity.

POTENTIAL SITES FOR CLOSED PERICARDIOCENTESIS
The potential sites for closed pericardiocentesis are as follows:

1. Subxiphoid. The needle is inserted directly inward at the left xiphocostal angle to the level of the inner rib cage and directed at about a 30-degree angle superiorly, posteriorly, and toward the left shoulder.
2. Apical. The needle is inserted in the fifth intercostal space about 2 to 3 cm lateral to the apex beat, or just inside the left border of cardiac dullness.
3. Left sternal border. The potential site is the fifth or sixth intercostal space, and the needle is directed medially.
4. Right-sided approach. If the effusion appears to be mainly on the right, one can insert the needle in the fourth intercostal space just inside the right border of cardiac dullness, directing the needle slightly medially.

POSSIBLE COMPLICATIONS OF CLOSED PERICARDIOCENTESIS
The possible complications of closed pericardiocentesis include entry into a cardiac chamber; arrhythmia; damage to the coronary artery, liver, stomach, or lungs; subepicardial hematoma; and infection from contamination. When bloody fluid is aspirated, rapid hematocrit determinations should be done to identify the source of the fluid. It should also be observed whether or not the fluid clots easily; pericardial fluid usually does not clot. The location of the catheter can also be determined by monitoring the pressure. If ventricular pressure is recorded, the catheter should be withdrawn.

THERAPY OF ACUTE HEART FAILURE OWING TO SEVERE SYSTEMIC HYPERTENSION

A sudden large increase in arterial blood pressure may precipitate left ventricular failure and acute pulmonary edema by increasing the resistance to left ventricular ejection and thereby decreasing stroke volume and increasing end-diastolic volume and pressure. The treatment of hypertensive heart failure and pulmonary edema is no different from the usual treatment of heart failure and pulmonary edema from any cause—namely, administration of oxygen, morphine, diuretics, and digitalis and use of rotating tourniquets and phlebotomy. One additional therapy that is important in the management of such patients is to attempt to decrease arterial pressure.

The diastolic arterial pressure may occasionally exceed 140 mm Hg in some of these patients. Blood pressure can be reduced rapidly with the use of diazoxide, phentolamine, trimethaphan, or nitroprusside.

DIAZOXIDE
Diazoxide (Hyperstat) is given intravenously in 300-mg doses as a bolus in a 10- to 15-second period. If only a slight reduction in arterial pressure occurs, or if the reduction is brief, i.e., 30 to 60 minutes instead of 8 to 9 hours, additional doses of 150 to 300 mg should be administered every 15 to 30 minutes until the desired effect is achieved and maintained. Because diazoxide tends to retain sodium, it should be combined with diuretics. Administration of phentolamine and nitroprusside has been described previously.

TRIMETHAPHAN
Trimethaphan camphor sulfonate (Arfonad), a tertiary amine ganglionic blocking agent, is administered in concentrations of 0.1 to 1.0 mg/ml intravenously at a rate of 3.0 to 4.0 mg/min. Hypotension is achieved within minutes, and blood pressure rises rapidly after discontinuation of the drug.

If the clinical situation is less acute, reserpine given intramuscularly (1- to 3-mg doses every 2–12 hr) or methyldopa (Aldomet) given intravenously (250–500 mg every 8 to 12 hr) may be used. Once the acute hypertensive crisis is under control, oral antihypertensive therapy should be instituted.

PUMP FAILURE SECONDARY TO BACTERIAL ENDOCARDITIS
Bacterial endocarditis may precipitate rapid and severe cardiac decompensation from valvular regurgitation. In addition to appropriate antibiotics to eradicate the infective organisms, antifailure drugs (digitalis and diuretics) should be started. In patients with severe mitral or aortic regurgitation associated with left ventricular failure, vasodilator agents (sodium nitroprusside, phentolamine, nitrates, or hydralazine) may improve cardiac function, and the signs and symptoms of heart failure may be controlled. There is, therefore, a potential role for vasodilator agents in addition to conventional antifailure treatment to tide the patient over a critical period until infection is under control. However, if heart failure cannot be controlled with pharmacologic agents, valve replacement should be considered, even in the presence of infection.

SELECTED READINGS
Abrams, E., et al.   Variability in response to norepinephrine in acute myocardial infarction. *Am. J. Cardiol.* 32:919, 1973.

Bezdek, W., et al.   Myocardial metabolic effect of ouabain in acute myocardial infarction (AMI). *Circulation* 46 (Suppl. 2):113, 1972.

Chatterjee, K., et al.   Beneficial effects of vasodilator agents in severe mitral re-gurgitation due to dysfunction of subvalvar apparatus. *Circulation* 48:684, 1973.

Chatterjee, K., et al.   Hemodynamic and metabolic responses to vasodilator ther-apy in acute myocardial infarction. *Circulation* 48:1183, 1973.

Chatterjee, K., and Parmley, W. W.   Vasodilator therapy in heart failure. *Prog. Cardiovasc. Dis.* 19:301, 1977.

Chatterjee, K., and Swan, H. J. C.   Hemodynamic profile of acute myocardial in-farction. In E. Corday and H. J. C. Swan (eds.), *Myocardial Infarction.* Baltimore: Williams & Wilkins, 1973. P. 51.

Cohn, J. N., et al.   Right ventricular infarction. Clinical and hemodynamic fea-tures. *Am. J. Cardiol.* 33:209, 1974.

Crexells, C., et al.   Optimal level of filling pressure in the left side of the heart in acute myocardial infarction. *N. Engl. J. Med.* 289:1263, 1973.

Dikshit, K., et al.   Renal and extrarenal hemodynamic effects of furosemide in congestive heart failure after acute myocardial infarction. *N. Engl. J. Med.* 288:1087, 1973.

Franciosa, J. A., et al.   Improved left ventricular function during nitroprusside infusion in acute infarction. *Lancet* 1:650, 1972.

Ganz, W., et al.   A new technique for measurement of cardiac output by thermo-dilution in man. *Am. J. Cardiol.* 27:392, 1971.

Goldberg, L. I., et al.   Newer catecholamines for treatment of heart failure and shock: An update on dopamine and a first look at dobutamine. *Prog. Cardio-vasc. Dis.* 19:327, 1977.

Lejemtel, T. H., et al.   Amrinone: A new non-glycoside, non-adrenergic car-diotonic agent effective in the treatment of intractable myocardial failure in man. *Circulation* 59:1098, 1979.

Mueller, H. S., et al.   Effect of dopamine on hemodynamics and myocardial metabolism in shock following acute myocardial infarction in man. *Circula-tion* 57:361, 1978.

Parmley, W. W., and Chatterjee, K.   Vasodilator therapy. *Curr. Probs. Cardiol.,* Vol. II, No. 12, 1978.

Sanders, C. A., et al.   Mechanical circulatory assist: Current status and expe-rience with combining circulatory assistance, emergency coronary angiog-raphy, and acute myocardial revascularization. *Circulation* 45:1292, 1972.

Swan, H. J. C., et al.   Catheterization of the heart with use of a flow-directed balloon-tipped catheter. *N. Engl. J. Med.* 283:447, 1970.

Walinsky, P., et al.   Enhanced left ventricular performance with phentolamine in acute myocardial infarction. *Am. J. Cardiol.* 33:37, 1974.

Joel D. Mittleman
Dwight L. Makoff

11. HYPERTENSION

Hypertension has traditionally been defined as an elevation of arterial pressure above 140 to 150/90 mm Hg. There is evidence, however, that no true cutoff point exists at which normal blood pressure proceeds to hypertension. Rather, there is a continuum of increasing systolic, diastolic, and thus mean blood pressure, which appears to represent ever-increasing risk factors in the development of target-organ damage. Hypertension is a proven risk factor for the development of atherosclerotic disease of the brain, kidney, and heart. Additionally, hypertension increases the workload on the heart and may lead to left ventricular hypertrophy and heart failure. Intracranial hemorrhage and aortic aneurysm dissection are more prone to develop in the setting of elevated blood pressure.

In approaching the critically ill hypertensive patient, it is important to consider the cause of the blood pressure elevation. Often, however, treatment must be instituted before a specific etiologic diagnosis can be made. Therapy should be selected based on the target-organs most prominently affected and the rapidity with which blood pressure control is required.

PATIENT EVALUATION

DIAGNOSIS

The diagnosis of a hypertensive disorder rests on the objective finding of an elevated systolic or diastolic blood pressure or both. A single blood pressure recording may be misleading because emotional factors may have a profound effect on the blood pressure of some people. Care must be taken to evaluate the blood pressure in both arms; proximal arterial stenosis may produce a spuriously lowered reading. A sphygmomanometer cuff with a bladder too short to encircle the arm may lead to erroneously elevated blood pressure recordings.

Isolated systolic hypertension occurs most frequently in elderly patients and reflects in part the lack of distensibility of vessels associated with the aging process. However, evidence indicates that systolic hypertension correlates independently from diastolic pressure with risks of stroke, ischemic heart disease, and congestive heart failure [17]. To what degree the risks associated with systolic hypertension can be lessened by antihypertensive therapy is uncertain. Any treatment offered to a patient with isolated systolic hypertension must be carefully monitored to avoid postural hypotension and cerebrovascular insufficiency.

CLINICAL STATUS

HISTORY

An attempt should be made in taking the history to establish the duration of hypertension, family history of hypertension, and presence of symptoms of disorders that cause hypertension. A statement should be included in the history noting when the pressure had last been normal, or whether or not the blood pressure had ever been measured previously. Age of onset of hypertension before 30 or after 55, as well as the absence of a family history of hypertension, increases the possibility of a secondary cause of blood pressure elevation.

Essential hypertension is best considered a disease with variable or no symptoms. Specifically, a history of headaches, epistaxis, or tinnitus has shown no relation to either systolic or diastolic blood pressure in a survey of a large number of adults [19].

VASCULAR EXAMINATION

Assessment of vascular damage caused by hypertension is a critical part of the patient examination. Funduscopic examination allows direct visualization of damage to small vessels. Narrowing of the arteriolar lumen correlates with the degree of hypertension. Hemorrhages, exudates, and papilledema reflect consequences of severe hypertension.

Larger vessels should be evaluated by careful palpation and auscultation of pulses, with particular emphasis on lower-extremity vessels and carotid arteries. Patients with significant cerebrovascular disease may not tolerate the postural drop in blood pressure that may be induced by certain medications. A bruit may be heard over the abdomen of patients with renovascular hypertension.

CARDIAC STATUS

Careful history and physical examination, electrocardiogram (ECG), and chest x-ray are crucial in every hypertensive patient to evaluate heart disease. Both coronary artery disease and left ventricular hypertrophy or failure are complications related to hypertension that may be detected by these means. Prominent left ventricular impulse, loud aortic component of the second heart sound, and S_4 gallop are cardiac findings that should be expected in severe hypertension.

RENAL ASSESSMENT

Hypertension can produce renal disease if it is sustained or severe. Conversely, intrinsic renal disease often produces hypertension: It is important to establish by history if the patient had hypertension prior to the development of renal disease. A patient who has had proteinuria, abnormal urine sediment, or azotemia before the onset of elevated blood pressure has intrinsic renal disease with secondary hypertension. Urinalysis and serum creatinine are the two most useful screening tests for renal disease.

BLOOD PRESSURE CONTROL
DETERMINANTS OF ARTERIAL PRESSURE AND ORGAN PERFUSION
Blood pressure is the product of the cardiac output times the mean arterial resistance. Cardiac output is determined by diastolic filling and intrinsic myocardial factors. Certain hypertensive states are associated with an increased cardiac output. Peripheral resistance is a function of arteriolar tone, which is influenced by neural, humoral, and intrinsic blood vessel factors. Stroke volume and arterial compliance affect mainly systolic blood pressure, whereas the state of arteriolar tone determines mainly diastolic blood pressure. Blood flow to an organ will be determined not only by the perfusion pressure, but also by the vascular resistance in that organ. In states in which there is a high peripheral vascular resistance in an organ due to increased vascular tone or pathologic fixed blood vessel narrowing, the arterial pressure must be high to perfuse the organ adequately.

RENAL FACTORS
The kidneys play a key role in blood pressure control by virtue of the release of certain humoral factors as well as through intrarenal mechanisms that are important in regulation of body fluid volume. Normally, sodium reabsorption in the proximal and distal renal tubules is regulated to maintain an optimal total extracellular fluid volume. Proximal tubular sodium reabsorption varies with the state of the effective arterial volume and is controlled by the distribution of blood flow within the kidneys, renal interstitial pressure, plasma protein concentration, and possibly a humoral factor or factors. Distal tubular sodium handling is controlled through the renin-angiotensin-aldosterone system, which itself is also intricately involved in the regulation of blood pressure.

In normal persons, a fall in pressure at the afferent glomerular arteriole will ultimately lead to release from the juxtaglomerular apparatus of renin, which activates two mechanisms that will serve to help restore blood pressure: (1) generation of angiotensin II, a potent vasoconstrictor, and (2) secretion of aldosterone, a mineralocorticoid which promotes sodium retention. Disturbances in sodium balance or alterations in the renin-angiotensin-aldosterone system may have a profound effect on blood pressure. Other, less well understood renal mechanisms involved in blood pressure regulation are control of the level of extrarenal pressor substances and renal production of a vasodilator substance, possibly a prostaglandin, present in high concentrations in the renal medulla (see Fig. 11-1).

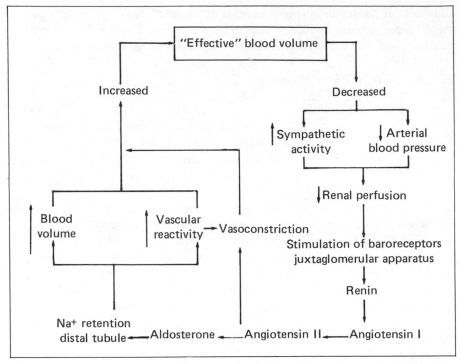

FIGURE 11-1. Renin-angiotensin-aldosterone system. "Effective" blood volume refers to intravascular volume as sensed by kidneys.

NEUROGENIC FACTORS

The autonomic nervous system is intimately involved with blood pressure regulation. Baroreceptors in the carotid sinus and aorta as well as stretch receptors in the cardiac atria and great veins provide information to the medulla in the brain about circulatory dynamics. Efferent sympathetic discharge controls constriction of resistance and capacitance vessels, cardiac output, and even the release of hormones such as catecholamines from the adrenal gland and renin from the kidney.

Despite the clear role of the autonomic nervous system in normal blood pressure regulation, a precise role for disordered nervous system regulation in most hypertensive states has not been found. It has been argued, however, that some patients labeled as having essential hypertension in fact have neurogenic hypertension [4]. These patients are characterized by adrenergic cardiovascular excitement with increased heart rate, cardiac index, total peripheral resistance, and shortened preejection index. Plasma norepinephrine concentration in this group is high, although not so high as characteristically seen in association with pheochromocytoma.

PRIMARY VASCULAR FACTORS

Intrinsic characteristics of the blood vessels themselves are important in blood pressure control because of their influence on peripheral vascular resistance. The capacitance of the vascular tree is reduced as a consequence of aging, and this reduced distensibility of vessels will tend to cause an elevation of blood pressure. Although pressor substances tend to increase vasomotor tone, the responsiveness of the vessels to these substances is variable and not completely understood. One factor that seems to alter reactivity of vessel walls is the sodium and water content of the vessel wall itself.

MISCELLANEOUS HUMORAL FACTORS

Glucocorticoid is necessary for normal function of the neurocirculatory homeostatic mechanisms. Hypotension occurs in instances in which there is primary glucocorticoid deficiency. Glucocorticoid excess, such as in Cushing's syndrome and adrenocorticotropic hormone (ACTH)–secreting tumors, is often associated with hypertension. Adrenal mineralocorticoids, primarily aldosterone, are needed for the maintenance of normal sodium balance. Hypertension secondary to mineralocorticoid excess occurs in primary aldosteronism due to an adrenal adenoma or hyperplasia, or to 11-hydroxylase or 17-α-hydroxylase deficiency.

Androgens, estrogens, and progesterone-like compounds may affect blood pressure through changes in sodium balance. Furthermore, estrogens may increase renin substrate and cause hypertension.

Although acromegaly may be associated with some increase in blood pressure, the role of growth hormone in blood pressure control has not been well studied. Parathyroid hormone has not been implicated as a regulator of blood pressure; however, ionized plasma calcium is of importance. Hypercalcemia is often associated with an increase in blood pressure. This is thought to represent either a direct effect of calcium on vascular smooth muscle or possibly a result of renin release stimulated by hypercalcemia.

THE CAUSES OF HYPERTENSION

Table 11-1 lists the causes of hypertension. Although the majority of patients with hypertension have what has been termed essential hypertension, the secondary causes of hypertension must be considered in each patient. A decision regarding what studies to perform in a particular patient will be dependent on the patient's age, the presence of target-organ damage, the severity of hypertension, at times the response to medical therapy, and clues from the history and physical examination regarding the possibility of a secondary cause of hypertension. It is beyond the scope of this chapter to discuss the tests to be performed to exclude all such causes.

TABLE 11-1. Causes of Hypertension

Essential hypertension
Renal hypertension
  Intrinsic renal disease
  Renovascular disease
  Renin-producing tumor
Adrenocorticoid hypertension
  Primary hyperaldosteronism
    Adrenal adenoma
    Bilateral adrenal cortical hyperplasia
  Cushing's syndrome
  Mineralocorticoid excess due to enzyme defects
    11-hydroxylase deficiency
    17-α-hydroxylase deficiency
Pheochromocytoma
Coarctation of the aorta
Toxemia of pregnancy
Oral contraceptives
Hypercalcemia

THERAPEUTIC CONSIDERATIONS IN HYPERTENSION
GOALS OF THERAPY
The treatment of the patient with hypertension who does not have immediate complications is aimed at maintaining a sustained lowering of blood pressure to prevent the long-term cardiovascular consequences of uncontrolled hypertension. Because of limitations in the medical therapy of hypertension, often it is not possible to normalize blood pressure in all positions and under all circumstances. One should attempt, however, to maintain a diastolic blood pressure less than 90 to 100 mm Hg in the standing position. Therapy can generally be initiated on an ambulatory basis unless a hypertensive emergency exists. The latter requires hospitalization and often initiation of therapy with parenterally administered agents.

RENIN PROFILE
Plasma renin activity (PRA) can be stimulated in normal individuals by low salt diet, upright posture, or diuretic drug administration. When patients with essential hypertension are compared with normal individuals after a standardized protocol of PRA stimulation, it is possible to identify low-, normal-, and high-renin essential hypertensives [10]. The mechanism accounting for hypertension may be different among these groups, although there may well be heterogeneity within the various groups.

There is no convincing evidence at present that renin has prognostic value or is a risk factor for end-organ complications independently of the degree of hypertension. Furthermore, renin profiling appears to be of limited value in guiding therapy by predicting response to various antihypertensive drugs [21]. For these reasons, empiric antihypertensive therapy in essential hypertension remains an acceptable standard of care.

PRACTICAL THERAPEUTIC PRINCIPLES

The patient with routine essential hypertension should be treated with the smallest dose of the fewest drugs possible to control blood pressure. The use of drug combinations in which small doses of each drug are used has rationale if side-effects are minimized by limiting the drug dose. In addition, one drug may enhance the action of another by blocking compensatory mechanisms that would otherwise come into play to limit blood pressure control. Consideration should be given to drug cost and convenience of administration, which are important factors in compliance to a long-term drug therapy program.

A stepped-care approach to empiric antihypertensive therapy has been developed by the Joint National Committee on Detection, Evaluation, and Treatment of High Blood Pressure [7]. The reader is referred to the report of this committee for a specific outline of an empiric approach to outpatient antihypertensive therapy that allows considerable individualization of the treatment plan.

HYPERTENSIVE EMERGENCIES

DEFINITION

Hypertensive emergencies include hypertensive encephalopathy, malignant hypertension, acute dissecting aneurysm of the aorta, hemorrhagic stroke, toxemia of pregnancy, and acute pulmonary edema associated with hypertension. Diastolic blood pressure sustained above 140 to 150 mm Hg carries an unacceptable risk, and therefore generally warrants urgent treatment even in the absence of symptoms. In any of these conditions, rapid lowering of blood pressure, often with the use of parenteral medications, may be needed (see Table 11-2).

ENCEPHALOPATHY

Hypertensive encephalopathy is a syndrome of diffuse cerebral dysfunction characterized by headache, somnolence, and sometimes coma and convulsions. Localizing sensory or motor defects may occur, but by definition they will be fleeting rather than fixed. Ultimately the diagnosis is confirmed by return to normal neurologic status after blood pressure is controlled.

Cerebral vessels normally are able to autoregulate by constriction to maintain blood flow constant; when blood pressure rises, cerebrovascular resistance rises. At some point, however, autoregulation fails as blood pressure rises and vasoconstriction cannot be maintained. Hyperperfusion

TABLE 11-2. Pharmacologic Agents for Parenteral Therapy of Hypertensive Crisis

| Drugs | Dosage | | | Onset of Action | Side-effects |
| | Intramuscular | Intravenous | | | |
		Single Dose	Continuous Infusion		
Direct vasodilators					
Hydralazine	10–50 mg q 2–6 hr	10–50 mg q 2–6 hr	100 mg/L 50–400 µg/min	IM: 30 min IV: 10 min	Tachycardia, flushing, headache, aggravation of angina
Sodium nitroprusside			50–200 mg/L 20–400 µg/min	Immediate	Sweating, muscular twitching, anxiety, thiocyanate intoxication
Diazoxide		50–300 mg (rapidly) q 3–10 hr		3–5 min	Tachycardia, flushing, nausea, aggravation of angina, hyperglycemia
Sympathetic blocking agents					
Ganglionic blockade					
Trimethaphan			1 gm/L 3–4 mg/min	IV: 5–10 min	Dry mouth, mydriasis, ileus, urinary retention
Selective sympathetic blockade					
Reserpine	0.5–5.0 mg q 4–12 hr			1–3 hr	Drowsiness, parkinsonism, unpredictable hypotensive response, peptic ulceration
Methyldopa		250–1,000 mg q 4–8 hr		2–3 hr	Drowsiness
Diuretics					
Furosemide	20–80 mg	20–200 mg q 4–6 hr		15–30 min	Electrolyte imbalance, hearing disturbances with large doses, volume depletion, hyperuricemia
Ethacrynic acid		50–100 mg q 4–6 hr		15–30 min	

occurs and results in cerebral edema. Initially this occurs in localized areas, but later it becomes diffuse and produces global cerebral dysfunction.

Chronically hypertensive individuals develop hypertrophy of arteriolar walls and are better able to autoregulate cerebrovascular resistance as blood pressure rises [16]. For this reason, hypertensive encephalopathy is more likely to develop in acutely hypertensive individuals and may appear at levels of blood pressure well tolerated by chronic hypertensives. Acute glomerulonephritis, toxemia of pregnancy, and ingestion of tyramine-containing foods by individuals taking monoamine oxidase inhibitors are three hypertensive disorders arising acutely in previously normotensive individuals that are frequently associated with encephalopathy.

MALIGNANT HYPERTENSION
Malignant hypertension is a clinical diagnosis made when severely elevated blood pressure, virtually always in excess of 125 to 135 mm Hg diastolic, has caused acute hypertensive retinopathy manifest by hemorrhages, exudates, and papilledema. Renal end-organ involvement with azotemia, proteinuria, and hematuria or central nervous system involvement with hypertensive encephalopathy may coexist. A semantic distinction may be made and the disorder termed *accelerated hypertension* when papilledema is absent but other features are present. The pathologic and clinical features are perhaps best considered as a continuum [8].

Hypertension of any etiology, either essential or secondary, may enter into an accelerated or malignant phase. Essential hypertension is the most common underlying disorder. Once a malignant phase is entered, the hypertension is self-perpetuating and will be fatal if not treated.

The pathologic hallmark of malignant hypertension is fibrinoid necrosis of arterioles. In addition, proliferative endarteritis may be seen. This characteristically affects afferent arterioles in the kidney and leads to glomerular obsolescence. Plasma renin activity is commonly elevated in malignant hypertension, sometimes to very high levels. The renin-angiotensin system may perpetuate the hypertension; however, activation of this system does not appear to be necessary to initiate malignant hypertension. Aldosterone levels are high, and hypokalemia often results.

Clinically, patients with malignant hypertension are likely to have pulmonary edema from high cardiac afterload. Neurological manifestations may be prominent. In some patients, oliguric renal failure with uremia may be present when the patient is seen initially. Microangiopathic hemolytic anemia related to microvascular disease is often present and may contribute to the renal failure.

Therapy of hypertensive encephalopathy and malignant hypertension is urgent blood pressure reduction to prevent life-threatening complications. Blood pressure need not be reduced to normal levels initially to control end-organ involvement. Anecdotal reports of stroke and myocardial infarction associated with blood pressure reduction below systolic pressures of 130 mm Hg suggest that reduction in blood pressure to the range of 150 to 160/100 mm Hg may be an appropriate goal for the first several days [15]. Nitroprusside is the agent most likely to rapidly achieve blood pressure control with least side-effects when facilities for continuous monitoring are present. Diazoxide has been used widely with success for malignant hypertension and encephalopathy and has the advantage of allowing treatment without requirements for continuous blood pressure monitoring. However, as discussed below, it has inherent risks related to its mode of action that make it an unacceptable drug in some clinical situations.

Some patients with accelerated hypertension who are asymptomatic and do not have the picture of rapid deterioration may be at greater risk from overly aggressive antihypertensive therapy than from immediate hypertensive complications. If a 12- to 24-hour delay in achieving blood pressure control is an acceptable risk, patients may be begun initially on other, less potent agents, such as parenteral or oral hydralazine combined with a β-adrenergic blocking agent. If adequate blood pressure control is not achieved within the specified time, then nitroprusside therapy may be instituted.

Because hypertensive patients retain sodium when blood pressure is reduced, diuretics are generally necessary adjuncts in drug therapy. In patients with malignant hypertension who have edema from heart or renal failure at the time of presentation, diuresis with a rapid-acting potent diuretic such as furosemide may be essential to normalize expanded plasma volume so that blood pressure can be controlled. There appears to be, however, a subset of patients with malignant hypertension who are characterized by intravascular volume depletion, probably related to augmented renal sodium excretion induced by severe systemic hypertension. These patients may have high plasma renin activity and may have tachycardia, postural hypotension, and signs of enhanced sympathetic tone (diaphoresis, tremor). Diuretic administration may actually make hypertension more difficult to control in these patients, presumably because further renin release and sympathetic stimulation are produced.

Renal function must be evaluated at the onset of therapy and followed very carefully. As blood pressure is lowered, there may be a decrease in renal function. At times, the impairment will be transient and improvement in renal function will occur as blood pressure is maintained under control. Dialysis may be needed transiently or permanently after blood pressure reduction, but overall patient survival is promoted by maintenance of controlled blood pressure [20].

Infrequently, bilateral nephrectomy must be undertaken in patients with end-stage renal failure because it is impossible to control the blood pressure until the kidneys are removed. The existence of this situation can generally be documented by finding markedly elevated plasma renin activity. Minoxidil is a vasodilator of extreme potency that offers a medical alternative to bilateral nephrectomy in some cases [14].

ACUTE DISSECTING ANEURYSM OF THE AORTA

Emergency medical treatment of dissecting aneurysm of the aorta is based on the objective of reducing blood pressure to diminish pulsatile forces within the aorta while maintaining perfusion to vital organs [11]. When clinical features suggest acute aortic dissection, aortography is required to confirm the diagnosis.

When the diagnosis is established, the decision regarding medical versus surgical management must take into account the success rate of surgical intervention in the institution in which the operation is to be done. In many centers, surgical therapy is carried out for acute dissection when there are no medical contraindications and when the origin of the dissection can be identified by angiography. Surgical therapy must, of course, be undertaken when there is acute aortic insufficiency, rupture of the aneurysm, or occlusion of a vital artery. Furthermore, surgical management appears to be more satisfactory than medical treatment when the dissection is in the proximal aorta just distal to the aortic valve. In distal dissection beyond the origin of the left subclavian artery, the results of medical and surgical therapy appear to be about the same.

Medical therapy is indicated for patients who are not suitable candidates for surgery because of advanced age or superimposed medical illness, particularly chronic obstructive pulmonary disease. Furthermore, if the dissection began more than 2 weeks before the patient is first seen, the therapy will often be pharmacologic lowering of blood pressure.

Drug therapy is initiated with continuous infusion of an agent that will lower systolic blood pressure to 90 to 130 mm Hg and diastolic blood pressure to 60 to 80 mm Hg. This can be done satisfactorily in most patients by continuous infusion of trimethaphan or sodium nitroprusside. Coincident with the beginning of titration of blood pressure by continuous infusion, the patient should be started on oral agents that can be used for long-term reduction in the blood pressure. Agents that reduce cardiac output and thus the propulsive forces of cardiac contraction are favored in the therapy of this condition. Among the pharmacologic agents for suitable therapy are parenteral reserpine, methyldopa orally or intravenously, propranolol, and oral guanethidine.

STROKE

Patients with severe hypertension who have markedly lateralizing, fixed neurologic signs usually have cerebrovascular thrombosis or intracranial hemorrhage rather than hypertensive encephalopathy. In both circumstances blood pressure reduction must be undertaken carefully.

Cerebrovascular thrombosis appears to impair cerebral blood flow autoregulation. Thus, hypertension may lead to hyperperfusion and cerebral edema, while systemic hypotension could enhance ischemic damage. The Clinical Management Study Group [2] suggests reduction of systolic pressure to no lower than 160 mm Hg as a reasonable goal in thrombotic stroke. Hydralazine is a useful drug in this situation since it does not decrease cardiac output and thus does not decrease cerebral blood flow. As an additional benefit, it does not cause sedation. Nitroprusside is an appropriate drug when precise blood pressure titration is needed. Sympatholytic agents such as trimethaphan or guanethidine are contraindicated because they reduce cerebral blood flow.

Both intracerebral hemorrhage and ruptured intracranial aneurysm are more likely to occur in the setting of hypertension. However, raised intracranial pressure from hemorrhage may lead to reflex hypertension. It is possible that to some extent this is a protective mechanism to restore blood flow. The optimal blood pressure in such clinical circumstances has not been defined. The Clinical Management Study Group has recommended a 20 to 30 percent reduction in systolic blood pressure in the setting of intracranial hemorrhage in patients with a systolic blood pressure greater than 200 mm Hg. Patients with less severe hypertension should have blood pressure reduced toward a goal of 160/100 mm Hg [2].

TOXEMIA OF PREGNANCY

Hypertension may complicate pregnancy and increase perinatal mortality. Women with underlying hypertension as well as those with chronic renal disease are susceptible to marked worsening of hypertension associated with pregnancy. Some women, particularly primigravidas, may develop toxemia of pregnancy in the last trimester characterized by hypertension and proteinuria. The disorder may progress to oliguria, neuromuscular irritability, and convulsions (eclampsia). The precise pathogenesis is unknown, although relative uteroplacental hypoperfusion is believed to be involved.

Toxemia is treated in the hospital with bed rest; magnesium sulfate may be useful in reducing neuromuscular irritability. Drug therapy is needed to counter the intense vasoconstriction if blood pressure does not fall steadily with bed rest alone. Hydralazine is the drug most frequently used in this setting. Diazoxide has been used in resistant cases. Ganglionic blockers may reduce uterine blood flow as well as produce meconium ileus in the fetus and are thus contraindicated. Because of depletion of effective intravascular volume in toxemia as well as evidence of adverse effects on placental circulation, diuretics are generally not recommended in modern obstetrical practice. Hypertension in toxemia resolves when the uterus is evacuated. Patients ill with toxemia with diastolic pressures greater than 100 mm Hg who fail to improve with drug therapy after 24 hours should have pregnancy terminated. If blood pressure and proteinuria improve with drug therapy in the hospital, it may be possible to allow gestation to continue to term.

ACUTE PULMONARY EDEMA
Although the initial therapy of pulmonary edema in the patient with an elevated blood pressure should continue to be the use of tourniquets, morphine, intermittent positive-pressure breathing, diuretics, and at times digitalization, there will occasionally be a place for reduction in arterial pressure. Frequently, improvement in pulmonary edema following the onset of diuresis will be accompanied by a prompt reduction in blood pressure. However, when blood pressure remains elevated, reducing the afterload by reducing diastolic blood pressure may be effective in improving the acute left heart failure. The drug of choice for prompt reduction in blood pressure in these instances is intravenous sodium nitroprusside. This drug has the additional advantage of reducing cardiac preload because of its effect on venous capacitance vessels.

ANTIHYPERTENSIVE DRUGS
Following is a discussion of the main antihypertensive drugs (see Table 11-3).

SODIUM NITROPRUSSIDE
Sodium nitroprusside (Nipride) has many characteristics that make it an ideal drug for hypertensive emergencies [12]. The drug acts specifically to relax vascular smooth muscle in arterial resistance as well as venous capacitance beds. It is direct acting and not mediated by the nervous system, so neither sedation nor ganglionic blockade occur. Its onset of action is within 1 to 2 minutes, and the effect of the drug disappears rapidly when infusion is discontinued. For this reason careful dosage titration—ideally, guided by direct intra-arterial pressure monitoring—is essential. With remarkable predictability, blood pressure of any magnitude can be titrated to the desired level at the desired rate.

Nitroprusside has been used with success in the treatment of malignant hypertension and hypertensive encephalopathy. Since both cardiac preload and afterload are reduced, the drug is useful in acute pulmonary edema with or without myocardial infarction when hypertension is present. Since it does not result in reflex cardiac stimulation, nitroprusside has an advantage over other direct acting vasodilators in this setting. Combined with propranolol to achieve myocardial depression, nitroprusside has been used successfully in the medical management of acute aortic dissection.

Dosage
The drug is available as a powder that can be diluted with sterile dextrose in water. The usual rate of infusion varies from 0.5 to 8 μg/kg/min. Pa-

TABLE 11-3. Pharmacologic Agents Commonly Used for Oral Therapy of Hypertension

Drug	Daily Dosage (mg)	Onset of Action	Duration of Action	Clinical Usefulness
Diuretics				
Hydrochlor-thiazide	25–100	2 hr	6–12 hr	Useful as initial therapy and in combination with other agents. All thiazide diuretics have equal antihypertensive potency.
Furosemide	20–400	30 min	6–8 hr	Potent agents that reduce intravascular volume. Useful to control sodium retention in hypertensive patients resulting from other agents, or from heart or kidney disease.
Ethacrynic acid	50–200	30 min	6–8 hr	
Spironolactone	25–400	2–3 days	18–20 hr	Major clinical usefulness is to minimize potassium loss produced by other diuretics. Contraindicated in renal failure.
Triamterene	100–200	Within 24 hr	6–12 hr	
Methyldopa	500–3,000	3–5 hr	8–12 hr	Effect additive to diuretic. Minimal effect on cardiac output. Useful in renal failure.
Hydralazine	40–400	1–3 hr	6–8 hr	Increases cardiac output. Better tolerated and more effective when combined with β blocking agent.
Propranolol	40–480	1 hr	8–12 hr	Useful alone or with diuretic in mild-to-moderate hypertension.
Metoprolol	50–450	1 hr	12 hr	In combination with vasodilator, useful in moderate-to-severe hypertension. Well tolerated in asthma or heart failure.

Table 11-3. (*Continued*)

Drug	Daily Dosage (mg)	Onset of Action	Duration of Action	Clinical Usefulness
Reserpine	0.1–0.25	3–6 days	2–6 wk	Useful in small doses in combination with a diuretic in patients not optimally controlled with diuretic alone. Risk of side-effects limits use at a higher dosage.
Clonidine	0.2–2.4	1 hr	12–24 hr	Usefulness similar to methyldopa. Can be combined with diuretic, β blocking agent, and vasodilator in resistant hypertension.
Guanethidine	10–125	48–72 hr	10 days	Small doses combined with a diuretic may be well tolerated in some patients with mild-to-moderate hypertension; free from sedative effect. Potent in higher doses, but limited by orthostasis.
Prazocin	3–20	1 hr	8–12 hr	Vasodilator free of reflex cardiac stimulation. Efficacy similar to that of hydralazine when used with β blocking agent.

tients on other antihypertensive agents may be very sensitive to the antihypertensive action of nitroprusside.

Prolonged administration of sodium nitroprusside can result in the accumulation of thiocyanate formed in the liver from cyanide liberated by the interaction of nitroprusside with sulfhydryl groups in red cells and tissue proteins. Nausea, fatigue, muscle twitching, and disorientation have occurred in association with elevated thiocyanate levels. If the drug is to be continued beyond 3 days, or if renal function is impaired, serum thiocyanate levels should be monitored. The drug should be discontinued if levels exceed 10 to 12 mg per 100 ml. A case of hypothyroidism associated with long-term nitroprusside administration has been reported.

DIAZOXIDE

Diazoxide (Hyperstat) is a nondiuretic thiazide derivative that is a potent, rapid-acting vasodilator [9]. Almost instantly after intravenous injection, arterial pressure falls rapidly to normal. Hypotensive overshoot is rare. Blood pressure may remain depressed for as long as 5 hours after a single dose. The subsequent rise in blood pressure is gradual and predictable.

Diazoxide acts directly on arteriolar smooth muscle to reduce vascular resistance. The drug has little effect on venous capacitance vessels and does not impair cardiovascular autonomic reflexes. Thus, the baroreceptors are activated as pressure falls, and a reflex increase occurs in heart rate, cardiac output, and left ventricular ejection velocity.

Hypertensive emergencies, including hypertensive encephalopathy, have been treated with diazoxide. The advantage of rapid action without the requirement for constant patient monitoring after treatment may be a tactical consideration in some situations. The drug should not be used in the treatment of aortic dissection or intracranial hemorrhage because of the danger of augmented mechanical shearing forces induced by the reflex cardiac response. Since the drug does not reduce cardiac preload, it is less useful than nitroprusside for the treatment of pulmonary edema associated with severe hypertension. Angina and myocardial infarction have been precipitated with diazoxide, presumably related either to increased myocardial oxygen demands resulting from reflex cardiac stimulation or to decreased coronary perfusion from abrupt blood pressure reduction. The drug should not be used in the setting of ischemic heart disease.

Dosage

The drug is given with the patient supine, usually as a bolus of 300 mg over a 10- to 30-second period. Mini-bolusing with doses of 50 to 100 mg until the desired effect is achieved may be safer than giving a full 300 mg in a single large bolus. Because diazoxide binds readily to plasma proteins, rapid injection produces higher levels of free drug to reach and activate arteriolar receptors. The drug loses effectiveness when given at slower infusion rates.

Side-Effects

Diazoxide will cause severe pain and cellulitis if extravasated during rapid injection. In addition to potential adverse effects related to rapid blood pressure lowering and cardiac stimulation, the drug commonly produces hyperglycemia and hyperuricemia. Renal sodium retention occurs with the drug; loop-acting diuretics such as furosemide are indicated when the drug is used.

HYDRALAZINE

Hydralazine (Apresoline) is a direct vasodilator which acts on smooth muscle in arterial resistance vessels. To a much lesser extent, it affects venous capacitance vessels. As peripheral resistance falls, reflex sympathetic stimulation occurs through activation of baroreceptor mechanisms. The resultant increase in cardiac output to some extent diminishes the antihypertensive action of the drug. When combined with a β-adrenergic blocking agent to control cardiac stimulation, the usefulness of hydralazine increases.

Blood flow to vital organs is not decreased by hydralazine. This makes the drug useful in the treatment of hypertension complicated by renal failure or vascular insufficiency, e.g., mesenteric insufficiency. It is particularly useful in toxemia of pregnancy, which, as discussed above, is thought to be related to uteroplacental ischemia. The tachycardia and increased velocity of cardiac contraction that occur with hydralazine limit the drug from use as sole therapy in patients with ischemic heart disease or acute aortic aneurysm dissection.

DOSAGE

When given orally, drug effect is usually observed within 1 hour. The initial oral dose of hydralazine is 30 to 40 mg per day in 2 divided doses. The dose can be titrated upward as needed. When given intramuscularly, drug levels can be titrated upward after an initial 10-mg dose in 10-mg increments at 2- to 4-hour intervals. In the past, the drug has been used by continuous intravenous administration, which requires constant monitoring, may lead to profound hypotension, or may fail adequately to lower blood pressure. Sodium nitroprusside appears to be preferable when continuous infusion therapy is desired.

SIDE-EFFECTS

Hydralazine used alone is limited by adverse effects. Throbbing headache, palpitations, and nausea may occur. These effects can be reduced by gradual upward titration of drug dosage and by concomitant administration of β-adrenergic blocking drugs.

Drug fever, skin rash, and peripheral neuropathy have been reported and appear more frequently with higher doses or in patients who are slow acetylators of the drug. Doses in excess of 300 to 400 mg per day sustained for several months have been associated with a lupuslike syndrome. Lupus erythematosus (LE) cells may appear in the blood, and an elevated antinuclear antibody titer may persist for several years. The syndrome is generally reversible when the drug is withdrawn, although resolution may be slow or require corticosteroid therapy.

METHYLDOPA

The antihypertensive action of methyldopa (Aldomet) was originally attributed to dopa decarboxylase inhibition, resulting in decreased norepinephrine stores at nerve terminals. This explanation has proved inadequate. Methyldopa appears to act by conversion in the central nervous system to

α-methylnorepinephrine, which exerts a direct α-sympathomimetic inhibitory action upon a brain stem vasomotor center. Blood pressure falls because of a decrease in peripheral vascular resistance. Renal perfusion is maintained. Cardiac output is not substantially affected. Plasma renin activity falls.

Use of methyldopa for hypertensive emergencies is limited by its sedative properties, delayed onset of action, and variable effectiveness. It is of use in settings where blood pressure control can safely be delayed for 4 or more hours and where drug-induced somnolence will not be confused with progression of an underlying neurologic condition. Relative freedom from adverse cardiac effects offers an advantage in the use of methyldopa in situations such as myocardial infarction.

DOSAGE
Gastrointestinal absorption of methyldopa varies. Maximal effects are seen 4 to 8 hours after an oral dose and within 4 hours after intravenous administration. The daily oral dose ranges from 500 to 3,000 mg given in divided doses. Patients with impaired renal function should be started on smaller doses, i.e., 250 to 500 mg daily, because of reduced clearance of the drug. Because of the fluid retention, refractoriness to methyldopa will often occur with continued use. For this reason, the drug should be administered with a diuretic agent.

SIDE-EFFECTS
Common side-effects are drowsiness, nasal congestion, and dry mouth. Less frequent reactions are Coombs' positive anemia, fever, hepatitis, and impotence.

β-ADRENERGIC BLOCKING AGENTS
Propranolol (Inderal) in low doses has a modest antihypertensive effect that can be correlated with the degree of renin suppression produced. At higher doses, blood pressure is lowered independently of changes in plasma renin activity by what is theorized to be a central nervous system effect [6]. In addition, β-adrenergic blockers allow utilization of vasodilators such as hydralazine and minoxidil at doses that might otherwise lead to intolerable symptoms related to reflex cardiac stimulation. By preventing a secondary rise in cardiac output, β-adrenergic blockers potentiate the antihypertensive effects of vasodilators.

Propranolol and metoprolol (Lopressor) are β-adrenergic blocking drugs currently available in the United States for clinical use. Metoprolol is more "cardioselective" than propranolol, causing less blockade of β-2-receptors of the bronchi and blood vessels. At doses necessary for treatment of hypertension, however, this advantage may be lost. The antihypertensive efficacy of the two drugs is similar.

DOSAGE

Propranolol can be initiated at doses of 40 mg per day and titrated upward to 480 mg per day in 2 or 3 divided doses if required. Metoprolol can be used in a daily dose of up to 450 mg.

SIDE-EFFECTS

Adverse effects of β-adrenergic blocking agents include symptomatic bradycardia. Congestive heart failure may be precipitated. Patients with decreased cardiac function in whom cardiac output is maintained by intense sympathetic tone are at the greatest risk for precipitation of congestive heart failure. Bronchospasm may occur even in those not previously diagnosed as asthmatic. Intermittent claudication may worsen in patients with peripheral vascular disease, presumably because of unopposed α-adrenergic vasoconstriction.

Mental depression, gastrointestinal disturbances, and Peyronie's disease have been reported with propranolol. The drug should be withdrawn gradually, since sudden withdrawal of propranolol has been reported to provoke angina pectoris in patients with ischemic heart disease.

GANGLIOPLEGIC AGENTS

Ganglioplegic drugs are potent antihypertensive agents, but their use is limited by side-effects. They reduce transmission of nerve impulses through the ganglia of the autonomic nervous system by interfering with the action of acetylcholine on the ganglionic cells. The major antihypertensive action of these drugs is to inhibit venous capacitance vessels from constricting and thus to reduce venous return. Cardiac output falls because sympathetic reflexes are blocked.

Unpleasant side-effects related to parasympathetic and sympathetic blockade have caused these drugs virtually to disappear from use in the treatment of chronic hypertension. The most rapidly acting ganglionic blocking agent, trimethaphan camsylate (Arfonad), has some use in certain acute settings. Because it reduces cardiac output, blood pressure, and cardiac contractility, it is useful as a single agent in the treatment of acute aortic dissection. Its use should never continue beyond several days.

DOSAGE

Trimethaphan camsylate is supplied in a 10-ml multidose vial containing 50 mg per ml. One vial should be diluted to 500 ml with 5% D/W to yield a concentration of 1 mg trimethaphan per ml. The solution should be administered intravenously at a rate of 3 to 4 mg per minute and titrated to achieve the desired drop in blood pressure. The onset of action is immediate, and the hypotensive effect of the drug disappears quickly when the infusion is discontinued. The blood pressure may fluctuate rapidly, so the rate of administration and blood pressure must be monitored constantly.

The patient should be placed in reverse Trendelenburg's position with the head of the bed on blocks to allow gravity to increase venous pooling.

SIDE-EFFECTS
Side-effects of autonomic blockade include dry mouth, blurred vision, constipation or paralytic ileus, impotence, and urinary retention.

CLONIDINE
Clonidine (Catapres) is a centrally acting drug of moderate potency available for oral administration. The drug appears to activate receptors in a cardiovascular control center in the medulla oblongata, resulting in a decrease in sympathetic neuronal stimulation of the heart, kidney, and peripheral vasculature [13]. Renin release is decreased because of depressed adrenergic tone to the juxtaglomerular apparatus through the renal nerves.

Clonidine has onset of action within 30 minutes after administration. It should be used with a diuretic agent to prevent fluid retention and loss of antihypertensive effectiveness. The action of clonidine is additive to that of a vasodilator and β-adrenergic blocking agent combination.

DOSAGE
Therapy with clonidine should be instituted with a low dose of 0.1 to 0.2 mg daily and increased slowly to minimized sedation. The maximum recommended daily dose is 2.4 mg.

SIDE-EFFECTS
Sedation and dry mouth are the major dose-related adverse effects of clonidine. Impotence and orthostatic hypotension occur with a frequency similar to that observed with methyldopa.

Patients should not abruptly discontinue clonidine therapy. Blood pressure may rise rapidly to pretreatment levels and possibly higher. A syndrome of adrenergic overactivity has been described after clonidine discontinuation. Its actual incidence is unknown. The syndrome can be treated by reinstitution of clonidine or by α-adrenergic blocking agents such as phentolamine. Clonidine is best avoided in unreliable patients. To prevent occurrence of this adrenergic overactivity in the perioperative period, clonidine should be withdrawn gradually prior to elective surgical procedures that will prohibit oral administration of clonidine.

GUANETHIDINE
Guanethidine (Ismelin) is taken up into the nerve endings and produces sympathetic blockade by depleting norepinephrine and also by blocking its release after nerve stimulation. Responsiveness of capacitance and resistance vessels is diminished. Venous return is reduced, and cardiac output is thus decreased. The effect on the venous capacitance vessels is responsible

for the orthostatic hypotension associated with guanethidine therapy. Sodium retention will occur with the drug and block its effectiveness unless plasma volume is regulated with a diuretic agent.

Guanethidine may be useful in patients with severe hypertension in combination with a diuretic and with a vasodilator and β-adrenergic blocking agent. In low doses the drug when combined with a diuretic may be well tolerated by patients with mild hypertension and provide the advantages of once daily dosage and freedom from psychic depression or sedation.

DOSAGE

Plasma concentrations of guanethidine at any given drug dosage vary a great deal from patient to patient because of complex drug metabolism. Drug dosage should be determined by titration. Because of a long half-life, patients with severe hypertension in whom blood pressure control is desired over a period of several days should receive a loading dose [22]. Outpatients with lesser degrees of hypertension may be started on 10 mg per day with increases at 2-week intervals. Doses of 60 mg or less per day may control patients with mild-to-moderate hypertension when given with a diuretic without disabling side-effects. Patients with severe hypertension may be treated with doses as high as 400 mg per day, although side-effects usually prevent administration of doses greater than 150 mg per day.

SIDE-EFFECTS

Common side-effects of guanethidine are orthostatic dizziness, syncope, failure to ejaculate, dry mouth, nasal stuffiness, and bradycardia. Azotemic patients may tolerate the drug poorly. Patients on tricyclic antidepressants or amphetamines will be resistant to guanethidine. Freedom from sedation, allergic reactions, and bone marrow or liver toxicity is a notable property of guanethidine.

RESERPINE

Reserpine depletes catecholamines from the sympathetic nerve endings, inhibits certain sympathetic reflexes, and lowers blood pressure. By acting primarily at postganglionic nerve endings, reserpine produces a selective blockade of the central nervous system without altering parasympathetic function. Reserpine may also deplete catecholamines and serotonin in the central nervous system. When given parenterally, it produces direct dilation of arterioles.

Reserpine may be effective in the treatment of mild hypertension, or it may be used in combination with other agents. Reserpine is sometimes given intramuscularly for the therapy of hypertensive emergencies. Administered by this route, the drug not only depletes catecholamines but also has a direct vasodilating effect on arterioles. However, the onset of action, effectiveness, and duration of effect of parenteral reserpine are unpredictable, and occasionally there may be a dramatic fall in blood pressure after very small doses. Since more predictable drugs are available for the treatment of hypertensive crisis, the value of parenteral reserpine is limited.

Dosage

Reserpine is the most potent of the rauwolfia alkaloids and the one most often used clinically. Reserpine should be started at a daily dose of 0.1 mg. The dosage may be increased slowly, but serious side-effects may be a problem at doses above 0.25 mg.

Reserpine may be used with a diuretic in the treatment of mild-to-moderate hypertension. It has the advantage of once-daily administration and low cost. When used parenterally, reserpine should be started at very low dosage, since hypotensive response may be marked at doses as small as 0.1 mg intramuscularly. The usual dose for control of hypertension is 2.5 to 5.0 mg initially, repeated every 4 to 12 hours as needed. In most instances, other parenterally administered agents are preferable in the treatment of hypertensive emergencies.

Side-Effects

The dose of reserpine is limited by the appearance of toxicity. The most dangerous complication of chronic reserpine administration is depression. Such effects are rare at daily doses of 0.25 mg or less. The risks of psychotic depression with suicide make use of higher dosages unjustified in the management of mild-to-moderate hypertension in view of the availability of other agents. Other side-effects include a tendency toward peptic ulceration, diarrhea, abdominal cramps, and nasal stuffiness. Most of these symptoms are related to sympathetic blockade with relative parasympathetic overactivity.

PRAZOCIN

Prazocin (Minipres) is a recently introduced quinazoline derivative that results in vasodilation through peripheral α-adrenergic blockade. Reflex tachycardia does not occur. Prazocin has been used in combination with a diuretic in mild-to-moderate hypertension. It has been used in association with a β-adrenergic blocking agent in more severe hypertension and has been shown to have an effectiveness similar to hydralazine in this role.

Dosage

To avoid a first-dose effect of syncope probably related to orthostatic hypotension, the drug should be initiated at a dose of 1 mg at a time when the patient can remain supine for at least 3 hours, e.g., bedtime. Dosage titration should be gradual to a maximum of 20 mg per day in 2 divided doses.

SIDE-EFFECTS
Postural hypotension with syncope, drowsiness, weakness, and anticholinergic effects may limit the use of prazocin. No rheumatologic syndromes have been reported with its use.

α-ADRENERGIC BLOCKING AGENTS

Phentolamine (Regitine) is an α-adrenergic blocker that is used in the treatment of hypertensive crisis in the setting of pheochromocytoma. It may also be useful in therapy of hypertensive crisis associated with tyramine ingestion in patients taking monoamine oxidase (MAO) inhibitors and in the hypertension of clonidine withdrawal.

The drug is given intravenously in a dose of 2 to 5 mg every 5 minutes until the blood pressure is controlled. The head of the bed should be elevated. If tachycardia produces symptoms, β-adrenergic blockers can be used. However, β-adrenergic blockers should not be used alone because blood pressure may become further elevated due to unopposed α-adrenergic vasoconstriction.

Phenoxybenzamine (Dibenzyline) can be given at a dose of 20 mg per day in 2 divided doses as an oral α-adrenergic blocker. Doses can be titrated upward slowly; the drug has a prolonged half-life and tends to accumulate. Phenoxybenzamine is used for the treatment of pheochromocytoma during stabilization for surgery or in patients with metastatic pheochromocytoma. It has limited usefulness in the treatment of patients with essential hypertension resistant to conventional therapy [5].

MINOXIDIL

Minoxidil is a potent oral vasodilator in the United States. It has a direct effect on smooth muscle of arterial resistance vessels. Cardiovascular reflexes are brought into play, and tachycardia and increased cardiac output occur.

Minoxidil is used in combination with propranolol for the treatment of severe hypertension refractory to conventional antihypertensive therapy. This combination will lead to vigorous sodium retention. Diuretics, generally furosemide, are required, sometimes in high doses. The potency of minoxidil exceeds that of hydralazine. In patients with renal disease and refractory hypertension, minoxidil may offer an alternative to bilateral nephrectomy [14]. Hirsutism is a troublesome adverse effect of the drug.

ANGIOTENSIN-CONVERTING ENZYME INHIBITORS

Both oral and intravenous agents that inhibit the enzyme that converts angiotensin I to angiotensin II are under clinical investigation. With the use of these agents peripheral resistance falls without significant changes in cardiac output and without tachycardia. Renal function may actually improve. There has been some use of converting enzyme inhibitors in patients with hypertensive emergencies [18].

DIURETICS

Diuretics are a firmly established component of the management of most hypertensive disorders. Diuretics are useful in the therapy of patients with mild-to-moderate hypertension and may suffice as single-agent therapy. Diuretics potentiate the effects of a variety of antihypertensive medications, including direct vasodilators, sympathetic blockers, and centrally acting drugs. In addition, diuretics can control sodium retention that occurs when blood pressure is reduced with other agents. Sodium retention of this type often leads to recurrence of hypertension after a period of initial blood pressure control.

There is some evidence that thiazide diuretics produce a decrease in peripheral vascular resistance. Interestingly, it is thought that the sodium content of the arteriolar wall may be a factor in determining vascular resistance. It may be that some of the effect diuretics have on peripheral vascular resistance is mediated by a decrease in the sodium content of the vessel wall. The major mode of action of diuretics in hypertensive emergencies, however, stems from the ability of these agents to reduce plasma volume.

Diuretics have their effect by interfering with reabsorption of filtered sodium. Thiazide diuretics work at a site in the distal tubule, the cortical diluting segment. Furosemide and ethacrynic acid are diuretics with action in the thick ascending limb of Henle's loop. They are of higher potency than thiazides and can be given intravenously. Aldosterone antagonists act on the distal nephron to inhibit the reabsorption of sodium and secretion of potassium and hydrogen ions. Since other factors can produce sodium retention even in the absence of aldosterone, agents acting in this segment of the nephron may lack sufficient potency.

Appropriate use of diuretics is an important skill in the management of hypertension, especially hypertensive emergencies. No predetermined dose of a diuretic may be invariably relied upon. The dose of each diuretic must be adjusted on the basis of underlying cardiac and renal function, sodium intake, and clinical evidence of hypervolemia. Assessment of the effect of the diuretic dose must be made by serial evaluation of edema, body weight, and orthostatic blood pressure change. Since significant plasma volume expansion may be present and may contribute to hypertension even in the absence of detectable edema, it may be necessary to augment diuretic dosage to achieve a negative sodium balance in a patient who appears refractory to antihypertensive therapy [3]. Observations must then be made to see if blood pressure control improves without the development of diuretic complications. If plasma volume is reduced excessively with diuretics, patients may develop weakness, orthostatic dizziness, and unacceptable degrees of azotemia. In some patients, blood pressure may actually become more labile because of stimulation of the renin-angiotensin system and catecholamines in response to the stress of volume depletion.

The thiazide diuretics all have a similar site of action and at equivalent natriuretic doses have equal antihypertensive action. At a daily dose of 100 mg of hydrochlorthiazide, the dose-response curve flattens and further dosage increase will add little to blood pressure control. Patients with diastolic blood pressures greater than 100 mm Hg will rarely be controlled with a thiazide diuretic alone.

Metalazone is a unique diuretic that retains its natriuretic potency even when renal function is significantly impaired.

The loop diuretics furosemide (Lasix) and ethacrynic acid (Edecrin) have considerable potency as natriuretic agents. Furosemide has the more linear dose-response curve of the two agents and can be titrated upward as needed to achieve the desired negative sodium balance even in patients who are refractory to thiazide diuretics or who have renal insufficiency. Because of their potency, inappropriate plasma volume depletion and prerenal azotemia may occur with loop diuretics. Although thiazide diuretics are preferred for routine use in uncomplicated essential hypertension, furosemide in doses of 20 to 200 mg may frequently be useful in the management of hypertensive emergencies.

Ototoxicity can occur with loop diuretics. High doses and rapid intravenous administration may predispose to hearing loss in some patients. The toxicity may be temporary, although with ethacrynic acid, permanent hearing loss has been reported. Allergic reactions of a hypersensitivity nature occur occasionally.

A variety of metabolic problems may develop with diuretic therapy. Hypokalemia occurs frequently. Symptomatic gout or asymptomatic hyperuricemia may occur during diuretic therapy. The thiazide diuretics may induce hyperglycemia. Another problem that has been seen with the various diuretic agents is hyponatremia related to a water excretion defect with inability to dilute the urine appropriately.

Spironolactone (Aldactone) may be successful in entirely correcting hypertension in primary hyperaldosteronism and in some metabolic disorders associated with mineralocorticoid excess. Its main use in the treatment of hypertensive states, however, is to control potassium wasting that can occur in association with the use of other diuretics. Spironolactone in doses up to 100 mg per day can be given for this purpose. It has a steroid nucleus, and estrogenic side-effects such as gynecomastia can occur with prolonged use. Triamterene (Dyrenium) is a nonsteroidal drug that blocks sodium reabsorption in the distal nephron independently of aldosterone. It can be used in a similar fashion in doses of 100 to 300 mg per day to control potassium loss caused by other diuretic agents. Fatal hyperkalemia can occur with either spironolactone or triamterene if given to patients with high potassium intake or with underlying renal failure.

REFERENCES

1. Chesley, L. C. *Hypertensive Disorders in Pregnancy.* New York: Appleton, 1978.
2. Clinical Management Study Group. Medical and surgical management of stroke. *Stroke* 4:273, 1973.
3. Dustan, H. P., et al. Dependence of arterial pressure on intravascular volume in treated hypertensive patients. *N. Engl. J. Med.* 286:861, 1972.
4. Esler, M. Mild high-renin essential hypertension. *N. Engl. J. Med.* 296:405, 1977.
5. Gifford, R. W., and Tarazi, R. C. Resistant hypertension: Diagnosis and management. *Ann. Intern. Med.* 88:661, 1978.
6. Hollifield, J. W., et al. Proposed mechanism of propranolol's antihypertensive action in essential hypertension. *N. Engl. J. Med.* 295:68, 1976.
7. Joint National Committee on Detection, Evaluation, and Treatment of High Blood Pressure. Report. *J.A.M.A.* 237:255, 1977.
8. Kaplan, N. M. *Clinical Hypertension.* Baltimore: Williams & Wilkins, 1978.
9. Koch-Weser, J. Drug therapy: Diazoxide. *N. Engl. J. Med.* 294:1271, 1976.
10. Laragh, J. H. Vasoconstrictor-volume analysis for understanding and treating hypertension: The use of renin and aldosterone profiles. *Am. J. Med.* 55: 261, 1973.
11. McFarland, J., et al. The medical treatment of dissecting aortic aneurysms. *N. Engl. J. Med.* 286:115, 1972.
12. Palmer, R. F., and Lasseter, K. C. Drug therapy: Sodium nitroprusside. *N. Engl. J. Med.* 292:294, 1975.
13. Pettinger, W. A. Drug therapy: Clonidine. *N. Engl. J. Med.* 293:1179, 1975.
14. Pettinger, W. A., and Mitchell, H. D. Minoxidil—an alternative to nephrectomy for refractory hypertension. *N. Engl. J. Med.* 289:167, 1973.
15. Richardson, D. W., and Raper, A. J. Management of complicated hypertension including hypertensive emergencies. In G. Onesti and A. N. Rest (Eds.), *Hypertension: Mechanisms, Diagnosis, and Treatment.* Philadelphia: Davis, 1978.
16. Strangaard, S., et al. Autoregulation of brain circulation in severe arterial hypertension. *Br. Med. J.* 1:507, 1973.
17. Tarazi, R. C. Clinical import of systolic hypertension. *Ann. Intern. Med.* 88:426, 1978.
18. Tifft, C. P., et al. Converting enzyme inhibitor in hypertensive emergencies. *Ann. Intern. Med.* 90:43, 1979.
19. Weiss, N. S. Relation of high blood pressure to headache, epistaxis, and selected other symptoms. *N. Engl. J. Med.* 287:631, 1972.
20. Woods, J. W., et al. Management of malignant hypertension complicated by renal insufficiency. *N. Engl. J. Med.* 291:10, 1974.
21. Woods, J. W., et al. Renin profiling in hypertension and its use in treatment with propranolol and chlorthalidone. *N. Engl. J. Med.* 294:1137, 1976.
22. Woosley, R. L., and Nies, A. S. Drug therapy: Guanethidine. *N. Engl. J. Med.* 295:1053, 1976.

William C. Shoemaker / 12. PATHO-PHYSIOLOGY AND THERAPY OF SHOCK STATES

Shock has been conveniently regarded as a low flow syndrome, since low cardiac output with high peripheral resistance is observed in both hemorrhagic and cardiogenic shock [5, 23]. According to this concept, therapy should be directed toward correction of the low cardiac output. However, the hemodynamic pattern of the anesthetized, exsanguinated dog and the patient with hypovolemic or myocardial infarction are not representative of most clinical shock syndromes [7, 10, 17, 24]. Further, shock is not a single entity to be treated properly by the principles of a simplified experimental model. Rather, shock is a complex group of syndromes with a wide variety of etiologic events; it is a stage in the pathways leading toward death from circulatory failure [10]. Physiologic changes vary as the syndromes evolve in time and are best described in terms of a sequential cardiorespiratory pattern which begins with the onset of the precipitating etiologic event, not when hypotension is recognized or when the patient is unresponsive to therapy. Therefore, it is incorrect both to characterize the shock states as a single disease entity in an oversimplified manner and to base therapy upon simplistic notions. In order to provide maximally effective therapy, it is essential to understand the natural history of the various shock syndromes and their pathophysiology. Shoemaker [10] has described the temporal cardiorespiratory patterns of shock following specific etiologic events—i.e., hemorrhage, trauma, sepsis, and cardiogenic causes—in order to understand the problems of patients with multiple circulatory problems.

PATHOPHYSIOLOGY

A systematic approach to pathophysiology was developed from the description of the common cardiorespiratory patterns that emerged from an analysis of over 10,000 sets of sequential cardiorespiratory measurements in 180 patients [9–21]. These data describe the natural history of various shock syndromes by serial cardiorespiratory events taken remote from therapy—i.e., before the therapy was given or after the immediate direct effects of therapy had worn off (Figs. 12-1–12-3).

The physiologic alterations were divided into early, middle, and late pe-

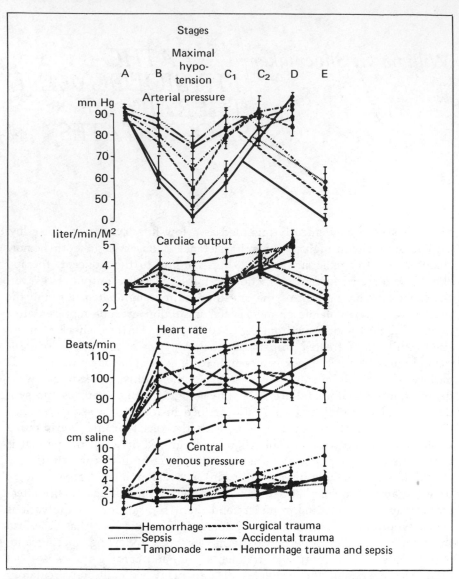

FIGURE 12-1. Serial hemodynamic changes at each temporal stage after various etiologic types of shock illustrating the sequential patterns. Means (dots) and standard error (SE) of the mean (vertical bars) are shown for mean arterial pressure, cardiac index, heart rate, and central venous pressure. Note the fall in cardiac index in the B and *low* stage after hemorrhagic shock and to a lesser extent after cardiac tamponade, while the cardiac index values of the other groups were normal or increased. Heart rates increased in all etiologic groups, but were greatest in the two groups with sepsis. The venous pressures were within the normal range except in the tamponade patients. (From W. C. Shoemaker and C. W. Bryan-Brown, Resuscitation and immediate care of the critically ill and injured patient. *Semin. Drug Treat.* 3:211, 1973. Reproduced by permission of Grune & Stratton.)

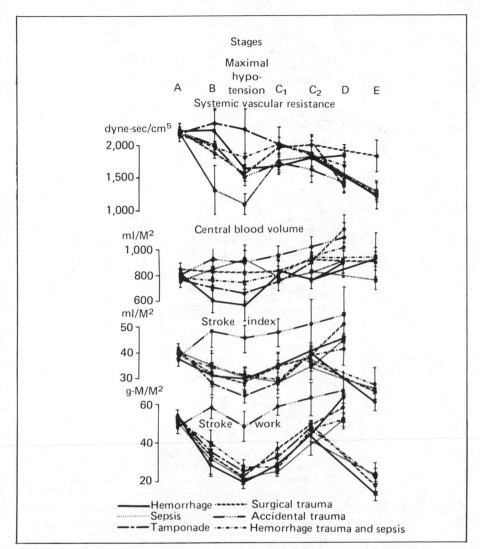

FIGURE 12-2. Sequential patterns of hemodynamic changes at each temporal stage for various etiologic types of shock showing systemic (peripheral) vascular resistance, central blood volume, stroke index, and left ventricular stroke work. Note the slight transient rise in peripheral resistance in the B stage after hemorrhage and tamponade and the subsequent progressive decrease with time in all categories. Also in the B and *low* stages of hemorrhage and tamponade patients, central blood volume values tended to be low, but the values of the other groups were normal or high. The stroke volume and stroke work increased progressively in accidental trauma, but these variables decreased in the B, *low*, and C_1 stages in the other groups. (From W. C. Shoemaker and C. W. Bryan-Brown, Resuscitation and immediate care of the critically ill and injured patient. *Semin. Drug Treat.* 3:211, 1973. Reproduced by permission of Grune & Stratton.)

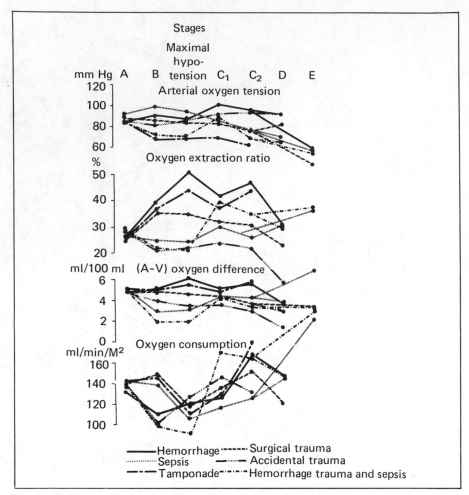

FIGURE 12-3. Sequential patterns in oxygen metabolism including arterial PO_2, oxygen extraction ratio, arteriovenous oxygen content difference and oxygen consumption after various etiologic types of shock. Note that PaO_2 values, although somewhat low, did not fall alarmingly until the late stages. The oxygen extraction ratios and to a lesser extent the $C(a-v)O_2$ rose in the hemorrhage and tamponade patients. The $C(a-v)O_2$ fell in the accidental trauma, sepsis, and hemorrhage-trauma-sepsis groups. Oxygen consumption fell in the early (B or *low* stage) period and rose in the middle periods in all groups. (From W. C. Shoemaker and C. W. Bryan-Brown, Resuscitation and immediate care of the critically ill and injured patient. *Semin. Drug Treat.* 3:211, 1973. Reproduced by permission of Grune & Stratton.)

riods by criteria of time and arterial pressure to analyze data from patients with different etiologic types of shock at comparable time periods. Criteria for staging are needed to analyze the data at comparable periods since physiologic events unfold at different rates of time and some patients go through their circulatory failure more rapidly than others [9–17]. The stages were defined as follows: stage A, the pre-illness control period; stage B, the initial period of falling arterial pressure immediately after the etiologic event; stage *low*, the lowest initial arterial pressure, which separates stage B from stage C, the middle period; stage C, divided into C_1 and C_2 by the point in time at which arterial pressure returns halfway to control values; stage D, the late or recovery period for surviving patients, started when arterial pressures return to control values; and stage E, the preterminal period in patients who subsequently died.

Physiologic mechanisms underlying the early cardiorespiratory events have pathogenic significance, while those of the late stage primarily reflect terminal mechanisms. Usually shock is first recognized by hypotension; by this time, however, the major pathophysiologic reactions have already occurred.

Cardiorespiratory measurements taken before, during, and after therapy were used to evaluate the effectiveness of therapy on the background of their natural physiologic history. The body's initial responses to different types of stress were quite variable, but within each etiologic category, the cardiorespiratory patterns were rather similar.

HEMORRHAGIC SHOCK

In the early period immediately after hemorrhage, the cardiorespiratory pattern usually consists of decreases in arterial pressure, cardiac output, central venous pressure (CVP), total blood volume, stroke volume, stroke work, oxygen delivery, and oxygen consumption ($\dot{V}O_2$), as well as increases in heart rate, systemic vascular resistance, arteriovenous oxygen content difference [$C(a\text{-}v)O_2$], and oxygen extraction (Figs. 12-1–12-3). The body's compensatory responses to hemorrhage consist of tachycardia, systemic and pulmonary metarteriolar vasoconstriction, and increased myocardial contractility [10].

With hypovolemia and low flow, the blood volume and flow are redistributed by metarteriolar vasomotor changes from increased sympathetic neural activity [10, 21]. This results in relatively greater percentages of blood flow to the heart and brain, but lesser flow to the kidney, gut, and skin [21]. Neural regulatory mechanisms also redistribute flow in the microcirculation within the various organs and tissues. When vasoconstriction is prolonged and intense, both flow and volume redistribution develop into maldistribution, the principal physiologic defect of shock states. The tissues extract oxygen more completely, because less blood is flowing more slowly; despite this compensation, the uneven flow results in inadequate tissue oxygenation and is manifest by reduced $\dot{V}O_2$. Metabolic acidosis occurs with hypovolemia and reduced blood flow; respiratory alkalosis is a compensatory mechanism to acidosis.

TRAUMATIC SHOCK

After acute injury, the early cardiorespiratory pattern usually consists of increased cardiac output, heart rate, central blood volume, stroke volume, stroke work, and oxygen delivery, as well as reduced arterial pressure, systemic vascular resistance, oxygen extraction, $C(a-v)O_2$, and $\dot{V}O_2$ (Figs.12-1–12-3). In essence, acute injury produces a generalized increase in autonomic neural activity; the latter stimulates the cardiac and respiratory centers of the brain to increase heart rates, myocardial contractility, and alveolar ventilation [10, 13, 15, 16]. When hypovolemia is not present, the stroke volume and cardiac output increase—the former because of myocardial stimulation, the latter because of increased stroke volume and heart rate. Ventilatory increases without hypovolemia produce respiratory alkalosis without antecedent acidosis.

The initial physiologic responses to the various types of trauma and hemorrhage are mediated primarily by neural mechanisms; that is, the generalized autonomic neural tone may stimulate cardiac and respiratory centers of the brain to increase cardiac and ventilatory drives [9, 10]. But the duration and magnitude of these effects depend on many factors. For example, the stimulation of cardiac function increases cardiac output after trauma and sepsis, but this response may be limited by hypovolemia and impaired myocardial function. Further, the cellular breakdown products of direct tissue injury increase metabolic needs for tissue repair, and metabolic influences intensify the high flow and low resistance.

SEPTIC SHOCK

The early cardiorespiratory pattern in sepsis consists of hypotension, tachycardia, and normal or high cardiac output as well as decreases in systemic vascular resistance, stroke volume, stroke work, $C(a-v)O_2$, and $\dot{V}O_2$. Subsequently, the $\dot{V}O_2$ further increases with the appearance of hyperthermia and hypermetabolism. The body's response to sepsis consists of stimulation of the heart rate, myocardial contractility, and ventilation by neural mechanisms [9, 10, 24]. When blood volume is not reduced by dehydration, cardiac index subsequently increases markedly as heart rate and myocardial contractility are stimulated. Increased respiratory drive produces hyperpnea, tachypnea, and respiratory alkalosis [10].

CARDIOGENIC SHOCK

The early cardiorespiratory pattern in cardiogenic shock consists of hypotension, tachycardia, high CVP, and decreases in cardiac output, stroke work, oxygen delivery, and $\dot{V}O_2$. In cardiogenic shock, increased neural activity produces tachycardia and increased vascular resistance in the early stages of about one-third of the cases. Increased CVP results from failure of the heart to keep up with the venous return, increased venomotor tone from neural mechanisms, and fluids given in excess or given too rapidly [10, 14].

COMMON PHYSIOLOGIC DEFECT OF SHOCK STATES

In summary, the common physiologic denominator in the early period of the various shock states prior to the initial hypotension is not *low flow*, but inadequate oxygen transport, usually from maldistributed flow. The striking physiologic response of the various etiologic types of shock is the body's stress response—i.e., increased cardiorespiratory function manifest by increased heart rate, myocardial contractility, and alveolar ventilation. The first two increase cardiac output unless there is reduced blood volume or reduced myocardial function.

The increased cardiorespiratory function may arise from: (a) stimulation of cardiac centers of the brain stem by the stress response, which produces a generalized increase in autonomic nervous system activity; (b) cellular breakdown products, hyperthermia, vasoactive peptides, metabolic end-products, and endotoxins; and (c) increased metabolic needs of the peripheral tissues. The increased metabolic requirements are reflected by increased oxygen delivery and $\dot{V}O_2$, which are seen in the middle (C_1 and C_2) stages of survivors and nonsurvivors as well as the late (D) stage of survivors [10, 17]. Metabolic acidosis occurs when hypovolemia and inadequate perfusion are present; respiratory alkalosis occurs when they are not.

GOALS OF THERAPY

The shock syndrome should be recognized as early as possible to achieve maximally effective therapy directed toward underlying pathophysiologic mechanisms. The normal hemodynamic values are not the optimal goals of therapy, since the compensatory bodily responses to stress, like the etiologic event of shock, also produce departures from the normal values. The major problem in the therapy of shock states is to define the therapeutic goals in terms of optimal physiologic criteria that result in reduced mortality and morbidity.

The cardiorespiratory patterns of survivors and nonsurvivors were described in a large series of critically ill patients subjected to major surgical procedures for life-threatening conditions [17]. The data obtained remote from therapy were analyzed by the conventional statistical approach (mean ± standard error of each variable) and by a nonparametric multivariate method to analyze differences in the distributions of survivors' and nonsurvivors' values for each variable (Fig. 12-4). This was done: (a) to define therapeutic goals from the patterns of the survivors, (b) to provide early warning of circulatory deterioration and death, (c) to evaluate the impor-

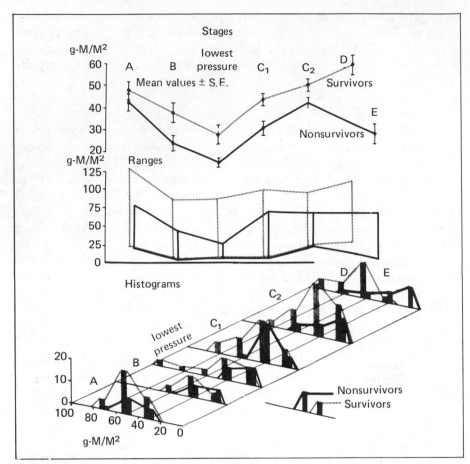

FIGURE 12-4. Sequential changes of survivors and nonsurvivors for a representative variable, left ventricular stroke work, by three different analyses: (1) (*upper section*) conventional statistics with mean and standard error of each group at each stage: (2) (*middle section*) ranges of each group at each stage; and (3) (*lower section*) histogram of frequency distributions of each group at each stage. (From W. C. Shoemaker et al., Physiologic patterns in surviving and nonsurviving shock patients. *Arch. Surg.* 106:630, 1973.)

tance and usefulness of each variable by its capacity to predict outcome, and (d) to evaluate the severity of illness by means of a predictive index that relates all the values of each variable to mortality [16].

The data of these variables are summarized in Table 12-1, and some of the methods for analysis of these data are illustrated in Figures 12-4 to 12-7 [19, 20]. In general, there were marked differences between the patterns of survivors and nonsurvivors, despite a wide variety of illness and operations. In the early period, cardiac index, left ventricular stroke work, systemic vascular resistance, hematocrit, blood volume, O_2 delivery, and $\dot{V}O_2$ were greater in the survivors. The mean arterial pressures, CVP, heart rate, wedge pressure, arterial oxygen tension (PaO_2), and mixed venous oxygen tension ($P\bar{v}O_2$) values of the two groups were not significantly different in the early period; these variables were poor predictors and therefore not very useful except as screening tests. In the early period, nonsurvivors had slightly higher pulmonary arterial pressures, markedly higher pulmonary vascular resistance, and lower pH, than did survivors [17].

Wide differences in the distribution of pulmonary vascular resistance, oxygen delivery, $\dot{V}O_2$, left and right ventricular stroke work, PCO_2, pH, and mean transit time made them useful as predictors even though no single variable was found to be capable of completely separating the groups.

The distributions of survivors' and nonsurvivors' values were compared and an algorithm developed which quantified the distance of each observed value of each cardiorespiratory variable from a single classification point that maximally separated the nonsurvivors' and survivors' values [19]. A predictive index was determined as the weighted average of all of these distances for all variables; this was found to be a reasonably sensitive, specific, and accurate predictor of outcome. It may be used to assess the severity of illness, to track the patient's cardiorespiratory status, and to evaluate the relative efficacy of alternate types of therapy.

The capacity of each cardiorespiratory variable to predict outcome correctly is a reasonable criterion of its biologic significance as well as its usefulness in clinical management. For example, if a variable is unable to differentiate the dying patient from the patient who survives, it may not be useful or relevant. However, if it is an excellent predictor of outcome, it may be related to essential pathophysiologic mechanisms and, therefore, a useful criterion for therapeutic decision-making. The percentages of correct predictions of outcome for each cardiorespiratory variable average over all stages are shown in Table 12-2. The poorest outcome predictors were frequently the commonly measured variables.

Table 12-3 lists the cardiorespiratory variables with the largest and smallest capability of predicting outcome at each stage expressed as the percentage of correct predictions. These percentages change, sometimes markedly, from stage to stage, indicating their stage-specificity. For example, pulmonary vascular resistance is a good predictor in the early stages (B, *low*), but not in the middle or late stages. Mean arterial pressure is a poor predictor in the early stages, but good in the late stages. Obviously, in the late stage, most variables predict outcome with a high degree of probability, but at this time clinical judgment also may be rather good so there is less need for prediction.

No one variable was entirely reliable as a predictor and no one problem was responsible for all postoperative deaths, since patients may succumb primarily from hypovolemia; cardiac, pulmonary, peripheral perfusion prob-

TABLE 12-1. Cardiorespiratory Variables

Variables	Abbreviations	Units	Measurements or Derived Calculations	Normal Values	Preferred Values
Volume-related					
Mean arterial pressure	MAP	mm Hg	Direct measurement	82–102	>84
Central venous pressure	CVP	cm H_2O	Direct measurement	1–9	<5
Central blood volume	CBV	ml/M^2	CBV = MTT × CI × 16.7	660–1,000	>925
Stroke index	SI	ml/M^2	SI = CI ÷ HR	30–50	>48
Hemoglobin	Hgb	gm/dl	Direct measurement	12–16	>12
Mean pulmonary arterial pressure	MPAP	mm Hg	Direct measurement	11–15	<19
Wedge pressure	WP	mm Hg	Direct measurement	0–12	>9.5
Blood volume	BV	ml/M^2	BV = PV ÷ (1 − Hct)[a] × surface area	men 2.74 women 2.37	>3.0 >2.7
Red cell mass	RCM	ml/M^2	RCM = BV − PV	men 1.1 women 0.95	>1.1 >0.95
Flow-related					
Cardiac index	CI	liter/min · M^2	Direct measurement	2.8–3.6	>4.5
Mean transit time	MTT	sec	Direct measurement	12–18	<13
Left ventricular stroke work	LVSW	g · M/M^2	LVSW = SI × MAP × .0144	44–68	>55
Left cardiac work	LCW	kg · M/M^2	LCW = CI × MAP × .0144	3–4.6	>5
Mean systolic ejection rate	MSER	ml/sec · M^2	MSER = SI ÷ duration of systole	580–980	>1,100
Tension time index	TTI	mm Hg · sec/cm	TTI = MAP × HR × duration of systole	270–470	>342
Right ventricular stroke work	RVSW	g · M/M^2	RVSW = SI × MPAP × .0144	4–8	>13
Right cardiac work	RCW	kg · M/M^2	RCW = CI × MPAP × .0144	0.4–0.6	>1.1
Stress-related					
Systemic vascular resistance	SVR	dyne · sec/cm^5 · M^2	SVR = 79.92 (MAP − CVP)[b] ÷ CI	1,760–2,600	<1,450

Parameter	Abbrev.	Units	Formula / Method	Normal range	
Pulmonary vascular resistance	PVR	dyne·sec/cm^5·M^2	PVR = 79.92 (MPAP − WP)[b] ÷ CI	45–225	<226
Heart rate	HR	beat/min	Direct measurement	72–88	<100
Rectal temperature	temp	°F	Direct measurement	97.8–98.6	>100.4
Oxygen-related					
Arterial hemoglobin saturation	SaO$_2$	%	Direct measurement	95–99	>95
Arterial CO$_2$ tension	PaCO$_2$	torr	Direct measurement	36–44	>30
Arterial pH	pH	...	Direct measurement	7.36–7.44	>7.47
Mixed venous O$_2$ tension	PvO$_2$	torr	Direct measurement	33–53	>36
Arterial-mixed venous O$_2$ content difference	C(a-v)O$_2$	ml/dl	C(a-v)O$_2$ = CaO$_2$ − C$\overline{v}$O$_2$	4–5.5	<3.5
O$_2$ delivery	O$_2$ deliv	ml/min·M^2	O$_2$ deliv = CaO$_2$ × CI × 10	520–720	>550
O$_2$ consumption	V̇O$_2$	ml/min·M^2	V̇O$_2$ = C(a-v)O$_2$ × CI × 10	100–180	>167
O$_2$ extraction rate	O$_2$ ext	%	O$_2$ ext = (CaO$_2$ − CvO$_2$) ÷ CaO$_2$	22–30	<31
Perfusion-related					
Red cell flow rate	RCFR	...	RCFR = CI × Hct	0.6–1.8	>1.3
Blood flow/volume ratio	BFVR	...	BFVR = CI ÷ BV	0.6–1.8	>1.7
O$_2$ transport/red cell mass ratio	OTRM	...	OTRM = V̇O$_2$ ÷ RCM	0.06–18	>0.25
Tissue O$_2$ extraction ratio	TOE	...	TOE = C(a-v)O$_2$ ÷ RCFR	1.8–6.6	>5.7
Efficiency of tissue O$_2$ extraction	ETOE	...	ETOE = C(a-v)O$_2$ ÷ RCM	0.06–18	>1.3
O$_2$ transport/red cell flow ratio	OTRF	...	OTRF = V̇O$_2$ ÷ RCFR	1–7	<3

[a] Hct corrected for packing fraction and large vessel hematocrit/total body hematocrit ratio.
[b] Venous pressures expressed in mm Hg.

Source: Reprinted with permission of Technicon Instruments Corporation, Tarrytown, New York.

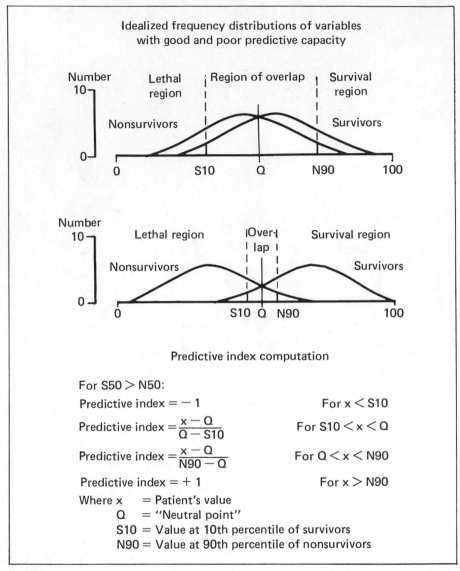

FIGURE 12-5. Idealized frequency distributions of survivors and nonsurvivors of a variable with wide overlap (*upper figure*) and with good separation (*lower figure*) showing the 10 percentile value of survivors (S_{10}), the 90 percentile value of non-survivors (N_{90}), and the classification point, Q, which maximally separates survivors and nonsurvivors. The algorithm for calculation of the predictive index is given at the lower section. (From W. C. Shoemaker et al., Cardiorespiratory monitoring in postoperative patients. *Crit. Care Med.* 7:237, 1979.)

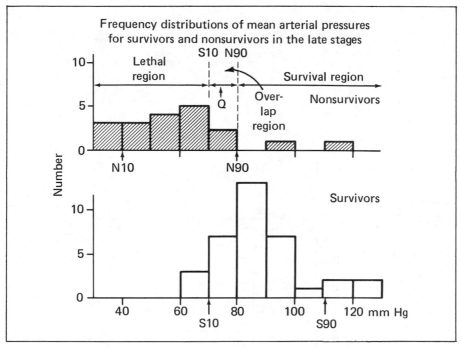

FIGURE 12-6. Frequency distributions of mean arterial pressures for nonsurvivors (*upper section*) and survivors (*lower section*) in the late (recovery) stage showing 10 and 90 percentile values for both groups. (From W. C. Shoemaker et al., Cardiorespiratory monitoring in postoperative patients. *Crit. Care Med.* 7:237, 1979.)

lems; shock; sepsis; or various combinations of these. In general, the perfusion-related variables were the best predictors, probably because they reflect interrelationships of oxygen transport with volume and flow. These perfusion variables represent not just oxygen transport, blood flow, or volume by themselves, since each of these was also assessed separately by individual variables. Rather, the perfusion variables express the interactions of oxygen transport per unit of red cell flow and red cell mass, and so on. These variables estimate the peripheral perfusion in shock, i.e., the adequacy of tissue oxygenation relative to flow and volume. On the basis of these data, we have proposed a tentative list of preferred or "optimal" therapeutic goals in terms of cardiorespiratory variables (Table 12-1).

The therapeutic implications of this analysis were integrated with data comparing and contrasting cardiorespiratory effects of various therapeutic agents, together with clinical experience in managing various types of shock and trauma states. The general principles are briefly reviewed below.

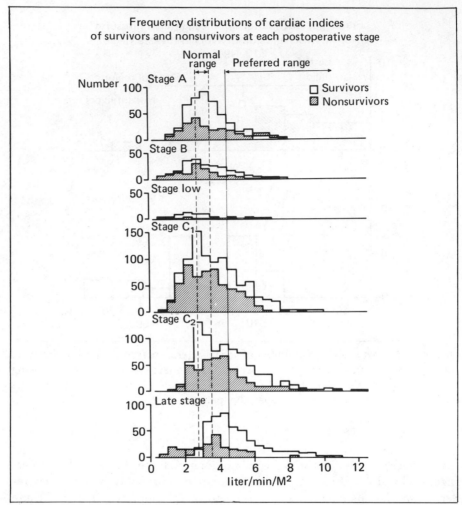

FIGURE 12-7. Frequency distributions of cardiac index values in the preoperative control period and at successive stages throughout the critical postoperative period in a series of high-risk surgical patients. Normal values are shown by the vertical dashed lines and the preferred range, represented by the median value of survivors in their late (recovery) stage. (From R. Bland et al., Physiologic monitoring goals for the critically ill patient. *Surg. Gynecol. Obstet.* 147:833, 1978. By permission of *Surgery, Gynecology & Obstetrics*.)

TABLE 12-2. Rank and Percentage of Correct Predictions for Each
Cardiorespiratory Variable Averaged over All Stages

Rank	Variable	% Correct	No. of Patient Stages*
1	ETOE	82	64
2	RCM	69	88
3	OTR	58	64
4	PVR	53	91
5	LCW	52	269
6	BVD	52	88
7	MAP	52	270
8	O_2 avail	51	178
9	BFVR	50	88
10	TOE	50	150
11	pH	47	178
12	LVSW	47	269
13	STTI	46	214
14	RCFR	43	175
15	MTT	42	221
16	OTRF	42	150
17	CI	40	270
18	RVSW	40	94
19	WP	39	95
20	$\dot{V}O_2$	38	175
21	$PaCO_2$	38	179
22	O_2 ext	37	174
23	RCW	37	94
24	$C(a-v)O_2$	36	174
25	PvO_2	35	175
26	MPAP	35	95
27	SaO_2	34	169
28	SI	34	269
29	MSER	31	214
30	Hgb	31	199
31	Temp	27	168
32	CVP	24	270
33	SVR	24	270
34	CBV	22	221
35	HR	19	269

* The number of patient stages is defined as the number of patients in whom the variable was measured during each stage; a variable measured in 1 patient throughout 1 stage constitutes 1 patient stage.

TABLE 12-3. Outcome Predictions for Cardiorespiratory Variables >75% and <67% in Each Stage*

Stage B	Stage Low	Stage C_1	Stage C_2	Stages D, E, F
OUTCOME PREDICTIONS >75% CORRECT				
ETOE	ETOE ⎫	ETOE	ETOE ⎫	ETOE ⎫
PVR	RCM ⎭	TOE	OTR ⎭	BVD ⎭
O_2 avail	BFVR		RVSW	RCM ⎫
RCM	OTR			BFVR ⎬
TOE	OTRF			OTR ⎭
WP	TOE			MAP
	TTI ⎫			LCW
	pH ⎭			TTI
	O_2 avail ⎫			LVSW
	O_2 ext ⎭			O_2 avail
	LCW			CI
	PVR			pH
	$P\bar{v}O_2$			RVSW
				RCFR
				$\dot{V}O_2$
				SI
				MTT
				$P\bar{v}O_2$
				$PaCO_2$
OUTCOME PREDICTIONS <67% CORRECT				
RCW	RVSW	$PaCO_2$	O_2 ext ⎫	CBV
RVSW	CBV	MPAP	$C(a\text{-}v)O_2$ ⎭	
CBV	CVP	LCW	CVP	
$P\bar{v}O_2$	SVR	SaO_2	SI	
SI	HR	SVR	TTI	
HR	PM	Hg	TOE	
		TR	$P\bar{v}O_2$	
		pH	O_2 avail	
		CVP	RCFR	
		HR	$PaCO_2$	
		CBV	TR	
			HR	
			SVR	

* Braces indicate variables with the same weight. The largest weights are at the top of each column; the smallest, at the bottom.

THERAPY

Hemorrhage and upper airway obstruction are two correctable, life-threatening emergencies that are readily apparent from the foot of the bed. Hypovolemia is associated with pallor, tachycardia, hypotension, semicoma, and oliguria; patients with upper airway obstruction have cyanosis or ashen gray appearance, dilated alae nasae, suprasternal and intercostal retraction, and agitation. Both of these catastrophic problems must be treated immediately.

The patient resuscitated from hypotensive shock with restoration of blood pressure becomes a critically ill patient with multiple vital organ failures and high mortality. This requires a well-integrated, systematic, coherent plan based on physiologic criteria for each potential vital organ or system failure. The following is a general outline for the most common problems of resuscitation and subsequent management of the acutely ill or shock patient in rough order of priorities [12, 21].

BLOOD VOLUME REPLACEMENT AND
VOLUME LOADING

In hemorrhagic shock, the first and most important principle is rapid restoration of blood volume with blood transfusions and other fluids. Similarly, volume replacement is the first line of defense in traumatic and septic shock associated with hypovolemia and dehydration; about 25 percent of patients with acute myocardial infarction have significant hypovolemia.

Maldistribution of blood volume and blood flow are common derangements in shock states; therefore, volume loading is required to make up for the circulation of those tissues and organs which were compromised. Administration of additional blood or plasma expanders is often needed after blood volume deficits have been replaced to open up vasoconstricted circuits by the force of added fluids and transfusions.

Volume loading in shock patients increases both blood volume and blood flow. Figure 12-8 illustrates the changes in plasma volume plotted against the changes in cardiac index after administration of whole blood and various oncotically active plasma expanders. The data suggest that for each increase in plasma volume, there are roughly comparable increases in flow. The blood volume over and above the expected norm tends to dilate the constricted capillary networks that persist from the earlier hypotensive stage. Most noncardiac patients who are, or recently were, in severe hypotensive shock tend to do better with blood volumes 500 to 1,000 ml in excess of their predicted norm, provided this increased volume does not increase the wedge pressure more than 18 mm Hg [17]. Excessive amounts of saline remain only transiently in the plasma volume and may overload the interstitial fluid (ISF) [10, 12].

Initially, during early resuscitation of patients with massive hemorrhage and severe hypotension, volume replacement should be given rapidly and

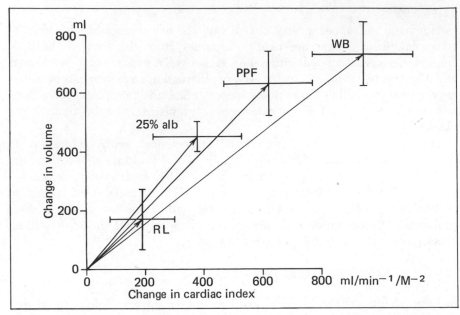

FIGURE 12-8. Change in volume plotted against the corresponding change in cardiac index after 1,000 ml Ringer's lactate (RL), 100 ml 25% albumin (25 gm), 500 ml 5% plasma protein fraction (PPF), and 500 ml whole blood given over a 60-min period. Vertical bars represent standard error (SE) of volume changes; horizontal bars represent SE of flow changes. (From C. J. Hauser et al., Oxygen transport responses to colloids and crystalloids in critically ill surgical patients. *Surg. Gynecol. Obstet.* 150:811, 1980. By permission of *Surgery, Gynecology & Obstetrics*.)

in sufficient quantities to restore systolic pressures above 100 mm Hg and mean arterial pressures above 80 mm Hg in previously normotensive patients. Subsequently, the volume and rate of fluid administration should be guided by arterial and venous pressures, heart rate, hematocrit, wedge pressure, blood volume, and cardiac output determinations [10, 12].

The main limiting factor in the rate of fluid administration is elevation in CVP and pulmonary precapillary wedge pressures. During initial resuscitation of blood volume, if elevations in the wedge pressures from normal values of 0 to +6 to over 20 mm Hg occur, it is likely that: (a) the fluids were given in excess or too fast; (b) there is continued peripheral vascular failure from the metarteriolar vasodilatation, pooling of the venous blood, and opening up of peripheral arteriovenous shunts; or (c) there was reduced cardiac function. The latter may represent myocardial insufficiency or inability of the heart to keep up with the increased metabolic and circulatory demands of the critically ill postoperative patient (as opposed to frank myocardial failure) [12, 21].

Tachycardia is a compensatory reaction that increases flow in the face of limited stroke volume. This response, when excessive or prolonged, may lead to decompensation because of reduced myocardial $\dot{V}O_2$ especially in the presence of increased cardiac work. Decreased myocardial oxygenation occurs when tachycardia reduces the diastolic time interval and thereby severely limits myocardial blood flow. Thus, tachycardia may improve cardiac output, but at great cost. When protracted, tachycardia may result in decompensation with reduced cardiac output, followed by bradycardia and cardiac arrest. Heart rates should be kept below 140 beat/min, if at all possible. When tachycardia occurs with reduced ventricular filling, volume loading may be indicated; digitalis and other cardiotonic agents also should be considered [12, 21].

In the initial period of resuscitation, when the primary objective is rapid replacement of blood losses, arterial pressure is the most readily available criterion for assessing the adequacy of transfusion therapy, and progressive elevation of CVP is the most readily available criterion for overtransfusion. Sooner or later the inevitable question arises, When should transfusions be slowed or stopped? At this time, reliable blood volume measurements have their greatest usefulness to titrate volume therapy. The most definitive assessment of the blood volume deficit is an accurate blood volume measurement [12, 21].

With hemorrhagic, traumatic, and septic shock, the blood volume is redistributed—i.e., pooled in the liver, splanchnic region, and postcapillary venules throughout the body [8, 22]. Under these conditions, more blood volume should be replaced than is lost; that is, after resuscitation, the optimal blood volume is about 500 to 1,000 ml greater than the predicted norms to make up for the ineffectively circulating (pooled) blood [17]. The advisability of additional volume expansion may be determined operationally by a trial of therapy (Fig. 12-9). In cardiogenic shock, the goal of optimal blood volume may be limited by diminished myocardial function. However, packed cells may be given judiciously when hematocrits fall below 32 percent in order to provide for the oxygen-carrying capacity of whole blood and to maintain myocardial oxygenation [12, 21].

In summary, successful resuscitation of circulatory shock involves restoration of four major elements: arterial pressure, blood flow, blood volume, and oxygen transport. Changes in the rate of $\dot{V}O_2$ reflect the overall changes of both body metabolism and tissue perfusion [19, 20]. Therefore, in most conditions, changes in $\dot{V}O_2$ may be a useful way to assess the relative effectiveness of alternate types of therapy. Figure 12-10 illustrates changes in plasma volume plotted against changes in cardiac index and $\dot{V}O_2$ during the infusion of 500 ml of colloids in a series of shock patients. These data suggest that the increased blood volume increased flow; but this increase may merely reflect increased flow through peripheral shunts. However, increased volume and flow associated with increased $\dot{V}O_2$ after volume

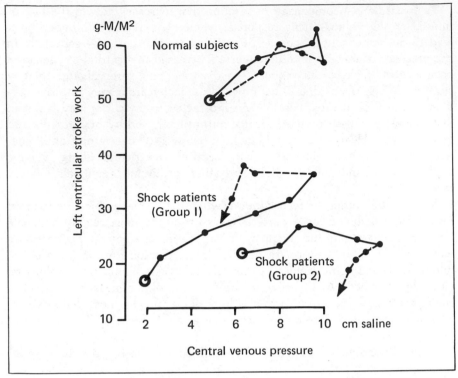

FIGURE 12-9. Evaluation of volume loading responses with modified cardiac function curves; left ventricular stroke work values plotted against inflow (central venous) pressure values before, during, and for 2 hr after administration of 500 ml dextran 40 infused over a 1-hr period. Solid line represents mean values taken at 10-min intervals after each 100 ml infused; dotted line represents the 2-hr postinfusion period. Comparison is made of normal subjects, group 1 shock patients who responded to the volume load with marked flow increases (59% of the cases studied) and group 2 shock patients (19%) who did not respond to volume loading with appreciable flow increases. (From P. A. Mohr et al., Sequential cardiorespiratory events during and after dextran 40 infusion in normal and shock patients. *Circulation* 39:379, 1969. By permission of The American Heart Association, Inc.)

loading suggests improvement in the peripheral perfusion associated with the correction of maldistribution problem of shock. The degree of increase in $\dot{V}O_2$ to plasma expansion is a measure of the correction of the fundamental perfusion defect and therefore an excellent criterion of the effectiveness of therapy [19, 20].

CORRECTION OF WATER DISCOLORATIONS

Rapid hemorrhage and hypovolemia limit cardiac output and oxygen transport to the tissues. Compensatory transcapillary migration of interstitial

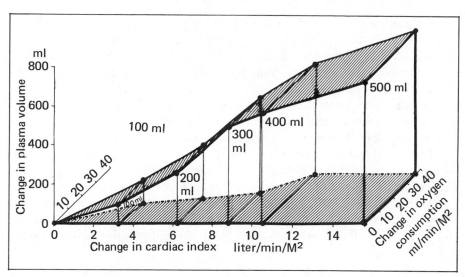

FIGURE 12-10. Volume flow–oxygen transport responses to volume loading. Data represent mean values of a group of shock patients who responded to 500 ml dextran 40 given over a 1-hr period. Changes in plasma volume are shown on the ordinate; corresponding changes in cardiac index are shown on the abscissa; and changes in oxygen consumption are shown on the third dimension represented by the scale at a 45-degree angle from the horizontal. Measurements were made after infusion of each 100 ml of dextran 40. (From W. C. Shoemaker and C. W. Bryan-Brown, Resuscitation and immediate care of the critically ill and injured patient. *Semin. Drug Treat.* 3:249, 1973. Reproduced by permission of Grune & Stratton.)

fluid into the intravascular space lowers hematocrit values, but this takes up to 24 hours for completion. Postoperative patients often do better with moderate hemodilution, i.e., to hematocrits of about 33 percent; this reduces viscosity and improves microcirculatory flow. In general, we use the following guidelines:

1. Rapid hemorrhage requires plasma expanders and whole blood transfusions, whereas hemorrhage occurring slowly over 6 to 24 hours or more usually requires predominantly whole blood or packed cells.
2. When hematocrit values are greater than 33 percent, or the red cell mass is greater than 1,080 ml/M² for men or 960 ml/M² for women, plasma expanders are more efficacious than whole blood.
3. When hematocrits are less than 33 percent, whole blood or packed red cells should be used for volume replaced.
4. When high CVP wedge pressure and myocardial failure limit transfusion therapy, packed cells should be used judiciously to maintain the oxygen-carrying capacity of the blood [19–21].

After whole blood and colloids administration, the plasma volume expansion persists for hours or in some instances for days, but crystalloids and electrolytes are more rapidly redistributed into the interstitial space. If excessive sodium-rich crystalloids are given, they may contribute to peripheral as well as pulmonary edema. The most common iatrogenic postoperative fluid electrolyte problem is water overload, which may produce expanded ISF in the face of contracted plasma volume [18]. The immediate therapeutic goal is to restore normal plasma volume, albumin concentrations, and colloidal osmotic pressures without overexpanding the ISF, particularly in the lung, since this may precipitate pulmonary edema [19–21].

The kidney may not excrete the excess ISF readily when the plasma volume is low. By giving oncotically active agents, such as 25% albumin, the ISF refills the plasma volume in accordance with Starling's law of the capillaries. As the plasma volume is expanded, more water is available for urinary excretion and as water is excreted, the plasma albumin concentrations increase—thus cycling water from the ISF to the plasma to the urine [12].

ESTABLISH PATENT UPPER AIRWAY AND ADEQUATE VENTILATION

Acute airway obstruction and ventilatory failure are readily recognized by cyanosis, gasping, stridor, suprasternal retraction, tachypnea, flaring of the nasal alae, restlessness, anxiety, agitation, diaphoresis, fatigue from muscular exertion, hypoxemia, hyperpnea, and respiratory acidosis. Nasopharyngeal obstruction commonly occurs in postoperative patients with postanesthetic depression that results in posterior displacement of the tongue. Pooling of blood and secretions in the posterior nasopharynx may occur after acute maxillofacial injury, and in the depressed or comatose patient; this often leads to vomiting and aspiration. Fractures of the larynx or trachea from direct injury and acute infections, such as croup, epiglossitis, and diphtheria, may produce airway obstruction. Inadequate ventilation may occur with pneumothorax, hemothorax, asthma, chronic obstructive lung disease, pleural effusion with multiple rib fractures with flail chest, and inadvertent insertion of an endotracheal tube into a main stem bronchus [1, 5].

Patent airway and adequate ventilation are of equal urgency to the replacement of blood volume in the resuscitation of acutely ill patients. The following maneuvers are used to restore ventilation:

1. Manually, remove nasopharyngeal obstructions, including dentures, foreign bodies, and so on.
2. Pull the mandible forward; insert an oral airway tube.
3. Intubate trachea.
4. Suction and ventilation with an Ambu bag.

If adequate spontaneous ventilation does not return after correction of these abnormalities, institute mechanical ventilation promptly with enriched O_2 sufficient to maintain PaO_2 greater than 80 torr.

RESPIRATORY CARE
A program of respiratory care should be undertaken in all patients with severe injuries, massive blood loss, extensive surgery, sepsis, and other acute life-threatening catastrophes to prevent pulmonary complications [1, 5].

1. Frequent stimulation of coughing.
2. Turning of the patient from side to side every 2 hours.
3. Endotracheal suctioning.
4. Postural drainage.
5. Humidification of inspired air.
6. Avoid overadministration of parenteral fluids, especially excessive salt.
7. Chest physical therapy.
8. Give oxygen by nasopharyngeal catheter or mask when PaO_2 values are low; enrichment of the inspired air with humidified oxygen may elevate alveolar oxygen concentrations to about 35 to 40 percent. The nasopharyngeal catheter is not suitable for long-term therapy and should be avoided in mouth breathers and comatose patients.
9. When this type of oxygen enrichment is inadequate to maintain arterial oxygen tensions above 60 torr or when the patient is exhausted by breathing, intubate the trachea and mechanically ventilate with increased fractional inspired oxygen (FiO_2). Intermittent mandatory ventilation (IMV) should be started as soon as the patient is able to tolerate it [17]. Positive end-expiratory pressure (PEEP) may be tried in small (3 cm of water) increments if blood volume has been restored. The patient must be carefully watched for reductions in arterial pressure or flow and the PEEP reduced promptly when this occurs to avoid severe circulatory deterioration and arrest, especially when hypovolemia is present.

High inspired oxygen concentrations required for prolonged periods may produce oxygen toxicity. Therefore, only FiO_2 levels required to maintain PaO_2 at about 80 torr or 90 to 95 percent saturation need be used [1, 5]. Inadequate oxygen delivery to peripheral tissues due to maldistribution of microcirculatory flow places an added burden on the heart. When there is maldistribution of flow, anemia, low hemoglobin saturation, or major pulmonary shunting, the heart must compensate by pumping at greater rates in order to supply the tissues with equivalent amounts of oxygen. When there is inadequate oxygen delivery to the heart itself because of maldistributions of the coronary circulation, anemia, hypoxemia, or low flow, the heart may be unable to compensate.

CORRECTION OF ACID-BASE PROBLEMS
Maldistribution of blood flow and inadequate oxygenation produces metabolic acidosis, but this may correct itself when circulatory deficits are corrected and blood volumes optimized. However, with continued peripheral circulatory impairment, acidosis increases and may further compromise cardiorespiratory function. After correction of circulatory deficiencies with plasma volume expanders, base deficits should be corrected by sodium bi-

carbonate or ⅙ molar sodium lactate. Ringer's lactate has 28 mEq/liter of sodium lactate; because it is racemic, only half is metabolized. Therefore, Ringer's lactate is inadequate to prevent or neutralize even moderately severe acidosis; it may give a false sense of security if used primarily to prevent acidosis. For example, in a 70-kg patient with a base deficit of 15 mEq/liter, the amount of base needed is estimated by multiplying the base deficit by the extracellular fluid volume (15 mEq/liter $\times$ 20 liter = 300 mEq); complete neutralization would require over 20 liters of Ringer's lactate, a dangerous amount of salt and water for most patients. This condition is better corrected with 4 ampules of sodium bicarbonate, 44 mEq/ampule (about half the estimated deficit) given over a 1- to 2-hour period; the remainder may be given more slowly, at 1 mEq/min, while pH values are rechecked at frequent intervals. It is necessary to titrate carefully the effect of the last part of the calculated dose to avoid metabolic alkalosis, which may be equally dangerous.

Respiratory acidosis is commonly associated with hypercarbia, hypoxia, and depressed ventilation; it is seen in postanesthetic states, obstructive lung disease, asthma, drug overdose, coma, and comparable conditions. It may be corrected by endotracheal suction and adequate ventilation, which may require mechanical ventilation.

Respiratory alkalosis is frequently thought to be a compensatory response to metabolic acidosis from hypovolemia and low flow. However, for respiratory alkalosis to be compensatory, there must be an antecedent metabolic acidosis. Moreover, the compensation may return the pH toward the normal range, but if it is truly a compensation, it should not drive the pH into the alkalotic range. For example, when the pH rises above 7.4, the alkalosis cannot be a compensatory response to presumed metabolic acidosis; other explanations must be sought. Respiratory alkalosis more often results from increased respiratory drive that increases alveolar ventilation in compensation for hypoxemia. Thus, increased autonomic neural activity associated with the stress response is a major stimuli for the increased respiratory drive that tends to restore PaO_2. Respiratory alkalosis usually may be treated effectively by properly adjusting the mechanical ventilation and by adding tubing to increase the external dead space. On occasion, 2 or 3 percent CO_2 with various proportions of oxygen and room air may be used in the inspired gas. With this approach, it is necessary to monitor CO_2 concentration of the expired gas or to measure arterial blood gases frequently to warn of hypercarbia.

Metabolic alkalosis may occur under the following circumstances:

1. Prolonged gastric suction.
2. With prolonged vomiting, such as pyloric obstruction.
3. In 6 to 12 hours after massive transfusion therapy, when the citrate (in acid citrate dextrose anticoagulant) has been metabolized, leaving sodium ions

(about 15 mEq per unit of blood) which are then buffered by the bicarbonate–carbonic acid system.
4. Overadministration of sodium bicarbonate following resuscitation from shock or cardiac arrest.
5. Massive steroid administration or marked stress in the absence of perfusion abnormalities.
6. Low serum K^+.
7. Failure of the kidney to exchange urinary HCO_3^- for Cl^-.

Correct metabolic alkalosis when it is greater than +10 mEq/liter with ammonium chloride or HCl. Lysine HCl is often used, but it is less effective and requires larger volumes of fluid to produce the same effect. Ammonium chloride or HCl should be given intravenously slowly, i.e., 0.25 to 0.5 mEq/min. Frequent pH measurements are needed to warn of overcorrection. Concomitantly, serum potassium abnormalities also should be corrected [21].

CARDIAC PROBLEMS IN SHOCK
There are four distinct clinical settings of shock with central pump failure, as follows:

1. Myocardial failure (valvular disease, myocardial infarction, congenital abnormalities, etc.).
2. Cardiac tamponade, from penetrating wounds or accidental perforation of the right atrial appendix or right ventricle during cardiac catheterization or central venous catheterization.
3. Bradyarrhythmias and tachyarrhythmias.
4. Patients with noncardiogenic shock who subsequently develop significant degrees of apparently impaired myocardial function from increased myocardial demand. The latter is a common pattern in the terminal stages of patients with postoperative and posttraumatic shock. Most of the patients we studied in each of the above subsets of cardiogenic shock had low cardiac output and about a third had high resistance in the early stage [14].

Cardiac tamponade represents a special subset of cardiogenic shock, failure from mechanical factors that limit ventricular filling and produce low stroke volume; in part, high CVP values compensate for the reduced effective filling pressure. Although high CVP values in most other kinds of shock warn of possible fluid volume overloading, fluid loading in tamponade improves ventricular filling, stroke volume, and cardiac output without producing pulmonary edema. Thus, high CVP in tamponade does not contraindicate fluid volume loading. The therapeutic goal is not to produce normal hemodynamic values, but to optimize the functional interactions that will reestablish circulatory integrity [19, 20].

Patients with shock from noncardiogenic etiologic events (hemorrhage, trauma, and sepsis) may develop impaired myocardial performance because

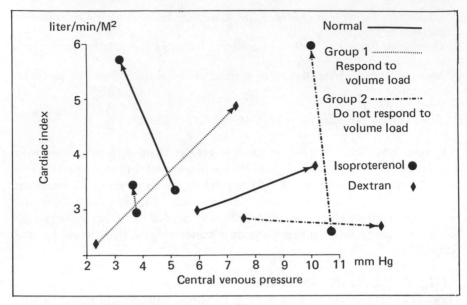

FIGURE 12-11. Evaluation of cardiac and peripheral vascular functional reserve with modified cardiac function curves. Cardiac index values are plotted against central venous pressures before and after volume loading with dextran 40 and isoproterenol administration in the same three groups shown in Figure 12-9. The solid lines represent the average responses of normal patients to each agent. The dotted lines of group 1 shock patients illustrate the pronounced flow response to the volume load, but minimal response to isoproterenol; this indicates peripheral circulatory failure responsive to volume therapy. The dashed lines of group 2 shock patients show failure of flow response to dextran 40 but pronounced response to isoproterenol; this indicates reduced myocardial function, which is responsive to inotropic agents. (From W. C. Shoemaker and C. W. Bryan-Brown, Resuscitation and immediate care of the critically ill and injured patient. *Semin. Drug Treat.* 3:249, 1973. Reproduced by permission of Grune & Stratton.)

of prolonged periods of increased cardiac work which may be associated with tachycardia, limited coronary blood flow, and reduced myocardial oxygenation (Fig. 12-11). Inotropic agents, such as digitalis and dopamine, may be used for impaired ventricular contractility. Digitalization should be considered in the elderly patient with preexisting cardiac failure, pulmonary edema, atrial fibrillation, sinus tachycardia, and comparable problems. Contraindications include conduction abnormalities such as partial or complete heart block, ventricular ectopic beats, and other evidence of myocardial irritability. The decision to digitalize should be reached early in the course of the shock syndromes, since the anoxic myocardium of the late stages of shock is more susceptible to dysrhythmias.

ISOPROTERENOL

Isoproterenol may be considered in patients with noncardiogenic shock. It is usually contraindicated in patients with acute myocardial infarction because it increases the work of the heart and the myocardial oxygen requirements. When given in low doses (1–4 μg/min for a 70-kg man), isoproterenol produces an inotropic effect which increases cardiac index about 0.5 liter/min/M^2 or more. Usually at this dose chronotropic effects are minimal [3, 4]. At this dose, cardiac output often increases promptly, but arterial pressures and urine outputs gradually improve, while the CVP falls; thus, as blood flow increases from direct action of the drugs, the patient achieves a better physiologic set (Fig. 12-11). Larger doses (5–10 μg/min) frequently produce tachycardia and dysrhythmias without appreciably improving flow. Also, if the patient is started on the low dose, it may be more easily increased when tachyphylaxis occurs.

BLOCKING AGENTS

Blocking agents (such as phentolamine, nitroprusside, nitroglycerine, hydralazine, and chlorpromazine) have a place in the treatment of shock, especially in the patient in whom volume loading is desired but venoconstriction with high CVP is also present. Blocking agents allow more fluids to be given with less harm in that they provide protection from mild degrees of fluid overloading [11]. Phlebotomy, ultrafiltration, or dialysis may be needed when fluid overload is large and unresponsive to diuretics, fluid and salt restriction, and other conservative measures.

SYMPATHOMIMETIC AGENTS

Sympathomimetic agents should be considered as a last resort when whole blood, plasma expanders and other fluids, correction of respiratory and acid-base problems, ventilator readjustments, cardiotonic agents, and other supportive measures have failed to restore arterial pressure and circulatory homeostasis. The use of sympathomimetic agents—such as dopamine, epinephrine, norepinephrine, and Aramine—should be regarded as an admission of defeat. Sympathomimetic agents should never be used as a substitute for blood volume replacement, nor are they appropriate as a temporary measure while blood is being typed and cross-matched, since it is just as easy to administer fluids intravenously. In essence, shock is not primarily a levophed-deficiency disease; volume restoration, not artificial elevation of arterial pressure, is the objective [3, 4, 19, 20].

CORRECTION OF FLUID OVERLOAD AND OLIGURIA

In the shock and trauma patient, volume loading is urgently needed to restore and maintain blood volume, arterial pressure, and circulatory homeostasis in the immediate posttraumatic and postoperative period. Subsequently, after circulatory stability has been achieved, pulmonary complications, sepsis, interstitial fluid overload, and renal failure may become the most serious life-threatening conditions. Therapy of conditions associated with interstitial fluid overload include:

1. Restriction of fluid and salt.
2. Establishment of normal plasma volume with 25% albumin.
3. Administration of osmotic diuretic, such as 20% mannitol and 50% glucose, or loop diuretics, such as furosemide and ethacrinic acid, which may be given intravenously. The latter act by inhibiting tubular reabsorption of Na^+ and promoting the excretion of urinary Na^+. In contrast with mannitol, they can be given repeatedly, since they are rapidly metabolized, but they may be ineffective in the presence of hypovolemia.
4. Hemodialysis, ultrafiltration, and peritoneal dialysis. When normal albumin concentration and plasma volume are present, but diuretics are ineffective, it may be necessary to resort to dialysis to reduce excess water, high serum K^+ concentrations, urea, creatinine, and other metabolic breakdown products.

PARENTERAL NUTRITION
Patients with shock, multiple vital organ failures, sepsis, burns, and hypercatabolic states require adequate arterial pressure, increased blood flow, increased blood volume, and increased oxygen transport. Of equal importance is an increased need for oxidative substrates to support energy metabolism. Since the limited carbohydrate reserves are rapidly exhausted and fat is not available for glycolysis, protein reserves are broken down to supply the energy required for body metabolism. When the labile protein stores are depleted, the lean tissues are cannibalized to provide substrates for the high-priority Krebs' cycle metabolism [19, 20, 21].

The 5% glucose solutions inadequately provide nutrition. Since each liter of 5% glucose contains only 50 gm of glucose, or 200 calories, it would take at least 12 liters to meet the normal caloric needs. By contrast, 500 ml of 50% glucose has the equivalent of about 1,000 calories.

Intravenous alimentation may provide adequately for caloric needs as follows: give 500 ml 50% glucose, together with 200 ml 8% amino acid solutions, slowly by constant infusion over 8- to 12-hour periods through a central venous catheter; crystalline insulin may be added if blood sugars exceed 200 mg/dl or the urine sugars are 2+ or more. The dose should be titrated carefully on the basis of frequent blood and urinary glucose as well as osmolarity determinations. Plasma protein fraction (albumin) solutions are used to maintain the oncotic pressure and plasma volume, but they are eventually broken down to individual amino acids and metabolized in the tissues. The immediate advantage of albumin is to redistribute water from the interstitial space to the plasma volume, but albumin also provides for some nitrogen metabolism and trace elements.

SUPPORT OF THE UNCONSCIOUS PATIENT

Cerebral edema may be minimized by diuretics, avoidance of extracellular fluid overload, fluid and salt restriction, high doses of steroids, parenteral alimentation to meet nutritional needs, dialysis for correction of uremia, correction of extracellular and intracellular hypoosmolarity, and other supportive measures.

Patients who are semiconscious may be nursed in the semiprone swimmer's position with—or, if possible, without—an endotracheal tube. The completely unconscious patient with long-term prognosis usually requires tracheostomy and mechanical ventilation to ensure adequate respiratory function.

CONTROL OF INFECTION

Abscesses should be drained, and adequate débridement of devitalized tissue and wound care should be provided in infected and contaminated cases. Wound, blood, sputum, urine, and other body fluids should be cultured, and the appropriate antibiotics given. Prophylactic antibiotic coverage in noncontaminated cases is not recommended. However, antibiotics may be used with obvious gross contamination when it is not advisable to wait for the results of bacterial cultures and sensitivities.

SUMMARY

A concept of the pathophysiology of the various shock states should be based upon descriptions of the natural physiologic history of the various shock syndromes obtained from sequential cardiorespiratory measurements during periods remote from the therapeutic interventions. Despite the wide variety of illnesses, there are characteristic sequential cardiorespiratory patterns of postoperative survivors and nonsurvivors of life-threatening illness. The early, common hemodynamic alteration in shock is not low cardiac output and high peripheral resistance; rather, it is a tissue oxygenation defect from uneven blood flow—that is, flow is not necessarily low (it may be normal or high), but it is maldistributed. Moreover, tissue oxygenation measured by $\dot{V}O_2$ is not necessarily low; it may be normal or high but inadequate for the increased metabolic needs. Since the most critical function of the circulation is the transport of oxygen, circulatory failure may be measured in terms of the developing patterns of oxygen transport variables.

The imbalance between neurohumoral vasoconstriction and metabolic vasodilation is the major factor leading to maldistribution of flow at the microcirculatory level. In tissues with high flow, more oxygen is carried through the wide-open metarteriolar-capillary networks, but blood oxygen is less completely extracted because cells adjacent to the open capillary channel are able to extract only that amount that they themselves utilize, while the oxygen supply to cells at a distance from the open capillaries is limited by diffusion of the gas across tissues. This perfusion defect is manifest by low $C(a-v)O_2$, low oxygen extraction, and low or inadequate oxygen consumption in the presence of normal or high flows and normal or high oxygen delivery. Tissue perfusion as well as the overall bulk oxygen transport may be adversely affected by decreased PaO_2 from pulmonary insufficiency, anemia with low arterial oxygen content, and rheologic abnormalities. The perfusion defect is self-perpetuating, and in many instances a negative feedback system develops whereby poor perfusion and oxygen transport to the heart, for example, curtail myocardial function and result in further circulatory deterioration. Thus, a common peripheral perfusion defect is produced by interrelated combinations of uneven vasoconstriction, metabolic vasodilation, redistribution of blood flow, redistribution of blood volume, and rheologic alterations including cellular aggregation. The net result is inadequate oxygenation relative to increased tissue requirements.

Since inadequate oxygen transport is the major pathophysiologic defect in circulatory shock syndrome, improved oxygen transport to peripheral tissues is physiologically the most important goal. Cardiorespiratory measurements also are useful in evaluations of the relative effectiveness of various types of therapy in the shock patient. Furthermore, frequent intermittent or continuous monitoring of cardiorespiratory variables permits trend analysis and early warning of inadequate responses that may signal impending disaster.

Predictors of death and survival were defined by frequency distributions of each variable and used as quantitative measures of the severity of illness; a high percentage of patients may be classified in the early period. The relative frequency with which changes in each of the physiologic variables identify survival or nonsurvival reflects the relevance of each of the variables to the pathophysiology of acute circulatory failure. When the therapeutic goals are defined appropriately by the cardiorespiratory pattern of survivors, treatment can be arranged by priorities according to the life-threatening capability of each cardiorespiratory derangement. Then, a therapeutic program may be developed with each therapy precisely titrated to the optimal goals and with due consideration for the unique aspects of each patient.

REFERENCES

1. Bendixen, H. H., et al. *Respiratory Care.* St. Louis: Mosby, 1965.
2. Bland, R., Shoemaker, W. C., and Shabot, M. M. Physiologic monitoring goals for the critically ill patient. *Surg. Gynecol. Obstet.* 147:833, 1978.
3. Brown, R. S., et al. Comparative evaluation of sympathomimetic amines in clinical shock. *Circulation* 34:260, 1966.
4. Carey, J. S., et al. Cardiovascular function in shock. *Circulation* 35:327, 1967.
5. Comroe, J. H., Jr., et al. *The Lung* (2nd ed). Chicago: Year Book, 1965.

6. Courand, A., et al. Studies of the circulation in clinical shock. *Surgery* 13: 964, 1943.
7. Del Guercio, L. R., et al. Pulmonary arteriovenous admixture and the hyperdynamic cardiovascular state in surgery for portal hypertension. *Surgery* 56:57, 1964.
8. Mohr, P. A., et al. Sequential cardiorespiratory events during and after dextran-40 infusion in normal and shock patients. *Circulation* 39:379, 1969.
9. Shoemaker, W. C. Cardiorespiratory patterns in complicated and uncomplicated septic shock. *Ann. Surg.* 174:119, 1971.
10. Shoemaker, W. C. Pathophysiologic basis of therapy for shock and trauma syndromes. *Semin. Drug Treat.* 3:211, 1973.
11. Shoemaker, W. C., and Brown, R. S. The dilemma of vasopressors and vasodilators in the therapy of shock. *Surg. Gynecol. Obstet.* 132:51, 1971.
12. Shoemaker, W. C., and Bryan-Brown, C. W. Resuscitation and immediate care of the critically ill and injured patient. *Semin. Drug Treat.* 3:249, 1973.
13. Shoemaker, W. C., et al. Hemodynamic patterns after acute anesthetized and unanesthetized trauma. *Arch. Surg.* 95:492, 1967.
14. Shoemaker, W. C., et al. Hemodynamic alterations in acute cardiac tamponade after penetrating injuries of the heart. *Surgery* 67:754, 1970.
15. Shoemaker, W. C., et al. Sequential hemodynamic events after trauma to the unanesthetized patient. *Surg. Gynecol. Obstet.* 132:651, 1971.
16. Shoemaker, W. C., et al. Sequential oxygen transport and acid-base changes after trauma to the unanesthetized patient. *Surg. Gynecol. Obstet.* 132:1023, 1971.
17. Shoemaker, W. C., et al. Physiologic patterns in surviving and nonsurviving shock patients. *Arch. Surg.* 106:630, 1973.
18. Shoemaker, W. C., et al. Body fluid shifts in depletion and post stress states and their correction with adequate nutrition. *Surg. Gynecol. Obstet.* 136:371, 1973.
19. Shoemaker, W. C., et al. Cardiorespiratory monitoring in postoperative patients. *Crit. Care Med.* 7:237, 1979.
20. Shoemaker, W. C., and Czer, L. S. C. Evaluation of the biologic importance of various hemodynamic and oxygen transport variables. *Crit. Care Med.* 7:424, 1979.
21. Shoemaker, W. C., and Walker, W. F. *Fluid-Electrolyte Therapy in Acute Illness.* Chicago: Year Book, 1970.
22. Slater, G., et al. Sequential changes in the distribution of cardiac output in various stages of experimental hemorrhagic shock. *Surgery* 73:714, 1973.
23. Wiggers, C. J. *Physiology of Shock.* New York: Commonwealth Fund, 1950.
24. Wilson, R. F., et al. The usage of dibenzyline in clinical shock. *Surgery* 56:172, 1964.

Robert L. Berger
Gideon Merin

13. MECHANICAL SUPPORT OF THE FAILING LEFT VENTRICLE

The intra-aortic balloon pump (IABP) is a left ventricular assist device. The system consists of an inflatable balloon mounted on a vascular catheter and deployed in the descending thoracic aorta through the femoral artery. The balloon is inflated and deflated by an extracorporeal power unit, and timing of the cycle is triggered from the electrocardiogram (ECG) or arterial pressure tracing. The balloon is inflated during ventricular diastole, augmenting aortic diastolic pressure. It is deflated during ventricular systole and thereby lowers systolic pressure. In substance, then, the patient with an intra-aortic balloon has two functional systemic ventricles: the biologic left ventricle, which ejects blood during systole, and the intra-aortic balloon, which exerts its principal pumping function during diastole (Fig. 13-1).

PHYSIOLOGY OF INTRA-AORTIC BALLOON COUNTERPULSATION

During diastole, the arterial tree is essentially a closed, distensible, fluid-filled system. The seal is provided by the coapted aortic valves at one end and the small peripheral vasculature at the other. Displacement of a volume of blood by the inflated balloon during diastole raises the pressure in the entire systemic circuit (diastolic augmentation). Deflation of the balloon during systole results in lowering of aortic pressure (systolic unloading).

The three benefits of diastolic augmentation are: (1) improved tissue perfusion, (2) a decrease in left ventricular workload, and (3) increase in coronary blood flow. Improved tissue perfusion is accomplished by augmentation of arterial pressure during diastole with only a small decrement in systolic pressure. The decrease in systolic pressure reduces left ventricular afterload, which, in turn, lowers myocardial oxygen requirement. The increase in coronary flow is achieved by the striking elevation in perfusion pressure during diastole, when most of the coronary blood flow is delivered.

The beneficial effects of intra-aortic balloon counterpulsation (IABP) on hemodynamics and myocardial metabolism during experimental canine studies are shown in Figure 13-2. In man, the hemodynamic changes in response to IABP include a rise in diastolic and fall in systolic arterial pres-

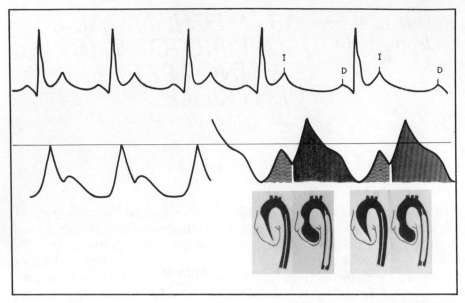

FIGURE 13-1. Graphic representation of intra-aortic balloon counter pulsation. Top row depicts electrocardiographic signal; below is the arterial tracing. Bottom drawings indicate state of balloon inflation. Horizontal stippling in arterial tracing represents systole, and vertical lines correspond to arterial diastole (I = inflation; D = deflation).

sures, a fall in left atrial pressure, and an increase in cardiac output as well as in coronary blood flow. Additionally, in the experimental animal, diastolic augmentation reduces infarct size, presumably by reclaiming ischemic but viable myocardium at the periphery of the frankly infarcted muscle. Although this observation has not been documented clinically, it is likely that a similar phenomenon occurs in man.

INDICATIONS FOR INTRA-AORTIC BALLOON COUNTERPULSATION

The indications for IABP are reasonably well-established, although some aspects remain controversial. The device has been employed in the following conditions:

1. Cardiogenic shock following acute myocardial infarction.
2. Complicated myocardial infarction.
3. Unstable anginal syndrome.
4. Extension of acute myocardial infarction.
5. Postcardiotomy cardiogenic shock.
6. Prophylaxis in cardiac surgery in patients with poor left ventricular reserve.
7. Prophylaxis in cardiac surgery in patients with high-risk anatomy (left main stenosis).

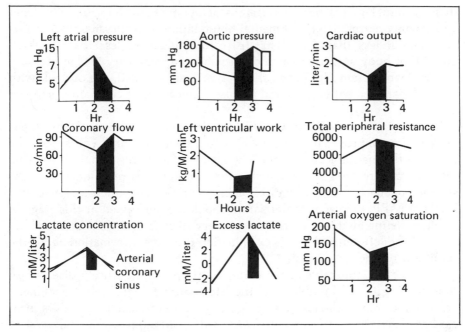

FIGURE 13-2. Influence of counterpulsation on hemodynamics and myocardial metabolism. Left ventricular failure in dogs was produced by serial ligation of coronary arteries. The animals were then observed for 2 hr, followed by counterpulsation for 1 hr (solid bars). (From J. Rosenzweig and K. Chatterjee, Restoration of normal cardiac metabolism and hemodynamics after acute coronary occlusion. *Ann. Thorac. Surg.* 6:146, 1968.)

8. Prophylaxis during noncardiac surgery in patients with severe cardiac disease.
9. Septic shock.
10. Induction of pulsatile flow during cardiopulmonary bypass.

CARDIOGENIC SHOCK FOLLOWING ACUTE MYOCARDIAL INFARCTION (CS-MI)

Approximately 10 percent of patients with acute myocardial infarction slip into refractory cardiogenic shock from power failure of the left ventricle. Postmortem studies show that destruction of at least 40 percent of the left ventricular muscle mass is necessary to produce forward failure. With medical therapy, the mortality rate in myocardial infarction complicated by cardiogenic shock is 85 to 95 percent.

The diagnosis of refractory cardiogenic shock should not be made until serious arrhythmias, volume deficits, and metabolic abnormalities are corrected. Once this is accomplished, the following criteria for defining cardiogenic shock are generally used: (1) documented acute myocardial infarction (chest pain, ECG, myocardial specific enzymes); (2) systolic pressure less than 80 mm Hg; (3) peripheral signs of sympathetic hyperactivity (cold and clammy extremities); (4) mental obtundation or restlessness; (5) a urinary output less than 25 ml/hr; (6) cardiac index of less than 2 liters/min/M^2 of body surface area, and (7) pulmonary capillary wedge pressure greater than 15 mm Hg. When these criteria are fulfilled, the outlook with medical management is grim and the use of mechanical circulatory support is justified.

The response to IABP in CS-MI is variable. A small proportion of patients fail to improve; they follow a progressively downhill course and die while on the mechanical support. The majority, however, show a favorable response and reach a stable circulatory state within a few hours after institution of mechanical assistance. Since it is safe under the protective umbrella of IABP, cardiac catheterization should be performed at this stage in order to define anatomy of coronary artery disease and the functional reserve of the left ventricle. This examination provides information about the feasibility of operative repair.

Patients are inoperable if the coronary arteries are diffusely diseased so that grafting is not feasible or if the left ventricle is diffusely hypokinetic and without any well-contracting segments. Approximately 24 hours after cardiac catheterization, weaning from IABP is attempted. If withdrawal of IABP is not possible, the outcome is usually fatal. Those who can be weaned still have a poor prognosis and usually die within weeks to months.

Patients are regarded as operable if the coronary arteries have localized proximal disease with patent distal vessels and the left ventricle has at least two well-contracting segments. Bypass grafting of the obstructed vessels is performed on an urgent basis. Overall survival is modestly improved by operative intervention. Because of the questionable benefits, the use of IABP in CS-MI is not widely practiced.

COMPLICATED MYOCARDIAL INFARCTION

Complicated myocardial infarctions—such as rupture of the ventricular septum with left to right shunt, or papillary muscle disruption with severe mitral regurgitation—are associated with a grim outlook, and the mortality rate approaches 90 percent following the first 6 weeks of the acute attack. The few survivors are usually critically ill and suffer from refractory congestive heart failure. Shock may or may not be present. In these two conditions, IABP provides specific hemodynamic benefits in addition to support of the general circulation. In the case of ruptured ventricular septum, the IABP-induced fall in aortic systolic pressure is transmitted to the left ventricle. The gradient between the two sides of the heart is reduced, and the left-to-right shunt through the defect is decreased. With ruptured papillary muscle, lowering of the aortic systolic pressure reduces impedance to left ventricular ejection and the degree of mitral regurgitation is reduced.

In complicated acute myocardial infarction, IABP is inserted following the appearance of refractory congestive cardiac failure. Counterpulsation is continued until the patient's condition stabilizes, and cardiac catheterization is performed. If the clinical diagnosis is confirmed and the left-to-right shunt is significant or the mitral regurgitation is massive, the appropriate surgical corrective measure is performed. In addition to repair of the mechanical deficit, the stenosed coronary arteries are bypassed. IABP support is continued during the surgical procedure and usually for several days postoperatively.

UNSTABLE ANGINAL SYNDROME
The intermediate syndrome is initially treated with bed rest, sedation, nitrates, and β blockade. Many patients respond to this therapy, and the symptoms abate. During the quiescent period, cardiac catheterization can be accomplished on a semielective basis, and if the coronary anatomy and left ventricular function are favorable, appropriate surgical therapy is performed during the same hospital admission. The results are excellent, with a mortality of about 2 to 5 percent.

A large number of patients, however, do not respond to intensive medical measures but can be controlled by intra-aortic balloon counterpulsation. Once the balloon is in place, cardiac catheterization is safe and should be performed. If left ventricular function and coronary anatomy are suitable, operative correction should be accomplished under IABP protection. Diastolic counterpulsation is usually continued postoperatively. Available evidence indicates that these patients can undergo cardiac repair with a low mortality (3–5%).

EXTENSION OF MYOCARDIAL INFARCTION
Extension of uncomplicated myocardial infarction is manifested by recurrence of ischemic pain and usually occurs several days or even weeks after the initial attack. If the pain persists in spite of maximal medical therapy, employment of IABP is indicated. With balloon support, the pain subsides in 80 percent of the patients, and cardiac catheterization can be performed. Weaning is attempted; if the pain does not recur, the balloon catheter is removed. Corrective surgery is performed approximately 4 to 6 weeks after the infarct. However, if weaning from IABP precipitates recurrence of the ischemic pain, full diastolic augmentation is resumed, and operative revascularization is performed on an urgent basis.

POSTCARDIOTOMY CARDIOGENIC SHOCK
Open heart surgery with the aid of the pump oxygenator is frequently followed by depression of myocardial function. The postcardiotomy myocardial depression can be transient and reversible, especially if the heart is supported during the critical period of impaired function. Frank myocardial infarction can also occur during cardiac operations, and the resultant

left ventricular failure may necessitate the temporary use of mechanical circulatory assist. Severe myocardial depression is usually first appreciated during unsuccessful attempts to discontinue cardiopulmonary bypass support as it becomes apparent that the heart cannot tolerate discontinuation of cardiopulmonary bypass support. The indication for balloon pumping in postcardiotomy cardiogenic shock during the early years of IABP usage was limited to clear-cut dependence on the pump oxygenator. With increasing experience, it became apparent that intra-aortic balloon pumping is simple and relatively safe. The use of IABP has therefore been extended to left ventricular failure of lesser severity than suggested by the above rigid criteria. Thus, mild-to-moderate left ventricular decompensation at the conclusion of cardiopulmonary bypass may be an additional indication for IABP. In our own experience, this practice has contributed to a smoother postoperative course and better survival rates in critically ill patients.

Intra-aortic balloon counterpulsation has also been used for low output states in the early postcardiotomy period. Criteria for its use are not clearly defined but usually consist of refractory shock despite correction of serious arrhythmias, adequate volume replacement, and catecholamine therapy.

PROPHYLAXIS IN CARDIAC SURGERY IN PATIENTS WITH POOR LEFT VENTRICULAR RESERVE

Several surgeons advocate prophylactic balloon counterpulsation during open heart surgery for acquired heart disease in patients with poor left ventricular function. The precise criteria for IABP are lacking, but in general it is suggested that with severe left ventricular dysfunction, the operation may be safer under the protection of balloon counterpulsation. Usually the device is inserted under local infiltration anesthesia prior to induction of general anesthesia. Counterpulsation is continued during the operation. While on the pump oxygenator, the balloon is triggered from a pacemaker, and thereby the steady flow of the roller pump is pulsated. After the operation, diastolic augmentation is usually continued until hemodynamic stability is secure. The duration of postoperative balloon support varies from a few hours to a few days. It is well to mention that this prophylactic use of the intra-aortic balloon is not universally accepted.

PROPHYLAXIS IN CARDIAC SURGERY IN PATIENTS WITH HIGH-RISK ANATOMY (LEFT MAIN STENOSIS)

Several authors advocate the prophylactic use of the intra-aortic balloon during bypass grafting for left main coronary artery stenosis. Previous experience indicates that these patients do not tolerate fluctuations in arterial pressure during induction of anesthesia and during manipulation of the heart prior to institution of cardiopulmonary bypass. Some surgeons claim that the operation is safer when an intra-aortic balloon is inserted prior to the operation. The balloon in this situation is inserted prior to induction, and pumping is maintained until cardiopulmonary bypass is discontinued. If the hemodynamics are stable at the conclusion of the operation, the balloon catheter may be removed. The use of the IABP during performance of bypass grafting for left main stenosis is practiced only in a few centers. With the advent of more intensive intraoperative hemodynamic monitoring, this approach is gradually being abandoned.

PROPHYLAXIS DURING NONCARDIAC OPERATIONS IN THE PRESENCE OF SEVERE CARDIAC DISEASE

Occasionally, patients with critical heart disease require emergency or mandatory noncardiac operations that are associated with a high incidence of perioperative infarction and death. In general, when possible the cardiac lesion should be repaired first, followed by the noncardiac operation. However, if the cardiac pathology is not amenable to surgical therapy, or if the noncardiac condition is emergent and time does not permit correction of the cardiac lesion, prophylactic IABP during the extracardiac procedure may be beneficial. Among conditions requiring urgent operative treatment are massive gastrointestinal bleeding and bowel obstruction. The mandatory operations are usually resection of various malignant tumors. The cardiac indications for IABP support include unstable angina pectoris, myocardial infarctions within 6 weeks of the proposed operation, Classes III and IV cardiac failure due to poor left ventricular function, and inoperable complex cardiac lesion.

The IABP is inserted under local anesthesia prior to the operation. Diastolic augmentation should be provided during induction of anesthesia, performance of the operation, and for 1 or 2 days postoperatively until the hemodynamics are satisfactory without the mechanical support.

SEPTIC SHOCK

Sporadic use of IABP in refractory septic shock has been reported. The few successes to date have been in patients with septic shock who had associated background coronary artery disease and low cardiac output. IABP support has not been beneficial in conditions where circulatory collapse is associated with a high cardiac output. The experience with IABP in circulatory failure from sepsis is limited, and its usefulness has not been established. It should be employed, if at all, when all conventional measures fail.

INDUCTION OF PULSATILE FLOW DURING CARDIOPULMONARY BYPASS

Conventional cardiopulmonary bypass with a roller pump provides a steady, nonpulsatile flow. It has been suggested that the lack of pulsation may result in suboptimal tissue perfusion and impaired cellular metabolism. IABP can convert a nonpulsatile flow into a pulsatile one (Fig. 13-3). Insertion

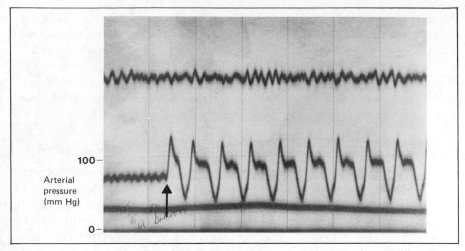

FIGURE 13-3. Arrow indicates initiation of intra-aortic balloon counterpulsation in a patient on total cardiopulmonary bypass. Change in pattern of arterial pressure is apparent.

of the balloon merely to pulsate the pump oxygenator flow may not be justified, but if the device is already in place, activation is a simple matter. If the heart is arrested, a pacemaker can provide satisfactory signal for triggering the balloon. We have employed this modality only in patients with indications for preoperative balloon pumping. The routine insertion of IABP for pulsating cardiopulmonary bypass flow is not indicated until the superiority of pulsatile over nonpulsatile flow is conclusively established. Several devices are now commercially available that pulsate the arterial line of the pump oxygenator with an IABP console without an intra-aortic balloon.

CONTRAINDICATIONS TO INTRA-AORTIC BALLOON COUNTERPULSATION

In the presence of moderately severe aortic regurgitation, the use of the device is contraindicated since intra-aortic balloon counterpulsation may distend the left ventricle by transmission of the augmented diastolic pressure through the incompetent aortic valve. In the failing heart, the muscle fibers are already stretched beyond the limit of optimal performance and the ventricle may be on the descending limb of the Frank-Starling curve. Any additional distension results in increased muscle fiber stretch and leads to deterioration of myocardial performance.

Insertion of the balloon catheter in the face of bilateral iliofemoral obstructive disease may not be feasible, and thus counterpulsation is not possible. However, if the chest is open, as is the case during cardiac surgery, the balloon can be inserted directly through the ascending aorta inside a prosthetic sidearm. Removal of the balloon can be accomplished at the subcutaneous level without reentering the mediastinum.

PATIENT MONITORING DURING INTRA-AORTIC BALLOON COUNTERPULSATION

The candidate for IABP is usually critically ill and requires intensive care. The following specific measures are indicated for safe management of the patient supported by the device:

1. Close monitoring of the clinical state and vital signs.
2. Continuous surveillance of the ECG is essential for detection of arrhythmias that may interfere with IABP triggering.
3. Direct arterial pressure monitoring through an indwelling catheter is essential for adjustment of balloon triggering.
4. A central venous line may be helpful for assessing right heart function.
5. A flow-directed, balloon-tipped pulmonary artery catheter can measure filling pressures on both sides of the heart. This information is essential to guide catecholamine infusion and fluid therapy. In addition, this catheter allows cardiac output determination by the thermodilution technique.
6. Measured hourly urinary output through a Foley catheter reflects renal function and overall tissue perfusion.

BALLOON CATHETER INSERTION
TECHNIQUE

The balloons for adults are manufactured in 20-, 30-, and 40-ml sizes. In the majority of patients, the largest size (40 ml) is employed. For patients weighing under 100 to 110 lb, the 30-ml balloon is more appropriate. If the iliofemoral artery does not accommodate the larger catheters, a 20-ml balloon with the smaller carrier may be used. The catheter is radiopaque so that its location can be verified by a portable chest x-ray film.

For optimal aseptic technique, it is preferable to insert the balloon catheter in the operating room or in the catheterization laboratory, but when transportation is not deemed safe, the procedure can be done with reasonable safety and ease at the bedside. An x-ray cassette is placed under the chest for subsequent verification of balloon position. The site of insertion is immaterial; usually, the femoral artery with the better pulse is selected. Local infiltration anesthesia can be supplemented by an intravenous sedative or analgesic.

A longitudinal incision is made over the femoral artery, with the groin crease as the midpoint. A 2-cm segment of the common femoral artery is isolated circumferentially. Proximal and distal control is obtained with vascular clamps, and 25 mg of heparin is injected into the distal femoral artery to prevent clotting beyond the site of the occlusion. An umbilical tape is passed around the femoral artery just above the proximal clamp, and a rubber tourniquet is slipped over the tape. A 1-cm longitudinal arteriotomy is made in the anterior wall of the isolated vessel segment. A woven tubular prosthesis, 8 mm in diameter and 5 to 6 cm in length, is beveled and slipped over the balloon catheter. The distance between Louis's angle and the femoral artery is marked by a tie on the balloon carrier to estimate the intravascular portion of the device.

The balloon is completely deflated with a syringe, and its tip is introduced through the femoral arteriotomy. It is advanced in a retrograde fashion to its position of function in the descending thoracic aorta, just distal to the left subclavian artery. The ligature marker on the balloon carrier should be outside the distal end of the graft. Once the balloon is beyond the femoral artery, the umbilical tape over the proximal artery is tightened to control bleeding. The catheter is connected to the console, and diastolic augmentation is initiated. The graft is sutured to the femoral artery with nonabsorbable sutures. Two heavy ligatures are tied around the graft, approximately 1.5 cm apart, to secure the catheter and to prevent leakage of blood. The distal vascular clamp and the proximal tourniquet are removed, thereby restoring flow to the extremity (Fig. 13-4). The presence of a femoral pulse distal to the insertion site is checked, and if absent, appropriate corrective measures are taken.

An alternate method is to suture the graft to the femoral arteriotomy, followed by introduction of the balloon-carrying catheter. This technique facilitates easier performance of the end-to-side anastomosis, but it does delay the initiation of counterpulsation. The recently developed percutaneous intra-aortic balloon catheter is now available and undergoing clinical trial [1]. If successful, this technique will offer another method of catheter insertion.

A portable chest x-ray film is obtained to check the location of the catheter tip, which should lie just distal to the aortic knob. If the position of the catheter is unsatisfactory, the fixation ligatures on the sidearm graft are loosened, and the catheter is repositioned. A second portable x-ray film may be necessary for visualization of catheter position. The groin wound is closed in layers. With an open chest, the position of the catheter can be determined by direct palpation of the aorta and the need for x-ray examination is obviated.

If resistance to balloon passage is encountered during insertion, the catheter is gently rotated. Forceful manipulation is not recommended, since it may lead to perforation or dissection of the aorta. If the femoral artery is unsuitable for cannulation, the incision is extended proximally, and the iliac artery is exposed through an extraperitoneal approach. If this step fails, introduction through the contralateral iliofemoral system is attempted. If peripheral insertion of the catheter is not possible, the ascending aorta can be used if the chest is open. This is accomplished by suturing an 8-mm

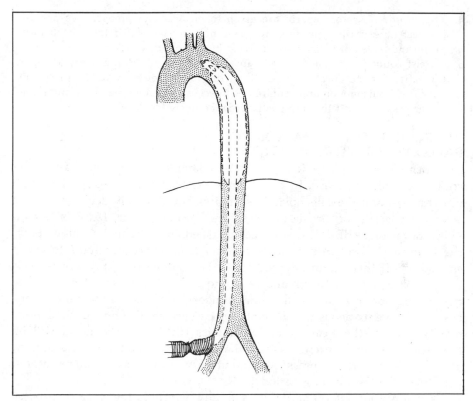

FIGURE 13-4. Position of intra-aortic balloon and method of graft fixation in femoral artery.

sidearm graft to the aorta and passing it parasternally through the right second or third interspace. The balloon is inserted through the graft and is advanced into the descending aorta. The position of the balloon can be verified by direct palpation of the aorta. Fixation ligatures on the sidearm grafts are applied at the subcutaneous level.

CARE OF THE PATIENT AFTER BALLOON INSERTION
Most patients on IABP are critically ill and require intensive supportive therapy and close monitoring. In addition, they need the following measures which relate specifically to the use of IABP:

1. Strict bed rest, with gentle restraint of the catheterized leg, in order to avoid kinking and obstruction of the catheter.
2. The dressing over the femoral incision is changed daily, and antibiotic ointment applied to the wound to prevent infection.
3. Low-molecular-weight dextran (10 ml/hr) is thought to protect against the excessive platelet destruction associated with IABP.

4. Therapeutic doses of heparin are given to medical and preoperative patients. For fear of excessive bleeding, we have not anticoagulated the postoperative group and have not noticed any increase in thrombotic complications.
5. Platelet count is obtained prior to insertion of the IABP and every 12 hours thereafter for the duration of IABP. A drop in platelets to 60,000 to 80,000/mm³ is not uncommon and requires no specific measures; platelet transfusions are necessary only if the count falls to dangerously low levels.

WEANING FROM INTRA-AORTIC BALLOON COUNTERPULSATION

In patients with cardiogenic shock, catecholamine therapy may have to be continued while on IABP. In successful cases, shock reverses, urinary output resumes, and the catecholamine requirement gradually decreases. After a variable length of circulatory stability, weaning from IABP is begun. Withdrawal of IABP is usually accomplished in a gradual fashion. First, the frequency of augmentation is reduced from every heartbeat to every second one. If this intermittent assistance is tolerated for 1 to 2 hours, then it is cut back to every fourth and finally to every eighth beat. This last frequency provides only minimal cardiac support, but it keeps the balloon mobile and prevents deposition of clots on its surface. Continued circulatory stability during the weaning period implies that balloon removal will be tolerated. It should be emphasized that the clinical state, cardiac output, atrial filling and arterial pressures, and urinary output have to be monitored closely during the weaning period.

Cardiac output determination is especially helpful in the weaning process from IABP. This measurement can estimate the contribution of the assistance and may establish the opportune time for its withdrawal. Paired measurements of cardiac output are made 5 to 15 minutes apart when the patient is on and off balloon pumping. IABP increases cardiac output initially, but as the heart recovers, the contribution of the mechanical assistance to cardiac output decreases and the left ventricle can maintain an adequate systemic flow. At this point the measured cardiac output values become similar whether balloon pumping is maintained or discontinued.

Although balloon pumping up to 30 to 40 days has been reported, in the overwhelming majority of patients the duration of support has been only several days.

REMOVAL OF THE BALLOON CATHETER

By the time removal of the balloon catheter is planned, the patient is usually stable, and transportation to the operating area is safe. The procedure is performed under mild sedation and local infiltration anesthesia. The groin wound is opened, proximal and distal control of the femoral artery is obtained, and the ligatures securing the catheter to the sidearm graft are removed. The balloon is deflated and the catheter is withdrawn. Fogarty embolectomy catheters are advanced through the stump of the graft both proximally and distally to remove any clots that may have formed in the iliofemoral system.

Repair of the arteriotomy can be handled in several different ways. The graft can be removed and the arteriotomy repaired by direct suturing. If primary approximation is likely to produce stenosis, an autologous vein patch harvested from the adjacent saphenous vein is inserted. A third possibility is amputation of the graft close to the artery and suture closure of the prosthetic stump. Although this last method is the simplest and appears attractive, it has the disadvantage of leaving a foreign body in a potentially infected wound. We use this method routinely unless the balloon catheter is inserted at the bedside or if wound infection is anticipated.

With ascending aortic insertion of the intra-aortic balloon, the device is removed by opening the skin incision about the balloon catheter. The fixation ligatures from the sidearm graft are released, the balloon is deflated, and the device is withdrawn. The graft is ligated, the stump is buried in the subcutaneous space, and the incision is closed.

The percutaneously inserted balloon catheter is removed by simple withdrawal of the deflated balloon. Finger pressure is applied to the insertion site for a prolonged period to insure adequate hemostasis.

COMPLICATIONS

The potential for complications of IABP are legion but, fortunately, in actuality they are not common. The following complications occur with varying frequencies.

RUPTURE OF THE BALLOON

Rupture of the balloon could be a very serious complication. Lack of reported cases implies that if it does happen, it must be extremely rare. Responsible quality control of the balloon must account for lack of rupture. In addition, the pumping system is equipped with built-in safety features to prevent overinflation and rupture.

PERFORATION OF THE AORTA

Forceful passage of the catheter during introduction can cause perforation of the aorta, and extreme caution should therefore be taken during this maneuver. With the appropriate technique, aortic perforation can be avoided.

FAILURE TO INTRODUCE THE BALLOON CATHETER

Even with a palpable femoral pulse, inability to pass the catheter is encountered in approximately 10 to 15 percent of patients. The obstruction is usually at the iliofemoral level or at the aortic bifurcation. Gentle rotation of the catheter may be helpful in overcoming the obstruction; forceful passage is ill-advised because of possible aortic perforation. Alternative sites for insertion have been mentioned in a previous section.

DISSECTION OF THE AORTA

A tear in the intima at the site of insertion can lead to dissection of the abdominal and thoracic aorta. Effective IABP can be carried out even in the false lumen and the complication may be recognized only at postmortem examination. Again, meticulous technique is the best prevention.

WOUND INFECTION

Wound infection is uncommon; in our experience it occurred in less than 5 percent of 300 cases. Fortunately, infection of the femoral artery or the prosthetic remnant has not been encountered.

Every effort should be made to avoid contamination and to adhere to sterile techniques, since an infection in the area may involve the femoral artery and result in rupture with exsanguination or eventual need to amputate the involved extremity. If a wound infection is detected while the balloon is in situ, it should be removed promptly. If continued cardiac assistance is mandatory, a new catheter may be introduced through the contralateral side after drainage of the infected wound and institution of antimicrobial therapy.

VASCULAR INSUFFICIENCY OF THE CATHETERIZED EXTREMITY

Since peripheral vascular disease is prevalent in the IABP population, an appreciable number of ischemic complications in the catheterized extremity can be anticipated. However, with meticulous technique during insertion and routine use of the Fogarty catheter during removal of the balloon, the incidence of ischemic changes can be reduced to acceptable levels. Amputation is rarely necessary, but vascular procedures for acute or chronic limb ischemia may be necessary in up to 20 percent of the assisted patients.

BLEEDING

Careful regulation of anticoagulation is essential for prevention of an iatrogenic bleeding diathesis. A decrease of platelet count is common during diastolic augmentation, but it rarely drops to levels that are associated with abnormal bleeding.

RESULTS

The hemodynamic effectiveness of IABP as a left ventricular assist device has been conclusively documented, both in experimental animals and in man.

In postinfarction cardiogenic shock, the reversal of the low output state has been gratifying but, unfortunately, in most instances the myocardium does not recover sufficiently to maintain life and the patient becomes balloon dependent. The majority of these patients die. Survival has been in the vicinity of 10 to 15 percent. Most of the survivors become cardiac cripples and succumb within weeks to months. A few return to a modestly active life. The addition of myocardial revascularization to balloon pumping may have increased salvage of these desperately ill patients slightly but it certainly has not been impressive; hence, it is not practiced widely in postinfarction cardiogenic shock.

Balloon support has been impressive in patients with ruptured interventricular septum or massive mitral regurgitation from papillary muscle dysfunction following acute myocardial infarction. In these situations, the IABP stabilizes the patients, facilitates safe cardiac catheterization, and provides substantial hemodynamic support before, during, and after surgical repair. The operative mortality rate in these patients has been reduced from approximately 70 to 80 percent to 25 to 30 percent.

Sporadic reports appear in the literature on the use of the intra-aortic balloon for patients with high-risk coronary anatomy and poor left ventricular function during cardiac surgery, but convincing evidence is lacking that the results are improved by this approach.

In unstable angina pectoris, diastolic augmentation controls ischemic pain in approximately 80 percent of the patients. Our present approach is to use IABP only when intensive medical therapy fails. In this group of patients, both the operative mortality and the perioperative infarction rate appear to be lower with the use of the intra-aortic balloon.

In postcardiotomy cardiogenic shock manifested by pump oxygenator dependence, the use of diastolic augmentation reduced mortality from near 100 percent to about 50 percent. It would also seem that when the balloon is inserted for lesser degrees of cardiac decompensation after cardiac operations, the postoperative course has been smoother and serious complications may have been ameliorated by the use of the intra-aortic balloon.

Mandatory or emergency extracardiac operations in patients with severe heart disease or recent myocardial infarction carry a high mortality rate, and prophylactic use of the intra-aortic balloon pumping may reduce the hazards of the procedure. We employed the intra-aortic balloon in 15 such patients without operative deaths or perioperative infarction. Further experience will be necessary in order to evaluate the effectiveness of this modality.

VENTRICULAR ASSIST DEVICES

Intense interest in mechanical circulatory support systems resulted in the development of a temporary left ventricular assist device (LVAD) that is much more powerful than the IABP and is capable of pumping total systemic blood flow. The LVAD underwent extensive evaluation in animals and has been used in clinical trials since 1975. By 1979, the device had been employed in approximately 60 cardiac surgical patients for pump oxygenator dependence, with 6 long-term survivors.

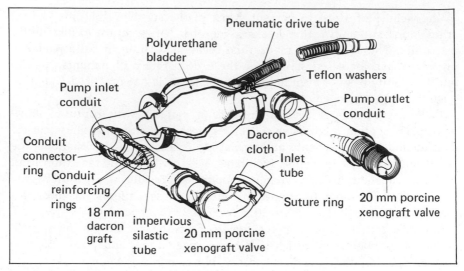

FIGURE 13-5. Schematic representation of the left ventricular assist device. The inlet tube is inserted into the left ventricle and the outlet graft is anastomosed to the ascending aorta in an end-to-side fashion.

There are several different designs available, but the ensuing remarks will be limited to the model developed by Bernhard and employed in our institution. The LVAD is a pneumatic pump with valved inflow and outflow conduits (Figs. 13-5–13-7). Power source and control console are external. Blood is drained from the left ventricle and pumped into the ascending aorta. The blood-contacting surfaces are flocked with 5- by 250-μ polyester fibrils in order to facilitate the rapid entrapment of autologous lining membrane. The pumping chamber consists of a trilobular, flexible polyurethane bladder housed inside a rigid cylindrical titanium shell. It connects with tubular Dacron inflow and outflow conduits, each incorporating a porcine aortic xenograft to ensure unidirectional flow. The inflow limb starts as a short, angled, metal tube and is inserted into the left ventricle through its apex. The distal end of the outflow tube is anastomosed to the ascending aorta in an end-to-side fashion. The bladder fills with blood from the left ventricle through the inflow conduit, is compressed by the introduction of carbon dioxide under pressure into the space between the rigid metal housing and the flexible polyurethane sac, and ejects into the ascending aorta. Pumping can be accomplished asynchronously or it may be synchronized with the ECG so that the bladder fills during ventricular systole and ejects during diastole. Maximal stroke volume and pumping rate are 80 ml and 100 per minute, respectively, so that the LVAD can handle up to 8 liter/min of blood.

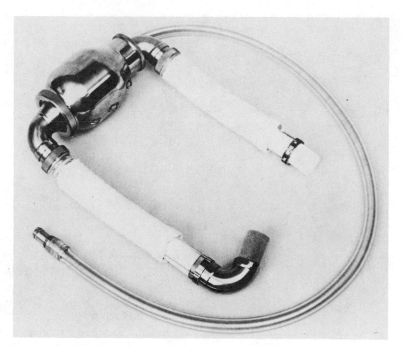

FIGURE 13-6. Photograph of the left ventricular assist device used in man. The metal elbow (*lower left*) is the left ventricular port. The metal casing houses the flexible pump bladder and the outflow conduit is on the upper right. The plastic tubing is connected to the pneumatic power console.

INDICATIONS FOR INSERTION OF LVAD

At the present time, the indication for the employment of the LVAD has been limited to cardiac surgical patients in whom satisfactory correction of the cardiac defect was accomplished and either cardiopulmonary bypass could not be discontinued (CPB dependence) or refractory cardiogenic shock developed during the first 72 hours postoperatively (CS-POP) in spite of correction of serious arrhythmias, adequate volume replacement, maximal pharmacologic support, and intra-aortic balloon pump assistance.

TECHNIQUE

The LVAD is inserted with the patient on conventional total cardiopulmonary bypass and a vented left ventricle. A 20-mm circular ring is sutured to the apex of the left ventricle. The outflow graft conduit is anastomosed to the ascending aorta in an end-to-side fashion inside a partially occlusive

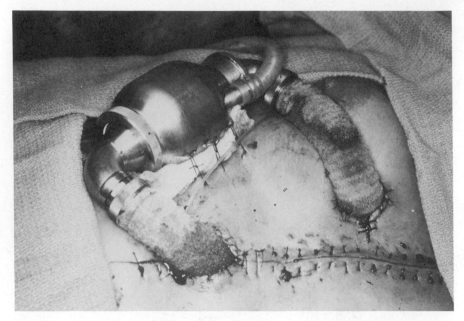

FIGURE 13-7. The left ventricular assist device in situ. The inflow conduit emerges from the lower pole of the sternotomy incision, the pump rests on the anterior right chest wall, and the outflow arm enters the mediastinum through a separate incision.

vascular clamp. Usually, even with several coronary bypass grafts and aortic cannulation for cardiopulmonary bypass, sufficient room is available on the ascending aorta for the LVAD outflow conduit. An 8- to 10-cm incision is made on the right anterior chest wall over the third intercostal space and a 2-in. segment of the third rib is resected. The outflow limb is passed out through this chest wall opening. A full-thickness core of the left ventricular apex is excised inside the previously placed ring and through this opening, the inflow arm is inserted into the left ventricle. It is channeled out through the lower portion of the sternotomy incision. The entire system is filled with fluid and the two conduits are attached to the pump through airtight screw-lock connectors. The system is de-aired, and pumping at low flows is commenced. Gradually, flow through the LVAD is increased, and simultaneously, pumping through the pump oxygenator is proportionately reduced. Catecholamine infusion is usually necessary to support the right ventricle. Once adequate flow (2 liter/min/M^2) through the LVAD is obtained, conventional cardiopulmonary bypass support is discontinued, the heart is decannulated, and heparin is neutralized with protamine. Since LVAD deployment is usually preceded by a relatively long pump oxygenator run, restoration of the clotting mechanism may be difficult and time-consuming, but nevertheless, it is crucial to obtain a relatively dry field prior to closure of the chest. If an IABP is in situ, it is removed after satisfactory LVAD function is established. Anticoagulation is not required during LVAD support.

In addition to the arterial, left atrial, and central venous pressure lines, use of a thermodilution pulmonary artery catheter for measurement of cardiac output is mandatory. The rate of pumping and the stroke volume are digitally displayed on the LVAD power console. The difference between the cardiac output value obtained by the thermodilution technique and LVAD flow represents a rough measure of left ventricular contribution to total systemic flow. In the early period of LVAD support, the two values are usually similar, reflecting both severe left ventricular failure and near total unloading of the chamber. Our experience with 9 patients indicates that in successful cases the myocardium recovers after 3 to 4 days of LVAD support; thus, uninterrupted pumping with full flows is practiced for this period. Weaning from LVAD is usually tried on the third or fourth day by gradual reduction of flow through the pump to 1 liter/min/M². If this is tolerated without significant fall in cardiac output and arterial pressure or without an appreciable rise in left atrial pressure, the period of reduced support is extended to 1 hr. Full pumping is resumed but the weaning trials are repeated at 4- to 8-hr intervals. If satisfactory cardiac function is maintained consistently during the weaning trials, the patient is prepared for removal of the device.

During the final weaning period, anticoagulation is instituted to prevent clot formation within the device during the low flow state. Gradual reduction of support continues for a 5- to 6-hour period until an LVAD flow of 0.5 to 0.6 liter/min is reached. If the hemodynamics remain satisfactory, the patient is returned to the operating room for removal of the LVAD.

Prior to withdrawal of LVAD support, an intra-aortic balloon is inserted through the femoral artery and diastolic augmentation is instituted in order to effect a gradual transition from total mechanical support to left ventricular independence. The inflow and outflow conduits of the LVAD are divided between occlusive clamps close to the chest wall, and the extracorporeal portion of the device is removed. The midsternal incision is reopened, the residual grafts are amputated close to the aorta and left ventricle, and the stumps are oversewn. Heparin is neutralized with protamine. The chest is closed in a routine fashion. Diastolic augmentation is continued for 24 to 48 hours; if hemodynamic stability continues, the balloon is removed.

The clinical experience to date clearly demonstrates that the LVAD can substitute effectively for total left ventricular function and provide sufficient systemic flow to maintain adequate total body perfusion. Vital organ function was satisfactory in all supported patients, and trauma to the formed elements of blood was minimal.

COMPLICATIONS

Excessive Bleeding

In the immediate postoperative period, excessive blood drainage is common. Although the LVAD does not consume the coagulation factors, the relatively long period on cardiopulmonary bypass necessitated by repair of the cardiac lesion, resuscitation to establish clearcut CIPB dependence, and the 45 to 60 minutes required for insertion of the LVAD are conducive to coagulopathy. It is anticipated that earlier implantation of the LVAD will be practiced in the future and pump oxygenator time will be shortened so that bleeding problems may be reduced.

Cardiac Tamponade

Excessive postoperative bleeding was almost invariably associated with the development of cardiac tamponade. Most of our assisted patients who survived for 12 to 24 hours after LVAD implantation had to be explored for compression of the heart. The hemodynamic manifestations of cardiac tamponade include a decrease in LVAD flow and a fall in arterial pressure with high left and right heart filling pressures. This hemodynamic constellation represents an absolute indication for reexploration and release of the tamponade.

Right Heart Failure

Seemingly irreversible right heart failure was another limiting factor in the early experience with LVAD. Our more recent cases suggest that the massive right ventricular dysfunction is frequently due to temporary myocardial depression rather than to irreversible infarction; aggressive therapy with catecholamines is usually effective.

Thus, the right heart appears to be less of a limiting factor than it was thought to be earlier, and biventricular pump is not necessary in most instances.

Infection

Mediastinal infections introduced through the inflow and outflow conduits had been of major concern prior to the clinical trials. This fear was initially allayed, since infections from the components of the assist device during the period of actual support (4–8 days) did not occur. However, in 2 of 4 surviving patients, the portion of the inflow conduit left behind in the left ventricle became infected 20 days and 16 months after discontinuation of support. In both patients, the LVAD remnant was removed without the use of cardiopulmonary bypass. Because of this experience, in the future, removal of the entire LVAD system is planned at the time the support is discontinued.

REFERENCES

1. Subramanian, V. A., Goldstein, J. E., Sos, T. A., McCabe, J. C., Hoover, E. A., and Gay, W. A., Jr.   Preliminary clinical experience with percutaneous intra-aortic balloon pumping. *Circulation* 62(Suppl. I):123, 1980.

SELECTED READINGS

McCabe, J. C., Abel, R. M., Subramanian, V. A., and Gay, W. A., Jr.   Complications of intraaortic balloon insertion and counterpulsation. *Circulation* 57: 769, 1978.

McEnany, M. T., Kay, H. R., Buckley, M. J., Daggett, W. M., Erdmann, A. J., Mundth, E. D., Rao, R. S., Detoef, J., and Austen, W. G.   Clinical experience with intraaortic balloon pump support in 728 patients. *Circulation* 58(Suppl. I):124, 1977.

Weintraub, R. M., Aroesty, J. M., Paulin, S., Levine, F. H., Markis, J. E., LaRaia, P. J., Cohen, S. I., and Kurland, G. F.   Medically refractory unstable angina pectoris. I. Long-term follow-up of patients undergoing intraaortic balloon counterpulsation and operation. *Am. J. Cardiol.* 43:877, 1979.

Kazi Mobin-Uddin

14. USE OF THE INFERIOR VENA CAVA UMBRELLA FILTER

Pulmonary embolism is a major threat to life in critically ill patients confined to bed on both medical and surgical services. It is estimated that pulmonary embolism causes approximately 200,000 deaths per year in the United States: it is the sole cause of death in 100,000 and is a major contributing cause in another 100,000 [6]. It has been estimated that a substantial number of deaths from pulmonary embolism are potentially preventable.

Barker and associates [1] have reported on the natural course of untreated thromboembolism in postoperative patients. Of 1,665 patients with pulmonary embolism, the first episode was fatal in 24.4 percent, and death occurred in 18.3 percent of the nearly one-third who had recurrent emboli. Based on the work of Murray [14], anticoagulation with heparin became the standard treatment for patients with thromboembolic disease. The effectiveness of anticoagulant therapy was documented by Barritt and Jordan [2] in a controlled study in which 5 of 19 patients given no treatment died from pulmonary embolism, and 5 other patients had further nonfatal recurrent emboli. No deaths and no further emboli occurred in 16 patients concurrently treated with heparin. Despite adequate anticoagulant therapy, recurrences of pulmonary embolism are not uncommon. The urokinase-pulmonary embolism trial phase 1 [15], a national cooperative study group, reported an 18 percent recurrence rate (9% fatal) in 60 patients treated with adequate anticoagulation.

Recurrent pulmonary embolism despite adequate anticoagulation is best prevented by interruption of the inferior vena cava (IVC). The operative mortality rate of IVC interruption in critically ill patients ranges between 20 and 50 percent, depending on the severity of the underlying cardiopulmonary disease and the extent of obstruction to pulmonary blood flow. In patients with right heart failure (cor pulmonale), either operative caval interruption is withheld or the lesser procedure of femoral vein ligation is performed, since the use of a general anesthetic poses too great a risk.

Transvenous interruption of IVC by the umbrella filter (UF) is performed under local anesthesia; it avoids a major surgical operation, maintains the

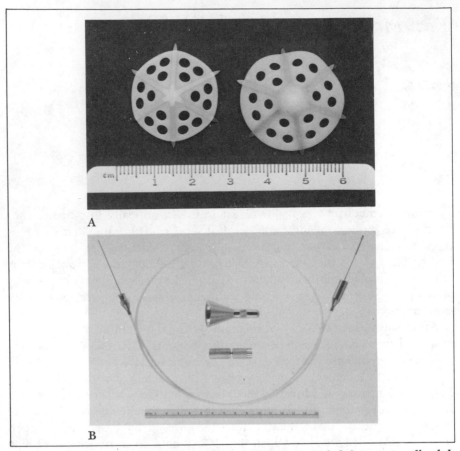

FIGURE 14-1. (A, right) The 28-mm filter now recommended for use in all adult patients. (A, left) The 23-mm filter may have an application in patients weighing less than 125 pounds. (B) Catheter used for umbrella filter implantation.

cardiac output, and at the same time protects the patients from potentially lethal pulmonary embolism [10–13]. This procedure can be done with minimal risk even in critically ill patients with acute pulmonary embolism.

OPERATIVE TECHNIQUE FOR UMBRELLA IMPLANTATION
The UF (Fig. 14-1A) consists of six spokes of stainless steel alloy radiating from a central hub and covered on both sides by a thin, circular sheet of silicone [8]. The spokes extend 2 mm beyond the silicone webbing, which has 18 perforations 3 mm in diameter. The original umbrella was 23 mm in diameter, but episodes of filter migration led to the development of a 28-mm device. At the end of the catheter (Fig. 14-1B) used for UF implanta-

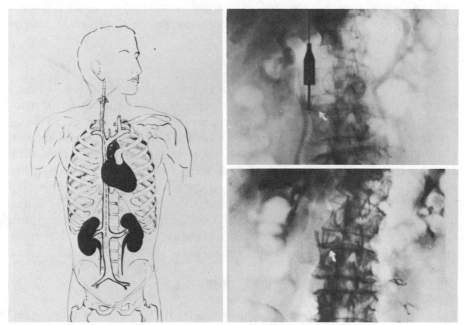

FIGURE 14-2. (*Left*) Applicator capsule containing collapsed umbrella filter has been inserted through right internal jugular vein into inferior vena cava (IVC) below renal veins. (*Top right*) Filter has been ejected from capsule into IVC. (*Bottom right*) Stylet has been unscrewed from filter, and applicator has been withdrawn.

tion, there is a metal capsule 6 mm in diameter and 32 mm in length. A threaded stylet fits inside the catheter and capsule.

The UF is folded into the catheter capsule with the help of a loading cone. Under local infiltration anesthesia, through a small incision in the neck, the catheter is inserted through a venotomy into the right internal jugular vein and advanced under fluoroscopic control into the infrarenal IVC (Fig. 14-2). The catheter capsule is generally advanced to the level of the bifurcation of the IVC and is then withdrawn, so that the distal tip of the capsule is positioned at the level of the midpoint of the third lumbar vertebra. By pushing the stylet, the umbrella is ejected from the capsule into the IVC, where it springs open. Firm upward traction is applied several times on the stylet to fix the filter securely in place. The stylet is unscrewed from the UF and is then withdrawn along with the catheter. The internal jugular vein is repaired before the incision is closed.

An inferior vena cavogram made before UF insertion is an invaluable adjunct. It demonstrates the level of renal veins and the size of the IVC and may reveal any unsuspected abnormalities of the IVC or of the renal veins. Any thrombus in the IVC that may interfere with placement of the UF can also be detected.

POSTOPERATIVE MANAGEMENT
Following UF implantation, anticoagulant therapy is withheld for 12 hours to minimize the possibility of bleeding in the neck or into the retroperitoneal space. Thereafter, intravenous heparin is resumed for 7 to 10 days, preferably by continuous infusion to maintain the partial thromboplastin time or the Lee-White clotting time at two times the control value. Oral anticoagulation with sodium warfarin is started on the third postoperative day and continued for 3 months. Patients with a continued predisposing factor such as cardiac failure, and those with chronic obstructive airway disease associated with microemboli and cor pulmonale, receive long-term anticoagulant therapy. Elevation, elastic support, and early ambulation are employed to prevent or control peripheral edema.

SELECTION OF PATIENTS FOR UMBRELLA IMPLANTATION
Pulmonary embolism is frequently unrecognized. The difficulty in diagnosis is partly due to the varied manifestations of the disease, and the diagnosis often depends on a high index of clinical suspicion. It may appear as unexplained dyspnea, pulmonary infarction, cor pulmonale, or acute cardiovascular collapse; or there may be worsening of the underlying heart or lung disease.

Radioisotope lung scanning is a valuable test for detecting abnormalities in the distribution of blood flow. A normal lung scan essentially rules out significant pulmonary embolism. Abnormal scans showing wedge-shaped defects with a clear chest x-ray film in areas other than the pulmonary infiltrate are highly suggestive of pulmonary emboli. The lung scans are difficult to interpret in the face of chronic obstructive airway disease, bronchial asthma, pneumonia, and congestive heart failure. Demonstration of deep venous thrombosis by phlebography may substantiate the diagnosis of pulmonary emboli. If phlebograms are negative, then pulmonary arteriography is usually required for diagnosis.

MASSIVE PULMONARY EMBOLISM
Patients with massive pulmonary embolism who have survived the acute insult can die from arrhythmias, low cardiac output, or recurrent pulmonary embolism. IVC interruption by the umbrella filter is usually recommended—reliance on anticoagulant therapy alone is not justified, since any additional embolization can be fatal. Bloomfield reported umbrella filter insertion in patients who had survived massive pulmonary embolism by 1 to 2 hours.

Of the 12 patients, 8 made uncomplicated recovery. Remarkable clinical and hemodynamic improvements have been observed in these patients within 2 to 12 hours following UF insertion, probably from prevention of pulmonary emboli [3–5].

Patients with massive pulmonary embolism, together with severe respiratory distress and sustained hypotension or shock that is refractory to intensive medical therapy, are treated by pulmonary embolectomy. Preoperative mechanical circulatory support with a pump oxygenator by peripheral cannulation of the femoral artery and vein under local anesthesia is imperative for a successful outcome [4]. Following embolectomy, the umbrella filter is inserted through the right atrial appendage [9].

FAILURE OF ANTICOAGULANTS
The umbrella filter insertion is recommended in patients in whom adequate heparinization has failed to prevent recurrent embolism. Pulmonary embolism is likely to recur in patients with a continued predisposition to pulmonary embolism, such as patients with chronic congestive heart failure, critically ill patients confined to bed, and patients with recurrent thrombophlebitis.

CONTRAINDICATION TO ANTICOAGULANTS
Contraindication to the administration of heparin may be absolute or relative. Treatment for each patient should be individualized and the need for therapy verified against the probable risk of hemorrhage. Usually heparin is not given to patients with recent cerebral vascular accidents, operation, or severe trauma or to those with recent history of actively bleeding lesions.

PRESENCE OF POTENTIALLY FATAL THROMBI
IN ILIOFEMORAL VEINS OR INFERIOR VENA CAVA
Nearly all emboli arise from thrombi in the lower extremities or pelvic veins. Major or fatal emboli come from the large deep veins of the thigh and pelvis. Vein thrombi of the lower leg may become significant if the thrombus extends into the popliteal vein. Clinical evaluation detects fewer than half the cases of deep venous thrombosis, and pulmonary embolism is often the first manifestation of the disease. At our institution, phlebography is used as part of the work-up in patients with pulmonary embolism to determine the extent of residual venous thrombosis. It is apparent that heparin in adequate doses may prevent thrombus formation or propagation but cannot prevent fragmentation or detachment of a nonadherent thrombus. A fresh, nonadherent thrombus appears as a radiolucent defect within the vein with the contrast medium lining the vein wall (Fig. 14-3). It is our practice to recommend IVC interruption by the UF in patients who have potentially fatal thrombi in the iliofemoral veins.

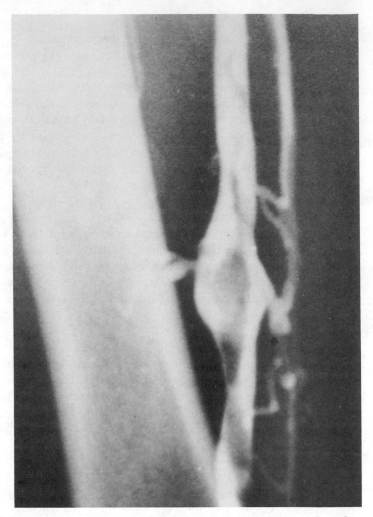

FIGURE 14-3. Phlebogram demonstrating potentially lethal, nonadherent thrombus in femoral vein.

PROPHYLACTIC

Thromboembolism continues to be a major cause for morbidity and mortality in elderly patients with hip fracture. The prophylactic use of the UF in patients with fracture of the proximal femur was evaluated in a controlled study group [7]. In 41 patients treated with the UF, there was no mortality from pulmonary embolism. In 59 patients in the control group, pulmonary embolism was the cause of death in 8 (13.5%).

In patients with fractured hips in whom surgery is delayed for more than 36 to 48 hours, development of deep venous thrombosis is the rule rather than the exception. Fatal pulmonary embolism is likely to occur in these patients if the hip operation is done in the presence of recent thrombi in the lower extremity or pelvic veins. At our institution, IVC interruption by the UF is performed prior to hip surgery if there is clinical or venographic evidence of peripheral deep-vein thrombosis.

RESULTS
A discussion of the results of clinical filter implants in 6,454 patients (3,123, 23 mm; 3,331, 28 mm), as reported by the evaluating physicians follows.

MORTALITY
Since transvenous interruption of the IVC by the UF can be performed with minimal risk even in critically ill patients with pulmonary embolism, the mortality is now more closely related to the underlying disease.

RECURRENT EMBOLISM
Recurrent embolism has been reported in 2 percent of patients who had clinical filter implants (fatal in 0.5%). In 3 patients a blood clot from the proximal surface of the filter was implicated as the source of pulmonary embolism. In an attempt to resist or prevent thrombus formation on proximal surface of the filter, the umbrella filters have now been treated with the tri-dodecylmethyl ammonium chloride–heparin complex. Moreover, postoperative anticoagulant therapy is continued for 3 months if there is no contraindication for its use. These measures may prevent thrombus formation and allow for growth of endothelium between the fenestrations of the filter. In my own experience with patients in whom the newly available heparin-treated umbrella was used, the patency rate in 20 patients followed with repeated venograms up to 3 years is 60 percent.

FILTER PERFORMANCE
FILTER MIGRATION
The original caval umbrella was 23 mm in diameter, but episodes of migration (1%) led to the development of a 28-mm device. With the use of the 28-mm umbrella, the incidence of migration has been reduced to 0.4 percent. Manufacturing and marketing of the 23-mm filter have been discontinued.

The migrated filter may lodge in the supra-renal IVC, right atrium, right ventricle, or in the pulmonary artery. The main causes of filter migration have been inadequate seating of the filter or an exceptionally large IVC. Umbrella filter insertion is not recommended if the transverse diameter of the IVC is more than 3 cm as shown by venography.

FILTER DISLODGMENT WITHOUT MIGRATION
Partial dislodgment of the UF without migration has been reported in 20 patients. To prevent migration, the 28-mm filter was implanted just above

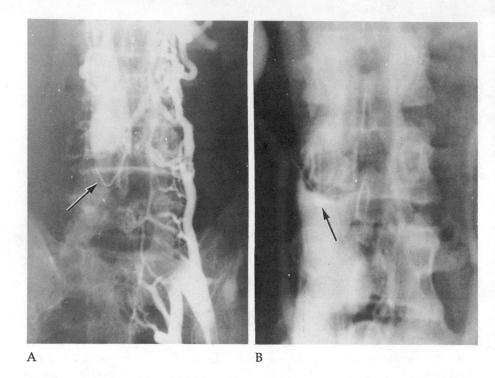

A   B

FIGURE 14-4. (A) Angiogram of inferior vena cava (IVC) in patient 5 days after umbrella implantation. Note complete thrombotic occlusion of IVC and development of collateral circulation. (B) Angiogram of IVC 3 months after implantation of heparin-impregnated umbrella filter. Note free flow of blood through filter.

the previous filter in 6 patients. In the remaining patients, either nothing was done, or surgical interruption of the IVC was performed with or without removal of the filter.

MISPLACEMENT OF THE FILTER
The UF has been improperly placed in the suprarenal IVC, right renal vein, and right iliac vein. In 3 patients in whom the UF was accidentally extruded into the suprarenal IVC, the filters could be pushed downward with the applicator capsule into the IVC below the renal veins. In 2 of these patients, a second filter was implanted proximal to the first because the latter became tilted. Of the 7 patients in whom the UF was inadvertently misplaced in the right renal vein, the UF was removed and the IVC interrupted by direct surgical approach in 3. The UF was mistakenly placed in the right iliac vein in 20 patients; they were treated either by removing the filter with interruption of the IVC or by implanting an additional filter in the IVC.

STASIS SEQUELAE

Significant clinical edema of the lower extremities not previously present developed in 5.1 percent of patients, and thrombophlebitis developed post-operatively in 1.5 percent. The majority of these patients improved with standard medical management. Edema of the lower extremities after umbrella insertion has not been a significant problem; occlusion of the filter occurs gradually and apparently allows sufficient time for the development of collateral circulation, thus avoiding acute hemodynamic changes.

OTHER COMPLICATIONS

Significant retroperitoneal bleeding has been reported in 5 patients, right recurrent laryngeal nerve injury in 2, and perforation of duodenum and ureter in 1 patient each. Air embolism during filter insertion has occurred in 2 patients and was fatal in 1.

SUMMARY

For prevention of pulmonary embolism, transvenous interruption of the inferior vena cava by the umbrella filter can be accomplished with minimal risk even in critically ill patients. Most investigators report satisfaction with the simplicity of the procedure and the results achieved. As physicians have gained experience with the technique, the complication rate has significantly decreased. A large number of physicians are now using the umbrella procedure as the method of choice for caval interruption.

REFERENCES

1. Barker, N. W., et al. Statistical study of post-operative venous thrombosis and pulmonary embolism. Incidence of various types of operative procedures. *Mayo Clin. Proc.* 15:769, 1940.
2. Barritt, D. W., and Jordan, S. C. Anticoagulant drugs in treatment of pulmonary embolism: Controlled trial. *Lancet* 1:1309, 1960.
3. Beller, B. M., et al. Nonsurgical inferior vena cava obstruction for prevention of pulmonary emboli. *J.A.M.A.* 220:973, 1972.
4. Berger, R. L. Pulmonary embolectomy with pre-operative circulatory support. *Ann. Thorac. Surg.* 16:217, 1973.
5. Bloomfield, D. A. The Use of Intracaval Umbrella Filters in Massive Pulmonary Embolism. In K. Mobin-Uddin (Ed.), *Pulmonary Thromboembolism.* Springfield, Ill.: Thomas, 1974.
6. Dalen, J. E., and Alpert, J. S. Natural history of pulmonary embolism. *Prog. Cardiovasc. Dis.* 17:257, 1975.
7. Fullen, W. D., et al. Prophylactic vena caval interruption in hip fractures. *J. Trauma* 13:403, 1973.
8. Grode, G. A., et al. Bio-compatible materials for use in the vascular system. *J. Biomed. Mater. Res.* 6:77, 1972.
9. Huse, W. M. Vena cava umbrella filter insertion during pulmonary embolectomy. *Arch. Surg.* 106:737, 1973.

10. Mobin-Uddin, K., et al.   Caval interruption for prevention of pulmonary embolism: Long term results of a new method. *Arch. Surg.* 99:711, 1969.
11. Mobin-Uddin, K., et al.   Intravenous caval interruption for pulmonary embolism in cardiac disease. *Circulation* 41(Suppl. 2):153, 1970.
12. Mobin-Uddin, K., et al.   Present status of the inferior vena cava umbrella filter. *Surgery* 70:914, 1971.
13. Mobin-Uddin K., et al.   Transvenous caval interruption with umbrella filter. *N. Engl. J. Med.* 286:55, 1972.
14. Murray, G.   Anticoagulants in venous thrombosis and prevention of pulmonary embolism. *Surg. Gynecol. Obstet.* 84:665, 1947.
15. Sasahara, A. A., et al. (Ed. Comm.).   The urokinase pulmonary embolism trial. A national cooperative study. *Circulation* 47(Suppl. 2):1, 1973.

Samuel R. Powers, Jr. | ## 15. FLUID AND ELECTROLYTE MANAGEMENT

DEFINITION OF THE PROBLEM
Fluid management for an otherwise normal patient who requires parenteral therapy is an exercise in fluid balance.

Example
The usual postoperative patient with an uncomplicated course.

Management of the fluid and electrolyte requirements for critically ill patients, on the other hand, is an exercise in optimizing physiologic function.

Example
A patient with multiple trauma, complicated by peritonitis and respiratory distress.

Disorders of fluid and electrolyte metabolism are manifested by functional abnormalities in one or more organ systems, and it is these abnormalities that the therapist strives to correct. Laboratory values of water and electrolyte quantity and composition should be used as guideposts toward the optimization of physiologic function, but they are not ends in themselves. Single determinations of serum electrolyte concentrations are among the least useful bits of data that are available from the laboratory. Daily water and salt balance sheets are useful in the management of the critically ill patient, but more often than not, an hourly imbalance of fluid and electrolyte intake and output is optimal therapy; intake must eventually balance output, but a transient imbalance is often the proper course.

The problem of fluid and electrolyte management in the critically ill must be considered as an exercise in how best to optimize the physiologic function of the various disordered organ systems on an hour-to-hour basis. Different electrolyte therapy may be required to optimize the patient's physiologic state at some later period of his clinical course. The management of water and electrolyte problems in a critically ill patient is modified by three axioms.

Axiom I

Proper replacement therapy depends on both the absolute level of the fluid and electrolyte disorder and on the clinical state of the patient at the time the disorder was observed.

Example

The appropriate program for management of a patient with a serum sodium of 122 mEq/liter who has had a low sodium intake for a prolonged period is entirely different from the management of a patient with the same laboratory values whose serum sodium was 145 mEq/liter 12 hours before. In the first patient, physiologic function of the various organ systems is probably close to optimal. In the second situation, the patient's central nervous system will be markedly hyperirritable, and the patient may be having a convulsion. The administration of sodium solutions in the former case would be likely to result in the onset of congestive heart failure. The withholding of sodium solutions in the latter case could well result in profound cerebral edema.

Functionally important disturbances in fluid and electrolyte metabolism are manifested by characteristic clinical findings. It is the clinical evidence of functional abnormality that should be treated rather than attempting to restore a series of laboratory values to some preconceived normal level.

Axiom II

The absolute value of serum electrolytes at any point in time is of less importance than the direction of change of these values between two points in time. The term *trajectory* is useful for describing this concept. *Trajectory* implies both the direction of change and the rate of change. The trajectory is of much greater importance than the absolute value.

Axiom III

The tolerance for error in the critically ill is much less than in the usual hospital patient. Normally functioning kidneys and a normal cardiovascular system will generally correct a therapeutic miscalculation. In the critically ill, these organs are functionally depressed and cannot be depended on to salvage fluid misman-agement. Sophisticated monitoring and accurate interpretation of the changing physiologic state are necessary in the case of the critically ill.

THE ESSENTIAL VOCABULARY

The concentration of solutes within the various body fluid compartments are described in units of either milliequivalents per liter or milliosmoles per liter. The language of fluid and electrolyte management cannot be under-stood until the essential vocabulary is mastered.

ELECTROLYTES

Electrolytes acquired their name because in aqueous solutions they conduct an electric current. For an electric current to pass through a solution, charged ions are required, and it is this ionic dissociation that gives electrolytes their particular properties. Positively charged ions, such as sodium, potassium, and calcium, are referred to as *cations* because they migrate toward the cathode when an electric current is passed through the solution. In similar fashion, chloride and sulfate ions are referred to as *anions* because they will migrate toward the anode. Solutions containing a mixture of anions and cations must maintain electrical neutrality by having the same number of positive and negative charges. Another way to state this is that the number of positively charged ions must be matched with an equivalent number of negatively charged ions. Chemically, the amounts of anions and cations are 1 equivalent when each is present in an amount equal to its atomic weight.

Example
A solution of sodium chloride, which contains 23 gm of sodium (atomic weight 23) and 35 gm of chloride (atomic weight 35) meets the requirement of electrical neutrality.

Equivalent amounts are those amounts equal to their atomic weights, and the solution described above is defined as having 1 equivalent of sodium ion and 1 equivalent of chloride ion. When the amount of dissolved material is in milligrams rather than grams, the concentration is described as 1 milliequivalent (mEq) of sodium ion and 1 mEq of chloride ion.

Example
If a solution contains 230 mg of sodium ions dissolved in 1 liter, then its concentration is $230/23 = 10$ mEq/liter. An equivalent amount of chloride ion is 350 mg, which is $350/35$ or 10 mEq/liter.

Certain ions, such as calcium and magnesium, have two positive charges rather than one and will therefore combine with, or be equivalent to, twice the number of single-charged anions.

Example
40 mg of calcium (atomic weight 40) will combine with 70mg of chloride ions (atomic weight 35).

One atomic weight of calcium is equivalent to two atomic weights of chloride. To calculate the number of milliequivalents of calcium or magnesium ions, it is necessary to take the atomic weight in milligrams and divide by 2.

THE OSMOLALITY OF BODY FLUIDS
If two solutions containing solutes at different concentrations are separated by a membrane that allows water to move freely from one solution to the

other but does not permit the movement of solute across the membrane, water will move across the membrane until the osmolality on the two sides is identical. Solutions are said to have the same osmolality when the number of dissolved particles per unit volume is the same in both solutions. The number of particles is proportional to the weight of each substance in milligrams divided by its molecular weight.

Example
180 mg of glucose (molecular weight in milligrams) has exactly the same osmotic pressure as 23 mg sodium ion.

The unit 1 milliosmole (mOsm) is defined as the number of milligrams of a substance that is equal to its molecular weight dissolved in a liter of water. Notice that 1 molecular weight of sodium chloride dissociates into 1 equivalent of sodium ion and 1 equivalent of chloride ion, thereby producing 2 mOsm. On the other hand, 1 molecular weight of glucose remains in solution as glucose and provides only 1 mOsm. Proteins may have molecular weights in the thousands, with thousands of milligrams required to make 1 mOsm of protein.

THE INITIAL CONDITIONS

The term *initial conditions* refers to the composition and distribution of water and electrolytes in a particular patient just prior to the institution of fluid therapy. In some patients, such as those with a routine postoperative status, these conditions will be identical with those in an average healthy person of the same body mass. These average values are given in Table 15-1. On the other hand, a critically ill patient may well have been in an abnormal state at the time the critical event occurred, and the values for initial conditions in such a patient may be different from those provided in Table 15-1. The table of normal values should be considered as a rough first estimate of a particular patient's initial fluid and electrolyte composition.

Example
A truck driver who has been driving for 12 hours without stopping for food or water will have a strikingly different set of initial conditions when he sustains a fracture of the femur than will the town drunk, who has been drinking beer and eating pretzels for several hours prior to the same injury. The fluid and electrolyte management of these two patients will be different because their initial conditions were different, even though the traumas were identical.

Example
A patient who is prepared for abdominal aneurysmectomy by optimizing his initial conditions with an intravenous infusion of isotonic sodium chloride during the several hours prior to surgery will have a different postoperative course from

TABLE 15-1. Composition of 70-Kg Man

Component	Plasma	Extracellular Inter-stitial Fluid	Intra-cellular	Bone	Total
Body water (kg or liter)	3.5	10	33	3.5	50
% body water	7	20	66	7	100
% body weight	5	15	50	5	71
mOsm/liter	290	290	290		
Na^+ (mEq)	500 (10%)	1,400 (30%)	600 (15%)	2,000 (45%)	4,500 (100%)
K^+ (mEq)	15 (<1%)	40 (1%)	3,300 (94%)	145 (4%)	3,500 (100%)
Ca^{++} (mEq)	18 (<1%)	50 (<1%)	100 (<1%)	59,900 (99%)	60,000 (100%)
Mg^{++} (mEq)	7 (<1%)	20 (<1%)	1,073 (50%)	1,000 (48%)	2,100 (100%)
Cl^- (mEq)	350 (15%)	1,000 (45%)	350 (15%)	500 (25%)	2,200 (100%)
$H_2PO_4^-$ and $HPO_4^=$ (mM)*	4 (<1%)	12 (<1%)	2,800 (14%)	17,000 (85%)	20,000 (100%)

* Because of different valence states, mass is expressed as millimoles (mM).

a patient prepared for the same operation by withholding all fluids after 8 P.M. the evening before surgery.

A careful history of the events prior to the onset of the critical illness is essential for evaluating the initial conditions. The exact magnitude of the initial derangement will in turn determine in large measure the response to a particular stress. Whenever possible, the initial conditions should be optimized (not necessarily normalized) prior to a critical event.

FLUID AND ELECTROLYTE MANAGEMENT WHEN THE INITIAL CONDITIONS ARE NORMAL

INPUT-OUTPUT IMBALANCE

FLUID LOSS FROM THE BODY

INSENSIBLE LOSS. Insensible fluid loss occurs principally through the lungs and skin. Inspired room air is low in water content, whereas expired air is saturated with water vapor at body temperature. This loss occurs as distilled water and amounts to a net loss of approximately 600 ml/24 hr. This figure is increased a small amount if the body temperature is increased (50 ml/24 hr/°F elevation) or if the respiratory minute volume is increased. This is the only mechanism for losing distilled water from the body, and it should be replaced by solutions that do not contain electrolytes (5% D/W) in an amount equal to 600 ml/24 hr. Ordinarily, there is no way the body can lose more distilled water than this amount. Therefore, the provision of intravenous replacement of 5% D/W in quantities greater than this may result in dilution of the electrolyte composition of the body. Under extreme situations, the total loss from the lungs and through the skin may equal 1.5 liters/day. The loss of water is balanced to some extent by the water of oxidation that results from the conversion of glucose into carbon dioxide and water and equals approximately 300 ml/day. Patients who are in a catabolic state, due either to starvation or to crushing injury, will release intracellular water, as much as 500 ml/day. Water is released from the cell when carbohydrate and protein within the cell are broken down and excreted. Water moves out of the cell to maintain normal osmotic balance.

URINARY LOSSES. Metabolism of a normal diet results in approximately 600 mOsm/day of solute. Healthy kidneys operating at a peak effort can concentrate urine to about 1,200 mOsm/liter. Therefore, 500 ml of urine is the absolute minimal volume that will maintain a normal internal environment; 1,000 ml/24 hr is a better standard, and this is best expressed as 40 ml/hr. *Oliguria is defined as a urine volume of less than 600 ml/24 hr* and is indicative of a functional deficit in extracellular fluid (ECF) of approximately 30 percent. Urinary electrolyte losses will vary considerably. In the severely stressed patient, urine contains almost no sodium, but under conditions of sodium loading, concentrations of up to 80 mEq/liter may be present. There is an obligatory loss of at least 30 mEq of potassium per day, but the loss may be as much as 60 to 80 mEq/day.

GASTROINTESTINAL LOSSES. Fecal water loss is less than 100 ml/day in a normal person. Patients who are suffering from vomiting or diarrhea or who have an enterostomy lose fluid that has essentially the same composition as ECF. Gastrointestinal secretions are slightly hypotonic, and their electrolyte composition varies somewhat in various portions of the gastrointestinal tract, but a good approximation for replacement therapy is fluid with a composition like that of ECF. The average composition of the various gastrointestinal fluids is given in Table 15-2. When the initial conditions are normal, 5% D/W and isotonic electrolyte solutions are the only ones that should be used to maintain balance. *Fluids should be replaced in the same form in which they are lost* (see Tables 15-3 and 15-4).

TABLE 15-2. Composition of Gastrointestinal Drainage and Replacement Solutions

Source of Drainage	Na⁺ (mEq/ liter)	K⁺ (mEq/ liter)	Cl⁻ (mEq/ liter)	HCO₃⁻ (mEq/ liter)	pH	Average Total Daily Secretion in Adult (ml)	Replacement Solution
Saliva	25	20	30	15	7.0	1,500	Multielectrolyte solution in 5% D/W
Acid-producing stomach	40–80	5–10	60–130	0	1–4	2,500	0.85% NaCl
Bile	120–140	5–15	90–100	15–30	7.4–7.6	500	Ringer's lactate
Pancreatic fistula or upper jejunum	120–140	5–15	60–90	15–30	7.4–7.6	700–1,500	Ringer's lactate
Lower ileum ileostomy, or rectal diarrhea	120–140	5–15	90–100	15–30	7.4–7.6	1,000–1,500	Ringer's lactate

TABLE 15-3. Proper Solutions for Replacement of Body Fluid Losses

Insensible loss (distilled water)	5% D/W. Maximum daily replacement 1,000 ml.
Gastrointestinal losses (extracellular fluid)	Isotonic saline or Ringer's lactate. Replace measured loss.
Urinary losses (approximates 5% D/W with 40 mEq K$^+$/liter)	5% D/W with 40 mEq K$^+$/liter. Replace measured loss.

REDISTRIBUTION OF FLUID AND ELECTROLYTES WITHIN THE BODY

Fluid may remain within the body but be redistributed within the various body compartments as a result of disease processes. Such fluids are functionally lost from the ECF, even though they remain within the body. The electrolyte composition of this redistributed fluid is invariably identical with that of ECF. The magnitude of these losses is frequently much greater than losses due to input-output imbalance but more difficult to recognize. Redistribution of fluid within the body does not appear as a change in the patient's weight or in the input-output fluid balance sheet. These losses can be detected only by physiologic changes in organ function.

SEQUESTRATION IN THE GASTROINTESTINAL TRACT

Patients suffering from mechanical intestinal obstruction or from adynamic ileus may sequester large quantities of ECF equal to many liters.

Example

The presence of air fluid levels on an upright abdominal x-ray film is generally indicative of a minimum of 1,500 ml within the lumen of the gut.

FLUID SEQUESTRATION IN PERITONITIS AND OTHER INFLAMED OR TRAUMATIZED AREAS

The peritoneal surfaces are equal to many square meters. A 1-mm thickness of edema fluid is the equivalent of several liters of fluid loss. Edema fluid is ECF and should be replaced only with fluid having the composition of ECF. Attempts to correct these deficits with hypotonic solutions, such as 5% D/W or ½ normal saline, will inevitably result in clinically significant hyponatremia.

MAINTENANCE OF FLUID BALANCE WHEN THE INITIAL CONDITIONS ARE NORMAL

Normally functioning kidneys will tend to correct disturbances of the initial conditions and restore them to normal as long as adequate salt and water are provided. The most reliable guide for the quantity of fluid replacement is the functional response of the various organs. Once the insensible loss

Table 15-4. Composition of Common Replacement Electrolyte Solutions

Solution	Na$^+$ (mEq/liter)	K$^+$ (mEq/liter)	NH$_4^+$ (mEq/liter)	Cl$^-$ (mEq/liter)	HPO$_4^=$ or H$_2$PO$_4^-$ (mEq/liter)	Carbonate, Lactate, or Acetate (mEq/liter)	mOsm/liter
0.85% NaCl	147			147			294
5.8% NaCl	1,000			1,000			2,000
0.25% KCl		34		34			68
NH$_4$Cl[a]	60	20	70	150			300
1.9% Na lactate (M/6)	167					167	334
Ringer's lactate[b]	130	4		109		28	274

[a] Not commercially available.
[b] Also includes 3 mEq/liter of calcium.

has been replaced (with 1,000 ml D/W) and the urinary loss is corrected (5% D/W with 40 mEq K), the remaining fluid replacement should be provided as Ringer's lactate. If the kidneys are normal, a sustained urine volume of >40 ml/hr is the best indication of adequate replacement. A transient increase in urine volume following the rapid administration of a small volume of intravenous fluid does not indicate adequate replacement. Satisfactory urine volume for a period of several hours is the best guide.

FLUID AND ELECTROLYTE MANAGEMENT WHEN THE INITIAL CONDITIONS ARE ABNORMAL

THE PRIMARY PROBLEM

The most common and often the most difficult problems associated with disorders of fluid and electrolyte metabolism in a critically ill patient are those associated with abnormalities of fluid volume. Such a patient has often lost most or all of the control mechanisms that ordinarily regulate fluid volume. There may be damage to the area of the central nervous system that controls thirst and therefore the quantity of water that is ingested; or to the gastrointestinal tract, which permits ready absorption of water; or to the kidneys, which facilitate the control of water excretion; or all may be collectively damaged. The solution to the problem is obscured by a lack of any direct laboratory tests that will measure the quantity of either ECF volume or total body water.

Indirect tests, such as serum electrolyte determinations, which are useful in the patient with intact control mechanisms, may be of no value in the critically ill patient and may in fact be misleading. The absolute concentration of serum electrolytes will not provide an estimate of the total fluid volume. Imagine a drinking glass full of isotonic saline, whose sodium concentration is 150 mEq/liter. If one-half of this glass is poured down the sink, the sodium concentration in the remaining half is still 150 mEq/liter. The measurement of electrolyte concentration fails to provide the slightest clue that the tumbler is half empty. To make matters worse, there are no data that define what a "normal" fluid volume should be for the myriad of clinical situations seen in the intensive care unit. Normal values, which are listed in Table 15-1, are called normal because they represent the mean of a large number of determinations carried out on healthy young persons under basal conditions. Little is known about what the optimal fluid volume would be for a variety of critically ill patients suffering from different disorders. One thing is certain: the optimal value for the fluid volume of a critically ill patient will rarely, if ever, be the normal value observed in healthy persons.

HOW TO ASSESS THE ADEQUACY OF FLUID VOLUME IN THE CRITICALLY ILL PATIENT

The definition of an adequate fluid volume in the critically ill patient is the volume that provides optimal physiologic activity for all organ systems—a

TABLE 15-5. Signs of Fluid Volume Depletion

System	Signs
Central nervous system	Apathy, weakness. A patient who has been previously optimistic about his recovery suddenly becomes depressed. Barbiturate-like effect.
Gastrointestinal tract	Anorexia, nausea, abdominal distension, and ileus
Cardiovascular system	Postural hypotension; thin, weak pulse
Renal system	Urine volume low, with a high osmolarity and a low urinary sodium. The serum blood urea nitrogen–creatinine ratio is probably the best clinical guide to volume depletion; specific gravity should not be used, since the presence of protein material (either albumin, which is passed out in the urine, or—more often in the seriously ill patient—the presence of bacteria) will give a false impression. Although it is possible to remove protein by boiling the urine, I have found that it is best just to avoid use of specific gravity entirely.
Skin	Loss of skin turgor and decreased ocular tension
Serum electrolyte changes	None

fluid volume that provides optimal function for the kidneys may result in less than optimal function for the lungs. The art of caring for the critically ill patient is to weigh the relative importance of each organ system on an hour-to-hour basis and to optimize the functioning of each system in turn as the changing clinical condition of the patient warrants.

CLINICAL EVIDENCE OF ABNORMAL ORGAN FUNCTION SEEN IN PATIENTS WITH VOLUME DEPLETION. Clinical signs of volume depletion (Table 15-5) will become apparent when volume depletion has progressed to a severe degree. In the well-managed patient, these signs will never be allowed to appear. The ECF volume must be decreased by 25 to 30 percent below optimal value before clinical signs become readily apparent.

CLINICAL SIGNS OF DISTURBED ORGAN FUNCTION
SEEN WITH FLUID VOLUME EXCESS
Skin. Edema is the classic sign of fluid volume excess. In the critically ill patient, this sign is frequently of little value in indicating volume excess and may be misleading. Volume excess is only one of the factors predisposing to the development of edema. Numerous other factors may lead to

edema in the critically ill patient. These include: hypoproteinemia; direct damage to tissues, such as contusions, burns, and pancreatitis; damage to capillary permeability, with leakage of protein into the interstitial space, which may occur following periods of profound hypotension or hypoxia; and localized venous obstruction, as is seen in thrombophlebitis. All of these may result in visible edema in the absence of fluid excess. To put this another way: the fluid volume necessary to provide adequate organ profusion in the critically ill patient may also be sufficient to produce edema. Edema in and of itself is not dangerous; its only importance is the suggested indirect evidence that cardiac failure may have taken place.

Cardiovascular system. When the neck veins are distended and dyspnea is present, overload of the vascular space has occurred, and under these circumstances, the presence of edema is significant. Edema in the absence of other evidence of vascular overload must be considered to be due to some other cause.

Kidney. Volume excess is manifested by a high urine volume. A urine volume of 40 to 50 ml/hr is desirable. Urine volume much above this—for example, in the range of 100 to 120 ml/hr—indicates that the body is trying to restore an overexpanded ECF. With few exceptions, a high urine volume should not be matched by an equally high fluid replacement; it is an indication to reduce the rate of intravenous fluid administration rather than to increase it. Volume excess may not produce a high urine volume in the presence of congestive heart failure or renal disease, in which the glomerular filtration rate may be markedly reduced. Conversely, in high-output renal failure, in which the resorptive power of the tubules is damaged, a high volume represents pathologic function of the kidneys, and the urine volume must be replaced. Congestive heart failure and renal disease can be suspected by other clinical signs.

ACHIEVEMENT OF OPTIMAL EXTRACELLULAR FLUID VOLUME
Optimal ECF volume has been achieved when the distribution of fluid between the vascular bed and the interstitial space results in sufficient venous return to the heart to assure adequate filling of the left ventricle and optimal cardiac stroke work. Evidence for an adequate cardiac stroke work is adequate organ perfusion, manifested by optimal organ function.

ESTIMATION OF LEFT VENTRICULAR FILLING PRESSURE. The filling pressure of the left ventricle can be obtained from the pulmonary wedge measurement with a Swan-Ganz catheter. It can be indirectly estimated in many situations with a central venous pressure (CVP) catheter near the right side of the heart. The Swan-Ganz catheter is a balloon-tipped, flow-directed device that will automatically position itself in the wedge position of the pulmonary artery without requiring the transportation of the patient from his room or the use of a portable image intensifier (see Chapter 10). Intravascular pressures developed at the tip of the catheter are monitored with a pressure transducer and an oscilloscope display device. This equipment should be a part of every critical care facility. Because of its ease of insertion and the high reliability of the information obtained, the pulmonary wedge pressure measurement is vastly superior to the CVP measurement and should supplant it in most situations.

INTERPRETATION OF PULMONARY WEDGE PRESSURE DETERMINATIONS. The stroke work of the left ventricle is related to left atrial pressure. The pulmonary wedge pressure is, in almost all situations, identical with left atrial pressure. However, it will not be identical when pulmonary hypertension is present, as evidenced by an increased pulmonary artery pressure, or when positive end-expiratory pressure is being used in association with a volume-cycled ventilator.

Estimation of stroke work is difficult, since the required measurements include stroke volume and mean aortic pressure. A useful approximation of stroke volume can be obtained from the peripheral arterial pressure line. Under steady-state conditions, left ventricular stroke volume is closely proportional to the central aortic pulse pressure, that is, the difference between systolic and diastolic pressure. If pulse pressure is multiplied by mean aortic pressure, a number roughly proportional to stroke work is obtained.

Increases in pulmonary wedge pressure associated with increases in the product of the pulse pressure times mean aortic pressure suggest that ventricular stroke work is improving and intravenous therapy is achieving the desired effect. An increase in pulmonary wedge pressure associated with a fall in the product of pulse pressure times mean aortic pressure indicates fluid overload and left ventricular failure. Pulmonary edema is imminent. Large increases in the product of pulse pressure and mean aortic pressure following relatively small increases in pulmonary wedge pressure suggest that the patient is volume-depleted, and further intravenous fluids should be provided. Fluid depletion is present if the pulmonary wedge pressure is less than 7 mm Hg, especially if associated with a pulse pressure less than 30 mm Hg.

OVEREXPANSION OF THE EXTRACELLULAR FLUID. Overexpansion of the ECF is suspected when pulmonary wedge pressure is in excess of 15 mm Hg. A pulse pressure and mean aortic pressure above the patient's normal levels may occur with volume overload and a compensated heart. Volume overload is treated with diuretics.

INTERPRETATION OF URINE VOLUME. Normal renal function not only implies normal kidneys but also indicates adequate perfusion of the renal mass and, by inference, of other solid organs. A high urine volume is the body's way of informing us that the ECF is overexpanded, just as a low urine volume suggests ECF depletion. Urine volumes in excess of 80 ml/hr should not be balanced; on the contrary, the rate of intravenous fluid administration should be reduced until the urine volume falls to a more appropriate level (around 40–60 ml).

How to Manipulate the Fluid Volume to an Optimal Level

VOLUME DEPLETION. Volume loss is shared by the entire extracellular fluid compartment and replacement should therefore reflect both the crystalloid and colloid composition of the vascular and extravascular space. Three parts of saline to one part of colloid is a good rule if the loss is from the vascular bed. Gastrointestinal losses, edema, peritonitis, and functional deficits should be replaced by a colloid-free solution with a composition similar to that of ECF. Crystalloid solutions are distributed between the vascular and the interstitial space; protein-containing solutions remain in the vascular bed and thus should not be used if large volumes are required for fluid replacement. Colloid solutions are particularly dangerous when they are administered rapidly in an attempt to correct a diminished plasma protein concentration in a patient whose vascular volume has already been expanded to optimal size with electrolyte solutions. The amount of water moving from the interstitial space into the vascular bed as a result of the increased oncotic pressure of the plasma may exceed the excretory ability of the kidney. Fluid overload and pulmonary edema may ensue. On the other hand, it is almost impossible to produce pulmonary edema by saline infusion when the myocardium is normal. In a critical situation, the safest program is rapid replacement with crystalloid solution to optimize fluid volume, followed by slowly administered plasma or albumin solution to correct the plasma protein concentration. Plasma protein concentration should be increased only to that level where organ function is adequate. Restoration of plasma protein concentrations to a preconceived normal value is unwarranted and may be hazardous.

VOLUME EXCESS. The optimal vascular volume for an emergency situation will frequently represent an excessive volume as the patient recovers. Treatment of peritonitis may require many liters of saline in excess of normal body composition, but as recovery takes place, this saline will be resorbed into the circulation and must be excreted. In most cases, the kidney will correct this volume excess by appropriate diuresis. When the vascular volume rises to dangerous levels, a diuretic is required to optimize cardiac function. Furosemide in small doses is the ideal agent. The judicious use of diuretics at the proper moment is a mark of the skilled intensive care physician.

DISTURBANCES OF ELECTROLYTE CONCENTRATION
Measurement of the serum electrolyte concentrations provides information on the relative proportion of water to salt and nothing more. It does not indicate whether a deficit or an excess of a particular electrolyte is present. The hyponatremia that may be seen in congestive heart failure is associated with excess total body sodium, not with a sodium deficit. Misinterpretation of serum electrolytes with ill-advised attempts to correct the serum sodium concentration by administering sodium chloride solution will only make the edema worse. On the other hand, the provision of an adequate fluid intake to a patient with normally functioning kidneys will result in self-correction of any electrolyte abnormality. The administration of intravenous solutions other than Ringer's lactate and 5% D/W should therefore be restricted to those rare instances in which disturbed electrolyte composition has resulted in organ function failure.

DISTURBANCES OF SODIUM CONCENTRATION
HYPONATREMIA. Hyponatremia is the most frequently observed electrolyte concentration disturbance in most intensive care units (ICUs). Its importance is that it almost invariably represents an error in management. The only common clinical states in which hyponatremia may occur spontaneously are adrenal insufficiency and inappropriate secretion of antidiuretic hormone (ADH). In all other situations, the lowered serum sodium concentration results from the loss of isotonic fluids and their replacement with hypotonic or sodium-free solutions. If intravenous fluids are administered as described in the earlier portion of this chapter, hyponatremia should not occur. Isotonic saline is generally the treatment of choice for volume depletion. When edema is present along with hyponatremia, the proper treatment is water restriction, not the administration of additional salt.

Water intoxication. Water intoxication is an extreme form of hyponatremia and deserves special mention because it may require radical replacement therapy. Water intoxication occurs when large quantities of electrolyte-free water are provided to the body at a time when there is a loss of isotonic fluids. This can occur when gastrointestinal losses are replaced by 5% D/W, or occasionally by the repeated use of large-volume tap water enemas.

Water intoxication should be suspected when confusion, stupor, muscle twitching, or grand mal seizures suddenly develop in a patient. Confirmation of the diagnosis is a serum sodium concentration of 115 mEq/liter or less. Correction of this disorder is obtained by administering 5.8% sodium chloride (1 mEq/ml) in an amount sufficient to relieve the central nervous system symptoms. An estimate of the sodium deficit is obtained by multiplying the patient's estimated total body water by the difference between the observed and desired sodium concentration. One-half this quantity should be administered slowly until the symptoms abate. The remainder of the replacement therapy should be provided as isotonic sodium chloride.

Example
A 70-kg male with serum sodium concentration of 115 mEq/liter
Total body water = (body weight) × 0.6
0.6 × 70 = 42 liter
(140 − 115) 42 = 1,050 mEq
One-half this amount = 500 ml 5.8% NaCl

Inappropriate antidiuretic hormone secretion. Inappropriate antidiuretic hormone secretion may occur in a wide variety of situations but is usually seen in association with cerebral injury or pulmonary disease. The syndrome is characterized by hyponatremia resulting from water retention and sodium excretion. The diagnosis is confirmed when the urine is found to contain large amounts of sodium and is hypertonic to plasma (i.e., inappropriately concentrated). Since the hyponatremia is secondary to water retention, the appropriate therapy is to restrict the intake of water below that of the insensible loss. Insensible loss will concentrate the serum sodium and correct the disorder.

HYPERNATREMIA. Hypernatremia is rarely seen in the critically ill patient and is almost invariably the result of an error in management.

Example
The use of osmotic diuretics, which results in large urine volume losses that are poor in sodium, combined with replacement of these losses by isotonic crystalloid solutions.

If the kidneys are normal and are permitted to function without interference, hypernatremia will not develop so long as a reasonable fluid volume is provided. Urine composition approximates 5% D/W in water with 40 mEq of potassium, and should be replaced as such. Osmotic diuresis either due to deliberate attempts to induce increased urine flow or due to the administration of high-protein tube feedings may result in urine volumes of several liters. If this is replaced as 5% D/W, hypernatremia will not occur.

Clinical evidence for hypernatremia is scant and may consist only of otherwise unexplained fever. Hypernatremia is invariably associated with a decrease in intracellular fluid volume, irrespective of whether the hypernatremia is due to water restriction or to excessive sodium intake. Intracellular dehydration results from the hypertonic ECF that draws fluid from the cells. Therapy in any case is therefore the administration of solute-free water.

The simplest method of calculating water deficit is to multiply the ratio of normal serum sodium to the observed serum sodium by the estimated normal volume of body water. This number provides an estimate of the patient's actual total body water. If this number is then subtracted from the estimated body water, the difference represents the approximate deficit. As in all other replacements of severe fluid and electrolyte losses, an amount of solute-free water equal to only half the estimated loss should be provided. Frequent reassessment of the serum sodium concentration is necessary to prevent a conversion of hypernatremia to water intoxication.

Example
A 70-kg patient with a serum sodium of 160 mEq/liter
Estimated current body water = 0.9 × 42 liters = 37.8 liters
Normal serum Na$^+$ = 140 mEq/liter
144/160 = 0.9
Estimated current body water = 0.9 × 42 liters = 37.8 liters
Estimated water deficit = 42 − 37.8 = 4.2 liters

DISTURBANCES OF POTASSIUM CONCENTRATION
HYPOKALEMIA. Decreased concentration of serum potassium is likely to occur in patients on prolonged intravenous fluid therapy. Isotonic saline solution contains no potassium, and even Ringer's lactate contains only 4 mEq/liter. To match the daily loss of 30 to 40 mEq, it would be necessary to administer 6 to 10 liters of Ringer's lactate per day. Total body stores of potassium for a 70-kg man are 3,500 mEq. Losses of 20 to 30 mEq/day can therefore be tolerated for a relatively prolonged period. Clinically significant hypokalemia becomes manifest in the presence of either significant gastrointestinal fluid losses or in the presence of an alkalosis. Hypokalemia begets alkalosis, and vice versa.

Signs of hypokalemia. The signs of hypokalemia are all related to disturbance of contractility of skeletal, smooth, and cardiac muscle. The observed signs progress from muscle weakness to flaccid paralysis and diminution or loss of the deep tendon reflexes. Smooth-muscle abnormality is evidenced by paralytic ileus, and cardiac muscle abnormality, by increased sensitivity to digitalis.

Treatment of hypokalemia. Initial management of hypokalemia consists in elimination or reduction of excessive potassium loss. If the losses cannot be corrected, accurate estimation of their magnitude must be carried out. Special clinical settings in the ICU of particular importance are those involving the use of diuretics or corticosteroids, both of which will result in increased potassium loss.

Hypokalemia rarely, if ever, requires emergency massive replacement therapy. Serum potassium levels above 2 mEq/liter are lethal, and the use of potassium replacement solutions containing 40 to 60 mEq/liter are, therefore, potentially hazardous. A safe concentration for administering potassium is 60 mEq/liter, and this should not be given at rates exceeding 500 ml/hr. Concentrated potassium solution should never be administered until an adequate urine volume has been obtained. The safest program is to start replacement therapy with a liter of Ringer's lactate, and when the urine volume achieves 40 ml/hr or more, the more concentrated potassium solution can be administered. Do not administer potassium in glucose-containing solutions, since the glucose may cause a further fall in serum potassium level with ensuing cardiac arrhythmias.

HYPERKALEMIA. Hyperkalemia in the ICU is generally seen only in patients with acute renal failure (see Chapter 21). Moderate hyperkalemia may be seen in association with prolonged hypoperfusion states. Increased tissue destruction associated with the metabolic acidosis of inadequate perfusion will result in the endogenous release of large amounts of potassium. If renal function is normal, however, serum potassium will never reach dangerous levels.

The single most important maneuver in managing hyperkalemia is to eliminate all potassium intake. Intravenous solutions such as Ringer's lactate contain potassium ion, as do many of the juices and broths permitted on a liquid diet. Penicillin G is a frequently forgotten source of potassium ion (17 mEq potassium per 10 million units of penicillin G).

DISTURBANCES OF CALCIUM METABOLISM
Evaluation of the significance of the serum calcium level requires a simultaneous measurement of the serum albumin. Approximately 50 percent of calcium is bound to albumin, so that any reduction in the serum albumin concentration will be reflected by a decrease in serum calcium. An approximate rule of thumb is that the serum calcium changes 1 mg/100 ml for each change in albumin of 1 gm/100 ml.

Hypocalcemia is essentially confined to patients with hypoparathyroidism. Hypercalcemia is rarely a problem but may present with clinical manifestations in patients who are on prolonged bed rest. This is particularly likely to occur in adolescent patients who have suffered long-bone fractures. Because of the rapid turnover rate of calcium in these patients, the kidneys may not be able to maintain plasma levels within the normal range, and hypercalcemia may result. The symptoms are usually anorexia, nausea, vomiting, and abdominal pain, progressing to dehydration, mental disturbance, and finally coma.

The most important therapeutic regimen for the correction of hypercalcemia is large quantities of intravenous sodium chloride, since this increases urine flow, allowing the excess calcium to be excreted. In addition, the sodium inhibits tubular resorption of calcium, further increasing calcium excretion. Corticosteroids may be useful in the management of hypercalcemia when the elevated calcium is not related to an increased level of circulating parathyroid hormone. Examples of such situations would include hypercalcemia secondary to cancer with bone metastasis. The usual therapeutic, not pharmacologic, doses are adequate. The use of edetate (EDTA) and mithramycin has generally been abandoned, since they are not so effective as the other methods described.

HYPOPHOSPHATEMIA

Hypophosphatemia is seen in patients receiving intravenous hyperalimentation, as well as in many others who are chronically ill. As many as 35 percent of patients in ICUs are probably suffering from hypophosphatemia.

The clinical significance of hypophosphatemia is the resulting left shift of the oxyhemoglobin dissociation curve, with increased affinity for oxygen. Phosphate levels below 2.7 mg/100 ml may be significant. Phosphate replacement corrects the shifted oxyhemoglobin dissociation curve.

MAGNESIUM DEFICIENCY

Magnesium deficiency is most frequently seen in clinical situations where the normal dietary intake is reduced. It may develop in patients being maintained on intravenous feedings or on hyperalimentation programs that do not include added magnesium. In addition, patients suffering from malabsorption syndromes or who have protracted losses of gastrointestinal fluid, such as may occur with intestinal fistulas or protracted diarrhea, may have magnesium deficiency.

The symptoms of magnesium deficiency are generally similar to those of calcium deficiency and include hyperactive tendon reflexes, muscle tremors, and eventually tetany. The key to the diagnosis of this condition is an awareness of the clinical setting in which it may occur. The diagnosis is confirmed by measurement of serum magnesium levels, with demonstration of a concentration less than 1.5 mEq/liter.

Treatment consists of the intravenous administration of magnesium sulfate at a concentration of 80 mEq/liter. This solution should be administered cautiously over a 2- to 4-hr period, since rapid administration may lead to cardiac arrest. Magnesium should be administered with the same precautions as used in the administration of potassium. Patients who are dehydrated or severely oliguric should be given only very small doses of magnesium until an adequate urine flow can be established.

SELECTED READINGS

Canizaro, P. C., and Shires, G. T. Fluid and Nutritional Management. In S. I.
 Schwartz (Ed.), *Principles of Surgery.* New York: McGraw-Hill, 1974. Vol. 2.
Moore, F. D. Homeostasis: Bodily Changes in Trauma and Surgery. In D. C.

Sabiston, Jr. (Ed.), *Davis-Christopher Textbook of Surgery* (10th ed.). Philadelphia: Saunders, 1972. Pp. 26–64.

Moore, F. D., et al. *Body Cell Mass and Its Supporting Environment: Body Composition in Health and Disease*. Philadelphia: Saunders, 1963.

Pitts, R. F. *Physiology of Kidney and Body Fluids*. Chicago: Year Book, 1963.

Schwartz, W. B., and Pelman, A. S. A critique of the parameters used in the evaluation of acid-base disorders. *N. Engl. J. Med.* 268:1382, 1963.

Wacker, W. E. B., and Parisi, A. F. Magnesium metabolism. I, II, III. *N. Engl. J. Med.* 278:658, 712, 772, 1968.

Frank E. Gump / # 16. ACID-BASE DISTURBANCES

The subject of acid-base physiology is of importance in many fields of medicine but nowhere more so than in the setting of the intensive care unit (ICU). Disorders of acid-base balance are commonplace in the critically ill, and the classic clinical syndromes are often modified by special techniques used in treating organ failure. It is obviously essential for all ICU physicians not only to recognize acid-base abnormalities but also to understand the underlying disturbance in order to formulate effective treatment. Unfortunately, many physicians consider the subject to be a particularly difficult and perplexing one. Acid-base physiology draws heavily and directly on certain disciplines of basic science, especially physical chemistry, which are poorly represented in the traditional medical school curriculum. Furthermore, despite decades of theoretical and developmental investigation, the goal of providing a simple quantitative evaluation of the nonrespiratory component of acid-base disturbances remains elusive.

A number of methods of acid-base blood analysis are available and will be discussed because the intensive care physician requires sufficient understanding of the principles underlying these methods to make intelligent use of them in caring for critically ill patients. The first part of this chapter will review certain troublesome concepts and compare the currently employed methods of acid-base blood analysis. The remaining subject matter has been organized along traditional lines, but an effort has been made throughout to focus special attention on problems that are unique to the intensive care setting.

CONCEPTS AND TERMS
Contemporary acid-base theory defines an acid as a substance that can donate hydrogen ions. This, of course, does not take into account the manner in which electroneutrality is maintained, but the need for cations to be balanced by an equal number of anionic negative charges is important. The need for balancing of a particular cation against a particular anion in blood and interstitial fluid will be considered later in relation to the electrolyte structure of plasma.

The reaction indicated below shows the dissociation of an acid into a hydrogen ion (or proton) and its associated (conjugate) base.

$$HA \rightarrow H^+ + A^-$$

It is important to appreciate that the tendency of the acid to donate a hydrogen ion is counterbalanced by an opposing tendency toward accepting a proton. A better way to show the reaction is as follows:

$$HA \rightleftharpoons H^+ + A^-$$

At equilibrium, every acid in solution dissociates to a greater or lesser degree. A fully dissociated acid will be able to donate more protons and is thus considered to be strong, while in the case of a weak acid, its conjugate base shows a greater affinity for protons, thus limiting dissociation.

The term *pH* represents the concentration of free hydrogen ions in solution; the pH value is inversely proportional to the concentration of hydrogen ions in the solution. The addition of a strong acid to water will obviously lower pH, but the presence of buffers will modify these changes. Buffering is critical in the physiology and pathophysiology of acid-base, but the precise chemical mechanisms need not concern us here. Rather, it is far more valuable to look at the effect of body buffers and how these systems operate in conjunction with the kidney and lung to maintain the pH of extracellular fluid at 7.4.

In vivo pH is held in the normal range primarily by maintaining plasma concentration of two substances: HCO_3^- at 24 mM/liter and CO_2 near 1.2 mM/liter. This represents the normal 20 : 1 ratio of HCO_3^-/CO_2. While it might be arbitrary to focus on the concentrations of HCO_3^- and CO_2 when there are many other buffer pairs present in plasma, the important point is that the organism exercises acid-base homeostasis by controlling arterial carbon dioxide tension ($PaCO_2$) and HCO_3^- levels.

There are two principal reasons for the primacy of HCO_3^- among the buffers of extracellular fluid (ECF); one is physicochemical, and one is physiologic. First, because of the open-ended system resulting from pulmonary control of $PaCO_2$, plus the evolutionary selection of 7.4 as the pH of ECF, the HCO_3^- and CO_2 buffer system accommodates more nonvolatile acid accumulating in ECF and yields more protons to added base than all the other buffers present collectively. This is even true in whole blood, despite the contribution of hemoglobin. As indicated, the second reason for the importance of HCO_3^- among the extracellular buffers is physiologic. Fluctuation of plasma HCO_3^- is the principal normal stabilizer of plasma pH as the acid-base load varies, because the change in plasma HCO_3^- affects urine pH in such a way that a steady state of zero acid-base balance normally is always approximated.

A number of other nonvolatile buffers require consideration. Ammonia (NH_4^+ and NH_3) is of great importance in the urine but of less importance in ECF because ammonia is in low concentration there. On the other hand, circulating protein, the principal plasma buffer, and inorganic phosphates are important in plasma, while hemoglobin in both its oxygenated and deoxygenated forms constitutes the primary whole blood buffering agent.

Although these buffers play a role in the regulation of pH, it is important to remember that pulmonary control of CO_2 and the renal bicarbonate mechanism determine survival, except over very short time periods. A diseased lung can result in an abnormally high level of PCO_2, but unless this lung can bring CO_2 excretion into line with production and thus stabilize $PaCO_2$, a fatal situation will develop rapidly. Similarly, a diseased kidney may allow plasma HCO_3^- to fall to very low levels, with an associated decline in pH; but the excretion of nonvolatile acids must quickly be brought into line with production, or a fatal outcome will follow. These pathophysiologic considerations are of importance in considering the use of buffering agents, a subject that will be considered in greater detail later.

Probably the most important role played by the nonvolatile buffers relates to the protection they provide against sudden respiratory failure with an abrupt rise in PCO_2. Renal compensation requires many hours to be effective, and during this interval the buffering capacity of whole blood provides an immediately effective defense against serious deviation of plasma pH. The same holds true to a lesser extent in sudden renal failure. Although respiratory compensation is more rapid, the nonvolatile buffers help the kidney to defend arterial plasma pH.

Returning to consideration of the plasma bicarbonate buffer system: the 20 : 1 ratio of HCO_3^- to H_2CO_3 has already been mentioned and points up the quantitative relationship between the concentrations of the dissociated and nondissociated constituents of a buffer pair. This can be expressed by an equation that sets forth the relationship between hydrogen ion concentration (H^+) and the ratio of the constituents of the bicarbonate (HCO_3^-)–carbonic acid (H_2CO_3) buffer system.

$$(H^+) = K \frac{(H_2CO_3)}{(HCO_3^-)}$$

K represents the equilibrium constant for this system. Since pH $(-\log [H^+])$ is used clinically instead of (H^+), the equation is rewritten:

$$pH = pK + \log \frac{(HCO_3^-)}{(H_2CO_3)}$$

In this form it is the familiar Henderson-Hasselbalch equation. This expression is applicable to the plasma bicarbonate system and is fundamental to any quantitative treatment of acid-base balance.

SYSTEMS OF ANALYSIS

Regardless of the clinical setting, acid-base analysis depends on examination of the blood. To diagnose, categorize, and eventually treat any abnormality, the physician will want to know (1) the pH of the blood, (2) what role the lung is playing, and (3) how much nonvolatile acid or base is present.

Present-day electrodes will provide rapid and accurate measurements of the pH of arterial, capillary, or venous blood. Measurements of pH quantitate the abnormality existing in the ECF. Similarly, electrodes designed to measure PCO_2 provide information regarding the role of the lung. $PaCO_2$ gives unequivocal information regarding the functional contribution of the lung, for PCO_2 is directly controlled by this organ, and there is no way that $PaCO_2$ can be misleading in this context. However, as Hills [4] has pointed out, there is no way in which the nonrespiratory constituent in any abnormality of the acid-base composition of ECF can be evaluated directly and quantitatively in the way the pulmonary constituent and arterial pH can be. Because of the dominant role of the HCO_3^-–CO_2 system, the plasma HCO_3^- concentration offers a useful index of the extent of accumulation of excess nonvolatile acid or base, but it does not represent a quantitative measure. Thus, much effort has been expended in the attempt to combine an accurate estimate of the nonrespiratory component with the evaluation of arterial blood pH and $PaCO_2$.

For many years, measurement of plasma HCO_3^- plus dissolved CO_2, which is referred to as plasma CO_2 content or total CO_2, served to estimate HCO_3^- concentration. Gamble [2] extended this work by utilizing total CO_2 in a graphic representation of the electrolyte partition of plasma. Gamble's bar diagrams (Figs. 16-1 and 16-2) show that total positive and negative charges must be equal to achieve electroneutrality. This analysis can be carried out on venous blood and is widely available. Interpretation relies on the fact that accumulation of nonvolatile base results in an increase in HCO_3^- concentration, and accumulation of acid results in a decrease in HCO_3^- concentration. Knowledge of the behavior of other ions, such as Na^+, Ca^{++}, and Cl^-, is also helpful in differential diagnosis, but the system is incomplete in that knowledge of pH and the specific effect of the respiratory component is not provided.

Bicarbonate is, of course, not actually determined but is approximated from total CO_2. As a rule, this is effective because the concentration of dissolved CO_2 usually falls between 0.6 and 1.6 mM/liter. Therefore, the maximum error involved in considering plasma HCO_3^- equal to total CO_2 is less than 2 mM/liter. The percentage of error becomes important only in severe acidosis, but, even then, it does not invalidate the diagnostic utility of analysis of plasma electrolyte compartmentalization.

However, comprehensive acid-base analysis requires the inclusion of pH and PCO_2 measurements that should be done on arterial blood. Once again, the problem resides in the evaluation of the nonrespiratory component. Bicarbonate concentration is not a quantitative measure of the accumulation of nonvolatile acid or base because it is affected by changes in PCO_2. Efforts to improve on blood or plasma HCO_3^- as a *measure* of the nonvolatile acid base component have been based on in vitro equilibration against a CO_2 tension of 40 mm Hg. The principle underlying such CO_2 titration tech-

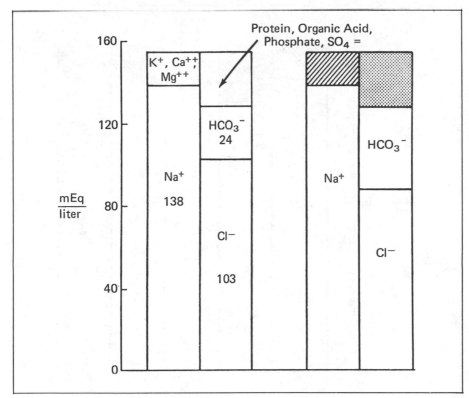

FIGURE 16-1. Normal electrolyte partition of plasma is shown on left; right-hand bars represent an example of metabolic alkalosis.

niques is that the bicarbonate concentration in the sample would then be identical to bicarbonate in the body when the PCO_2 was 40 mm Hg in vivo. Van Slyke and Cullen [7] popularized CO_2 combining power, which is simply total CO_2 of venous serum equilibrated at a PCO_2 of 40 mm Hg. Other systems based on CO_2 titration include buffer base (Singer and Hastings [6]), standard bicarbonate (Astrup et al. [1]), and base excess (Astrup et al. [1] and Siggaard-Andersen [5]). Base excess is the derived variable in general use in critical care medicine and will now be examined briefly.

When a blood sample is drawn, its pH is determined, and then the sample is equilibrated with two different CO_2–O_2 mixtures; pH is measured at the two known CO_2 tensions, and since two of the three variables of the Henderson-Hasselbalch equation are known, it is possible to calculate HCO_3^-. The Siggaard-Andersen curve nomogram shown in Figure 16-3 allows one to represent the pH and HCO_3^- of the sample as a function of PCO_2. The buffer strength of the blood sample determines the slope of the

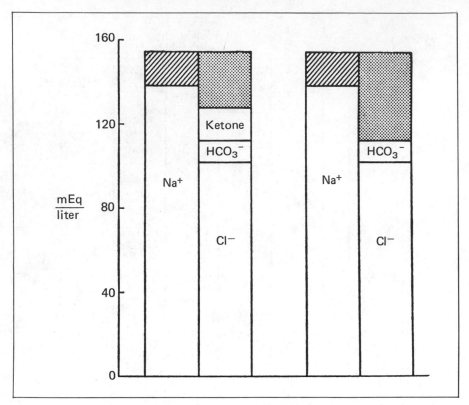

FIGURE 16-2. Metabolic acidosis. Diabetic acidosis is shown on left and renal failure on right.

CO_2 titration line. Given a value for buffering capacity, one can calculate how much acid or base would be needed to bring the HCO_3^- of the sample to 25 mM/liter. This is carried out at a PCO_2 of 40 mm Hg and is known as the base excess. Originally, this was expressed as a positive or negative value, but a negative base excess proved to be a difficult concept for many clinicians to accept, and is now often referred to as a base deficit. Since base excess quantitates accumulation of acid or base in the blood in terms of milliequivalents per liter of blood, it becomes theoretically possible to estimate how much mineral acid or alkali would have to be given to neutralize such abnormal accumulations therapeutically. In practice, however, such calculations are of limited value, because CO_2 titration in vitro is not the same as whole-body CO_2 titration resulting from manipulation of alveolar PCO_2. This is because in vivo exchanges of ions between multiple compartments cannot be reproduced by CO_2 titration of a blood sample that has been removed from the body.

The Siggaard-Andersen alignment nomogram shown in Figure 16-4 is

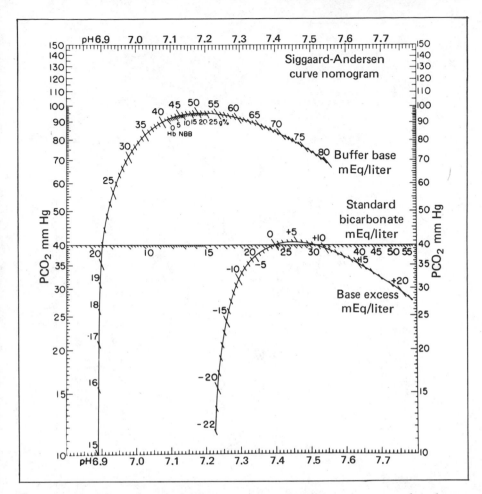

FIGURE 16-3. Siggaard-Andersen curve nomogram. (From O. Siggaard-Andersen and K. Engel, *Scand. J. Clin. Lab. Invest.* 12:177, 1960; O. Siggaard-Andersen, *Scand. J. Clin. Lab. Invest.* 14:598, 1962. Reproduced by permission of Radiometer A/S, Copenhagen, Denmark, and The London Company, Cleveland, Ohio. Copyright © 1959, 1962, 1967 by Radiometer A/S, Emdrupvej 72, DK-2400, Copenhagen NV, Denmark.)

simpler to use than the curve nomogram. If two of the three variables are measured, the third, along with the base excess, can be calculated.

The limitations that have been pointed out are important for proper application of data obtained from modern equipment. However, physicians today have a unique advantage over their predecessors: acid-base analysis has approached a technical and theoretical stage of development that makes its application far more convenient and useful than was the case even a few years ago.

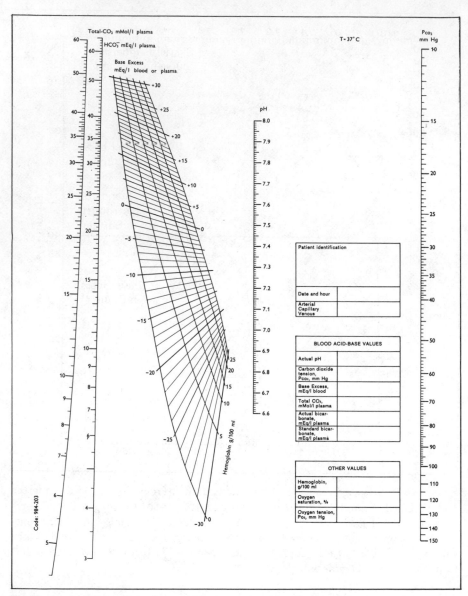

FIGURE 16-4. Siggaard-Andersen alignment nomogram. (From O. Siggaard-Andersen, *Scand. J. Clin. Lab. Invest.* 15:211, 1963. Reproduced by permission of Radiometer A/S, Copenhagen, Denmark, and The London Company, Cleveland, Ohio. Copyright © 1962, 1967 by Radiometer A/S, Emdrupvej 72, DK-2400, Copenhagen NV, Denmark.)

PULMONARY COMPONENTS OF
ACID-BASE BALANCE

The muscles of respiration are innervated by lower motor-neurons that are controlled by the respiratory center lying in the brain stem. The inspiratory center controls this activity, and alteration in the chemical composition of the blood will immediately influence respiration. Small changes in the concentration of CO_2 in the blood will affect respiration by a direct action on the respiratory center. Under normal circumstances, $PaCO_2$ can be regarded as stable at 40 mm Hg, and respiratory control functions to hold this parameter within narrow limits. A $PaCO_2$ value of 40 mm Hg implies that the ratio of rates of CO_2 production to alveolar ventilation are normal, since these two factors control the level of CO_2 in the blood. It is important to remember that CO_2 tension rather than total CO_2 is the controlling factor, and this is why current CO_2 electrodes are of such great clinical value.

Carbon dioxide production is increased in critically ill patients if they have sepsis, long-bone fractures, burns, or other conditions that increase metabolic expenditure. However, it rarely increases more than 50 percent and is only a small fraction of the CO_2 that normal lungs can excrete with large increases in metabolic expenditure, such as in exercise. Factors that decrease alveolar ventilation are more likely to raise $PaCO_2$ in the ICU. These will be dealt with in greater detail in the section on respiratory acidosis.

Increased alveolar ventilation is also common in the ICU, and a variety of causes can be listed. While hypoxia is often considered to be a factor, CO_2 tension is generally accepted as dominant in stimulating respiration. Certain peripheral receptors are sensitive to hypoxia, but, even here, CO_2 levels are important in potentiating the response. Since the effect on respiration of a change in the acid-base status of the blood is probably mediated through pH changes in the cerebrospinal fluid, the delay caused by the blood-brain barrier makes acute hypercapnia or hypocapnia of great importance.

METABOLIC OR NONRESPIRATORY COMPONENT
OF ACID-BASE BALANCE

Nonvolatile acid is constantly being produced in the body from neutral precursors. The recent concept of load is of great value because it defines the requirements that the kidney must meet if it is to maintain acid-base homeostasis. Although the load usually consists of dietary acid and alkali, as well as organic acids that result from metabolism, it is also important to realize that acid and base can be generated in ECF when there are extrarenal losses of base or acid.

In other words, loss of base from some nonrenal route causes proton transfer to the buffers of ECF and so generates acid in ECF. Similarly, base can be generated by loss of acid from a nonrenal route. This is especially important in the setting of critical illness, because the combination of impaired renal function and large-scale extrarenal losses so often coexist in these patients.

METABOLIC ACIDOSIS

Clinical problems involving metabolic acidosis fall into two broad categories: (1) conditions in which loss of base represents the primary mechanism, which can be loss from either the kidney or the gastrointestinal tract [4], and (2) conditions in which acidic compounds accumulate in the ECF.

GAIN OF ACID BY EXTRACELLULAR FLUID

DIABETIC ACIDOSIS

The classic example of organic acidosis is diabetic acidosis. In this severe metabolic disturbance, large amounts of glucose and β-oxybutyric acid accumulate in the blood, although lactic acid and free fatty acids may also contribute to the condition.

SHOCK

Shock is far more common in the ICU setting than diabetic acidosis, and although it remains an incompletely understood state, its association with lactic acidosis is well established. While hemodynamic parameters are generally employed as a guide in resuscitation, measurement of arterial pH is extremely helpful. Serum lactate levels can be measured directly, but this is not a standard determination in most hospital laboratories. Arterial pH will provide a reliable guide to the severity of the lactic acidosis; pH measurements are also important in evaluating the patient in shock, because not all patients in shock are acidotic. Routine administration of sodium bicarbonate to these patients without knowledge of arterial pH will result in severe alkalosis following the resuscitation stage.

RENAL FAILURE

Metabolic acidosis is associated with renal failure, since the latter involves retention of phosphate, sulfate, and organic acid anions. In addition, the failing kidney may be unable to regenerate bicarbonate, and this will also lead to metabolic acidosis.

METABOLIC ACIDOSIS WITH HYPERCHLOREMIA

Metabolic acidosis with hyperchloremia may be associated with therapy utilizing ammonium chloride. This dangerous effect of ammonium chloride is well known and is usually considered when administering this substance.

HYPERALIMENTATION OR TOTAL PARENTERAL NUTRITION

The possibility that acidosis may be associated with intravenous hyperalimentation is not generally appreciated. In early nutritional studies, the nitrogen source consisted of hydrolysates of either casein or fibrin, but more recently these formulations have been replaced by mixtures of synthetic L-amino acids. Such mixtures are considered to be more desirable in that a more reproducible amino acid intake is made possible. Acidosis was not encountered with the protein hydrolysates, but it has been observed with the synthetic amino acid mixtures. Heird et al. [3] have shown that the synthetic amino acid mixtures contain an excess of cationic amino acids in relation to anionic amino acids or other organic anions. Metabolism of these cationic amino acids results in a net excess of hydrogen ion, which makes the observed acidosis understandable.

A more dramatic acid-base problem associated with total parenteral nutrition (TPN) relates to the fact that the response to a carbohydrate load in excess of energy requirements is a rise in the nonprotein respiratory quotient (RQ) to 1.0 or greater. When the RQ is 1.0, it indicates that the main substrate being oxidized for energy is glucose. An RQ above 1.0 indicates conversion of exogenous glucose to fat. In either case there is an increased CO_2 production, and this will have to be excreted by the lungs. The actual increases, when measured, are striking, averaging about 35 percent in depleted patients receiving between 2,500 and 3,000 glucose calories and 19 gm of amino acid nitrogen a day. Carbon dioxide production is increased even further when similar TPN solutions are given to injured, septic patients. Increases in CO_2 production of 50 to 75 percent have been recorded when such patients are started on TPN. This obviously represents a significant acid load; in a patient with compromised pulmonary function, respiratory distress may be precipitated.

The rise in CO_2 production in the depleted patient is most marked when the RQ rises above 1.0 and net lipogenesis takes place. If a patient has compromised pulmonary function, the total glucose intake should be kept low to avoid the high CO_2 production associated with lipogenesis. Alternately, fat emulsions can replace glucose calories as a source of energy and thereby limit CO_2 production.

In the septic patient the RQ does not change so much with the institution of TPN because oxygen consumption also increases. However, the mild rise in RQ should not obscure the fact that even larger increases in CO_2 production may take place. Small amounts of glucose (50–100 gm) do not seem to cause this phenomenon, but levels used in even moderate intravenous feeding programs will have a marked effect on CO_2 production.

This is especially important in the ICU setting because the increase in CO_2 production may be a critical factor in weaning a patient who requires mechanical ventilation. Frequently patients requiring long-term mechanical ventilation will also require intravenous nutrition. The increase in CO_2 production may be a factor in failure to wean the patient from mechanical ventilation. Once again, fat emulsions which are oxidized with an RQ of 0.7 should prove useful under these circumstances.

LOSS OF BICARBONATE FROM EXTRACELLULAR FLUID

The second general mechanism underlying metabolic acidosis relates to loss of HCO_3^- from the extracellular space. Two major routes of loss must be considered: the kidney and the gastrointestinal tract.

RENAL LOSS

Renal loss of bicarbonate is more common in chronic than acute renal disease, and the term *renal tubular acidosis* has been applied to the condition. In these patients there is abnormal loss of HCO_3^- from the renal tubules, and this probably represents a specific tubular defect in the kidney, as opposed to the generalized renal disease seen in azotemic or renal failure acidosis. These patients are acidotic with a low serum HCO_3^- and a base deficit, but the urine is alkaline because of the HCO_3^- leaked from the tubules. The inappropriately alkaline urine with a pH above 7 has also been termed *paradoxical* and clearly identifies the condition.

LOSS OF SMALL-INTESTINE SECRETIONS

All gastrointestinal fluids have a HCO_3^- concentration that is higher than that in plasma. Gastric juice is the only exception, since it contains no HCO_3^- at all. Pancreatic juice contains by far the most HCO_3^-, so that fistulas in this organ will rapidly lead to acidosis. Bile and succus entericus contain less HCO_3^- but still more than is found in plasma. Diarrheal fluid represents a mixture of all these secretions, and thus diarrhea will obviously result in loss of HCO_3^-.

Many ICU patients have gastrointestinal tubes; some may vomit or have diarrhea. Intestinal fistulas also represent a common ICU problem. For these reasons, loss of HCO_3^- is a frequent cause of acidosis in the ICU.

DIAGNOSIS

Diagnosis of metabolic acidosis is not difficult. Definitive diagnosis requires that there be a decrease in total CO_2 and also in blood pH. Confusion is conceivable, since total CO_2 is low in both metabolic acidosis and respiratory alkalosis; however, the pH measurement will separate these conditions. If this determination should not be immediately available, it is worthwhile remembering that marked decreases in HCO_3^- concentration (below 15 mEq/liter) are almost always due to metabolic acidosis rather than compensation for respiratory alkalosis.

TREATMENT

The wide variety of disorders that have been described make it clear that the underlying disease process rather than simply the acid-base problem generally constitutes the first priority in treatment. A striking example would be use of Ringer's lactate in the treatment of hypovolemic shock. In many of these patients, shock is associated with lactic acid accumulation and clear-cut metabolic acidosis. At first glance, the infusion of additional lactic acid might appear to be irrational, but since fluid resuscitation corrects the volume deficit and restores tissue perfusion, it makes it possible for both endogenous and exogenous lactate to be cleared from the blood rapidly.

While the need to treat the underlying condition cannot be stressed enough, under certain circumstances it is necessary to treat the acidosis per se. When the blood pH is below 7.2, and when correction of the underlying condition will take an appreciable amount of time, it is best to initiate treatment of the acidosis. Sodium bicarbonate is the preferred agent and is usually available in ampules containing 44 mEq. Elaborate calculations utilizing the difference between measured and desired plasma HCO_3^- concentration and the extracellular distribution of HCO_3^- are seldom worthwhile, because hydrogen ion is buffered intracellularly as well as extracellularly. As a rule, in the crisis situation being described, 1 or 2 ampules of $NaHCO_3$ should be given intravenously and blood gas measurements repeated. A more gradual correction is also possible by adding several ampules to the intravenous solutions being administered.

Reversal of acidosis with $NaHCO_3$ should rarely be undertaken without giving some thought to possible body potassium deficits. Serum potassium will be elevated in the presence of acidosis and may mask marked deficits of this critical ion. Rapid correction of acidosis without replacing potassium deficits may result in dangerous manifestations of hypokalemia as a result of potassium's moving into the cells as pH responds to $NaHCO_3$ administration.

METABOLIC ALKALOSIS

The clinical setting of patients requiring intensive care explains why metabolic alkalosis is such a common abnormality in the ICU. Furthermore, its management is extremely difficult because the underlying mechanisms are not easily rectified. A number of factors play an important role—such as chronic diuretic use, loss of gastric juice from vomiting or nasogastric suction, liberal use of sodium bicarbonate in resuscitation, hypovolemia, and the administration of steroids. Diuretics and steroids both result in depletion of body potassium, which is the key metabolic derangement in this state. Hypovolemia triggers mineralo-corticoid release which will also result in renal potassium loss. Loss of hydrochloric acid will also affect body potassium while a large bicarbonate load will be more likely to result in severe alkalosis if potassium depletion interferes with the kidney's ability to excrete sodium.

Depletion of body potassium stores should not be confused with hypokalemia. Unfortunately, serum potassium levels are a poor reflection of total body potassium since it is primarily an intracellular ion. With no reliable clinical or laboratory guides that can quantitate total body potassium, the clinician must simply be alert to the factors that result in potassium loss. These have been mentioned above; in addition, nutritional depletion will also result in loss of intracellular potassium. Replacement of this ion (and chloride) is the key to treatment, and this will be dealt with below.

Even though whole body or intracellular potassium deficiency is the factor underlying metabolic alkalosis, it is often helpful to the clinician to categorize this abnormality into the gain of HCO_3 in the ECF or the loss of acid from the ECF.

GAIN OF BICARBONATE IN THE EXTRACELLULAR FLUID
ADMINISTRATION OF SODIUM BICARBONATE
Alkali ingestion in ulcer patients is ordinarily considered the most common method by which HCO_3^- can be increased in body fluids. In the ICU, however, treatment with sodium bicarbonate represents the usual reason for gain of bicarbonate in the ECF. $NaHCO_3$ may have been necessary to treat acidosis, but experience in many ICUs indicates that it is easy to overshoot the mark, and the administered sodium may not be readily excreted in the critically ill patient.

TRANSFUSION ALKALOSIS
A condition often labeled *transfusion alkalosis* represents a special form of increased bicarbonate in the ECF. Since the common anticoagulant used in banked blood is sodium citrate, massive transfusions will result in an appreciable sodium load (about 17 mEq/unit of blood). Provided that the citrate is metabolized, the sodium ion remains as $NaHCO_3$ and may contribute to metabolic alkalosis. Obviously, any impairment of renal function that limits urinary sodium excretion will aggravate alkalosis resulting from such conditions.

LOSS OF ACID FROM EXTRACELLULAR FLUID
GASTROINTESTINAL LOSS
Loss of HCl from the stomach, usually through a gastric tube, is obviously common in the ICU. If there is pyloric obstruction, the losses are markedly increased, and despite some bile staining, the material comes close to being pure gastric juice. Potassium depletion is often associated with the chloride depletion seen in pyloric obstruction, and severe alkalosis may result. Unless potassium is administered, it will not be possible to correct the alkalosis caused by loss of HCl from the stomach. Furthermore, loss of gastric and upper intestinal secretions due to suction or vomiting may result in deficits of sodium and water. Contraction of the ECF volume is itself a cause of alkalosis. Hypovolemia will depress the kidney's regulatory efficiency, including its normal ability to eliminate base as urinary HCO_3^-. Under these circumstances, aldosterone secretion is stimulated, and while

it helps to preserve body sodium and extracellular volume, it may well aggravate potassium depletion.

RENAL LOSS

Renal alkalosis, alkalosis caused by loss of potassium from the kidney, is common in the ICU because of the widespread use of diuretics. Diuretics that are especially likely to cause this problem are the thiazides, ethacrynic acid, and furosemide. While thiazides are the most commonly implicated, the contraction of ECF volume and resulting loss of sodium chloride and potassium are common effects of most diuretics. Hypermineralocorticism contributes to the alkalosis in most such patients; in fact, chronic corticosteroid administration in itself will lead to alkalosis.

DIAGNOSIS

Elevation of the total serum CO_2 is a clear-cut indication of metabolic alkalosis. Chronic respiratory acidosis will cause the same blood abnormality, but the underlying clinical conditions are usually readily identifiable and will allow one to differentiate between these possibilities. If necessary, pH and PCO_2 measurements can be done.

TREATMENT

The renal mechanisms that regulate potassium homeostasis tend to favor excretion, which helps to explain why clinical states involving potassium deficits are not only commonplace but also difficult to correct. Whereas it was once thought that potassium depletion was responsible for metabolic alkalosis by increasing renal bicarbonate absorption, we now know that potassium loss is a secondary event resulting from the effects of alkalosis on the kidney. The chloride ion also plays a critical role because the continued disparity between the demand for sodium conservation and the supply of reabsorbable anion (chloride), provides a relentless stimulus to continued potassium and hydrogen ion secretion. Therefore, the clinician must focus on the deficit of potassium and chloride; not only must KCl be given, but the magnitude of the deficit must be realized. Potassium deficits amounting to 300 to 500 mEq are commonly encountered in patients with metabolic alkalosis. However, the repair of these deficits must be carried out carefully. Since the severity of the deficit cannot be measured clinically, the exact amount required for replacement cannot be predetermined. The serum potassium level provides a limiting end point in that values above 5 mEq/liter suggest that replacement must be slowed even if they do not necessarily indicate that total body stores have been replenished. Since the clinician must strike a balance between the need for correcting important deficits and the risk of cardiotoxic serum concentrations, the rule would be to err on the side of caution and repair deficits slowly. When the need for more rapid replacement exists, potassium can be administered intravenously at rates up to 20 mEq/hr; as much as 150 to 200 mEq/day can be given safely. It is obvious that serum levels must be followed closely and ECG monitoring is necessary to detect early signs of hyperkalemia.

At times, patients with severe metabolic alkalosis do not respond to the administration of KCl or KCl cannot be safely administered. Increasing experience is now available in the use of 0.1 N HCl. Ammonium chloride and arginine hydrochloride serve a similar purpose but are difficult to use in patients with hepatic insufficiency. When properly diluted, HCl is safe but must be administered through a central vein, since it will cause phlebitis when used peripherally.

However, one should never lose sight of the fact that it is the underlying condition that requires treatment. Since volume depletion is often associated, correction with isotonic saline is important. The use of solutions that have more sodium than chloride (such as Ringer's lactate) are obviously contraindicated, and all replacement should be with saline. Saline administration alone is usually ineffective unless the associated potassium depletion has been ameliorated.

In the ICU setting, where many patients are being mechanically ventilated, one can also decrease pH by reducing minute ventilation. This will bring the pH toward normal while one is waiting for the kidneys to excrete the excess fixed (nonvolatile) base.

RESPIRATORY ACIDOSIS

Respiratory acidosis is due to retention of CO_2, with an increase in PCO_2 and carbonic acid. CO_2 is almost entirely eliminated in the expired air, and its concentration in the body depends on the relationship between metabolic production and alveolar ventilation. When the metabolic rate is normal, about 200 ml/min of CO_2 is being produced. Hypermetabolic states, especially those associated with sepsis and fever, will increase metabolic rate and CO_2 production.

PATHOGENESIS

Regulatory mechanisms in the respiratory center control ventilation and maintain $PaCO_2$ close to 40 mm Hg. A number of factors can depress the respiratory center; these are commonplace in the ICU setting and are dealt with in Chapter 8. Both acute and chronic CO_2 retention are seen, despite the fact that CO_2 is extremely soluble and diffusible. This means that its arterial concentration is in effect identical in alveolar gas and end-capillary pulmonary venous blood. Therefore, $PaCO_2$ levels accurately reflect alveolar ventilation. A decrease in alveolar ventilation will result in respiratory acidosis.

DIAGNOSIS

The diagnosis of chronic respiratory acidosis can frequently be made when there is elevation of the serum CO_2 content, provided, of course, that metabolic alkalosis is not responsible. More often, the diagnosis is established by an increase in $PaCO_2$ and a fall in pH as determined by analysis of blood gases. Changes in dissolved CO_2 have a marked effect on pH despite the presence of buffers. While the generation of HCO_3^- will limit the fall in arterial pH when dissolved CO_2 is increased, this takes hours to days. For this reason, acute respiratory acidosis cannot always be diagnosed by an elevation of total CO_2, and there is little doubt that it is essential to use arterial blood gas values of PCO_2 and pH in the ICU. $PaCO_2$ levels are usually significantly higher than the mild elevations seen as a compensatory mechanism for metabolic alkalosis.

TREATMENT
Treatment is obviously directed at improving minute ventilation. At times, this may require assisted ventilation, or a change in ventilator settings if the patient is already on a ventilator. Specific techniques for spontaneously breathing patients are also important, such as stabilizing a flail chest, improving the airway, or administering pain medication to a patient with a thoracic incision. It is hard to see how the administration of $NaHCO_3$ is ever necessary in respiratory acidosis. Since most patients in the ICU had adequate pulmonary function prior to the event that made them candidates for intensive care, respiratory acidosis is almost synonymous with alveolar hypoventilation, and prompt correction by increasing ventilation is totally effective. Acute respiratory failure or posttraumatic pulmonary insufficiency, a constant problem in all ICUs, is associated with hypoxemia and is difficult to correct. However, the high diffusibility of CO_2 assures that CO_2 retention will continue to respond to increased ventilation until the end stages of respiratory failure.

RESPIRATORY ALKALOSIS
Respiratory alkalosis is due to hyperventilation, with decreased $PaCO_2$ levels and an elevated pH.

PATHOGENESIS
Some degree of respiratory alkalosis is extremely common in the ICU, since hyperventilation is associated with many stressful conditions. In fact, hyperventilation characterizes the critically ill patient. Many hypermetabolic states result in hyperventilation, and it is extremely common in gram-negative sepsis and peritonitis. Peritoneal irritation of the lower side of the diaphragm, anxiety, and pain all stimulate respiration. Prolonged hyperventilation and respiratory alkalosis often characterize the early stages of acute respiratory failure. In some patients, the hyperventilation is related to inadequate oxygenation, but it does not appear that one common etiologic factor can adequately explain the abnormality in all instances.

When patients are on controlled ventilation, hyperventilation, as evidenced by a low $PaCO_2$, may be the result of excessive tidal volume or too rapid a respiratory rate. However, a high minute ventilation may be necessary to maintain arterial oxygenation, and even patients on assisted ventilation who can control rate if not tidal volume may show respiratory alkalosis.

DIAGNOSIS

The diagnosis of respiratory alkalosis rests on the demonstration of a decreased PCO_2 and an increase in pH. The total serum CO_2 does not change appreciably, and renal compensation for this abnormality is extremely limited.

TREATMENT

A marked degree of respiratory alkalosis is undesirable for a number of reasons. Patients with heart disease, especially if on digitalis or with a tendency toward arrhythmias, are exposed to increased risk under alkalotic conditions. The cerebral effects of hypocapnia and alkalosis represent another reason why alkalosis is poorly tolerated. Vasospastic changes produced by hypocapnia or alkalosis will contribute to cerebral ischemia, and this will be further accentuated in patients with generalized atherosclerosis. When $PaCO_2$ falls below 20 mm Hg, cerebral blood flow falls by almost a third; levels below 30 mm Hg should probably be treated. Once again, the underlying condition must be considered, and primary treatment must be directed toward the cause of the hyperventilation. However, in patients on ventilators, certain more direct approaches are useful. If $PaCO_2$ falls below 30 mm Hg, and minute ventilation cannot be reduced because of the high tidal volumes necessary to achieve blood oxygenation, it is possible to introduce dead space or some rebreathing elements into the airway and in that way bring $PaCO_2$ closer to the normal range. It is not necessary to maintain $PaCO_2$ at the normal value of 40 mm Hg in patients on mechanical ventilation, but efforts to keep this value above 30 mm Hg are clearly important.

MIXED ACID-BASE DISTURBANCES

Hemorrhagic, cardiogenic, and septic shock produce complex abnormalities of acid-base regulation, usually associated with hypoxia, increased ventilation, and hypocapnia. Alkalemia is often seen in the early stages, and acidemia may become predominant later on. In addition, some degree of lactic acidosis is generally present. Such patients make up much of the typical ICU population.

The complexity of these states, as well as poorly defined alterations involving the metabolism of heart, lung, brain, kidney, and peripheral tissues, produce acid-base disturbances that are often mixtures of the four basic abnormalities that have been described. Clinically it is common to see simultaneous respiratory and metabolic derangements. It is essential for the clinician not only to look at the arterial blood gases and associated derived acid-base values but also to evaluate the clinical setting carefully. Losses of acid or alkali are usually recognized, while gains related to therapy frequently receive less attention or are overlooked completely. Resolution of many complex acid-base problems depends on taking into account not only the underlying disease process but also its treatment. This is especially true in the ICU, where critical illness and vigorous therapy exist in combination.

As a general principle, compensatory mechanisms are incomplete, so that despite compensation, the abnormal pH remains abnormal and in the direction of the primary disturbance. In other words, if a patient loses HCO_3^- from a pancreatic fistula, pH and total serum CO_2 will decrease. The resulting metabolic acidosis will stimulate the respiratory center, and hyperventilation will reduce $PaCO_2$. Respiratory alkalosis thus compensates for the previously uncompensated metabolic acidosis, and pH tends to return toward normal. However, the pH would still remain below the normal value of 7.4, indicating that the primary disturbance is acidosis rather than alkalosis.

"Overcompensation" is possible under certain special circumstances that should be mentioned here. In patients with respiratory alkalosis with maximal compensation, abrupt correction of the hypocapnia will lead to acidosis. Overcompensation occurs because the rate of renal adjustment lags behind the respiratory correction. Similarly, overcompensation can develop in patients with long-standing CO_2 retention (respiratory acidosis) and maximal compensation if their hypercapnia is abruptly corrected. Once again, this is related to the time required for renal adjustments, which lag behind the rapid respiratory correction. Awareness of overcompensation is important in the ICU because mechanical ventilation provides the means for abruptly changing body CO_2 stores. As is the case in many other ICU problems, acid-base management requires not only careful consideration of the patient's underlying disease but also serial observations that make it possible to interpret evolving patterns that would otherwise be extremely confusing when considered in isolation.

REFERENCES

1. Astrup, P. K., et al.   Acid-base metabolism: A new approach. *Lancet* 1:1035, 1960.
2. Gamble, J. L., Jr.   *Regulation of the Acidity of the Extracellular Fluids: Teaching Syllabus.* Baltimore: Johns Hopkins University Press, 1966.
3. Heird, W. C., et al.   Metabolic acidosis resulting from intravenous alimentation mixtures containing synthetic amino acids. *N. Engl. J. Med.* 287:943, 1972.
4. Hills, A. G.   *Acid-Base Balance.* Baltimore: Williams & Wilkins, 1973.
5. Siggaard-Andersen, O., et al.   Micro method for determination of pH, carbon dioxide tension, base excess and standard bicarbonate in capillary blood. *Scand. J. Clin. Lab. Invest.* 12:172, 1960.

6. Singer, R. B., and Hastings, A. B.   Improved clinical method for estimation of disturbances of acid-base balance of human blood. *Medicine* 27:223, 1948.
7. Van Slyke, D. D., and Cullen, G. E.   Studies of acidosis. I. Bicarbonate concentration of blood plasma; its significance, and its determination as measure of acidosis. *J. Biol. Chem.* 30:289, 1917.

SELECTED READINGS

Davenport, H. W.   *The ABC of Acid-Base Chemistry* (4th ed.). Chicago: University of Chicago Press, 1958.
Filly, G. F.   *Acid-Base and Blood Gas Regulation: For Medical Students Before and After Graduation.* Philadelphia: Lea & Febiger, 1971.
Siggaard-Andersen, O.   Titratable acid or base of body fluids. *Ann. N.Y. Acad. Sci.* 133:41, 1966.
Winters, R. W., et al.   *Acid-Base Physiology in Medicine.* London, Ontario, Can.: Talbot, 1967.

Josef E. Fischer | 17. NUTRITIONAL MANAGEMENT

The appearance of a chapter on nutrition in a book on intensive care illustrates how far the entire concept of nutrition has come in the past decade. In fact, as one looks back, it seems ridiculous for this not to have occurred sooner. Patients have been supported with sophisticated monitoring and other techniques with heroic measures for weeks—sometimes for months—on end without regard to nutritional needs. This situation often results in what is almost certainly death by starvation. The reasons for this occurring are not difficult to understand. Until recently, there were no practical methods available to provide adequate nutrition for seriously ill patients. It remained for the monumental contributions of Rhoads and Dudrick and their co-workers in parenteral nutrition, as well as Randall, Levenson, and others in the area of predigested and elemental diets, for it even to become possible to think about nutritional support in a sophisticated fashion.

Several statements about the gravity of the problem are in order. First, in any illness, a loss of 30 percent of the lean muscle mass, presumably catabolized for gluconeogenesis and energy, assures a fatal outcome. Second, in small-animal experiments, it has been shown that in addition to muscle catabolized for gluconeogenesis during the first several days of starvation, a significant additional source of protein is the rapidly turning over and (parenthetically) more recently synthesized protein from the metabolically active tissues. This includes some of the most critical tissues in the body, including the liver enzymatic protein, renal tubular enzymes, and the rapidly turning over gastrointestinal mucosa. The cannibalization of these critical proteins seems to make little sense from the point of view of body economy and perhaps may help explain why in prolonged starvation and sepsis, failure of individual or isolated organ systems, most frequently the kidney and liver, may determine the final outcome.

NUTRITIONAL NEEDS

NORMAL ADULT NEEDS

It seems appropriate at this point to review the normal nutritional needs of adult patients. This is perhaps artificial since most of what is known in nutrition has been derived from normal human volunteers or patients in a comparatively steady state. Thus, all of our "ideal" amino acid criteria, for example, are derived either from the ideal composition of a protein such as egg albumin, thought to be of high biologic value, or from the safe requirements of amino acids, such as those proposed by Rose, which have again been based on investigations in well patients in the steady state.

Normal nutrition needs include a basal caloric expenditure rate of 1,800–2,000 calories/day. The protein contribution of this caloric expenditure is about 10 gm of nitrogen, in approximately 60 or 70 gm of protein, which is well within the range of the protein normally ingested in this country daily. The basal expenditure does not increase significantly following minor surgery (herniorrhaphy) or after minor trauma.

NUTRITIONAL NEEDS FOLLOWING INJURY (PATTERNS)

Following massive injury, with or without sepsis, there is a change in the energy consumption pattern, so that an increased fraction of the caloric needs is derived from protein. This results largely from the glucose intolerance that follows sepsis or major injury. This intolerance appears to be due to several additional factors, such as the release of catecholamines, the relatively high glucagon-insulin ratio, especially in the acutely injured septic patient, and the inability of tissues, especially the liver, to take up glucose from the plasma, resulting in the net release of glucose across the liver. This inability in turn may be the result, at the cellular level, of a deficiency of, or loss of efficiency in, the enzyme glucokinase, which, as it were, traps glucose within the liver by phosphorylation to glucose 6-phosphate, from which it is converted into glycogen. During the absence of exogenous glucose, as in starvation, the muscle and brain, among other tissues, will use either glucose derived from gluconeogenesis, derived in turn from muscle breakdown and proteolysis, or ketone bodies derived from free fatty acids generated from lipolysis. In addition, the muscle at least will utilize branched chain amino acids, valine, leucine, and isoleucine for energy. These substances, which also serve as sources for alanine for glucose-alanine cycle (and thus gluconeogenesis), are unique in that they may be oxidized for energy directly without the intervention of glucose. This unique property makes them more valuable in trauma and sepsis.

In sepsis and severe trauma, glucose intolerance, decreased ability of the liver to manufacture ketone bodies, and perhaps impaired utilization of fatty acids all conspire to increase the energy demands and increase breakdown of lean body mass to provide the caloric supply for vital organ function.

Numerous direct effects of injury or of major surgery increase caloric needs. These include fever; tissue damage blood, plasma, and protein loss; plasma exudation by damaged capillaries into the surrounding tissues; and the metabolic requirements for clearance of the damaged tissues. The plasma lost at injury is often not replaced, and increased synthesis of albumin and other proteins by the liver is an additional metabolic drain in the early postinjury period. Additional metabolic requirements may be secondary to the increased work of breathing and respiratory function. Fever remains the most significant factor in the increase in caloric needs. It is estimated that each degree of fever brings about a 10 to 13 percent increase in oxygen consumption. The caloric equivalent of a 10 to 13 percent increase in oxygen consumption has not been demonstrated exactly, but one may calculate approximately 500 to 1,000 calories for each degree of fever (Fahrenheit). This may not take into account the increased loss of water vapor with the diaphoresis and tachypnea that occurs with fever.

Whether or not we assume that parenteral nutrition is helpful in the prevention of complications that may be due to debility, such as hypostatic pneumonia and decubiti, clinical evidence from our own institution suggests that the incidence of suture-line leaks may be decreased in the depleted patient who is operated on after having been repleted with hyperalimentation. For example, following colon bypass in depleted patients with esophageal carcinoma, the incidence of leaks from the sophagocolostomy has all but disappeared. In rats, intestinal suture-line strength is increased by hyperalimentation. Patients subjected to total colectomy after hyperalimentation for ulcerative colitis may have a shorter postoperative hospital stay than those not treated, even though the patients who were treated with parenteral nutrition were more gravely ill. These data, however, are merely suggestive, and it is not known with certainty how long a patient can be subjected to starvation without suffering deleterious effects. Presumably, this occurs before the 30 percent loss of lean body mass that results in death.

EFFECTS OF STARVATION
How long should patients be allowed to go without nutrition? In my own experience, it has worked well to follow an age-dependent rough time sequence, after which parenteral nutrition should be recommended if the patient is not able to resume taking oral nourishment. In a patient in the seventh decade, the time is approximately a week to a maximum of 10 days; in a patient in the sixth decade, it is about 14 to 17 days. Some form of nutritional intervention is appropriate much earlier.

The nonspecific deleterious effects of starvation include wound disruption, poor healing, and decreased anastomotic strength; lack of mobility leads to an increased tendency to phlebitis and skin breakdown, with formation of decubiti (also aided and abetted by poor skin nutrition). There are nonspecific effects on the central nervous system as well. Patients become less alert. They sleep more and cooperate in their care to a lesser extent and have a decreased ability to clear secretions. It is not established whether these central nervous system effects are mediated by the lack of caloric intake for the brain and resulting decreased brain function or by other nonspecific toxic factors, including the accumulation of products from the breakdown of muscle. It is known that some of the transmitter functions of the central nervous system are influenced by the concentration of certain amino acids in the serum and that these amino acids compete at the blood-brain barrier for entry into the brain and in turn determine the neuro-transmitter profile of the brain. In liver disease and perhaps renal disease, amino acid imbalances may contribute to the decreased alertness. It is there-fore possible that some of the effects of starvation on the central nervous system may be mediated to the brain by the known alterations in plasma amino acid patterns.

As starvation goes on and muscle is utilized for gluconeogenesis, the pa-tient may ultimately reach a point where so many intercostal and upper ab-dominal muscles are compromised that insufficient muscle mass remains to perform the work of breathing. This is one common reason for the inabil-ity to wean patients who have been on the respirator for a prolonged pe-riod. The intercostal muscles of such a patient may have been so wasted away by starvation that, even if he is repleted and hyperalimented, respira-tory failure due to loss of muscle mass may become almost irreversible since the muscles are unable to hypertrophy with respiratory work. In ad-dition, there are data that clearly relate nonspecific host resistance to defi-cits in protein and perhaps the essential amino acids. Since death from sep-sis is common in starvation, loss of host resistance probably plays a greater role than we have heretofore been aware of.

Starvation in the presence of sepsis may contribute to multiple organ systems failure, such as the liver and kidneys. It has been previously noted that rapidly turning over proteins may be used for gluconeogenesis under certain circumstances and that these include the newly synthesized enzy-matic elements of both liver and kidney. To be sure, most instances of in-explicable hepatic and renal failure in patients who are overwhelmingly ill reflect generalized organ failure and the inability of the organism to pro-vide homeostasis. It is possible, however, that a significant contribution to hepatic and renal failure may be the cannibalization of useful functional elements for gluconeogenesis. As yet, there is little or no evidence to sug-gest this, but it has not been specifically investigated.

PARENTERAL NUTRITION
ALTERNATIVES IN PARENTERAL NUTRITION
There may be several different objectives relative to patients who require parenteral nutrition. Some patients only need supplementation because of a consistently poor oral intake and do not require completely parenteral maintenance.

Others, because of enteric disease or extensive bowel resection, may ben-efit from an elemental diet plus parenteral nutrition; and still others may require total parenteral nutrition.

One may not want to assume the risks of central catheter parenteral nu-trition, even though such risks may be small with good catheter care (the most critical factor in our experience) [10]. In this case, peripheral parenteral nutrition may be an alternative.

PERIPHERAL PARENTERAL NUTRITION

Peripheral parenteral nutrition is, as the name implies, the technique of supplying total intravenous nutrition through a peripheral vein using a fat emulsion as a principal source of calories, with some glucose, and a nitrogen source. This method avoids the use of hypertonic carbohydrate and the central venous catheter, the principal source of complications from the central parenteral technique. Although fat emulsions have been utilized successfully in Europe for the past decade, they have only recently become commercially available in this country.* The cornerstone of peripheral therapy is the use of approximately 1,500 ml of 10% fat emulsion (or, when available, 750 ml of 20%), providing approximately 1,500 calories, together with the use of large volumes of protein hydrolysate with glucose, fructose, and alcohol as carbohydrate caloric sources. This may be carried out sequentially over a 24-hour period, giving 10% glucose and amino acids for a 16-hour period and fat emulsion over an 8-hour period. Alternatively, solutions may be administered in Y fashion, giving fat and carbohydrate simultaneously.

LIMITATIONS

There are several limitations to the use of the peripheral technique as total support.

The amount of fat that can be given is limited to approximately 2 gm/kg/24 hr. Although occasional investigators have exceeded this amount, the incidence of thrombocytopenia and fat embolism increases significantly above the level of 2 gm/kg.

To date, only the 10% solution of the fat emulsions has been available (approximately 1 calorie/ml), although 20% emulsions exist. The amino acid solution, even if administered as 10% glucose, contains only 500 calories/liter. Thus, the total comfortably attainable by this technique is 3,000 calories (4,500 ml/24 hr). Some authorities have suggested the utilization of diuretics and the infusion of large volumes of 10% dextrose and amino acids in an effort to achieve 4,000 to 5,000 calories. Even at an infusion of 6 liters of 10% dextrose and amino acids, only 4,500 calories can be achieved. Most patients who are on respirators, for example, are kept somewhat fluid-restricted; the accumulation of body water and interstitial pulmonary edema would be injurious. It thus seems more logical to use a central technique, which can supply a greater number of calories in a smaller volume.

* Intralipid 10% fat emulsion, Cutter Laboratories, Inc., Berkeley, Calif., or Liposyn 10%, Abbott Laboratories, Chicago, Ill.

It is difficult to conceive of keeping peripheral intravenous lines in patients for a prolonged period of time, say 6 to 8 weeks, without an extraordinary amount of attention to intravenous technique. Prolonged peripheral administration may lead to loss of peripheral venipuncture sites in patients who are chronically ill. This may constitute a drawback, particularly if surgery is contemplated.

Nonetheless, the peripheral technique lends itself well to circumstances in which supplemental rather than total nutrition is desired, and when the risks of central total parenteral nutrition are great. Alternatively, when the patient resumes oral intake and one is not certain that gastrointestinal function will return rapidly, it may serve as an intermediate technique.

MONITORING

Frequent monitoring is necessary in patients on peripheral parenteral nutrition. Monitoring should be done daily for the first 3 days and should include triglycerides and cholesterol, which may not be cleared initially. In addition, frequent monitoring of blood sugar, electrolytes, calcium, phosphorus, and magnesium is also essential, although serious ionic deficiencies are less likely to occur than they are with central nutrition. Fat emulsions, however, will provide essential fatty acids, usually required after 1 week in patients totally maintained, and to a certain extent will decrease the need for phosphate replacement, since they contain phospholipids in abundance.

ADMINISTRATION

Fat emulsions are administered at a rate equivalent to 60 ml/hr during the first 24 hours. If tolerated, and if a blood sample taken the next day shows no increased milkiness in the serum and no substantial elevation of triglycerides and cholesterol, the amount can be increased to 500 ml/day and then given in increments of 500 ml during 24-hour intervals, provided cholesterol and triglycerides remain normal. A maximal infusion rate of 2 gm fat per kg over 24 hours may be achieved over the next 72 hours and may be held steady thereafter without undue concern about hyperglycemia, toxic reactions, or thrombocytopenia. Occasionally a febrile reaction will develop in a patient, but this usually occurs at initiation of therapy.

PROTEIN SPARING

The infusion of amino acids has been advocated by some as a means of decreasing the catabolism of lean body mass with subsequent reliance on endogenous caloric sources (i.e., fat). It is assumed that most patients for whom the possibility of parenteral nutrition is entertained are so catabolic that exogenous calories are required. The interested reader is referred to the work of Blackburn et al. [2] for a discussion of the protein-sparing effect of exogenous amino acid. Other authorities have clearly shown that the provision of glucose is beneficial. Whatever the practice, this technique is inadequate for the nutritional support of the sick patient.

CENTRAL PARENTERAL NUTRITION

There is little question that provision of large amounts of calories and proteins to seriously ill patients by central parenteral nutrition has already saved hundreds, perhaps thousands, of lives. Unfortunately, the method is not free of complications, and as with most complex therapy, some of the pitfalls are just now being appreciated. By far, the most serious of these complications are septic, generally catheter-related. It appears that even with an extremely rigid protocol, such as is in use in many institutions throughout the United States, a certain minimal level of septic complications appears to be unavoidable, at least with our present techniques. In our experience, catheter care is the most important of all factors involved in reducing the sepsis rate to 1 to 3 percent.

Let us now proceed to examine the types of solutions available, their conditions of use, their indications, and some of their complications.

STANDARD SOLUTIONS

CALORIC SOURCE. In the United States, the only solutions that are available for use contain glucose as the principal caloric source. In other countries, fructose and polyhydrate alcohols are also available, and the rationale for their use is to improve on the glucose intolerance present in posttraumatic patients, who may be more tolerant of fructose and alcohol in small amounts for the first 3 to 4 days following the injury. These advantages seem more apparent than real, since alcohols and fructose generate problems in turn, such as lack of physiologic control, difficulty in readily measuring blood excess of such carbohydrates, hepatic damage (in the case of xylitol), and lactic acidosis secondary to fructose. These must remain theoretical considerations, since it is unlikely that other carbohydrate sources will be commercially available in the future.

LIMITING FACTORS. There are several limiting factors in the amount of solution that can be administered to a given patient in 24 hours. Some of this is variable, depending on the patient's age, metabolic status, and endocrine reserve. The practical limit in the administration of glucose readily metabolized in the normal adult is approximately 800 to 1,000 mg/min. There are 1,440 minutes in a 24-hour period; the rate of glucose administration should not exceed approximately 800 mg/min, or 1,100 gm/24 hr, above which metabolic problems occur at greatly increased frequency. Most solutions currently available utilize a 23% glucose caloric source; the limit of administration is therefore approximately 5 liters/24 hr.

The calorie-nitrogen ratio is a magic number unsupported by hard data. The calorie-nitrogen ratio for efficacy of nitrogen utilization falls between

125 and 200 nonprotein calories per gram of nitrogen; there is little evidence of which this author is aware to suggest that any ratio higher than this offers any significant advantage. Most studies, including our own, have concluded that a calorie-nitrogen ratio of about 150 : 1 is appropriate.

HYDROLYSATES. Hydrolysates were the first solutions in use, the protein source being the hydrolysate of either casein or fibrin. There appears to be a small but theoretical advantage to casein, although fibrin gave excellent clinical results. The solution is generally used as a formulation of 30 gm protein to approximately 200 to 250 gm of glucose/liter. Only approximately 55 percent of the available nitrogen in casein hydrolysate, for example, is available as α-amino nitrogen. It is known that hydrolysis is not complete, and it is not known whether or not dipeptides and tripeptides can be efficiently utilized by the body. Thus, the wastage in this type of solution accounts for the small amount (approximately 2.2 gm of nitrogen/liter of solution) available to the patient for use in protein synthesis. There may be situations (e.g., burns) in which patients are extremely septic and their catabolic rate, even in the presence of parenteral nutrition, exceeds this figure. In such patients, rather than promoting anabolism, this solution may merely maintain the body at a near steady state. Nonetheless, results with each of the hydrolysates have been excellent for the most part, although a few patients may perhaps have done better with a synthetic amino acid solution. This discussion is presently of historical interest only.

SYNTHETIC AMINO ACID SOLUTIONS. The theoretical advantages to a synthetic amino acid solution are that its composition is known exactly, there are no dipeptides and tripeptides, and the amino acid composition may be varied with different situations. It has been demonstrated in a few patients that the smaller amount of protein in a synthetic amino acid solution and its slower rate of infusion as compared with a hydrolysate may be successful in promoting positive nitrogen balance.

Theoretical objections to these solutions include their amino acid composition. An amino acid imbalance appears to contribute to a metabolic acidosis, a problem that can be easily remedied by the administration of sodium as the acetate rather than as the chloride (Table 17-1). Hyperammonemia has been reported with Freamine, but this appears to be confined to neonates of low birth weight. No cases have been observed since the original report (R. Winters, personal communication). In our own studies, only slight increases in blood ammonia have been observed in large numbers of adults given Freamine.

INDICATIONS FOR PARENTERAL NUTRITION
Indications for the use of parenteral nutrition appear to vary from institution to institution and in general reflect both the current status of the pro-

TABLE 17-1. Ingredients of the Mixed Amino Acid Solution (Freamine)
Currently in Use at the University of Cincinnati Medical Center[a]

Ingredient	Amount
Protein equivalent (gm)	40
Nitrogen, utilizable (gm)	6.4
Nitrogen, total (gm)	6.4
Total calories	959
Potassium (mEq/liter)	40
Sodium (mEq/liter)	21
Chloride (mEq/liter)	8
Magnesium (mEq/liter)	8
Calcium (mEq/liter)	4.7
Phosphate (mM/liter)	13.4
Acetate (mEq/liter)	29
Insulin USP (units)	15[b]
Vitamins	B Group, C (A, D, E)

[a] There is a certain amount of variation in the ionic components that the pharmacy will mix at the physician's request. The pharmacy will prepare the following variations: low potassium, O; additional sodium, 50 mEq/liter (total).
[b] Optional.

cedure's safety in a given institution and the understanding and acceptance of this mode of therapy by the staff. It is a truism that in an institution with a low complication rate, a wider range of indications is used. Conversely, in institutions where the administration of parenteral nutrition by a central route is accompanied by a high complication rate, this treatment will be reserved for only the most seriously ill.

A generous list of indications will be given here, since the list reflects the widespread use of parenteral nutrition in our institution for indications that may be considered marginal in others. However, it also reflects our preoccupation with safety and a relatively low complication rate.

In its briefest statement, if parenteral nutrition is considered, it should with rare exceptions be initiated—"if you think of it, you probably should do it." This point of view is based on the fact that it is much easier to prevent the complications of starvation than to treat them once they have occurred. An argument could therefore be made for the immediate institution of hyperalimentation in any patient who is seriously injured with multiple organ systems involved and who is likely not to be able to resume oral intake for approximately a week to 10 days. Alternatively, patients with fractures, fat emboli, or fever, or patients who have had a laparotomy because of some abdominal injury are so catabolic that it would be in turn wise to institute hyperalimentation immediately. A radical view? Perhaps, but this is our current practice. In addition to the classic indications of inadequate gastrointestinal tract functions—including fistulas, prolonged ileus, retroperitoneal hematoma, and ileus associated with a spinal injury—any patient who is unlikely to resume oral intake in a week is placed on central nutrition. Those patients with extensive injury should be started on parenteral nutrition shortly after the hemodynamic status stabilizes.

PLACEMENT OF THE CATHETER IN INTRAVENOUS NUTRITION

SITE

Only two sites are acceptable for prolonged intravenous nutrition—the subclavian and internal jugular veins, terminating in the superior vena cava. Other sites (i.e., femoral vein, saphenous vein, and long arm lines) appear to be associated with too high an incidence of infection, or thrombosis, or both. Of the two, the subclavian approach is preferable, although it is accompanied by a slightly higher incidence of technical complications in placement. These complications decrease with experience, although even the most experienced personnel will occasionally cause a complication. The subclavian catheter is more easily cared for, the dressing is more easily carried out, and it is also more comfortable for the patient.

In our institution catheter placement is made easier by the prepackaging of kits for subclavian placement that include catheter, masks, gown, gloves, sterile towel, half sheets for draping of the patient, and simple instruments including a Kelly clamp, scissors, and forceps (Table 17-2). These are available on all floors and on special hyperalimentation carts placed at strategic locations throughout the hospital. In addition to the kits, the carts contain intravenous and "prep" solutions. Orders are available on each unit.

PROCEDURES

The procedure may be performed in the patient's room with the patient in bed. The area of catheter placement is shaved and prepared with a surgical "prep" solution, including acetone, iodine, and alcohol. In general, it is preferable to prepare both the subclavian and the internal jugular sites. Then, if one is not successful in passing a subclavian catheter, for example, an internal jugular placement may be attempted, and vice versa. A nurse experienced in the technique should be present. Fewer technical errors and breaches of technique will occur under these circumstances.

The patient is placed in bed with a towel roll between the shoulder blades to throw the shoulders back and the head of the manubrium sterni forward; the arm is at the side. The subclavian vein is more easily approached in this fashion. The landmarks I use are approximately midway along the clavicle, 1 cm medial and 1 cm caudad to the bend. The point of the needle is directed toward 1 fingerbreadth above the manubrium sterni (Fig. 17-1).

TABLE 17-2. Subclavian Intravenous Catheter Placement Set in Use at the University of Cincinnati Medical Center

Quantity	Item*
2	3-ml disposable syringe with 22-gauge needle
1	3-0 silk with straight needle (put on 3 × 3 sponge)
1	5-ml vial of lidocaine
1	Kelly "Pean"
1	Thumb forceps 5½"
1	B&S scissors 5½"
3	Towel clips
1	Folded half sheet
3	Flat towels
10	3 × 3 Topper sponges
1	Disposable precaution gown

* The instructions are as follows: place in Ekco tray, wrap in two 25 × 25 autoclave papers, and label. After set is autoclaved, put in a 12 × 20 Tower bag with a #16 Intracath 8" #3112, Betadine ointment, two filter masks, two pairs of size 7½ gloves. Seal. Date 2 months ahead. Flush equipment with distilled water before sterilizing for removal of pyrogens.

In general, I prefer to locate the subclavian vein with the #22 needle in which the lidocaine has been placed in the skin and infiltrated around the periosteum. When the vein is located, the large-bore needle through which the catheter is passed will then be directed in a similar direction (toward the manubrium sterni). It is important not to direct the needle more than 10 or 15 degrees to the horizontal (Fig. 17-2). One must recall that the subclavian vein is the most anterior of all the structures in the thoracic inlet; all the structures that can be damaged, including the subclavian artery, brachial plexus, and the apex of the lung, are posterior.

Once the needle is in place, the patient is asked to perform a Valsalva maneuver, and the catheter is passed through the open end of the needle. To avoid placing the catheter in the internal jugular vein, the hub of the needle is directed cephalad. The catheter is then sutured into place, and an infusion of 5% D/W is started, to continue until the catheter's position can be confirmed by a chest x-ray film; hypertonic solutions should not be administered before it is taken. A final 0.22-μ filter is inserted in the line.

With respect to the internal jugular percutaneous puncture, one must remember that the internal jugular vein is anterior and lateral to the carotid artery. The landmarks used here are a point 2 fingerbreadths above the clavicle at the posterior border of the sternocleidomastoid border. The patient's neck is turned to the opposite side, and the arm is alongside the body. Again, the vein may be located with a #22 needle containing lido-

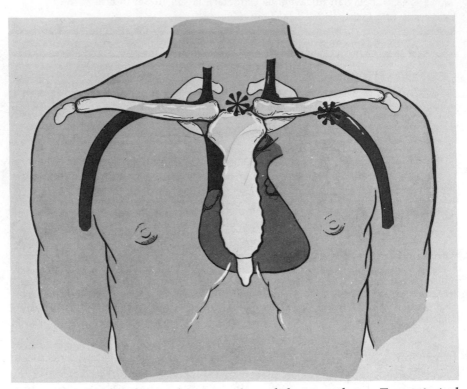

FIGURE 17-1. Landmarks in placement of a subclavian catheter. Two principal landmarks are midpoint of clavicle, 1 cm below and 1 cm lateral to point at which clavicle bends, and a point 1 fingerbreadth above manubrium sterni (toward which the needle should point).

caine, pointing toward the notch above the manubrium sterni. Here again, the catheter is sutured in place. It may be possible to pass the catheter subcutaneously under local anesthesia over the clavicle, so that the exit point is on the chest. This gives the additional protection of the subcutaneous tunnel, which should theoretically decrease the incidence of sepsis; it is our belief that sepsis occurs by bacteria growing along the site of the venipuncture from the skin into the vein. Also, dressing is easier in this position. Again, a chest x-ray is used to confirm the location of the catheter tip, which should be in the superior vena cava and not in the right atrium. Several cases of arrhythmia have been reported from placement of the catheter too close to the sinoatrial node.

AFTERCARE

The dressing is changed every 48 hours after the site has been cleansed with acetone iodine and alcohol solutions and an antifungal and a povidone

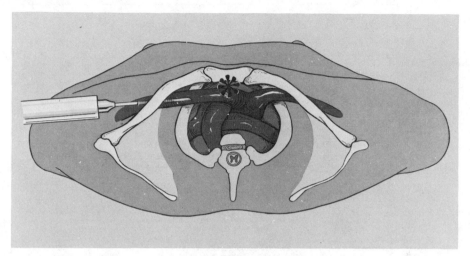

FIGURE 17-2. Position of subclavian vein in reference to clavicle. Note that subclavian vein is uppermost structure in thoracic inlet. All the other structures, including subclavian artery, brachial plexus, and apex of lung, lie inferior and, to a certain extent, caudad. Needle is kept horizontal. If it is inserted at an angle of no greater than 10 or 15 degrees to the horizontal, complications will be avoided.

ointment, is applied. The position of the catheter when the dressing is done should be such that it is directed toward the nipple over the chest and not over the arm, shoulder, or another point.

GUIDELINES FOR PARENTERAL NUTRITION
GENERAL GUIDELINES
The most frequent metabolic complications in parenteral nutrition occur following too rapid administration of hypertonic dextrose solutions when hyperalimentation is begun. Consequently, if the body is allowed time to equilibrate and if one allows an endogenous insulin response to build up, parenteral nutrition should be carried out safely and without hyperglycemia. The infusion is started at a rate of 60 ml/hr (assuming 23% dextrose as the caloric source). In older patients, this is increased by increments of 20 ml/hr every other day; or, if the patient is more depleted, at more frequent intervals, until a maximal rate of infusion of 165 ml/hr (4 liter/day) is reached. In younger patients, the infusion rate can be increased by increments of 20 ml/hr at 24-hour intervals. Insulin is added to the infusion in all patients over 30 years of age; this is my own preference and is not followed by many other investigators working in the area. Urine testing is carried out routinely, as shown in the printed orders (Fig. 17-3) that are with every patient's chart and are signed by the physician initiating the hyperalimentation. However, unless blood sugar is elevated, the presence of

PHYSICIAN'S ORDER FORM
Parenteral Nutrition - CENTRAL Formulation
STANDING ORDERS
KEEP WITH DAILY ORDERS AND FILE IN MEDICAL RECORDS

DATE_____ TIME _____

1. Infuse via new, sterile subclavian or internal jugular catheter terminating in superior vena cava, innominate or intrathoracic subclavian vein. X-ray confirmation of catheter position is mandatory. Infuse D₅W at a rate of 20 ml/hr until catheter tip location is documented in patient's chart.

2. Notify M.D. in event of clotted line or leakage from catheter or insertion site.

3. Test urinary sugar and acetone q 6 h with Tes-tape. For 3+ glycosuria, or greater, obtain **STAT** serum glucose and notify M.D.

4. Daily I & O, calorie count (please notify Dietician), and weight before 8 A.M. Save all I & O sheets. Vital signs and temperature q 6 h.

5. Care of dressing: Change q Mon., Wed., Fri., and p.r.n. Care of IV tubing and filter: Change q 24 h at 2 P.M. via Nursing Policy and Procedure Manual.

6. Infusion rate **must** be kept constant using an IV controller. Check every 30 minutes and reset to rate ordered. **DO NOT ATTEMPT TO CATCH UP.** Initiate any rate change at 2 P.M. with bottle # 1, unless otherwise specified. Please **NOTIFY** Pharmacy if any rate changes **must** be made.

7. If **CENTRAL** formulation is not readily available, D₂₀W should be infused at the **same** rate. If patient is receiving regular insulin in the **CENTRAL** formulation, ½ the total amount of regular insulin per bottle of **CENTRAL** formulation **must** be added to the **500 ml** bottle of D₂₀W before it is administered.

8. Blood Work: These are fasting bloods if the patient is not N.P.O. Obtain **before** initiating **CENTRAL** formulation and bi-weekly on Monday and Thursday: Na, K, Chloride, Total CO₂, Glucose, BUN, Creatinine, Total protein, Osmolality, Magnesium, Calcium, Phosphorous, Alk. Phosph., ɤ GT, Albumin, Bilirubin: Total and Direct, SGPT, SGOT, Ammonia, Platelets, PT, PTT, Hgb, Hct, WBC with diff.

9. Catheter **CANNOT** be used for other IV's, medications, blood sampling, or CVP readings.

10. Upon catheter removal, culture catheter tip immediately. Send to laboratory in culture tube **STAT**. Request C & S and **be sure** to **NOTE** on laboratory slip to "Smear on Plate Immediately", "Hold for Fungal Testing", and "Hyperalimentation Patient".

_____ M.D.

PARENTERAL NUTRITION SOLUTION
AMINO ACIDS *CENTRAL* FORMULATION

Each **1000ml** contains:
Amino Acids (4.25%)	42.5 Gm.
Dextrose (25%)	250 Gm.
Non-protein Calories	850 Kcal.
Total Calories	1000 Kcal.
Nitrogen	6.25 Gm.

VITAMINS - DAILY
< B Complex - 1ml
Ascorbic acid equiv. = 550mg.

in addition to above on
Monday
ONLY
< Multivitamins (B Complex, A, C, D & E)-2.5ml
Ascorbic acid equiv. = 250 mg.

Osmolarity 1900 mOsm. (standard formulation)

	* K	Na	Mg	Ca	P(mM)	Cl	Acetate	Regular Insulin (UNITS)
STANDARD	12	21	8	4.7	13.4	8	29	0
WITH ADDED SODIUM	12	51	8	4.7	13.4	24	43	0
WITH ADDED INSULIN	12	21	8	4.7	13.4	8	29	15
WITH ADDED SODIUM & INSULIN	12	51	8	4.7	13.4	24	43	15
WITH ADDED POTASSIUM	40	21	8	4.7	17.3	16	43	0
WITH ADDED POTASSIUM & SODIUM	40	51	8	4.7	17.3	32	57	0
WITH ADDED POTASSIUM & INSULIN	40	21	8	4.7	17.3	16	43	15
WITH ADDED POTASSIUM SODIUM & INSULIN	40	51	8	4.7	17.3	32	57	15

*Values expressed in mEq. liter unless otherwise noted.

NOTE: For maximum allowable concentrations of electrolytes please consult Allowable Additive Supplementation Sheet on reverse side.

FIGURE 17-3. Standard orders that must be inserted in chart of each patient receiving hydrolysate solution. For patients receiving renal failure solution or essential amino acids, an experimental solution, order must be placed by physician member of hyperalimentation team.

CGH-122a
12/78

University of Cincinnati Medical Center
Cincinnati General Hospital

PHYSICIAN'S ORDER FORM
Parenteral Nutrition - Central Formulation

DATE _____ TIME _____   ORDERS MUST BE IN THE PHARMACY BEFORE 9:30 A.M.

SOLUTIONS FROM PHARMACY
CHECK **ONE** FORMULA FOR EACH BOTTLE

ADDITIVES:

INDICATE **TOTAL** AMOUNT OF EACH ADDITIVE DESIRED PER BOTTLE (INCLUDE THE BASIC AMOUNT IN EACH BOTTLE PLUS THE ADDITIONAL DESIRED TO EQUAL THE **TOTAL**.)

BOTTLE	STANDARD	ADDED Na	ADDED INSULIN	ADDED Na & INSULIN	ADDED K	ADDED K & Na	ADDED K & INSULIN	ADDED K, Na & INSULIN
#1								
#2								
#3								
#4								
#5								

RATE _____ ML/HR _____ M.D.

DATE _____ TIME _____   ORDERS MUST BE IN THE PHARMACY BEFORE 9:30 A.M.

SOLUTIONS FROM PHARMACY
CHECK **ONE** FORMULA FOR EACH BOTTLE

ADDITIVES:

INDICATE **TOTAL** AMOUNT OF EACH ADDITIVE DESIRED PER BOTTLE (INCLUDE THE BASIC AMOUNT IN EACH BOTTLE PLUS THE ADDITIONAL DESIRED TO EQUAL THE **TOTAL**.)

BOTTLE	STANDARD	ADDED Na	ADDED INSULIN	ADDED Na & INSULIN	ADDED K	ADDED K & Na	ADDED K & INSULIN	ADDED K, Na & INSULIN
#1								
#2								
#3								
#4								
#5								

RATE _____ ML/HR _____ M.D.

DATE _____ TIME _____   ORDERS MUST BE IN THE PHARMACY BEFORE 9:30 A.M.

SOLUTIONS FROM PHARMACY
CHECK **ONE** FORMULA FOR EACH BOTTLE

ADDITIVES:

INDICATE **TOTAL** AMOUNT OF EACH ADDITIVE DESIRED PER BOTTLE (INCLUDE THE BASIC AMOUNT IN EACH BOTTLE PLUS THE ADDITIONAL DESIRED TO EQUAL THE **TOTAL**.)

BOTTLE	STANDARD	ADDED Na	ADDED INSULIN	ADDED Na & INSULIN	ADDED K	ADDED K & Na	ADDED K & INSULIN	ADDED K, Na & INSULIN
#1								
#2								
#3								
#4								
#5								

RATE _____ ML/HR _____ M.D.

FOR THIS ENTRY SEND YELLOW COPY TO PHARMACY

FOR THIS ENTRY SEND PINK COPY TO PHARMACY

FOR THIS ENTRY SEND GOLDENROD COPY TO PHARMACY

ALLOWABLE ADDITIVE SUPPLEMENTATION

ADDITIVES	AVAILABLE PRODUCTS	MAXIMUM ALLOWABLE TOTAL PER LITER BOTTLE
Calcium	* Calcium Gluconate Inj. Calcium Chloride Inj.	9 mEq.
Magnesium	Magnesium Sulfate Inj.	12 mEq.
Phosphate	* Sodium Phosphate Inj. Potassium Phosphate Inj.	21 mM.
Potassium	* Potassium Chloride Inj. Potassium Acetate Inj.	80 mEq.
Sodium	* Sodium Chloride Inj. Sodium Acetate Inj.	Patient tolerance and/or need
Chloride	* Sodium Chloride Inj. Calcium Chloride Inj. Potassium Chloride Inj.	Limited by amount of cation
	HCl Inj.	100 mEq.
Acetate	* Sodium Acetate Inj. Potassium Acetate Inj.	Limited by amount of cation
Insulin	Regular Insulin Inj.	50 UNITS

NOTE: With these electrolytes, unless otherwise specified on **PHYSICIAN'S ORDER FORM**, additives supplemental to the established formulas will be added as the asterisked (*) salt.

SOME POINTS TO REMEMBER

• Bicarbonate salts **must** not be added to parenteral nutrition formulations since they create a number of incompatabilities and are ineffective given in this manner.

• Medicinal agents not mentioned (such as all antibiotics, cardio-active agents, colloids, and electrolytes not specified as compatible) **must** not be admixed or administered with parenteral nutrition formulations due to resultant incompatabilities.

• Phosphate supplementation **must** be ordered in terms of millimoles (mM) of phosphate. Please note that phosphate is available only as the sodium or potassium salts and that when the potassium salt is used for "added" phosphate it must not exceed the maximum allowable concentration of potassium (i.e. 80mEq.)

CGH-268
(12/78)

University of Cincinnati Medical Center
Cincinnati General Hospital

PHYSICIAN'S ORDER FORM

Parenteral Nutrition - RENAL Formulation

STANDING ORDERS
KEEP WITH DAILY ORDERS AND FILE IN MEDICAL RECORDS

DATE_____ TIME _____

1. **INITIAL** order for **RENAL** formulation **must** be written by an M.D. from the Hyperalimentation Unit.

2. Infuse via new, sterile subclavian or internal jugular catheter terminating in superior vena cava, innominate or intrathoracic subclavian vein. X-ray confirmation of catheter position is mandatory. Infuse D_5W at a rate of 20 ml/hr until catheter tip location is documented in patient's chart.

3. Notify M.D. in event of clotted line or leakage from catheter or insertion site.

4. Test urinary sugar and acetone q 6 h with Tes-tape. For 3+ glycosuria, or greater, obtain **STAT** serum glucose and notify M.D.

5. Daily I & O, calorie count (please notify Dietician), and weight before 8 A.M. Save all I & O sheets. Vital signs and temperature q 6 h.

6. Care of dressing: Change q Mon., Wed., Fri., and p.r.n. Care of IV tubing and filter: Change q 24 at 2 P.M. via Nursing Policy and Procedure Manual.

7. Infusion rate **must** be kept constant using an IV controller. Check every 30 minutes and reset to rate ordered. **DO NOT ATTEMPT TO CATCH UP.** Initiate any rate change at 2 P.M. with bottle # 1, unless otherwise specified. Please **NOTIFY** Pharmacy if any rate changes **must** be made.

8. If **RENAL** formulation is not readily available, $D_{20}W$ should be infused at the **same** rate. If patient is receiving regular insulin in the **RENAL** formulation, ½ the total amount of regular insulin per bottle of **RENAL** formulation **must** be added to the **500ml** bottle of $D_{20}W$ before it is administered.

9. Blood Work: These are fasting bloods if the patient is not N.P.O. Obtain **before** initiating **RENAL** formulation and bi-weekly on Monday and Thursday: Na, K, Chloride, Total CO_2, Glucose, BUN, Creatinine, Total protein, Osmolality, Magnesium, Calcium, Phosphorous, Alk. Phosph., Y GT, Albumin, Bilirubin: Total and Direct, SGPT, SGOT, Ammonia, Platelets, PT, PTT, Hgb, Hct, WBC with diff.

   DAILY Bloods: Na, K, Glucose, BUN, Creatinine, Hgb, Osmolality.

   NOTE: Serum glucose levels should be drawn q 6 h for initial 48-72 hours, then twice daily or more frequently if indicated. They should not be drawn **less** frequently than daily.

10. Additional regular insulin, if required, should be added to the **RENAL** formulation or given S.C. according to the patient's **serum** glucose levels **only, NOT** according to urine glucose levels.

11. Catheter **CANNOT** be used for other IV's, medications, blood sampling, or CVP readings.

12. Upon catheter removal, culture tip immediately. Send to lab in culture tube **STAT**. Request C & S and be sure to **NOTE** on laboratory slip to "Smear on Plate Immediately", "Hold for Fungal Testing" and "Hyperalimentation Patient."

_____ M.D.

PARENTERAL NUTRITION SOLUTION
AMINO ACIDS *RENAL* FORMULATION

Each **750ml** contains:

Amino Acids (essential) (1.7%)	12.75 Gm.
Dextrose (46.6%)	350 Gm.
Non-protein Calories	1190 Kcal.
Total Calories	1250 Kcal.
Nitrogen	1.46 Gm.

VITAMINS

DAILY ⟨ Multivitamins (B Complex, A, C, D & E) - 2.5ml
      ⟨ Ascorbic Acid equiv. = 1250mg.

Osmolarity 2125 mOsm (standard formulation)

	* K	Na	Mg	Ca	P(mM)	Cl	Acetate	Regular Insulin (UNITS)
STANDARD	0	1.2	0	0	0	0	0	0
WITH INSULIN	0	1.2	0	0	0	0	0	15

*Values expressed in mEq./750ml unless otherwise noted.
NOTE: For maximum allowable concentrations of electrolytes please consult Allowable Additive Supplementation Sheet on reverse side.

CGH-268a
12/78

University of Cincinnati Medical Center
Cincinnati General Hospital

PHYSICIAN'S ORDER FORM
Parenteral Nutrition - Renal Formulation

DATE _____ TIME _____   **ORDERS MUST BE IN THE PHARMACY BEFORE 9:30 A.M.**

SOLUTIONS FROM PHARMACY
CHECK **ONE** FORMULA FOR EACH BOTTLE

ADDITIVES:

INDICATE **TOTAL** AMOUNT OF EACH ADDITIVE DESIRED PER
BOTTLE (INCLUDE THE BASIC AMOUNT IN EACH BOTTLE
PLUS THE ADDITIONAL DESIRED TO EQUAL THE **TOTAL**.)

BOTTLE	STANDARD RENAL	STANDARD RENAL WITH INSULIN	
#1			
#2			
#3			

RATE _____ ML/HR. _____ M.D.

DATE _____ TIME _____   **ORDERS MUST BE IN THE PHARMACY BEFORE 9:30 A.M.**

SOLUTIONS FROM PHARMACY
CHECK **ONE** FORMULA FOR EACH BOTTLE

ADDITIVES:

INDICATE **TOTAL** AMOUNT OF EACH ADDITIVE DESIRED PER
BOTTLE (INCLUDE THE BASIC AMOUNT IN EACH BOTTLE
PLUS THE ADDITIONAL DESIRED TO EQUAL THE **TOTAL**.)

BOTTLE	STANDARD RENAL	STANDARD RENAL WITH INSULIN	
#1			
#2			
#3			

RATE _____ ML/HR. _____ M.D.

DATE _____ TIME _____   **ORDERS MUST BE IN THE PHARMACY BEFORE 9:30 A.M.**

SOLUTIONS FROM PHARMACY
CHECK **ONE** FORMULA FOR EACH BOTTLE

ADDITIVES:

INDICATE **TOTAL** AMOUNT OF EACH ADDITIVE DESIRED PER
BOTTLE (INCLUDE THE BASIC AMOUNT IN EACH BOTTLE
PLUS THE ADDITIONAL DESIRED TO EQUAL THE **TOTAL**.)

BOTTLE	STANDARD RENAL	STANDARD RENAL WITH INSULIN	
#1			
#2			
#3			

RATE _____ ML/HR. _____ M.D.

CGH-274   University of Cincinnati Medical Center
(12/78)   Cincinnati General Hospital

PHYSICIAN'S ORDER FORM

Parenteral Nutrition - CARDIAC Formulation

STANDING ORDERS
KEEP WITH DAILY ORDERS AND FILE IN MEDICAL RECORD

DATE _____ TIME _____

1. **INITIAL** order for **CARDIAC** formulation **must** be written by an M.D. from the Hyperalimentation Unit.

2. Infuse via new, sterile subclavian or internal jugular catheter terminating in superior vena cava, innominate, or intrathoracic subclavian vein. X-ray confirmation of catheter position is mandatory. Infuse D_5W at a rate of 20 ml/hr until catheter tip location is documented in patient's chart.

3. Notify M.D. in event of clotted line or leakage from catheter or insertion site.

4. Test urinary sugar and acetone q 6 h with Tes-tape. For 3+ glycosuria, or greater, obtain **STAT** serum glucose and notify M.D.

5. Daily I & O, calorie count (please notify Dietician), and weight before 8 A.M. Save all I & O sheets. Vital signs and temperature q 6 h.

6. Care of dressing: Change q Mon., Wed., Fri., and p.r.n. Care of IV tubing and filter: Change q 24 h at 2 P.M. via Nursing Policy and Procedure Manual.

7. Infusion rate **must** be kept constant using an IV controller. Check every 30 minutes and reset to rate ordered. **DO NOT ATTEMPT TO CATCH UP.** Initiate any rate change at 2 P.M. with bottle # 1, unless otherwise specified. Please **NOTIFY** Pharmacy if any rate changes **must** be made.

8. If **CARDIAC** formulation is not readily available, $D_{20}W$ should be infused at the **same** rate. If patient is receiving regular insulin in the **CARDIAC** formulation, ½ the total amount of regular insulin per bottle of **CARDIAC** formulations **must** be added to the **500ml** bottle of D_xW before it is administered.

9. Blood Work: These are fasting bloods if the patient is not N.P.O. Obtain **before** initiating **CARDIAC** formulation and bi-weekly on Monday and Thursday: Na, K, Chloride, Total CO_2, Glucose, BUN, Creatinine, Total protein, Osmolality, Magnesium, Calcium, Phosphorous, Alk. Phosph., 𝛾 GT, Albumin, Bilirubin: Total and Direct, SGPT, SGOT, Ammonia, Platelets, PT, PTT, Hgb, Hct, WBC with diff.

   NOTE: Serum glucose levels should be drawn q 6 h for initial 48-72 hours, then twice daily or more frequently if indicated. They should not be drawn **less** frequently than daily.

10. Catheter **CANNOT** be used for other IV's, medications, blood sampling, or CVP readings.

11. Upon catheter removal, culture catheter tip immediately. Send to laboratory in culture tube **STAT**. Request C & S and be sure to **NOTE** on laboratory slip to "Smear on Plate Immediately", "Hold for Fungal Testing", and "Hyperalimentation Patient".

_____ _____ M.D

PARENTERAL NUTRITION SOLUTION
AMINO ACIDS *CARDIAC* FORMULATION

Each **UNIT** (860-880ml) contains:

Amino Acids (3.5%)	30.6 Gm.
Dextrose (40%)	350 Gm.
Non-protein Calories	1190 Kcal.
Total Calories	1320 Kcal.
Nitrogen	4.5 Gm.

Osmolarity 2500 mOsm. (standard formulation)

VITAMINS   DAILY { B Complex - 1ml / Ascorbic acid equiv. = 550mg.

in addition to above on Monday **ONLY** { Multivitamins (B Complex, A, C, D, & E) - 2.5ml / Ascorbic acid equiv. = 250mg.

	*K	Na	Mg	Ca	P(mM)	Cl	Acetate	Regular Insulin (UNITS)	Volume (ml)
STANDARD	0	3.6	8	0	3.6	0	16	0	860
WITH ADDED POTASSIUM	50	3.6	8	0	12.6	0	53	0	880
WITH ADDED INSULIN	0	3.6	8	0	3.6	0	16	15	860
WITH ADDED POTASSIUM AND INSULIN	50	3.6	8	0	12.6	0	53	15	880

*Values expressed in mEq./unit (860-880ml) unless otherwise noted.
NOTE: For maximum allowable concentrations of electrolytes please consult Allowable Additive Supplementation Sheet on reverse side.

CGH-274a
12/78

University of Cincinnati Medical Center
Cincinnati General Hospital

PHYSICIAN'S ORDER FORM
Parenteral Nutrition - Cardiac Formulation

DATE _____ TIME _____ ORDERS MUST BE IN THE PHARMACY BEFORE 9:30 A.M.

ADDITIVES:

SOLUTIONS FROM PHARMACY
CHECK **ONE** FORMULA FOR EACH BOTTLE

INDICATE **TOTAL** AMOUNT OF EACH ADDITIVE DESIRED PER
BOTTLE (INCLUDE THE BASIC AMOUNT IN EACH BOTTLE
PLUS THE ADDITIONAL TO EQUAL THE **TOTAL.**)

BOTTLE	STANDARD CARDIAC	ADDED POTASSIUM	ADDED INSULIN	ADDED POTASSIUM & INSULIN
#1				
#2				
#3				

RATE _____ ML/HR _____ M.D.

DATE _____ TIME _____ ORDERS MUST BE IN THE PHARMACY BEFORE 9:30 A.M.

ADDITIVES:

SOLUTIONS FROM PHARMACY
CHECK **ONE** FORMULA FOR EACH BOTTLE

INDICATE **TOTAL** AMOUNT OF EACH ADDITIVE DESIRED PER
BOTTLE (INCLUDE THE BASIC AMOUNT IN EACH BOTTLE
PLUS THE ADDITIONAL TO EQUAL THE **TOTAL.**)

BOTTLE	STANDARD CARDIAC	ADDED POTASSIUM	ADDED INSULIN	ADDED POTASSIUM & INSULIN
#1				
#2				
#3				

RATE _____ ML/HR _____ M.D

DATE _____ TIME _____ ORDERS MUST BE IN THE PHARMACY BEFORE 9:30 A.M.

ADDITIVES:

SOLUTIONS FROM PHARMACY
CHECK **ONE** FORMULA FOR EACH BOTTLE

INDICATE **TOTAL** AMOUNT OF EACH ADDITIVE DESIRED PER
BOTTLE (INCLUDE THE BASIC AMOUNT IN EACH BOTTLE
PLUS THE ADDITIONAL TO EQUAL THE **TOTAL.**)

BOTTLE	STANDARD CARDIAC	ADDED POTASSIUM	ADDED INSULIN	ADDED POTASSIUM & INSULIN
#1				
#2				
#3				

urinary glucose alone (at least within the first 48 hr) should not be used as an indication to administer insulin by test.

The ideal weight gain should be between ½ and 1 pound a day. A gain of over 1 pound almost certainly indicates fluid retention, and signs of fluid retention in legs or sacrum will be detectable.

It is our custom never to use a pump in patients who are not in intensive care situations; pumps generally tend to cause more problems than they solve. Of course, in cases in which fluid overload is critical, a pump is safe if supervised by a well-trained nurse, but this supervision rarely exists on a general hospital floor.

ION REQUIREMENTS

Ion requirements for patients on parenteral nutrition will vary from patient to patient, depending on previous body stores, renal function, and the primary disease for which the patient is being treated. However, it is possible to suggest approximate requirements. Since it is my own practice to carry patients on 4 liters of hyperalimentation solution a day, I shall suggest requirements for that infusion rate. These suggestions may be adjusted to patients with slower infusion rates.

POTASSIUM

Whole-body potassium stores are depleted in starved patients, potassium being the primary intracellular cation that tends to be lost in the urine as muscle is catabolized for gluconeogenesis. Thus, repletion of lean body mass is usually accompanied by a tremendous requirement for potassium, approximately 160 mEq/day. Its fate is varied; much enters intracellularly through repletion of protein and an anabolic state, some is lost in the urine, and some is lost in perspiration. Patients with compromised renal function will not tolerate 160 mEq of potassium, and a decreased dose is administered carefully. Potassium is generally determined twice weekly in patients who are stable. Potassium is administered as the chloride, phosphate, or acetate.

MAGNESIUM

The requirements for magnesium appear to vary with calcium and phosphorus metabolism. In patients with a normal serum phosphorus and normal bony stores of calcium, approximately 26 to 32 mEq/day of magnesium is reasonable. Magnesium is useful as a co-factor and much is taken up intracellularly. Again, patients whose renal function is impaired will have a lower requirement for magnesium than patients with normal renal function. Magnesium is administered as the sulfate.

PHOSPHATE

Hypophosphatemia is not a complication of hyperalimentation. It is a deficiency state, since most total parenteral nutrition solutions do not contain adequate phosphate. Unfortunately, numerous cases of hypophosphatemic coma occurred prior to the realization that phosphate, present in normal diets, had been omitted. The requirement for phosphate is approximately 90 to 100 mEq/24 hr; it is greater in very depleted patients. Much of this is utilized for membrane phospholipids, high-energy phosphate bonds, and perhaps some storage in the bone. Patients with renal impairment will excrete and require less phosphate than those with normal renal function. Phosphate is generally administered as the sodium or potassium salt.

CALCIUM

The requirement for calcium is approximately 10 to 20 mEq/day but may in fact be much higher. It will be increased if the patient is allowed to become hypophosphatemic or hypomagnesemic. Serum levels, of course, do not reflect total body stores, since bone contains vast calcium stores; rather, they reflect the levels of magnesium and phosphate. Calcium is administered as the chloride or gluconate.

SODIUM

One does not ordinarily think of sodium in terms of requirement. If sodium is not administered, urine excretion of water may be impaired, with resultant water retention and hyponatremia. It is currently my practice to administer approximately 100 mEq of sodium daily, even in patients in whom fluid retention is suspected and peripheral edema may be a problem. Paradoxically, the administration of sodium to these patients appears to enable them to excrete sodium along with water, and the incidence of peripheral edema and hyponatremia does not appear to be so high under these circumstances. Sodium may be administered in the form of chloride or as acetate, which will tend to counteract any metabolic acidosis in amino acid preparations.

Most patients on parenteral nutrition tend to become hypochloremic. Hypochloremia rarely becomes a problem. If there is a metabolic syndrome associated with hypochloremia, I have not recognized it. Approximately 50 to 100 mEq of chloride appears to be required. Its fate is uncertain; it may be stored in the bone or be lost in perspiration. Requirements for chloride will, of course, be increased if the patient has a large gastrostomy or nasogastric tube output; in this case, increased amounts of chloride may be given as potassium chloride or sodium chloride; both may be required.

IONIC COMPATIBILITIES

Even in patients with high and complex gastrointestinal losses, it should not be necessary to administer extra intravenous fluids to manage metabolic problems. Additives are sufficiently varied to enable management with hyperalimentation solution alone. A list of compatibilities is shown in Table 17-3.

TABLE 17-3. Allowable Additive Supplementation

Additives	Available Products	Maximum Allowable Total per Liter Bottle
Calcium	*Calcium gluconate inj. Calcium chloride inj.	9 mEq
Magnesium	Magnesium sulfate	12 mEq
Phosphate	*Sodium phosphate inj. Potassium phosphate inj.	21 mM
Potassium	*Potassium chloride inj. Potassium acetate inj.	80 mEq
Sodium	*Sodium chloride inj. Sodium acetate inj.	Patient tolerance or need
Chloride	*Sodium chloride inj. Calcium chloride inj. Potassium chloride inj.	Limited by amount of cation
	Hcl inj.	100 mEq
Acetate	*Sodium acetate inj. Potassium acetate inj.	Limited by amount of cation
Insulin	Regular insulin inj.	50 units

* With these electrolytes, unless otherwise specified on Physician's Order Form, additives supplemental to the established formulas will be added as the asterisked salt.

TRACE METALS

Knowledge about trace metals constitutes an extensive void. It is known, for example, that zinc is required in patients with severe surgical illness and that prolonged parenteral nutrition may be associated with a zinc deficiency. Estimations of zinc, while not technically difficult, are not often available, and are unreliable as a measure of total body zinc. Wound healing may be impaired in zinc deficiency.

However, there is no reason to assume that such deficiencies are limited to zinc alone. Although there are few data available on trace metals, it is perfectly clear that the administration of 2 units of plasma a week, originally recommended by Dudrick [4], is as inadequate in providing the necessary stores of trace metals as it is in providing adequate amounts of essential fatty acids. We need to know a great deal more about the effect of deficiencies of zinc and other related metals. In addition to zinc's effect on wound healing, deficiencies in trace metals may perhaps be associated with the anemia and some of the metabolic complications such as fatty liver that are seen during hyperalimentation. It appears that there soon will be commercially available mixtures of trace metals that may be administered once or twice weekly in hyperalimentation solutions. Until then, zinc as the sulfate or acetate may be given by gastrostomy or jejunostomy tube or orally; 10 ml of the 2% solution appears adequate.

ESSENTIAL FATTY ACIDS

Essential fatty acid deficiency in patients receiving prolonged parenteral nutrition was recognized as long ago as 1929 [3]. At present, however, the early lesions are difficult to recognize, but essential fatty acid deficiency probably has serious implications for the patient on prolonged parenteral nutrition. In addition to the skin lesions and anemia associated with fatty acid deficiency, it is clear that wound healing is adversely affected. Some have claimed that the correction or prevention of fatty acid deficiency prevents the fatty liver that results from parenteral nutrition and is associated with normalization of liver chemistries, but our limited experience has not proved this to be the case. However, it must be said that fatty liver and abnormal liver chemistries do not appear to have great short-term significance, i.e., the clinical picture in patients with fatty liver is not like that in patients with hepatic insufficiency.

Biochemical lesions suggesting essential fatty acid deficiency are manifested as a change in the ratio of unsaturated fatty acids and the appearance of eicosatrienoic acid in the serum, generally after 3 to 4 weeks without oral intake. Other biochemical lesions, such as failure of prostaglandin synthesis, manifest as decreased intraocular pressure, are present in a week after fat-free parenteral nutrition [8]. At 4 weeks, skin lesions begin to appear. Anecdotal reports on some patients have indicated that wound healing appears to improve with correction of essential fatty acid deficiency.

Essential fatty acid deficiency can be prevented by the administration of fat emulsions as approximately 4 to 5 percent of the caloric requirement daily, i.e., about 200 ml of 10% fat emulsion in the average patient. As an alternative, 50 gm of corn or safflower oil given daily through a gastrostomy or jejunostomy tube should be sufficient to prevent fatty acid deficiency.

VITAMINS

Although there are many data on the requirements for vitamins in normal patients, it is not clear whether or not these requirements are increased in patients who are stressed, injured, starved, or septic. There is some evidence that surgical patients require large amounts of vitamin C, and it is my practice to administer between 2 and 3 gm of vitamin C over 24 hours to such patients. A daily requirement for vitamin B appears to be easy to satisfy (see Table 17-4), and vitamin B toxicity has not been recognized. Clinical syndromes from overdosage with the fat-soluble of vitamins A and D have been recognized for some time in patients on prolonged parenteral nutrition. I have observed at least 2 cases of vitamin D toxicity and 1 case of vitamin A toxicity, the latter including eye and skin lesions and jaundice.

TABLE 17-4. Daily Vitamin Requirements[a]

Vitamin	Amount
Thiamine	5–10 mg
Riboflavin	4–5 mg
Niacin	8–20 mg
Pyridoxine	20 mg
Pantothenate	20 mg
Vitamin C	300–500 mg[b]
Vitamin A	2,500–5,000 IU
Vitamin D	400 IU
Vitamin E	10 IU

[a] This is one of several schemata for daily vitamin requirements. The exact requirements are not known, but this is a reasonable approximation.
[b] In injury and large wounds, up to 2 gm of ascorbic acid may be given. Evidence for efficacy is not well established.

With this in mind, our practice has been to give 5,000 units of vitamin A and 500 units of vitamin D on a weekly basis. This has been sufficient to prevent the appearance of clinical deficiency of these vitamins, and toxicity has not been observed. There is less knowledge about vitamin E, and the existence of a clinical vitamin E deficiency state is controversial. It is therefore appropriate to administer small amounts of vitamin E, together with the other fat-soluble vitamins. Folate, vitamin B_{12}, and vitamin K apparently are not stable within the solution, and thus we do not add them, but administer them parenterally.

MONITORING

Monitoring of a patient with hyperalimentation depends on the patient's overall stability. In patients who are stable without massive fluid requirements or shifts, it is sufficient to monitor urine glucose 4 times daily and to check sodium, potassium, chloride, bicarbonate, calcium, phosphorus, magnesium, total protein, blood urea nitrogen (BUN) and creatinine, blood sugar, ammonia, prothrombin time, and osmolality twice weekly or every 5 days. It is our practice to obtain only serum bilirubin and not serum glutaminic-oxaloacetic transaminase (SGOT) and alkaline phosphatase. Hepatic dysfunction, if it occurs, is transient, does not appear to bother the patient, and will only worry people if it is detected. Other aspects of monitoring are detailed in the standard orders (Fig. 17-3) that are included in each patient's record. More frequent determination of electrolytes and other parameters may be required by the patient's condition, especially if large amounts of fluid shifts occur or if gastrointestinal losses are high, such as in patients with fistulas or high-gastrostomy drainage.

COMPLICATIONS OF PARENTERAL NUTRITION

METABOLIC COMPLICATIONS

Significant metabolic complications that may occur include deficiency states, which are common. These include alterations in sodium, potassium, and, more commonly, magnesium and phosphorus, which are present in the normal diet in large amounts but are not thought of as being specifically required. Thus, the administration of adequate amounts of magnesium and phosphorus is of greatest importance. The requirements for sodium, potassium, and chloride will depend on the basic disease for which the patient is being treated.

HYPERGLYCEMIA

The appearance of hyperglycemia in a previously stable patient who has not been spilling glucose generally signals the onset of sepsis; the latter will usually become apparent within 12 to 18 hours. The appearance of a 4+ glucose urine in a patient whose urine was previously negative should provoke an intensive search for sources of sepsis before it assumes overwhelming proportions. Prompt treatment will result in subsidence of the tendency toward hyperglycemia.

One stage beyond the development of hyperglycemia is the symptomatic hyperosmolar nonketotic state leading to coma. This clinical syndrome, comprising fever, osmotic diuresis, obtundation, and finally death, may be recognized by the presence of large quantities of glucose in the urine and the change in the mental status of the patient, without symptoms that would suggest acidosis. Ketone bodies are not present in the blood or urine, but the blood sugar will range from 400 to 1,000 mg/100 ml. If this is not corrected, death follows rapidly. The serum sodium tends to be low if measured during the acute episode, but this is spuriously low secondary to hyperglycemia. With the correction of hyperglycemia, serum sodium will return to normal without the addition of exogenous sodium.

Therapy consists of prompt cessation of glucose infusions, administration of heroic quantities of insulin (up to 200 units intravenously every 4 hr), and administration of large volumes of glucose-free solutions. Potassium is also required.

HYPOGLYCEMIA

Hypoglycemia in patients receiving infusions of 4 liters of 23% dextrose a day is a curious metabolic complication.

Without further reflection, this would seem extremely unlikely. However, the amount of radioimmunoactive insulin present in patients receiving total parenteral nutrition is perhaps the highest seen in clinical practice. This is undoubtedly due both to glucose and to amino acid release of pancreatic insulin. It tends to occur in younger patients. When typical symptoms of hypoglycemia appear, even in the presence of steady infusions of glucose, the rate of infusion should be decreased. Although this would seem paradoxical, in practice it prevents the symptoms of hypoglycemia, and blood sugars that are usually in the range of 30 to 45 mg/100 ml of blood will rise to 55 to 65/100 ml.

HYPOMAGNESEMIA

Hypomagnesemia may be suspected clinically by complaints of tingling in the extremities and around the mouth. Agitation is also common. Serum magnesium will often be less than 0.6 mg/100 ml or undetectable. In patients with normal renal function, 26 mEq/day is generally required. However, during repletion states, particularly in patients with liver disease or with profound diarrhea, this may be exceeded. Magnesium can be replaced as the 10% sulfate in the solution or 50% sulfate in 2-ml intramuscular injections.

HYPOPHOSPHATEMIA

Hypophosphatemic coma was late in being recognized, merely because a clinical counterpart had previously not been seen often. It is not a complication of hyperalimentation per se but rather a deficiency state secondary to inadequate intravenous administration of phosphate. It is estimated that 90 mEq of phosphate is required normally. During periods of repletion, this may be exceeded. The symptomatology of hypophosphatemic coma is striking; having once observed it, one will not easily forget it. The earliest manifestations are lethargy and a slurring of speech; the patient says he has a "thick tongue." Thereafter, hypophosphatemia progresses to unconsciousness and coma. Anemia and abnormalities in phagocyte function and oxygen delivery have been attributed to hypophosphatemia.

TECHNICAL COMPLICATIONS

Complications secondary to catheter placement often occur with distressing frequency when hyperalimentation is initiated at a given institution. However, with increasing experience, the number of such complications should decrease. The most common complication in placement of internal jugular catheters is carotid artery cannulation or laceration, with secondary neck hematomas. Occasionally, respiratory obstruction may result and require urgent tracheostomy. Usually, however, an inadvertent carotid artery puncture will subside with pressure alone, except in patients with bleeding disorders.

Subclavian catheterization results in a much more interesting and varied group of complications. Technical complications may be largely avoided by keeping the needle near the horizontal plane, since the vein is most anterior. The most common complication by far is pneumothorax. Since many patients will be on the respirator when catheterized, it is my practice to take them off the respirator and hand-breathe them with a self-inflating bag, e.g., Ambu bag,* for the duration of the catheter insertion, since this will not hyperinflate the lungs to the same extent as the respirator does, and the apex of the lung remains posterior and inferior to the vein. Laceration of the subclavian artery for the most part is uncommon, and since the subclavian artery lies posterior to the subclavian vein, one will rarely strike it if the needle is kept at an angle no steeper than 15 degrees to the horizontal. Pressure above and below the clavicle will result in the cessation of hemorrhage. Another avoidable complication is administration of fluid intrathoracically, which occurs because x-ray confirmation of catheter position is imperfect. Infusion of hypertonic solutions will bring about a hydrothorax, recognizable by the development of pain, tachypnea, respiratory distress, and often shock. The chest film will confirm what has been detected by physical examination. This complication may be prevented by making certain before starting infusions that blood can be aspirated through the catheter.

Not all hydrothoraxes are secondary to catheter malposition. A rare and poorly understood complication is the development of "sympathetic effusion," in which the material infused does not enter the thoracic cavity, but a clear "sympathetic" exudate free of glucose is obtained. The reason for this complication is not known, although it may follow a mediastinal hematoma.

Many other mechanical complications have been described in the literature, covering virtually every situation imaginable, including thoracic duct fistula, bronchopleural cutaneous fistula, and superior vena cava bronchial fistula. Air embolism may be prevented at the time of insertion by having the patient perform a Valsalva maneuver as the catheter is passed. Some minimal technical complications appear to be unavoidable. Even physicians with extensive experience will occasionally cause a pneumothorax. However, the incidence can be decreased to an unavoidable minimum with experience.

SEPSIS

The most dreaded complication of parenteral nutrition is the development of bacterial or fungal sepsis. It is generally agreed that adherence to a strict protocol in the care of catheters and using catheters that are reserved only for parenteral nutrition will result in a decreased incidence of sepsis. This has been shown in our institution by a prospective study [11]. Although there are rare cases of hematogenous sepsis in patients with repeated bacteremias from other sources, by and large, most sepsis originates from the skin; this is borne out by epidemiologic studies in our institution. One cannot rely on the appearance of the catheter site; a septic catheter may appear perfectly benign.

My practice is as follows: if a fever develops in a previously afebrile pa-

* Air-Shields, Inc., Hatboro, Pa.

tient at the time when a new bottle is hung, the bottle is removed and replaced by another bottle, and the tubing is changed. If the fever does not subside within 3 to 4 hours and there is no other obvious source of fever— that is, an *obvious* source that would explain a fever of 103 to 104° F—the catheter is immediately removed following blood culture both through the catheter and of the peripheral blood; the tip is also cultured. Another catheter is not placed for an additional 24 hours, to allow the septicemia to subside.

When this protocol is followed, a large number of catheters that are ultimately shown to be sterile will be removed. However, if the line is septic, an endophlebitis will not be established, and the requirements for additional or new antibiotics or both will be minimal. It is much better to remove catheters when in doubt than to allow the development of a septic and thrombosed subclavian vein and superior vena cava.

If candidiasis develops, it is absolutely necessary not to reinstate glucose infusions until serial blood cultures have been demonstrated to be free of *Candida* organisms. It has been our experience that not all patients with blood cultures positive for *Candida* need to be treated with amphotericin B if cultures revert to negative. However, even after catheter removal and negative blood cultures for several days, *Candida* may appear in the bloodstream when hyperalimentation is resumed. If this is the case, hyperalimentation must be stopped, and the possibility of alternative means of nutrition, such as fat infusion or tube feedings, must be entertained.

The amphotericin flush technique does not appear to offer any significant advantage in the prevention of candidiasis. It results in further manipulation of the line, and in our experience, excessive manipulation of the line is by far the most frequent and common cause of sepsis. The way to prevent sepsis is to use a line that is reserved for parenteral nutrition alone and to be sure of rigid asepsis in the care of the line.

SUBCLAVIAN THROMBOSIS
The complication of subclavian thrombosis has been overlooked in the past. However, a recent study has suggested that the incidence is actually much more common than has been heretofore appreciated. In the study of Ryan et al. [11], pathologic examination of thrombosed subclavian vessels suggested that thrombosis does not necessarily originate at a point where the hypertonic glucose impinges against the vein; it appears to originate in any point where the catheter comes in contact with the vein (Fig. 17-4). Polyvinylchloride may be somewhat more reactive than the substance in the catheters being developed, which most investigators hope will be Teflon coated, Silastic-coated polyvinyl, or entirely Silastic or made of some other less reactive material.

Subclavian thrombosis may be the source of pulmonary emboli. If subclavian thrombosis occurs, the catheter should be removed immediately and

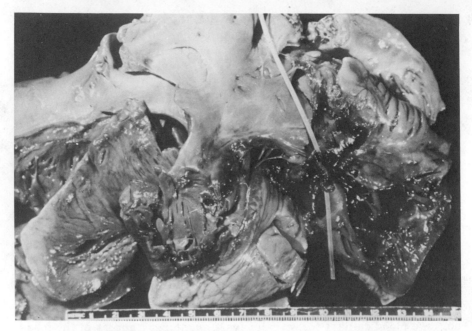

FIGURE 17-4. Pathologic specimen depicting thrombosis of subclavian vein. Note that catheter extends through thrombus and that thrombus originates from subclavian vein wall in an area of impingement but not necessarily an area where hypertonic solution runs into vein wall. This suggests that subclavian vein thrombosis, an overlooked complication, occurs because of catheter reactivity rather than because of impingement of hypertonic solution against the vein.

anticoagulation with heparin begun. If treatment is prompt, the arm swelling will usually decrease markedly, with minimal residual effect. A prominent venous pattern, however, will remain in the upper extremity and around the shoulder of the thrombosed subclavian vein. Occasionally, these will recanalize and allow the placement of another catheter. However, in our experience, this has almost never happened, and the affected side is lost for cannulation (Fig. 17-5).

SOLUTIONS FOR USE IN SPECIFIC ORGAN SYSTEM FAILURE
RENAL FAILURE
Although the use of specific solutions for organ failure is in its infancy, there has been sufficient experience with total parenteral nutrition in different disease states at our institution and others to suggest that specific diseases may require alterations in solution composition for greater efficacy. By far, the largest amount of information is available on the administration of essential amino acids and hypertonic dextrose to patients in acute renal

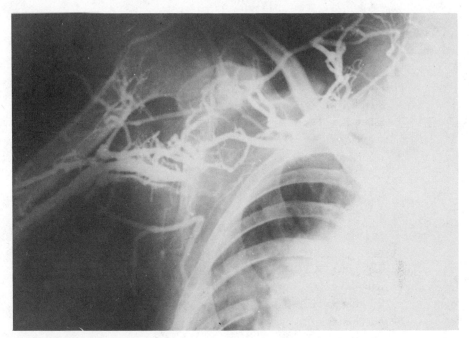

FIGURE 17-5. Venogram of vessels in shoulder area following thrombosis of sub-clavian vein. Note that there is complete obliteration of subclavian vein, which is replaced by a number of smaller vessels, none of which is suitable for cannulation.

failure. This solution, with which extensive experience has been gathered, is an intravenous modification of the Giordanno diet. Giordanno [9] had shown that in patients with chronic renal failure, positive nitrogen balance can be achieved, with lowering of the BUN and improved patient well-being, provided that essential amino acids primarily are given and that the amount of nonessential amino acids is limited. Under such circumstances, urea nitrogen, previously thought to have been an end-product in man, is split by gut bacteria to ammonia, reabsorbed, and made available for synthesis by transamination into nonessential amino acids. The combined essential and nonessential amino acids are then synthesized into protein. The entire process takes place at a lower protein intake than had been previously thought.

The first reports on the use of renal failure solution for patients who could not eat and required hyperalimentation were by Wilmore and Dudrick [13] at the University of Pennsylvania. The studies at the Massachusetts General Hospital have been carried out under the direction of Dr. Ronald Abel [1] and have had a slightly different emphasis. In our study, we have used a solution consisting of essential amino acids and 47% dextrose (Table

TABLE 17-5. Composition of 750-Ml Unit of Nephramine (Renal Failure Solution) in Use at the University of Cincinnati Medical Center*

Constituent	Amount
Essential amino acids	
L-Isoleucine	1.40 gm
L-Leucine	2.20
L-Lycine HCl	2.00
L-Methionine	2.20
L-Threonine	1.00
L Tryptophan	0.50
L-Valine	1.63
Total	13.13 gm
Vitamin content	
Thiamine HCl (B_1)	25 mg
Riboflavin (as phosphate) (B_2)	5 mg
Pyridoxine HCl (B_6)	7.5 mg
Niacinamide	50 mg
Dexpanthenol	12.5 mg
Vitamin A	5,000 USP units
Vitamin D (ergocalciferol)	500 USP units
Vitamin E (di-α-tocopheryl acetate)	2.5 IU
Ascorbic acid (vitamin C)	1.25 gm
Calories (47% dextrose)	1,400
Total nitrogen	1.46 gm
α-Amino nitrogen	1.3 gm

* This intravenous modification of the Giordanno diet is well within the tolerance of most patients, even those with oliguric or anuric renal failure.

17-5) as primary therapy for patients with acute renal failure. It was used both for the caloric sparing effect of glucose, at which there are apparently two break points, 800 and 2,200 calories, as was so well shown by Professor Henry Lee [10], and for the Giordanno effect, that is, to lower BUN. These effects have been confirmed by other investigators, and although the frequency of dialysis among our patients was not decreased, we observed a somewhat unexpected but statistically significant increase in survival, and renal failure was of shorter duration. Another beneficial effect was an improvement in the patients' ability to withstand complications. Although complications such as infection, gastrointestinal hemorrhage, and pneumonitis were not prevented, a higher patient survival followed if the complication occurred when the patient was receiving essential amino acids. A protective effect on uremic coma was observed as well.

We thus advocate the use of essential amino acids in 47% dextrose in all patients with acute tubular necrosis, either intravenously or as an elemental diet (Amin Aid*), which may be substituted for the intravenous form and which is discussed below. Since elemental diets must be started slowly, we generally start with intravenous infusion and gradually introduce the elemental diet if the patient's gastrointestinal tract is functioning.

The components of the solution are given in Table 17-5. Note that 47% dextrose is given in a small volume, so that even patients who are oliguric may receive a substantial number of calories. If there are gastrointestinal tract losses from a gastrostomy or nasogastric tube, an intake of 2,250 calories is easily achieved. The solution is started at 30 ml/hr and increased 10 ml/hr each day until a rate of 70 ml/hr is reached. Since urinary glucose is notoriously unreliable in renal failure, the blood glucose should be checked at least daily when therapy is started. Insulin is added to the bottle as necessary, since hyperglycemia tends to develop in these patients, particularly if hepatic malfunction is present. It is not clear that a rate of greater than 70 ml/hr offers any significant advantage, and the incidence of hyperglycemia increases markedly beyond this rate. Hypokalemia, hypomagnesemia, and hypophosphatemia occur regularly, and electrolytes should be checked every other day instead of twice weekly or every 5 days as with the standard solutions.

Although the use of this solution may forestall the need for dialysis, a statistically significant effect on the incidence of dialysis has not been observed in our series. If aggressive dialysis is undertaken, both essential and nonessential amino acids will be lost, and we would suggest that patients be then changed to a solution containing both essential and nonessential amino acids. This will cause a marked increase in blood urea. This type of solution is suggested only for patients who are dialyzed every other day regardless of their symptoms or blood urea nitrogen. If a more flexible schedule of dialysis can be undertaken, we suggest that the patient be given only essential amino acids and hypertonic dextrose in order to decrease the frequency of dialysis; dialysis in itself may be harmful, particularly in the elderly or in patients with unstable cardiovascular function. We have not observed more frequent sepsis or metabolic complications in patients with renal failure who receive total parenteral nutrition, perhaps because of the importance of the essential amino acids in nonspecific host resistance.

CARDIAC FAILURE
The patient with rheumatic heart disease, particularly with mitral stenosis and insufficiency, is often cachectic on the basis of long-standing anorexia

---

* McGaw Laboratories, Glendale, Calif.; division of American Hospital Supply Corporation.

and cardiac malfunction. If one adds cardiopulmonary bypass to an already nutritionally depleted patient, the complications most frequently seen (hepatic dysfunction, renal dysfunction, and respiratory insufficiency) undoubtedly have a significant nutritional component. Preliminary hyperalimentation of patients undergoing cardiopulmonary bypass may be beneficial, although this remains to be verified in prospective fashion. For such patients who frequently can tolerate only a limited fluid volume, a synthetic amino acid solution with 43% dextrose, known as Cardiac Hypercal for lack of a better name, is being utilized. This offers the advantage of a large number of calories in a small volume. Precautions in its administration are similar to those for the so-called renal failure solution. Infusion is started at 30 ml/hr and gradually increased by 10 ml/hr on a daily basis until the rate of 60 or 70 ml/hr is reached. If a patient can tolerate 1,500 ml, it is doubtful that the hypertonic glucose solution is required; and since it is not known whether or not such hypertonic solutions are well tolerated indefinitely (for example, is the incidence of subclavian thrombosis higher?), it would seem reasonable to change to a 23% dextrose solution in patients who can tolerate the volume.

Monitoring is carried out every other day as suggested with renal failure patients. The occurrence of hyperglycemia and other metabolic problems can be much more sudden in patients receiving 43% dextrose than in those receiving the 23% solution.

HEPATIC FAILURE

The patient with hepatic failure often manifests long-standing malnutrition. If one were able to replete the patient, liver regeneration might perhaps be promoted. However, the intolerance of patients with chronic liver disease to oral protein extends to a lesser extent to intravenous protein, and the administration of a large amount of intravenous protein to patients with hepatic failure will often produce hepatic encephalopathy.

Another problem is volume intolerance in the patient with ascites, edema, and excess body water. In patients with hepatic and renal insufficiency, essential amino acids have been used in the treatment of the uremic component; the amount of nitrogen administered is small. However, amino acid patterns following such infusions are grossly abnormal and suggest that the patient with severe hepatic impairment is incapable of synthesizing nonessential amino acids from the essential amino acids [5]. Furthermore, nitrogen balance is not restored. If one administers nonessential with essential amino acids, using an ammonia-free solution (i.e., Freamine), an abnormal amino acid pattern results as well and may in itself contribute to encephalopathy. A series of solutions are being investigated in our laboratory. They appear promising in animals as well as in human patients [6, 7, 12].

The patient with severe hepatic failure may tolerate 40 to 50 gm of intravenous protein in the form of synthetic amino acids, which may be helpful in bringing about clinical improvement, although definite positive nitrogen balance has not been observed. Glucose must be used as the energy source, and monitoring must be extremely careful, since there is a marked tendency for hyperglycemia and nonketotic coma to develop in patients with liver disease. Catheter insertion should be carried out with the greatest of care, since any mishap may lead to prolonged bleeding from venipuncture, and laceration of any of the large vessels around the thoracic inlet may result in death.

In spite of the dangers, parenteral nutrition in patients with chronic liver disease will be an important aspect of their therapy when a satisfactory parenteral solution is found and may be of therapeutic benefit in aiding hepatic regeneration.

THE USE OF THE GASTROINTESTINAL TRACT

Not all patients following severe trauma or in intensive care units have a paralytic or postoperative ileus, and since if parenteral nutrition were the preferred route, man would have been created with a natural subclavian catheter, the use of the gastrointestinal tract is preferable whenever possible. However, there are several theoretical objections to this route of administration. An indwelling esophageal tube in the presence of a tracheostomy cuff that may erode can result in a tracheoesophageal fistula. A Levine or feeding tube through the gastric cardia renders the cardia incompetent and may result in acid reflux, with subsequent esophageal stricture. A prolonged paralytic ileus may preclude the use of the gastrointestinal tract, as will fistulas and other intra-abdominal disasters.

STANDARD TUBE FEEDINGS

I see little advantage to starting patients on elemental diets when they will tolerate standard tube feedings. A #5 pediatric feeding tube or another small-lumen tube will not be subject to the erosion of a tracheostomy cuff and is of sufficient caliber to allow the passage of finely ground and diluted blenderized meals or tube-feeding formulas. Tube feedings should be begun slowly. My own practice is to offer 50 ml of an electrolyte solution every 2 hours on the first day and skim milk on the second day. If these are accepted, tube feedings diluted in water are begun (50 ml of tube feeding and 50 ml of water every 2 hr). These feedings should not be given in a bolus or forced in, but should be allowed to drip in slowly with a drip apparatus. The volume may then be increased until equal volumes of tube feeding and water are given (approximately 150 ml of each every 3 hr). It is unusual for patients to tolerate amounts greater than this, and gastric retention often becomes a problem if these volumes are exceeded, with vomiting and aspiration a potential hazard. Nor should tube feedings become more concentrated, since hyperosmolar, nonketotic coma with hypernatremia may result. We have tended not to use pumps, since they are inclined to immobilize patients, making them prone to other complications, such as decubiti, hypostatic pneumonia, and thrombophlebitis. Drop counters may be useful, however.

Tube feedings are much less expensive than elemental diets and are of equal caloric value. Thus, they should be used whenever possible. If prolonged tube feedings are planned, a gastrostomy or jejunostomy tube should be placed when the patient stabilizes.

ELEMENTAL DIETS

Chemically defined diets are for specialized situations and should not be used indiscriminantly. A well-balanced blenderized meal is probably more efficacious and has a better nitrogen-calorie ratio as compared with many elemental diets. Further, it may supply trace metals and X-factors, whose identity is, of course, unknown. The use of elemental diets should be reserved for patients with gastrointestinal fistulas or in whom ileus or partial obstruction precludes the administration of tube feedings. Chemically defined diets may be profitably used in the presence of renal failure when the patient is capable of oral intake (Amin-Aid*), or in patients with protein intolerance in liver disease (Hepatic-Aid*).

A profusion of chemically defined diets are available. In general, most are given by nasogastric tube using pumps, which, as noted, tend to immobilize patients. Many chemically defined diets are sufficiently palatable so that when patients are told the reason for administration, they will drink the diet over ice, overlooking the mildly objectionable taste. Osmolality is a critical factor, and a solution of 600 mM may be begun provided that 30 ml/hr is not exceeded. The patients sip material over an hour's time. The amounts are slowly increased to a maximum of 180 ml/hr, thereby providing (during waking hours) approximately 2,500 calories without the use of a nasogastric tube.

Chemically defined diets may be used in combination with parenteral hyperalimentation, since it is often approximately 10 days to 2 weeks before the patient will take calorically adequate amounts of elemental diets. Continued use of both hyperalimentation and elemental diet will enable the patient to get up to 6,000 calories without metabolic difficulty and will often result in closure of a fistula, for example, more rapidly than with either method alone.

MONITORING AND COMPLICATIONS

In addition to the previously mentioned complication of tubes, other complications of enteral feeding are basically metabolic.

---

* McGaw Laboratories, Glendale, Calif.; division of American Hospital Supply Corporation.

It is rare for hyperglycemia to result in patients given elemental diets cautiously, in reasonable amounts and with proper safeguards. However, hyperosmolality can occur due to the administered glucose and can lead to osmotic diuresis and diarrhea, which in turn may result in acidosis, hypernatremia, convulsions, and death, particularly when the diet is started suddenly and without acclimatization of the gastrointestinal tract. In summary, the chemically defined diet may have great usefulness in the presence of gastrointestinal fistulas, ileus, and bowel preparation for colonic surgery. With a slightly different amino acid composition (Amin-Aid), it can also be used in renal failure. A new branched-chain amino acid–enriched diet (Hepatic-Aid) is also available for patients with hepatic impairment with protein intolerance. Under such circumstances, if parenteral nutrition through a central catheter is not desirable, the use of elementally defined diets may be of extreme value to these patients. Since most available preparations are palatable, one can hope that such a patient will be able to receive adequate nutrition without the use of an indwelling tube or pump.

REFERENCES

1. Abel, R., et al.   Improved survival from acute renal failure after treatment with intravenous essential L-amino acids and glucose. *N. Engl. J. Med.* 288: 695, 1973.
2. Blackburn, G. L., et al.   Protein sparing therapy during periods of starvation with sepsis of trauma. *Ann. Surg.* 177:588, 1973.
3. Burr, G. O., and Burr, M. M.   A new deficiency disease produced by the rigid exclusion of fat from the diet. *J. Biol. Chem.* 82:345, 1929.
4. Dudrick, S. H., et al.   Long-term total parenteral nutrition with growth, development, and positive nitrogen balance. *Surgery* 64:137, 1968.
5. Fischer, J. E., et al.   Plasma amino acids in patients with hepatic encephalopathy. *Am. J. Surg.* 127:40, 1974.
6. Fischer, J. E., et al.   The role of plasma amino acids in hepatic encephalopathy surgery. *Surgery* 78:276, 1975.
7. Fischer, J. E., et al.   The effect of normalization of plasma amino acids on hepatic encephalopathy in man. *Surgery* 80:77, 1976.
8. Freund, H., et al.   Essential fatty acid deficiency in total parenteral nutrition. *Ann. Surg.* 190:139, 1979.
9. Giordanno, C.   Use of exogenous and endogenous urea for protein synthesis in normal and uremic subjects. *J. Lab. Clin. Med.* 62:231, 1963.
10. Hyne, B. E. B., et al.   The effect of caloric intake on nitrogen balance in chronic renal failure. *Clin. Sci.* 43:679, 1972.
11. Ryan, J. A., Jr., et al.   Catheter complications in total parenteral nutrition. *N. Engl. J. Med.* 290:757, 1974.
12. Smith, A. R., et al.   Alterations in plasma and CSF amino acids, amines, and metabolites in hepatic coma. *Ann. Surg.* 187:343, 1978.
13. Wilmore, D. W., and Dudrick, S. J.   Treatment of acute renal failure with intravenous essential L-amino acids. *Arch. Surg.* 99:669, 1969.

Harold C. Neu / # 18. ANTIMICROBIAL AGENTS AND INFECTION

Infection remains a significant problem in the management of patients within the intensive care unit (ICU). Although many of the important improvements in patient care achieved in the ICU prolong patient survival in terms of respiratory function or nutrition, they contribute significantly to the development of serious infections. Furthermore, since many patients admitted to ICUs have sustained injuries that have significantly damaged normal body defenses, they are ideal hosts for opportunistic pathogens. Therapy of infection in such patients must be directed at particular infecting organisms, with an eye to balancing the toxicity seen with use of the particular agent against its relative merits and remembering the interaction of antimicrobial agents with other pharmacologic agents being used concurrently.

INFECTING ORGANISM

In many situations it is necessary to initiate treatment before the results of cultures are available. Thus, it is important to know what agents are probable in different infections. Such knowledge must be based on consideration of the past hospital history of the patient, since in many instances the ICU patient will be admitted to the unit following a prolonged stay either in another hospital or in a different area of the same hospital. Organisms prevalent in one area of the hospital may not be those characteristically seen in another.

Knowledge of the replacement of one type of organism by another is important. For example, the patient with extensive burns is infected with *Staphylococcus aureus* or *Streptococcus pyogenes* (group A streptococcus) in the first 3 or 4 days; later, by *Pseudomonas aeruginosa* or *Proteus*. Treatment of such patients with either topical or systemic antimicrobial agents prevents these bacterial infections, but viral infections, such as herpes simplex or fungal infections with *Candida, Torulopsis,* or *Phycomycetales* may develop.

A positive culture result does not necessarily mean that the patient is infected with that particular microorganism. All patients become colonized with microorganisms within a few days of entry into the ICU. It is imperative that the physician differentiate between colonization and invasion.

This is a simple matter when considering positive blood cultures, but complex when faced with culture reports of gram-negative bacilli from tracheal suction.

DETERMINATION OF INFECTING ORGANISM BY CULTURE AND GRAM STAIN

Therapy should be initiated only after adequate attempts have been made to determine the possible etiologic agents. In each instance this will depend on pertinent clinical information regarding the suspected site of infection, type of infection, duration of infection, and antimicrobial agents previously administered.

Appropriate cultures should be obtained from all patients in whom one suspects an infection. Gram stains of secretions frequently will aid in the decision about selection of the proper antimicrobial agents. Common errors in performance of gram stains are underdecolorization due to excessive thickness of material, interpretation of precipitated stain as gram-positive cocci, or inadequate samples. The absence of leukocytes in a specimen may suggest that previous culture results indicate colonization and not infection.

Blood should be taken for culture from any patient thought to have bacteremia. Venous blood is adequate, but the technique used to obtain the culture is critical. The site must be prepared adequately, preferably with 2% iodine in 70% alcohol or an iodophor. Blood cultures should not be obtained through existing intravenous lines except when the line is to be discontinued. Blood should be cultured both aerobically and anaerobically in any appropriate system.

Sputum cultures should be obtained from coughed-up specimens. If that is impossible, they should be obtained through the use of transtracheal aspirates. In patients who have either nasotracheal, orotracheal, or tracheostomy tubes, cultures should be obtained through a suction trap. This material should be cultured immediately for both aerobic and anaerobic bacteria. Anaerobic cultures should not be performed on sputum, since it is uniformly contaminated with mouth contents that contain anaerobic flora.

Wound cultures should be placed into a suitable transport medium and immediately taken to the laboratory where they can be processed for aerobic and anaerobic bacteria. Aspiration of closed-space infections, such as would occur with a thoracentesis, paracentesis, or an abscess, provides material that can be best transported to the laboratory in a sterile syringe that has been capped with a sterile cork. By this means it is possible to obtain adequate cultures of anaerobic organisms that otherwise would die in transit to the laboratory.

Other useful techniques in making a diagnosis of infection come into play with fungal infections. Scrapings of the oral pharynx or of wound sites for fungi should include examination of the material following potassium hydroxide treatment. The presence of mycelial forms suggests invasion. Debilitated patients, particularly those who are immunosuppressed, may be infected with rare microorganisms, fungi, and parasites in a critical care area. Biopsy specimens must be adequately stained with periodic acid-Schiff and silver methenamine to reveal such microorganisms. Funguria in the absence of an indwelling urethral catheter should suggest disseminated candidiasis.

ANTIBIOTIC SUSCEPTIBILITY

The antibiotic susceptibility of organisms will be investigated routinely by the microbiology laboratory. Sensitivity determinations on organisms such as pneumococci, group A streptococci, and α-hemolytic streptococci are not necessary. The majority of laboratories determine antimicrobial sensitivity by the Kirby-Bauer method of disk testing. This technique utilizes a single antibiotic impregnated disk and provides information about the sensitivity of the particular invading organism in relation to usually obtainable concentrations of the drug. But the physician should always consider the site of the infection, since a given drug might be inadequate because of its poor penetration to that site. In many situations it is not necessary to know the actual minimal bactericidal concentration; in the treatment of sepsis, it may be helpful to have such information. This is particularly true when using aminoglycoside antibiotics or when dealing with multiresistant organisms. It is possible to obtain serum bactericidal levels; this refers to the minimal dilution of serum necessary to inhibit the infecting microorganism. A dilution of serum of 1 : 8 or higher is usually effective. The serum concentrations that may be expected following the administration of usual doses of antibiotics are given in Table 18-1.

KNOWLEDGE OF SUSCEPTIBILITY PATTERNS

It may take several days before the results of sensitivity tests are available, since they must be performed on pure cultures. It is thus useful to have knowledge of the sensitivity patterns of organisms in your particular situation. This can be obtained from your microbiology laboratory. A typical listing for our institution is given in Table 18-2. These results usually are based on organisms isolated from patients in the entire institution. It is helpful for the ICU physician to have his laboratory select the sensitivity patterns of organisms isolated in the unit. These data are particularly important in controlling problems of cross-contamination of patients in an area of high use of antibiotics, such as occurs in most ICUs. It is useful to keep a line listing of microorganisms isolated from patients in the ICU; an example is given in Table 18-3. This allows one to anticipate cross-contamination among patients and to prevent nosocomially associated outbreaks such as have occurred in intensive care areas. With certain microorganisms, it is further necessary to perform either serotyping or bacteriocin typing to determine if a particular strain is an endemic one.

TABLE 18-1. Dosage of Antibiotics to Be Used in the Treatment of Severe, Life-Threatening Infection[a]

Antibiotic	Total Daily Dose (gm)	Interval Between Doses (hr)	Serum Concentrations (μg/ml)[b]	Average Concentration (μg/ml) Needed to Inhibit Susceptible Organism[c]	
				Gram-Positive	Gram-Negative
Penicillin G	10–12 × 10^6 MU	4	4–10	0.05–0.5	0.5–8
Amikacin	15–20 mg/kg	8	15–25	0.1–1	1–10
Ampicillin	12	4	10–40	0.05–0.5	
Methicillin	12–16	4	6–10	0.3	
Oxacillin, nafcillin	8–12	4–6	5–20	0.1–0.3	
Carbenicillin	24–40	4	100–200	0.1–1.0	1–150
Cephalothin	8–12	4	10–30	0.05–1.0	1–16
Cefazolin	4–8	6	20–80	0.05–1.0	1–12
Cefamandole	4–12	6	20–70	0.1–1	1–25
Cefotaxime	2–9	6	20–70	0.1–4	0.01–6
Moxalactam	1.5–12	8–12	30–120	0.1–8	0.01–16
Cefoxitin	4–12	6	20–70	0.5–4	1–25
Erythromycin	2–4	6	5–15	0.05–1.0	
Lincomycin	4–8	6	2–20	0.5–1.0	
Clindamycin	2–5	6	2–20	0.02–1.5	
Tetracycline	2	6	2–10	0.5–1.0	0.5–3.0
Chloramphenicol	50 mg/kg	6	10–20	0.5–2.0	1–10
Kanamycin	15 mg/kg	8–12	15–30		1–10
Gentamicin	3–6 mg/kg	8	4–12		0.5–6
Tobramycin	3–6 mg/kg	8	6–10		0.5–6
Vancomycin	2	6	6–20	0.5–6.0	

[a] Based on normal renal function.   [b] Based on intermittent therapy program.
[c] Clindamycin is active against *Bacteroides*. Gentamicin and kanamycin are effective against staphylococci. Enterococci (*Strep. fecalis*) should not be considered sensitive at gram-positive concentrations.

TABLE 18-2. Antimicrobial Susceptibilities[a]

Antibiotic	Percent Susceptible																							
	α-Hemolytic Streptococci	Strep. pyogenes	Enterococci	Pneumococci	Peptostreptococcus	Staph. aureus	Staph. epidermidis	Peptococcus	Clostridium	E. coli	Klebsiella	Enterobacter	Serratia	P. mirabilis	Proteus Indole-positive	Ps. aeruginosa	Other Pseudomonas Species	Salmonella	Shigella	Acinetobacter	Hemophilus	Neisseria	Bacteroides	Listeria
Penicillin G	100	100	20	100	100	25	20	60	100													100	35	100
Ampicillin	100	100	98	100	100	25	20	60	100	75	10	15	10	90	10	0	0	75	50	20	90	100	40	100
Methicillin and oxacillin		100	5	100		95	80	75															5	
Carbenicillin	100	100		100	100	25	25	50	100	75	10	70	25	98	80	80	30	75	50	70	90	100	75	
Cephalothin	100	100	0	100	95	90	95	89	100	85	85	5	0	95	2	0	0	95	95	5	80	100	5	
Cefazolin	100	100	0	100	95	90	95	89	100	85	85	5	0	95	2	0	0	95	95	10	80	100		
Cefamandole	100	100	0	100	100	95	95	95	90	95	95	75	20	95	70	0	0	95	95	10	95	100	50	
Cefotaxime	90	100	0	100	90	95	90	90	95	100	100	95	85	100	90	50		100	100	20	95	100	40	0
Cefoxitin	100	100	0	100	100	95	95	95	90	98	98	10	50	95	85	0	20			10	95	100	90	
Erythromycin	98	98	75	100	85	94	85	80	95														25	85
Clindamycin	98	98		100	90	96	93	90	95														90	
Tetracycline	85	88		87	80	80	83	80	90														50	
Chloramphenicol	95	98	75		85	88	80	80	90									95					99	95
Streptomycin						80				70	80	85	10	90	25	5								
Kanamycin						90				90	92	95	52	98	40	5								
Gentamicin[b]						90				95	95	90	70	98	90	80	20			80				
Amikacin						90				98	98	98	98	98	95	98	90			90				
Polymyxin B or E										99	99	97	10	2	5	99	15			90				
Vancomycin	100	100	95		80	95	95	85	95														25	

[a] Agents of choice are given in Table 18-5. Normally, sensitivities of some of the gram-positive cocci are not determined. These are listed, since they are common in wound infections.
[b] Tobramycin has similar sensitivities.

Table 18-3. Sample Monthly Intensive Care Report

Diagnosis	Days Prev. Hosp.	Colonized			Infected				Type of Infection	Antibiotic Before Infection	Days Used	Days in Unit	Contributing Factors
		Resp. Tract	Wound	Urine	Resp. Tract	Wound	Urine	Blood					
Colectomy	5				Pseudomonas, Klebsiella			Candida	Acquired	Clindamycin, chloramphenicol	8,1	22	Tracheostomy, hyperalimentation
Aneurysm	0							E. coli	Acquired	None		7	Urinary catheter
Prostatectomy	6		Enterococci					Enterococci	Acquired	Kanamycin	5	3	Urinary catheter
Intestinal bypass	27	Candida						E. coli, Staph. epidermidis	Acquired	Cephalothin	10	16	IV catheter, urinary catheter

ANTIMICROBIAL AGENTS

GENERAL CONSIDERATIONS

Antimicrobial agents may be divided into groups on the basis of their mechanism of action on the bacterial or fungal microorganism. Agents interfere with (1) cell-wall biosynthesis, (2) cytoplasmic membrane function, (3) protein synthesis (either transcription or translation), (4) nucleic acid metabolism, and (5) intermediary metabolism within the microorganism. Agents may be bactericidal, killing the microorganism, or bacteriostatic, preventing continued proliferation of the microorganism only while present within the microorganism. In many situations, a bacteriostatic agent is as successful as a bactericidal agent would have been. On the other hand, the patient in the ICU, because of the nature of his particular illness or the length of his illness, may be at a special disadvantage. Phagocytic function in critically ill patients is often less effective than in healthy persons. Antibody function may be decreased secondary to the administration of other agents. The presence of foreign bodies makes eradication of infecting organisms more difficult with a bacteriostatic agent than with a bactericidal agent.

The mechanisms of action of currently available antimicrobial agents are given in Table 18-4.

It is frequently stated that bactericidal and bacteriostatic agents should not be used together. This proscription applies to a well-defined infection caused by a single agent, for example, pneumococcal meningitis. Mixed infections, such as those in abdominal wounds, abscesses of the liver, and so on, have been effectively treated with combinations of penicillin and chloramphenicol, or clindamycin and gentamicin. The reason for the success in such situations is that each agent treats a specific problem. Nonetheless, a single agent should be used whenever possible. Table 18-5 lists the agents of choice in serious infections requiring intravenous therapy.

The indications for the use of more than one antimicrobial agent are as follows:

1. In the prompt treatment of desperately ill patients when it is impossible to determine precisely which pathogen is the most probable infecting agent.
2. In mixed infections.
3. To delay the emergence of microbial mutants resistant to one drug, such as may occur in chronic infections.
4. To achieve true bacterial synergism.

The disadvantages of antibiotic combinations are that they lead to a false sense of security, decrease efforts toward specific diagnosis of the infecting agent, and pose a greater risk of side-effects and superinfection with drug-resistant bacteria or fungi than does a single agent.

Once the etiologic agent is known, it is wise to discontinue the agents that are not necessary. The old clinical maxim that one should continue

TABLE 18-4. Mechanisms of Action of Antimicrobial Agents

Antimicrobial Agent	Site of Action	Mode of Action
Penicillins	Cell wall	Bactericidal
Cephalosporins	Cell wall	Bactericidal
Bacitracin	Cell wall	Bactericidal
Vancomycin	Cell wall	Bactericidal
Aminoglycosides (streptomycin, neomycin, kanamycin, gentamicin)	Protein synthesis, ribosomes	Bactericidal
Polymyxins	Cytoplasmic membrane	Bactericidal
Tetracyclines	Protein synthesis, ribosomes	Bacteriostatic
Chloramphenicol	Protein synthesis, ribosomes	Bacteriostatic
Erythromycin	Protein synthesis, ribosomes	Bacteriostatic
Lincomycins	Protein synthesis, ribosomes	Bacteriostatic
Rifampin	Protein synthesis, RNA polymerase	Either bactericidal or bacteriostatic
Sulfonamides	Competition PABA	Bacteriostatic
Trimethoprim	Dihydrofolate reductases	Bacteriostatic
Nystatin	Cytoplasmic membrane	Either bactericidal or bacteriostatic
Amphotericin	Cytoplasmic membrane	Bactericidal

therapy that is working does not always apply. If a single agent will control the situation, that agent should be used, and the use of the other agent or agents also started as presumptive therapy should be discontinued.

PHARMACOLOGIC CONSIDERATIONS

The physician has available a vast array of antimicrobial agents. The following comments are to alert the physician to specific problems that should be considered in the choice of an antimicrobial agent.

The patient's age should be considered. Renal excretion is decreased in the neonate and in elderly patients who have diminished filtration rates. Utilization of only the blood urea nitrogen (BUN) may be misleading. Total body size in terms of distribution of the drug in lipid may be important. Body size is a particular consideration in the patient whose body mass may have decreased significantly. Genetic defects are important in the metabolism of certain compounds, for example, glucose 6-phosphate dehy-

TABLE 18-5. Antibiotics to Use in Serious Infections Requiring Intravenous Therapy*

Antibiotic	α-Hemolytic Streptococci	Streptococci Groups A, B, C	Strep. fecalis (enterococci)	Pneumococci	Staph. aureus (penicillinase-neg)	Staph. aureus (penicillinase-pos.)	Hemophilus	N. meningitidis	E. coli	E. coli (hosp.-acquired)	Klebsiella	Klebsiella (hosp.-acquired)	Enterobacter cloacae	Enterobacter aerogenes	Serratia	Citrobacter	P. mirabilis	Proteus, Indole-Positive	Pseudomonas	Acinetobacter	Salmonella	Clostridium	Candida	Bacteroides
Penicillin G	1	1	1	1			1	1														1		
Ampicillin	1	1	1	1			1	1	1								1				1	1		
Methicillin					1	1																		
Oxacillin and nafcillin					1	1																		
Carbenicillin, ticarcillin													1					1	1	2				2
Cephalothin	2	2		2	2	2	3	3	1	1	1	2					2							
Cefazolin	2	2		2	2	2	3	3	1	1	1	2					2					2		
Cefotaxime	2	2		2	2	2	1	2	1	1	1	1	2				1	1						
Moxalactam						3	1		1	1	1	1	1	1	2		1	1	3	3		2		3
Cefoxitin									1	1	1		1	1	1	1	1	2	2			3		2
Erythromycin	3	3		3	3	3		3																
Clindamycin	3	3		3	3	3																		1
Tetracycline HCl							3		3		3											2		
Chloramphenicol							2	2														3		1
Amikacin									1	1	1	1	1	1	1	1	3	1	1	1	1			
Gentamicin, tobramycin									1	1	1	1	1	1	1	1	3	1	1	1				
Vancomycin			2			3																		
Amphotericin																							1	

* Where more than one agent is listed, either could be used, although circumstances might make one drug preferable. Therapy should be changed to the least toxic agent as soon as susceptibilities are known.

Note: 1 = first choice; 2 = second choice; 3 = third choice.

drogenase (G-6-PD) deficiency. Concurrent disease, allergy, and the type of microbial flora that the physician hopes to retain to prevent superinfection must also be considered.

It is important to realize that fever may not necessarily be due to infection and that the etiology of the slightly elevated temperature will not be solved by the addition of new or more potent antimicrobial agents. Finally, therapy may fail if an improper dose of antibiotic is used. This occurs when considerations of distribution of the agent have not been made prior to therapy. Most important, however, therapy may fail because of failure to use measures such as the drainage of an unsuspected abscess or because a new nosocomial infection has developed.

The agents that will be discussed will be those ordinarily used in an ICU. A number of preparations that produce blood levels inadequate for serious infections will not be mentioned. Oral therapy may be used if that is the only method available for administration of a particular compound, or if it is clear that the patient has normal gastrointestinal absorption. Patients in a cardiac ICU may be able to take oral therapy, but the majority of patients in either a medical or a surgical ICU will not be. In the presence of hypotension or alterations of normal blood flow, drugs should be administered intravenously. Administration of drugs intravenously demands careful attention to the half-life and period of time during which serum concentrations will be adequate. Although it is possible to treat a patient with pneumococcal pneumonia with an injection of 300,000 units of procaine penicillin twice a day, such patients must have normal host defenses. Such a situation does not occur in the patient who has hypogammaglobulinemia or decreased phagocytic ability and will not be able to utilize these defenses to halt microorganism growth during the periods when antibiotic levels are low. Attention must also be given to other agents being used (Table 18-6).

PENICILLINS

PENICILLIN G (BENZYLPENICILLIN)

SPECTRUM. Penicillin G is effective against most gram-positive cocci, including anaerobic streptococci, *Neisseria, Hemophilus,* and *Proteus mirabilis,* but not against staphylococci that produce β-lactamase (penicillinase). Penicillin G is less active than ampicillin against gram-negative microorganisms.

PREPARATIONS, DOSAGE, AND ADMINISTRATION. Penicillin is available as a crystalline aqueous solution, Na or K salts, procaine suspension, and benzathine salt. Intramuscular (IM) injections of crystalline penicillin G produce peak blood levels of 1 to 2 units/ml for each 1 million units/day; a single IM injection of procaine penicillin produces peak levels in the range of 0.75 unit/ml or less. Procaine penicillin provides moderate levels for periods of 12 to 24 hours; crystalline penicillin is almost totally removed from the

TABLE 18-6. Drug Interactions

Type of Interaction and Antibiotic	Affected or Displaced by—	Effect
SERUM CARRIER DISPLACEMENT		
Sulfonamides	Tolbutamide	Hypoglycemia
	Bishydroxycoumarin	Bleeding
	Warfarin	Bleeding
	Bilirubin	Kernicterus
INTERACTION AT TISSUE SITE		
Polymyxins	Curare	Apnea
Aminoglycosides (kanamycin, neomycin, gentamicin)	Succinylcholine	
Aminoglycosides	Polymyxins	Nephrotoxicity
Aminoglycosides	Ethacrynic acid, furosemide	Ototoxicity
Cephaloridine	Furosemide	Nephrotoxicity
COMPETITION FOR BINDING SITES		
Sulfonamides, chloramphenicol	Tolbutamide, chlorpropamide	Hypoglycemia
Sulfonamides, chloramphenicol	Bishydroxycoumarin	Increased anti-coagulation
Chloramphenicol	Bilirubin	Jaundice of the newborn
Isoniazid	Rifampin	Liver toxicity
Isoniazid	Phenytoin	Neurotoxicity

body in 3 to 4 hours. Increasing the individual dosage of procaine penicillin G above 600,000 units prolongs the duration of plasma level but does little to increase peak plasma levels. Probenecid administered prior to a dose of penicillin will increase the blood levels 1½ times and prolong excretion.

Penicillin G is widely but unevenly distributed, with high concentrations in the kidney, blood, liver, bile, and intestine and low concentrations in the brain, bone marrow, and muscle. Penetration into wounds is good if the wound area is well vascularized, but it is poor into avascular areas. Inflammation normally enhances the movement of penicillin into areas such as the spinal fluid, joint spaces, and peritoneum. Penicillin normally is not destroyed in the body but is excreted by active proximal tubular secretion. It can be destroyed in abscesses.

It is still uncertain whether or not intermittent therapy is to be preferred to sustained blood levels. We recommend that penicillin G be administered intravenously (IV) over a 30-minute period every 4 hours, providing adequate peak and trough levels.

USE. Penicillin G is used for pneumococcal and streptococcal infections and uncomplicated aspiration pneumonia.

TOXICITY. Penicillins are the least toxic antimicrobial agents. Allergic responses occur in 5 to 10 percent of patients but are exceedingly rare in very young children. Reactions may be immediate or delayed. Anaphylaxis is the most severe and the most uncommon reaction, composing only 0.1 percent of immediate reactions. Before administering penicillin, always question a patient about a history of reaction to penicillin or penicillin analogs. If the patient had a delayed reaction, which is the case in approximately 95 percent of instances, penicillin can be administered if the situation is life-threatening, since anaphylaxis is exceedingly rare in these situations. If the patient had an immediate anaphylactic reaction, penicillin should never be administered. Skin tests with penicillin G are unreliable. Skin testing with benzylpenicilloyl-polylysine and penicilloic acid is useful. Treatment of penicillin allergy with penicillinase is to be condemned; it is ineffective and may sensitize the patient to this foreign protein. The other side-effects are uncommon. They include (1) myoclonic seizures, seen only with very high doses, particularly in patients receiving probenecid who have reduced renal function, and (2) interstitial nephritis, a rare complication heralded by fever, oliguria, decreased renal function, and eosinophilia.

AMPICILLIN

SPECTRUM. Ampicillin, a semisynthetic penicillin, is active against the same organisms as is penicillin G, but it is more effective against enterococci, *Escherichia coli. Proteus mirabilis, Salmonella,* and *Shigella. Enterobacter,* and *Serratia* are resistant, as are the penicillinase-producing staphylococci.

ADMINISTRATION, DOSAGE, AND PROPERTIES. Ampicillin is available in oral, IM, and IV forms. In the ICU, oral treatment should be avoided. The body distribution is similar to that of penicillin G. In the presence of obstruction of the common or cystic duct, ampicillin levels in the gallbladder and bile are markedly decreased.

TOXICITY. The toxic effects of ampicillin are similar to those seen with penicillin G. The precautions are also the same. Rash unrelated to penicillin allergy occurs twice as frequently with ampicillin as with penicillin; the mechanism of the rash is unknown. Superinfections with resistant gram-negative organisms, such as *Klebsiella,* occur more frequently than with narrower spectrum penicillins.

USE. Ampicillin is used in the treatment of *P. mirabilis* infections, infections due to enterococci, selected sensitive biliary tract infections, and selected urinary tract infections. A significant proportion—40 percent of hospital-acquired *E. coli* infections—will be ampicillin-resistant. In view of the number of resistant bacteria, it should rarely be the agent of initial therapy in the ICU patient.

CARBENICILLIN

SPECTRUM. Carbenicillin has gram-positive activity similar to that of penicillin G and ampicillin. It is less effective against enterococci than is ampicillin but more effective against anaerobic microorganisms. It is active against many *Pseudomonas aeruginosa*, *Enterobacter*, indole-positive *Proteus* (*P. vulgaris*, *M. morganii*, *P. rettgeri*), and selected *Serratia* strains. *Klebsiella* organisms are uniformly resistant, and the compound is inactivated by staphylococcal penicillinase. The inhibitory concentrations required to kill *Pseudomonas* are high, necessitating administration of a large amount of the drug. Most *Bacteroides* organisms are killed by these high concentrations.

PREPARATIONS, DOSAGE, AND ADMINISTRATION. The compound is available in IM and IV forms. IM usage is only for patients with moderate infections. The current program of administration of carbenicillin is 4 to 5 gm administered over a ½- to 1-hour period every 4 hours. Children below age 12 can be treated with doses of 400 to 500 mg/kg/24 hr, administered in a similar fashion. Blood levels can be further raised by the concomitant administration of 0.5 gm of probenecid given ½ to 1 hour before a dose of carbenicillin.

Carbenicillin shows the wide general body distribution of other penicillins, but carbenicillin's excretion by the kidney is altered in the presence of decreased renal function or decreased hepatic function. The normal half-life is 1 hour, which increases to 15 hours in the presence of anuria and hepatic dysfunction further increases the T ½ to 30 hours.

TOXICITY. The toxicity is similar to that of other penicillins in terms of hypersensitivity reactions. It is a disodium salt (4.7 mEq Na/gm), and sodium intake must be monitered to avoid congestive failure. Administration of doses in the range of 24 to 40 gm occasionally results in severe hypokalemia. Bleeding disorders have occurred that appear to be due to platelet dysfunction.

USE. Therapeutic indications for the use of carbenicillin are in patients with sepsis due to *Pseudomonas*, *Proteus*, or *Enterobacter*, especially patients with granulocyte counts below 1,000. It is also useful in aspiration pneumonia which has developed in the hospital and in certain *Bacteroides* infections.

TICARCILLIN

SPECTRUM. Ticarcillin has in vitro activity similar to carbenicillin, but is twice as active against *Pseudomonas aeruginosa*. It can be used interchangeably with carbenicillin.

DOSAGE. Ticarcillin is available in IM and IV forms. IM usage is only for urinary infections. The usual dosage is 3 gm administered over ½ to 1 hour every 4 hours. Doses of 300 to 500 mg/kg/24 hr have been used. The drug accumulates in the presence of renal failure, and dose adjustments should be made. Further adjustment is required if the drug is given to an individual with combined renal and hepatic failure.

TOXICITY. The toxicity of ticarcillin is similar to that of carbenicillin. Sodium and potassium levels must be monitored.

USE. Therapeutic use of ticarcillin is to treat susceptible infections due to *Pseudomonas, Proteus,* or *Enterobacter*. It may be beneficial in treatment of hospital-acquired pneumonitis due to a mixed aerobic-anaerobic flora. It has also been shown to be effective therapy for abdominal or gynecologic infections due to mixed flora, but in this situation it should be combined with an aminoglycoside.

OTHER ANTIPSEUDOMONAS PENICILLINS

Azlocillin, mezlocillin, and piperacillin are available in other countries and may become available in the United States when this volume is in use. The agents are more active in vitro against *Pseudomonas* than is carbenicillin. Mezlocillin and piperacillin also inhibit many strains of *Klebsiella pneumoniae* resistant to carbenicillin.

The pharmacologic properties of the compounds are more like those of ampicillin than of carbenicillin. They accumulate to only a small degree in the presence of renal failure. Normal half-life of the agents is 1 hour. They are administered in IV doses of 200 to 300 mg/kg/day as divided doses every 4 to 6 hours. There is as yet no data to establish that these agents are clinically more effective than the older agents.

ANTISTAPHYLOCOCCAL PENICILLINS

METHICILLIN

SPECTRUM. Methicillin is active against staphylococci that are resistant to penicillin G and produce penicillinase. It should be used only for the treatment of staphylococcal infection, since it is inferior to penicillin G against other gram-positive microorganisms. Methicillin-resistant staphylococci are uncommon in the United States, although they are a problem in some intensive care units. Such staphylococci are resistant to all other semisynthetic penicillins and to the cephalosporins as well.

DOSAGE. Methicillin should be administered IV in doses of 2 to 3 gm every 4 hours (12 gm or more per day in severe infections); in children, at a dose of 150 to 300 mg/kg/day. Methicillin is relatively unstable in acid solutions and should be prepared just prior to use. It is less protein-bound than all other antistaphylococcal semisynthetic penicillins. This may be important in occasional closed-space infections.

TOXICITY. The toxic reactions seen with methicillin are similar to those seen with penicillin G. Interstitial nephritis, however, heralded by fever, oliguria, nitrogen retention, and eosinophilia, appears more frequently than with penicillin G.

OXACILLIN

SPECTRUM AND DOSAGE. Oxacillin has an antibacterial spectrum similar to that of methicillin, is more active on a weight basis, and is more highly bound to serum proteins (94%). Although oxacillin is available as an oral preparation, it should be used IM or IV as a 1- to 2-gm dose every 4 to 6 hours, for a total dosage of 6 to 12 gm/day; in children, the dosage is 100 to 250 mg/kg/day.

TOXICITY. The side-effects of oxacillin are similar to those seen with penicillin in terms of hypersensitivity reactions. Renal toxicity and hepatic toxicity have also been seen. Oxacillin should be considered as the parenteral penicillin to use when staphylococci are suspected as possible etiologic agents, since most hospital-acquired and nonhospital-acquired staphylococci currently are resistant to penicillin G.

NAFCILLIN

Nafcillin has a spectrum similar to that of oxacillin and is slightly more effective against streptococci and pneumococci. Oral absorption is erratic, but good blood levels can be achieved and maintained with IM or IV administration. The daily dosage is 0.5 to 2.0 gm every 4 to 6 hours. Since nafcillin has a significant biliary excretion, it may be useful in the treatment of staphylococcal biliary and hepatic infections. Its toxic effects are the same as those of other penicillins.

ORAL THERAPY WITH SEMISYNTHETIC PENICILLINS

Either cloxacillin or dicloxacillin should be used for oral therapy with semisynthetic penicillins, since their absorption is superior to that of the other agents available. Dosage is in the range of 0.5 to 1.0 gm every 6 hours in the adult and 50 to 100 mg/kg/day in children, preferably 30 to 60 minutes before meals. Since the absorptive states of patients in ICUs may be erratic, it may be unwise to utilize these agents with critically ill patients. Dicloxacillin is currently available as an IM preparation, but in this form it has no more merit than oxacillin or nafcillin.

CEPHALOSPORINS
Cephalothin
SPECTRUM. Cephalothin is active against many gram-positive cocci and penicillinase-producing staphylococci but less active than ampicillin against enterococci, anaerobic coccal organisms, and *Hemophilus influenzae*. It is active against many strains of *E. coli, P. mirabilis,* and *Klebsiella* but inactive against *Enterobacter*, which frequently are seen as colonizers in patients being treated with cephalothin. Cephalothin is inactive against all *Pseudomonas* and *Bacteroides* species. Staphylococci resistant to methicillin are resistant to cephalosporins.

ADMINISTRATION, DOSAGE, AND PROPERTIES. For all practical purposes, cephalothin can be administered only IV; IM administration is too painful. The normal dosage is 1 to 2 gm every 4 to 6 hours in adults and 40 to 100 mg/kg/day in children. The solution should be dissolved in 100 ml of 5% D/W and administered over a 30-minute period. Neutralization of the solution with bicarbonate may decrease the incidence of phlebitis as a side-effect.

Cephalothin is rapidly excreted by the kidney tubular mechanism, and has a half-life of ½ hour. About a third is converted to a desacetylcephalothin in the liver, and this compound is one-half to one-eighth as effective as the parent compound. The distribution is wide, but biliary levels can be low, and cerebrospinal fluid distribution is poor.

TOXICITY. Allergy to the cephalosporins is exceedingly uncommon. Cross-allergenicity between the cephalosporins and penicillins occurs in less than 5 percent of patients. The majority of patients allergic to penicillin can tolerate cephalosporins. Individual allergy to cephalosporins can develop in the absence of allergy to penicillin. Superinfection with resistant gram-negative bacilli, such as *Pseudomonas* and *Enterobacter*, is a complication of long-term therapy with this agent. Patients frequently have a positive direct and indirect Coombs' test result, but true hemolytic anemia is rare. False-positive reactions for glucose are seen in the urine because of the reducing abilities of the compound. Phlebitis is common.

USE. Cephalothin is an alternative to penicillin in the penicillin-allergic person. It is particularly useful in the treatment of staphylococcal, ampicillin-resistant *E. coli,* and *Klebsiella* infections.

Cephapirin Sodium
Cephapirin sodium has an antibacterial spectrum similar to that of cephalothin and a half-life of ½ hour. The blood levels produced by IM or IV use of the agent are similar to those achieved with cephalothin. It can be used interchangeably with cephalothin.

CEPHRADINE

Cephradine (Velosef) has an antibacterial spectrum similar to the other cephalosporins. Blood levels achieved after IM or IV use are similar to those achieved with cephalothin and cephapirin. Cephradine is excreted unchanged in the urine. Probenecid slows tubular excretion and increases serum concentrations. The compound is also available as an oral preparation that is equivalent to cephalexin in antimicrobial activity and pharmacologic properties. The side-effects of cephradine are similar to those that follow use of any of the other cephalosporins.

CEPHALEXIN

The antibacterial spectrum of cephalexin (Keflex) is similar to that of cephalothin, with lower activity against staphylococcal strains. Cephalexin is administered orally in a dose of 0.25 to 1.0 gm every 6 hours. Absorption is considerably impaired if given after a meal. Indications for the use of cephalexin are urinary tract infections with organisms not susceptible to other agents, or for gram-positive coccal infections in patients allergic to penicillin. It should not be considered a first-line drug in the patient in the ICU. Indeed, following treatment with cephalothin or cefazolin, the physician, prior to embarking on a follow-up course of cephalexin therapy, should determine whether or not the patient truly needs further chemotherapy. This is particularly important to avoid the development of cephalosporin-resistant gram-negative organisms in the unit.

CEFAMANDOLE

SPECTRUM. Cefamandole inhibits gram-positive bacteria at concentrations similar to those required for cephalothin. It is β-lactamase stable, and inhibits many *E. coli* and *Klebsiella* resistant to cephalothin and cefazolin. It also inhibits many *Enterobacters*. It is not active against *Bacteroides fragilis* nor *Pseudomonas*.

DOSAGE. Cefamandole may be administered by the IM or IV route every 4 or 6 hours at doses of 0.5 to 2 gm. Blood levels are higher than those achieved with a comparable dose of cephalothin. It produces high biliary levels. Cefamandole accumulates in the presence of renal failure and is removed by dialysis. Its toxicities are similar to those of the other cephalosporins. The precise role of this agent in the ICU patient is not established.

CEFOXITIN

SPECTRUM. Cefoxitin is a cephamycin which is β-lactamase stable. It is less active than older cephalosporins against staphylococci with concentrations of up to 4 μg/ml needed to inhibit some isolates. It inhibits most cephalothin-resistant *E. coli*, *Klebsiella*, and *Proteus*, but not *Enterobacter*. It also inhibits indole-positive *Proteus* and some *Serratia*. It inhibits most *B. fragilis*, but not *Pseudomonas*.

DOSAGE. Cefoxitin is best given intravenously in doses of 1 to 2 gm every 4 to 6 hours. It has a slightly longer half-life than cephalothin. Like other β-lactam compounds, it is cleared by renal excretion. It is not metabolized. In the presence of renal failure it accumulates, and dosage adjustments must be made.

USE. Cefoxitin has been shown to be excellent therapy for pulmonary, abdominal, and pelvic infections due to mixed bacteria. It is an alternative to the combination of an aminoglycoside and clindamycin or chloramphenicol provided Pseudomonas is not involved. When Pseudomonas is present, it should be combined with an aminoglycoside. There is no evidence that there is increased toxicity when it is used with aminoglycosides.

CEFOTAXIME

SPECTRUM. Cefotaxime is an iminomethoxy aminothiazolyl cephalosporin which is β-lactamase stable. It is less active than older cephalosporins against staphylococci with up to 4 μg/ml needed to inhibit some isolates, but is as active as penicillin G against Streptococcus pyogenes and S. pneumoniae. It is the most active agent against Escherichia coli, Klebsiella and Proteus, inhibiting most strains at concentrations below 0.25 μg/ml. Indeed it inhibits Enterobacters, Citrobacters, Morganella and indole-positive Proteus, including bacteria resistant to cefamandole, cefoxitin and gentamicin. It also inhibits many Serratia, some Pseudomonas and some Bacteroides at high concentrations, 16–32 μg/ml.

ADMINISTRATION, DOSAGE, AND PROPERTIES

Cefotaxime is given intramuscularly or intravenously in dosages of 0.5 gm to 1 gm every 6 to 8 hours, but it can be given in doses up to 9 to 12 gm per day. It is metabolized but the metabolite, desacetylcefotaxime, is also more active than older antibiotics. The metabolite does not inhibit Pseudomonas nor Morganella. It does not accumulate in renal failure although the metabolite does.

USE

Cefotaxime can be used in pulmonary, abdominal and pelvic infections. It is an alternative to aminoglycoside therapy. It can enter the CSF and may be useful in selected cases of gram-negative meningitis.

MOXALACTAM

SPECTRUM. This agent is an oxa cephem with an extremely broad range of antibacterial activity. It is less active against pneumococci and staphylococci than older cephalosporins. But it inhibits β-lactamase producing E. coli, Klebsiella and Proteus at concentrations below 0.5 μgm/ml. It also inhibits Bacteroides and Pseudomonas at concentrations of 8 to 32 μgm/ml.

ADMINISTRATION, DOSAGE, AND PROPERTIES
Moxalactam can be used in a wide dosage range from 250 mg twice daily to 9 gm per day in four divided doses. It has a longer half-life (2 hours) than older agents. Urine levels are high as are biliary levels. It also enters the CSF.

USE
This is a broad spectrum agent which can be used in life-threatening infections of a pulmonary or abdominal nature since it covers such a wide range of bacteria. It can be used for meningitis and ventriculitis caused by *E. coli* and *Klebsiella*. It can cause antabuse reactions if a patient drinks alcohol up to 48 hours after receiving the agent, and it also can cause prolongation of prothrombin time and bleeding. Thus prothrombin levels should be checked. The drug accumulates in renal failure and dosage adjustments are necessary.

CEFOPERAZONE
SPECTRUM. Most gram-positive and negative bacteria including *Pseudomonas* are inhibited. It is not as β-lactamase stable as cefotaxime and moxalactam so there are resistant *E. coli*, *Klebsiella* and *Bacteroides*.

ADMINISTRATION, DOSAGE, AND PROPERTIES
Cefoperazone has a 2 hour half-life so the usual dose is 2 gm every 12 hours although in very serious situations the dosage can increase to 2 gm every 8 hours. The drug is excreted in the bile, only 25% is in the urine and it does not accumulate in the presence of renal failure. In the presence of biliary obstruction, it is excreted by the kidney.

USE
Pulmonary, abdominal and gynecologic infections due to susceptible organisms.

CEFTIZOXIME, CEFTRIAXONE, CEFTAZIDIME, CEFMENOXIME
Ceftizoxime, ceftriaxone, ceftazidime, and cefmenoxime are broad spectrum aminothiazolyl cephalosporins which will become available in the next few years. They are β-lactamase stable and have certain differences in antibacterial spectrum and pharmacology from the aforementioned agents. None of these agents nor the aforementioned inhibit enterococci, *Streptococcus faecalis*.

VANCOMYCIN
Vancomycin is a bactericidal (cell-wall action) antibiotic effective against most gram-positive but not against gram-negative bacteria. It is useful in the patient who is allergic to both penicillins and cephalosporins.

ADMINISTRATION, DOSAGE, AND PROPERTIES

Vancomycin is not absorbed from the gastrointestinal tract but is active there. It is administered by the IV route. Its half-life is 6 hours, with 80 percent excreted by the kidney. It poorly enters the bile and cerebrospinal fluid. The normal dose in an adult is 0.5 gm every 6 hours (some use 1 gm administered every 12 hr), which must be adjusted in renal failure (Table 18-7). The dosage for children is not well established but is usually 20 to 40 mg/kg/day in 2 doses.

TOXICITY

Phlebitis is the most common side-effect, followed in frequency by rash, chills, and fever. The most serious side-effect is deafness, which occurs with excess doses or if the dose is not adjusted in the presence of decreased renal function.

USE

Vancomycin may be used in the treatment of enterocolitis due to *Clostridium difficile* by administering 125 mg orally every 6 hours. It is the drug of choice in the treatment of serious staphylococcal or streptococcal infections in patients allergic to penicillin and cephalothin.

ERYTHROMYCIN

SPECTRUM. Erythromycin is a bacteriostatic agent which inhibits most gram-positive cocci such as streptococci, staphylococci, mycoplasma, *Chlamydia*, and *Legionella pneumophilia*. It also inhibits oral anaerobic species and intestinal anaerobes such as *Bacteroides* at higher concentrations.

ADMINISTRATION, DOSAGE, AND PROPERTIES

Although erythromycin is used primarily as an oral agent, it can be used intravenously at doses of 1 to 2 gm per day in four divided doses. It does not accumulate in renal failure and has no major toxicities. It does produce phlebitis.

USE

Erythromycin is used to treat aspiration pneumonitis in some patients. It is the drug of choice to treat Legionnaires' pneumonia. It is useful as an oral agent in preparation for colon surgery.

TETRACYCLINES
SPECTRUM

The tetracyclines may be discussed as a group since antimicrobial activity is very similar. They are active against many gram-positive and gram-negative bacteria, rickettsiae, and *Mycoplasma*. Hospital-acquired staphylococci often are resistant to tetracyclines, as are some group A β-hemolytic streptococci. Many anaerobic cocci, particularly *Bacteroides fragilis*, are resistant to the tetracyclines.

ADMINISTRATION, DOSAGE, AND PROPERTIES

The tetracyclines may be administered orally, IM, or IV, but the IM route is not desirable. Tetracycline HCl, oxytetracycline, and chlortetracycline can be administered orally in a dosage of 250 to 500 mg every 6 hours to patients with normal renal function, or in a 500-mg dose every 12 hours through a slow IV drip. Minocycline is given in an initial dose of 200 mg, followed by 100 mg every 12 hours. Doxycycline is given in 3 initial doses of 100 mg every 12 hours. Then, 100 mg is given daily. Intravenous tetracycline should not be used in a dosage greater than 2 gm/day at any one time. Doxycycline or minocycline can be administered at 100 mg over 1 to 4 hours every 12 hours. The tetracyclines are widely distributed in the body including bone, liver, and nervous system.

TOXICITY

Minor toxic side-effects with tetracyclines are nausea, vomiting, upper gastrointestinal tract distress, rash, and thrombophlebitis. Superinfection with fungal organisms or with drug-resistant bacteria are more important side-effects. In addition, plasma prothrombin activity may be depressed, so that patients receiving anticoagulants may require lower doses. All the tetracyclines, with the exception of doxycycline, accumulate in the presence of decreased renal function (Table 18-7). Of the tetracyclines, only doxycycline should be used if renal function is abnormal.

Since the administration of tetracyclines results in increased urinary losses of nitrogen and sodium, their use must be considered carefully in a patient with significant metabolic problems, such as the severely injured patient who has remained for a long period in an ICU.

USE

The tetracyclines do not have a major use in the intensive care patient except in those with biliary tract disease caused by susceptible organisms. Doxycyline may be of value in treatment of some anaerobic infections.

CHLORAMPHENICOL

SPECTRUM

Chloramphenicol is active against many gram-positive and gram-negative bacteria, particularly anaerobes, including *B. fragilis.* Some *Salmonella typhosa* strains are resistant. The resistance of staphylococci is dependent on the extent to which the agent is used in a particular locale.

ADMINISTRATION, DOSAGE, AND PROPERTIES

Chloramphenicol is well absorbed orally, but not by IM injection. The oral dosage is 0.5 to 1.0 gm every 6 hours for an adult or 50 to 100 mg/kg/day in 4 divided doses for a child. The IV dosage of chloramphenicol is identical; usually 3 to 4 gm/day is administered to seriously ill patients. Each dose may be administered in 50 ml of solution over a 15-minute period. Vitamin preparations should not be in the same bottle. Chloramphenicol is

TABLE 18-7. Use of Antibiotics in Renal and Hepatic Disease

Antibiotic	Removed from Body by—	Serum Half-Life (hr)		Toxicity in Uremia	Intervals Between Doses with Various Creatinine Clearances			Dose Altered by Dialysis			Dose in Hepatic Failure
		Normal	Oliguria		Normal (100 ml)	Renal Failure		Hemo-dialysis	Peritoneal	Added to Dialysate	
						Moderate (24–40 ml)	Severe (<10 ml)				
Penicillin	K-T	0.5	2–4	CNS	4 hr	NC	1×10^6 MU/6 hr	1×10^6 MU/6 hr	No		NC
Amikacin	K	2	50	Renal, ear	2 hr	Use nomogram		Check serum level			NC
Ampicillin	K-T	0.5	8	CNS	4 hr	NC	1 gm/8 hr	0.5 gm/6 hr	No		NC
Oxacillin	K-T	0.5	2	None	4–6 hr	NC	1 gm/8 hr	No	No		NC
Methicillin	K-T	0.5	4	None	4 hr	NC	1 gm/8 hr	No	No		NC
Carbenicillin	K-T, L	1.0	15	CNS, bleeding	4 hr	NC	2 gm/8 hr	1 gm/4 hr	Yes	100 µg/ml	Decreased if renal failure also present
Cephalothin	K-T	0.5	15	None	4 hr	NC	1 gm/8 hr	1 gm/6 hr	Yes	20 µg/ml	NC
Cefotaxime	K	1	2	None	6–8 hr	NC	1 gm/12 hr	Yes	No		Decrease dose
Moxalactam	K-G	2	19	?	8–12 hr	12–24	24 hr	Yes			
Cephaloridine	K-G	1.5	22	Renal	6–8 hr	Do not use	Do not use	Yes			NC
Cefazolin	K-T	1.9	30	None	6–8 hr	NC	24 hr	Yes	Unknown		NC
Cephalexin	K-T, G	1	20	None	6 hr	8 hr	24 hr	Yes			NC
Erythromycin	L	1.5	4–6	None	6 hr	NC	NC	Slight	No		Do not use
Tetracycline-HCl	K-G, L	8.5	100	Renal, hepatic	6 hr	Do not use	Do not use	No	Slight		Do not use
Oxytetracycline	K-G, L	9	70	Renal, hepatic	6 hr	Do not use	Do not use	Yes			Do not use

Minocycline	K-G, L	15	35	Renal hepatic	12 hr	Do not use	Do not use	Yes		5–10 µg/ml	Do not use
Doxycycline	L	17	17	None	12 hr	12 hr	NC	No	Yes		Do not use
Chloramphenicol	L	1.0–2.5	3–5	None	6 hr	NC	NC	Yes	No		Decrease dose
Lincomycin	L	4–5	10–13	None	6 hr	NC	10 hr	No	No		Decrease dose
Clindamycin	L	2.5	10	None	6–8 hr	NC	10 hr	No	No		Decrease dose
Polymyxin B	K-G	4–7	72	Renal, CNS	6–8 hr	24–36 hr	4 days	No	No		NC
Colistimethate	K-G	2–3	72	Renal, CNS	6–8 hr	24–36 hr	4 days	No	No		NC
Streptomycin	K-G	2–4	100	Ear, renal, CNS	12 hr	Do not use	Do not use	Yes	Yes		NC
Kanamycin	K-G	2–4	85	Ear, renal, CNS	8–12 hr	Use nomogram or serum levels		Yes			NC
Gentamicin	K-G	2–3	70	Ear, renal, CNS	8 hr	Use nomogram or serum levels		Yes	Yes		NC
Tobramycin	K-G	2	70	Ear, renal	8 hr	Use nomogram or serum levels		Yes	Yes		NC
Vancomycin	K-G	5	240	Ear, renal	6–12 hr	2½ hr	4–6 days	No	No		NC
Isoniazid	K-L	1–4	8	None	24 hr	NC	Decrease dose	Yes	Yes		Decrease dose
Ethambutol	K	4–6	30	Visual	24 hr	Decrease dose	Do not use	Yes	Yes		NC
Rifampin	L, K	1.5–5.0	3–5	None	24 hr	NC	NC	No			Decrease dose
Nalidixic acid	K	1.5	20	None	6 hr	NC	Do not use	Unknown			NC
Sulfisoxazole	K	6	12	Renal	12 hr	24 hr	Do not use	Yes	Yes		NC
Trimethoprim	K	10	15–40	Marrow	12 hr	24 hr	48 hr				NC
Amphotericin B	K	24	48–72	Renal	24 hr	3 days	5 days	No	No		NC
5-Fluorocytosine	K	3–8	20	Marrow	6 hr	12–24 days	2 days	25 mg/kg			NC

Note: NC = No change; K = kidney; G = glomerular; T = tubular; L = liver.

well distributed to all parts of the body, including the liver, bone, and cerebrospinal fluid.

TOXICITY

Bone marrow depression of one or all cellular elements may occur. Careful observations of the patient's white cell and differential count, noting the development of granulocytopenia, will help one avoid this problem. Similar attention should be given to a decline in reticulocyte count. Rare idiosyncratic aplastic anemia is unrelated to dosage. Any patient receiving chloramphenicol should have a complete blood count done at frequent intervals.

Diarrhea occurs in some patients, and fungal or bacterial superinfection occurs rarely. The hazard of toxicity may be greater in patients with impaired liver function.

USE

The use of chloramphenicol is not contraindicated in the patient with a hematologic disorder if it is the best drug for the particular infection. Areas of use are in anaerobic infections caused by *Bacteroides*, in meningitis in the penicillin-allergic patient, and in ampicillin-resistant *Salmonella*.

CLINDAMYCIN AND LINCOMYCIN

SPECTRUM

The activity of clindamycin (Cleocin) and lincomycin (Lincocin) is similar. Both are active against gram-positive coccal organisms, including most strains of *Staph. aureus*. However, clindamycin is active against both anaerobic cocci and bacilli, except some *Fusobacterium varium* and clostridial strains. Clindamycin has particularly high activity against *B. fragilis*.

ADMINISTRATION, DOSAGE, AND PROPERTIES

Both clindamycin and lincomycin may be administered orally, IM, and IV. The oral dosage of clindamycin is 150 to 300 mg every 6 hours; the IM dosage is 600 to 1,200 mg/day in 2 to 4 equal doses, and the IV dosages range from 600–2,400 mg/day in four equal doses. Dosages as high as 4.8 gm/day have been used in critically ill patients. Normally, clindamycin should be diluted to a concentration of no more than 300 mg/50 ml and administered at a rate not faster than 300 mg over 15 minutes.

Lincomycin can be administered in doses of 600 mg every 12 hours IM or at 600 mg every 6 to 8 hours IV. Dosages up to 8 gm/day have been given to critically ill patients. However, at these high dosages the drug should be diluted to no more than 1 gm/100 ml and infused over an hour.

TOXICITY

Pseudomembranous colitis has developed in patients who have received clindamycin or lincomycin either orally or IV. The incidence of colitis is 2 to 10 percent. Erythema multiforme occurs rarely. Excretion of clindamycin may be delayed in patients with severe liver disease. Development of severe diarrhea should prompt discontinuance of the drug and proctoscopy to look for pseudomembranous colitis.

USE

Clindamycin is an excellent alternative to chloramphenicol in the treatment of serious anaerobic pulmonary or abdominal infections. It is a useful alternative to semisynthetic penicillins or cephalosporins in the treatment of staphylococcal osteomyelitis. Since clindamycin has no activity against the Enterobacteriaceae and Pseudomonads in the treatment of certain mixed infections, another agent, such as gentamicin or amikacin, should be used with it.

AMINOGLYCOSIDE ANTIBIOTICS

AMIKACIN

SPECTRUM. Amikacin is effective against many gram-positive and gram-negative bacteria. It is ineffective against enterococci, *S. pneumoniae*, and anaerobic species. It is resistant to inactivation by most gram-negative bacteria resistant to gentamicin and tobramycin. Hence, it will inhibit gentamicin-tobramycin resistant *E. coli, Klebsiella,* indole-positive *Proteus, Serratia,* and *P. aeruginosa* that cause infection in intensive care areas. Although in vitro studies show that amikacin is less active than other aminoglycosides on a weight basis, the higher doses and higher serum levels obtainable without increased toxicity make the in vitro differences negligible.

ADMINISTRATION, DOSAGE, AND PROPERTIES. Amikacin may be given IM or IV in 2 or 3 equal doses in a daily dosage of 15 to 20 mg/kg/day depending upon renal function. Adjustment of dosage should be based upon calculated creatinine clearance adjusted for age and weight. The normal half-life of the drug is 2 hours, but it accumulates in renal failure. It can be removed by either hemodialysis or peritoneal dialysis. Amikacin, like the other aminoglycosides, does not yield adequate cerebrospinal fluid levels.

TOXICITY. Nephrotoxicity and ototoxicity are the most frequent complications in the use of amikacin. The incidence of toxicity is similar to that encountered with the other agents.

USE. Amikacin would be the agent of choice in treatment of unknown sepsis in an ICU in which there is a significant bacterial resistance problem. In hospitals with low gentamicin resistance, it seems reasonable to use gentamicin or tobramycin and reserve amikacin for resistant organisms.

KANAMYCIN

SPECTRUM. Kanamycin is effective against many gram-positive and gram-negative organisms. However, it is either relatively or totally ineffective against many streptococci, particularly enterococci, pneumococci, anaerobes, and *Pseudomonas*. Resistance of gram-negative organisms such as *Klebsiella* and E. coli varies with the use of the agent within the institution. In certain areas of the United States, this has been a serious problem.

ADMINISTRATION, DOSAGE, AND PROPERTIES. Kanamycin is not absorbed from the gastrointestinal tract, although it exerts antibacterial activity there. It may be administered IM or IV at a dosage of 15 mg/kg/day in 2 or 3 divided doses; IV infusion should be given over at least 1 hour. Dosage should be adjusted in the presence of decreased renal function, as is noted in Table 18-7.

TOXICITY. Renal toxicity and ototoxicity occur. In most patients, nephrotoxicity is heralded by the presence of albuminuria and hematuria. Most lesions are reversible if therapy is stopped, although recovery takes 4 to 6 weeks.

Both branches of the eighth nerve may be involved in the ototoxicity, but it is primarily auditory function that is impaired. Decreased hearing is related to total dosage, height of blood levels, duration of therapy, degree of impairment of renal function, and preexisting auditory status. Loss of high tones occurs prior to subjective hearing loss. Patients over the age of 50 should not receive more than 20 gm of kanamycin in one therapeutic course. It can produce a neurotoxic effect through binding at the neuromuscular junction.

Rarely, after peritoneal lavage injection or rapid IV administration, respiratory paralysis may develop. This often can be overcome by administration of neostigmine or calcium gluconate. Kanamycin can be removed by dialysis. This method should be considered in the treatment of a patient in whom symptoms of toxicity develop.

USE. The use of kanamycin in the ICU has been replaced by the use of gentamicin, tobramycin, or amikacin.

GENTAMICIN

SPECTRUM. Gentamicin is active against most gram-negative bacteria; 95 percent of Pseudomonas species are inhibited. Many staphylococci are inhibited, but it is not the drug of choice for staphylococcal infections. Although Serratia and indole-positive Proteus are usually sensitive, some isolates of Providencia stuarti and Serratia are resistant. Enterococci, pneumococci, and anaerobes are resistant to readily obtainable concentrations.

ADMINISTRATION, DOSAGE, AND PROPERTIES. Gentamicin may be given IM or IV in 3 equal divided doses in a dosage of 3 to 6 mg/kg/day, depending on renal function. Adjustment of dosage with decreased renal function (Table 18-7) should be on the basis of serum creatinine or, better, creatinine clearance. When a patient has reduced renal function, the dosage of gentamicin is often kept constant at 1.0 to 1.5 mg/kg, but the interval between doses is lengthened. A simple way to calculate the interval is to multiply the se-rum creatinine by 8. For example, a patient weighing 70 kg with a creati-nine of 2 mg/100 ml would receive 105 mg every 16 hours. The problem with this method is that it may produce unduly high peak levels and pro-longed trough levels, which result in periods of inadequate therapy. An al-ternative method is given in the section on the use of drugs in the presence of decreased renal function. It should be stressed that the optimal way to adjust gentamicin dosage is by assay of serum levels. A number of methods are currently available and applicable to diagnostic laboratories.

The body distribution of gentamicin is variable, although it enters most body spaces. Concentrations in the spinal fluid are inadequate. Patients in whom peritonitis develops during dialysis should receive intraperitoneal in-jections, since concentrations from IM or IV administration will be inade-quate. In the treatment of meningitis due to *E. coli, Klebsiella,* or *Pseudo-monas,* the drug must be administered by intrathecal injection. The dosage would be 5 to 10 mg in 10 ml, administered slowly by barbotage on a daily basis. The new cephalosporins (moxalactam or cefotaxime) would be better choices.

TOXICITY. Untoward reactions and hypersensitivity are rare with gentamicin. Nephrotoxicity appears to be the most important toxic side-effect and is re-lated to the state of renal function, amount of drug given, duration of drug therapy, and use of other nephrotoxic drugs at the same time. Currently, there is discussion about whether or not nephrotoxicity is seen more fre-quently during the concomitant administration of gentamicin and cephalo-thin. We also have seen renal toxicity when large doses of gentamicin and furosemide are used together. This nephrotoxicity may or may not be reversible.

Ototoxicity occurs less frequently (in less than 2%) than with kanamy-cin and is primarily vestibular. It is related to renal function.

USE. Gentamicin has been a drug of choice in the treatment of sepsis of un-known etiology, especially if *Pseudomonas* or *Serratia* organisms are sus-pected and especially in the treatment of sepsis that develops in burn patients or patients with underlying neoplastic disease receiving chemotherapy. It is useful in the treatment of *Pseudomonas* urinary tract infections.

NEOMYCIN

Neomycin's spectrum of activity is almost identical with that of kanamycin. This is an important fact, since the use of neomycin may cause build-up of kanamycin-resistant bacteria. The drug can be used orally at a dosage of 1 gm administered every 6 hours, or as a topical solution containing 5 mg/ml. It should be used with caution, since large volumes of irrigating fluid or prolonged administration may permit enough absorption to cause toxicity; nephrotoxicity, nerve deafness, neuromuscular blockade, and an intestinal malabsorption syndrome similar to sprue have followed. The use of neomycin orally to prevent hepatic coma in patients who also have decreased renal function may allow accumulation of enough of the drug to cause some hearing loss. In addition, the physician should realize that when culture reports list an organism resistant to kanamycin, it is likely that the organism is also resistant to neomycin; hence, neomycin irrigation solutions should not be used.

TOBRAMYCIN

SPECTRUM. Tobramycin (Nebcin) is active against most gram-negative bacteria. It is active against some *Ps. aeruginosa* strains resistant to gentamicin, but it is not active against the Enterobacteriaceae—i.e., *E. coli, Serratia,* and indole-positive *Proteus,* which are resistant to gentamicin. *Bacteroides,* enterococci, and pneumococci are also resistant.

ADMINISTRATION, DOSAGE, AND PROPERTIES. Tobramycin may be given IM or IV in doses of 1 mg/kg every 8 hours in serious infections and up to 1.66 mg/kg every 8 hours in life-threatening infections. As with all of the aminoglycoside antibiotics, dosage must be reduced in the presence of decreased renal function. A suggested formula to use if the serum creatinine is available is 1.5 mg/kg given every 6 times the serum creatinine. Serum levels should be obtained if possible to achieve peak levels of 4 to 8 μg/ml at a half hour after administration. Levels obtained just prior to the next dose of the agent will reveal accumulation and toxicity earlier than does a rise in the serum creatinine.

TOXICITY. Nephrotoxicity, the most important side-effect, is related to the state of renal function. Avoid simultaneous use of other nephrotoxic drugs. Obtain serum creatinine daily. The result of ototoxicity is primarily high tone loss and occurs in patients with depressed renal function.

USE. Tobramycin is an alternative to gentamicin in the treatment of sepsis of unknown etiology, particularly if sepsis due to *Pseudomonas* is suspected. It is not useful in the treatment of anaerobic infections. It appears to cause less nephrotoxicity than gentamicin.

OTHER AMINOGLYCOSIDES

SISOMICIN. Sisomicin is similar in activity to gentamicin, but is more active against *Pseudomonas* and *E. coli.* It is inactivated by enzymes which inactivate gentamicin. The dosage of sisomicin would be 3 to 4.5 mg/kg/day given as 3 equal doses. Its clinical efficacy is similar to that of the other aminoglycosides.

NETILMICIN. Netilmicin has a spectrum of activity similar to that of gentamicin, but it is the most active agent against *E. coli, Citrobacter,* and *En-*

terobacter. It also inhibits gentamicin-resistant *E. coli, Klebsiella,* and *Enterobacter*, but not gentamicin-resistant *Serratia* or *Pseudomonas*.

The half-life, volume of distribution, and renal excretion of netilmicin are similar to those of gentamicin. Although the agent is less toxic than other aminoglycosides in animals, this has not been established in man. It should be given at a dose of 6 mg/kg/day in 3 equal doses with adjustment made for decreased renal function.

POLYMYXINS: POLYMYXIN B AND COLISTIMETHATE
SPECTRUM
Polymyxin B and colistimethate (polymyxin E) have identical antibacterial activity. They are effective against most gram-negative bacilli but ineffective against gram-positive microorganisms and *Proteus* species.

ADMINISTRATION, DOSAGE, AND PROPERTIES
Both polymyxin B and colistimethate may be administered IM, IV, or orally. They are not absorbed from the gastrointestinal tract in adults, but there is absorption in newborn children. There is no appreciable absorption from the skin or mucosal surfaces. Administered IM or IV, the drugs are widely distributed but diffuse poorly into body cavities and tissue. In neither case does any of the drug enter the central nervous system. Polymyxins are bound in the body to lipid membranes, particularly in the kidney, and are only slowly disassociated to be excreted, sometimes requiring 2 to 3 days for total elimination.

Current dosage schedules for polymyxin B are 2.5 mg/kg/day given IM or IV in 3 divided doses. No person should receive more than 200 mg/day, and each dose should be administered slowly over a 60- to 90-min period. The dose of colistimethate is 5 mg/kg/day in divided doses, usually every 6 hours. The dosage of both agents must be reduced in the presence of renal disease (Table 18-7), and since there are no currently available methods of adequately monitoring serum or tissue levels of the compounds, the use of these agents in the presence of renal disease is exceedingly dangerous.

Polymyxin B sulfate has been used as an aerosol administered every 4 hours at a dosage of 2.5 mg/kg/day in patients with endotracheal tubes or tracheostomies and has been advocated to prevent the development of respiratory tract infections in hospitalized patients. The results have been conflicting, since superinfection with staphylococci or *Proteus* has developed. Thus, at this time, this type of prophylaxis cannot be recommended for the patient in the ICU. The drug occasionally will produce asthmalike attacks in patients when used as an aerosol.

Polymyxin B is also available as an irrigating solution for indwelling urinary catheters, with 200,000 units of polymyxin and 40 mg of neomycin added to 1 liter of saline. This system is successful only if used as a continuous irrigation and for periods of less than 2 weeks. Longer use usually results in colonization or infection with *Candida*.

TOXICITY

Nephrotoxicity manifested by the development of renal insufficiency or acute tubular necrosis can occur. Toxicity is related to the total dose and the state of renal function and is often reversible. Neurotoxicity presents with paresthesias, weakness, and respiratory paralysis and is entirely reversible. Neither agent can be removed by dialysis.

USE

Polymyxin B and colistimethate are unique for the treatment of serious gram-negative infection when the use of other agents is not possible. They are rarely used today.

SULFONAMIDES

Sulfonamides have a wide spectrum of activity, but are less useful in the type of patient encountered in the ICU because they are bacteriostatic. In addition, their effectiveness is reduced by the presence of necrotic tissue, a large inoculum of organisms, and fibrin barriers that occur in abscesses.

The two compounds that might be used currently are either sulfadiazine or sulfisoxazole (Gantrisin). Sulfisoxazole has a greater solubility than sulfadiazine, and renal precipitation has not been a problem. The only major use for these compounds in the ICU, aside from use in urinary tract infections, would be in the treatment of nocardial infections. Infection with *Nocardia asteroides* occurs in patients with underlying defects of immunologic function. It is seen particularly in the renal transplant patient on immunosuppressive therapy or in leukemia or lymphoma patients.

The dosage of intravenous sulfadiazine or sulfisoxazole is 1 to 2 gm every 4 to 6 hours. There are many untoward reactions to sulfonamides: rash, drug fever, and occasionally severe vasculitis and blood dyscrasias. Renal function should be monitored, and crystallization should be prevented through the use of alkalization and increased water intake. Hematologic problems range from hemolytic anemia seen in the G-6-PD–deficient patient to methemoglobinemia. In addition, sulfonamides compete for plasma protein-binding sites with oral anticoagulants, oral antihypoglycemic agents, and methotrexate. The dosage of the compound should be reduced in patients with markedly reduced renal function.

TOPICAL SULFONAMIDES

MAFENIDE. Mafenide (Sulfamylon) is used as a 10% cream applied twice daily. Unlike other sulfonamides, it is not inactivated by para-aminobenzoic acid and hence is effective in the presence of necrotic tissue. It has a low degree of sensitization when used topically. This agent is of value in the treatment of burn infections due to *Ps. aeruginosa*. However, when it is used in the treatment of burns with a large area of infection, hyper-chloremic acidosis can develop.

SILVER SULFADIAZINE. Silver sulfadiazine (Silvadene) has excellent activity against many gram-positive and gram-negative microorganisms and certain nonfilamentous fungi, such as *Candida*. Silver sulfadiazine is a topical oint-ment in the treatment of burn infections. It is somewhat better tolerated than mafenide and does not cause as much pain when dressings are changed.

TRIMETHOPRIM-SULFAMETHOXAZOLE

Trimethoprim-sulfamethoxazole (Bactrim, Septra), a combination antimi-crobial agent, is effective against a wide range of microorganisms with the exception of *Ps. aeruginosa*. The compound is rapidly absorbed following oral administration and has been used for the treatment of recurrent urinary tract infections administered in a dose of 2 tablets twice a day. The adverse reactions seen with the compound are those that are normally expected with sulfonamides. In certain situations this combination agent may be use-ful in treating serious infections produced by agents resistant to the major-ity of common antimicrobial drugs currently available. The dosage should be altered in patients with decreased renal function. This agent may be use-ful in the treatment of urinary infections in the ICU because hospital-acquired strains still have a low level of resistance.

Trimethoprim-sulfamethoxazole is the therapy of choice for *Pneumocys-tis carinii* infections given at a dose of 20 mg trimethoprim (TMP) and 100 mg sulfamethoxazole (SMX) per day for 2 weeks.

A parenteral preparation, extremely useful to treat serious pulmonary and urinary infections in ICU patients when the organisms are resistant to other compounds, should be used at doses of 3 vials in 100 ml of 5% dex-trose in water. It should be administered slowly over ½ to 1 hour every 12 hours. Dosage adjustment is necessary in renal failure so that a loading dose is given and subsequent doses are at a reduced level.

ANTITUBERCULOSIS AGENTS

ISONIAZID

Isoniazid is highly effective against most *Mycobacterium tuberculosis* strains encountered in the United States. The compound is well absorbed after oral or IM administration and may be administered as a single 300-mg dose orally to adults; for patients with extensive or disseminated tuberculosis, 10 to 15 mg/kg/day in 3 divided doses can be given. The compound is well distributed into all body tissues including the cerebrospinal fluid. Reactions to isoniazid are uncommon, although hepatitis develops in some patients. This is a delayed hypersensitivity reaction with symptoms similar to those of viral hepatitis, but, in general, it is reversible. Toxicity may develop in some patients receiving diphenylhydantoin and isoniazid concomitantly, since the agents compete for inactivating enzymes. Isoniazid would be used as therapy in any patient with tuberculosis in the isolation area of an ICU.

ETHAMBUTOL

Ethambutol can only be administered orally. The dosage is 15 mg/kg/day administered either as a single dose, or divided into 2 doses if that is more convenient. At this dosage, optic neuritis is rarely seen. This toxicity is heralded by loss of visual acuity and loss of ability to discriminate colors. Vision usually returns to normal. Ethambutol cannot be given parenterally.

RIFAMPIN

Rifampin is a highly effective antituberculosis agent also effective against many gram-positive and gram-negative microorganisms, though resistance develops rapidly in gram-negative organisms and staphylococci. Rifampin is used only for treating tuberculosis in the U.S. It is available orally and is well absorbed from the gastrointestinal tract. The average dosage for adults is 600 mg/day, though dosages as high as 900 to 1,200 mg have been used in fulminant tuberculosis patients. The compound is excreted through the biliary system and has a large enterohepatic circulation that maintains blood levels. A microbiologically active metabolite is also excreted in the bile. Decreased renal function has little effect on blood levels.

Untoward effects are uncommon with rifampin, but hepatic dysfunction is seen in patients receiving both rifampin and isoniazid. Lysis of fever in a patient treated with rifampin does not signify that the patient was infected with tuberculosis, since the drug is effective against other microorganisms.

ANTIFUNGAL AGENTS

NYSTATIN

Nystatin (Mycostatin) is a polyene antifungal agent that is fungistatic against *Candida* species and certain yeasts. It is poorly absorbed from the gastrointestinal tract, skin, and mucous membranes. It is virtually nontoxic. It is available as a powder, which can be suspended as a cream and ointment. As a solution, it is stable for about a week. Nystatin is useful as an oral suspension in patients with oral thrush. A dose of 100,000 units (1 cc) in 30 ml of water, gargled and then swallowed, can be used 4 times a day. Treatment of *Candida* esophagitis should be with 1,000,000 units daily, in 4 doses, for 7 to 10 days and intravenous amphotericin B or oral ketoconazole. Thrush and esophagitis may develop in patients receiving large doses of broad-spectrum antibiotics.

Topical perineal use is beneficial in patients on antibiotics who have indwelling catheters, since it decreases the concentration of organisms in the area. Use at indwelling intravenous catheter sites may also decrease fungal infections, but this is not proved.

AMPHOTERICIN B

Amphotericin is effective against most fungi. Its marked toxic side-effects limit its use to serious systemic infections. It is not absorbed from the gastrointestinal tract or body surfaces. It is administered by the IV route and has a half-life of 24 to 48 hours. Amphotericin is the agent of choice in the treatment of systemic candidiasis, fungal endocarditis, aspergillosis, cryptococcosis, and generalized histoplasmosis.

ADMINISTRATION, DOSAGE, AND PROPERTIES. Formerly, the dosage of amphotericin was increased daily by extremely slow increments, and it was administered over a 6-hour period. This has been altered. We administer an initial dose of 3 to 5 mg and double the daily dosage until we reach 50 mg (5, 10, 20, 50). Thereafter, we administer 50 mg on alternate days. The solubility of amphotericin is poor (1 mg/10 ml). The first 5 mg is put in 100 ml of 5% D/W; saline or solutions with cations cannot be used. This is administered over 1 to 2 hours. Subsequent doses are given in appropriate volumes over 2 to 3 hours.

If the patient sustains a high fever and chills after the first dose, we give 600 mg of aspirin 2 hours before infusion and infuse 30 mg of hydrocortisone immediately before starting the amphotericin. Heparin can be added to the fluid without inactivation of the drug. Exposure to light for up to 12 hours does not cause inactivation. If nausea develops, the administration of 50 mg of chlorpromazine before infusion will prevent recurrence. Some reactions are prevented by administration of intravenous meperidine.

Patients who have candidemia that fails to resolve with the removal of indwelling lines and do not have a recognized site of infection, i.e., endocarditis or renal lesions, can be successfully treated with a short course of therapy (e.g., a total of 300–500 mg). Other indications for use usually require total dosage in the range of 2 gm.

TOXICITY. Side-effects occur in all patients ranging from chills, fever, and emesis to nephrotoxicity, the latter avoided by watching creatinine clearance. Transaminase elevations occur, but hepatitis is rare. Anemia is common.

5-FLUOROCYTOSINE

5-Fluorocytosine (Ancobon), a pyrimidine derivative, is effective in treatment of selected *Candida* and cryptococcal infections. It should be used only to treat systemic infections in which an organism is sensitive. Half the routine *Candida* isolates are resistant, and resistance can develop in cryptococci. Filamentous fungi, *Aspergillus*, and others are resistant. This agent would not be considered when *Candida* organisms are isolated from sputum or urine, since these mostly represent only colonization.

MICONAZOLE NITRATE

An antifungal agent, this drug is available for IV use at doses of 200 to 400 mg every 8 hr. Used to treat *Candida*, cryptococcal, and *Coccidioides* infections with a modicum of success, its role is still unclear. Phlebitis, nausea, rash, arthralgias, and lipoprotein abnormalities have followed its use.

KETOCONAZOLE

Ketoconazole is an oral antifungal drug effective against *Candida*, cryptococci and topical fungi. It is given in daily doses of 100 to 400 mg depending on body size. Its role in the treatment of fungal infections is not yet fully established.

THE USE OF ANTIBIOTICS IN THE PRESENCE OF DECREASED RENAL FUNCTION

Many antimicrobial agents are eliminated from the body through renal excretion, by glomerular filtration, or by active renal tubular secretion. The margin between antimicrobial effectiveness and toxic levels is large for some agents and small for others. It is in the latter instances that special consideration must be given to the adjustment of the dose of the compound. The renal elimination rate of many substances is proportional to the glomerular filtration rate. The creatinine clearance is thus a useful means of estimating glomerular filtration rate. It is not always necessary to have a 24-hour urine volume to estimate the creatinine clearance; shorter periods may be used successfully. Also, there are methods that permit a rough evaluation of creatinine clearance, such as that of Jelliffe. Utilizing these techniques, it is possible to maintain blood levels of antibiotics in patients with kidney disease that are the same as those obtained in normal persons.

Kunin has recommended that the anuric patient receive a full loading dose with subsequent administration of the agent at half that dose at intervals corresponding to the mean half-life of the drug in the anuric patient. Although this is acceptable with the penicillins and cephalosporins, the use of such a program with the aminoglycoside antibiotics kanamycin and gentamicin presents difficulties at very low creatinine clearances. It is extremely important to remember that it is impossible to predict absolutely whether a drug level will be adequate or nontoxic. If at all possible, serum levels of the agent should be determined. There are available a variety of microbiologic, chemical, and immunologic methods to determine the precise blood level of an antibiotic.

Table 18-7 presents suggested adjustments of antibiotic dosages in the presence of decreased renal or hepatic function.

Gentamicin, tobramycin, and netilmicin should be given as a loading dose of 2 mg/kg followed by a percentage of maintenance dose of 1 to 1.5 mg/kg every 8, 12, and 24 hours as desired. Amikacin should be given as a loading dose of 8 mg/kg followed by a percentage of a 5 mg/kg maintenance dose.

Creatinine Clearance (ml/min)	% of Dose		
	8 Hr	12 Hr	24 Hr
>80	100	100	
80	80	90	
70	75	88	
60	70	85	
50	65	80	
40	55	70	95
30	45	65	85
20	35	50	75
15	30	40	65
10	25	35	55

Blood levels should be obtained whenever renal function is changing to validate the use of the tabulation.

Creatinine clearance is based on the formula:

$$C_r = \frac{(140 - \text{age}) \text{ weight in kg}}{72 \times \text{serum creatinine}}$$

Since many agents are bound to protein or to red cells to varying degrees, higher levels than usual of free drug may occur in a debilitated patient with marked hypoproteinemia and marked anemia. Adjustment of drug dosage for renal dysfunction does not take into account the possibility that metabolites may accumulate even on reduced dosage schedules.

Antibiotics are removed to varying degrees by peritoneal and hemodialysis, so that doses must also be adjusted in patients undergoing dialysis (Table 18-7).

Finally, a patient with decreased renal function on a reduced dose may have inadequate concentrations of antibiotic in the urine, making eradication of urinary tract infection difficult.

TREATMENT OF INFECTIONS

The choice of antibiotic is only one of the important therapeutic measures that should be instituted to treat serious infections. Removal of foreign bodies, drainage of abscesses, removal of obstructions, and correction of metabolic abnormalities are often equally important. Continued attention must be given to the development of nosocomial infections. These are a major problem in patients hospitalized in ICUs because of the large number of intravenous lines and respiratory equipment needed to maintain life in ICU patients. Treatment of infections should be for an adequate period of time. Antibiotics should be discontinued as soon as the patient has clinically recovered from the particular infection that provoked the initial treatment, since continuation of antimicrobial agents will result in superinfection and overgrowth of opportunistic microorganisms.

PNEUMONIA

PNEUMONIA ACQUIRED OUTSIDE THE HOSPITAL

Pneumonias should be divided into those acquired outside the hospital versus those acquired within the institution. Pneumonia acquired outside the hospital occurs in otherwise healthy persons and is usually caused by viruses, pneumococci, or mycoplasmas and much less frequently by *H. influenzae, Klebsiella pneumoniae*, and *Staph. aureus*. Anaerobic mouth flora contributes significantly to pneumonitis in patients admitted to the ICU who are obtunded due to a drug overdose. Thus, anaerobic and microaerophilic streptococci and *Bacteroides* and *Fusobacterium* species would be considered. Organisms such as *Legionella* should be considered if the patient has gastrointestinal, mental, and renal symptoms and clear sputum.

Diagnosis is determined in all cases by examination of an adequate amount of sputum or tracheal material. Gram stain of saliva is of no value. In the absence of adequate sputum, transtracheal aspiration should be performed. Cultures and gram stain of suctioned material should be done in patients intubated prior to admission to the unit. The subsequent development of pneumonitis may be caused by microorganisms found on this initial aspiration. The selection of proper antibiotics and alternative antibiotics, depending on the possible agents, is given in Table 18-5.

Intravenous therapy should be utilized in the patient ill enough to be admitted to the ICU. Arterial blood gases should be analyzed to determine the degree of deoxygenation and CO_2 retention. Suppression of cough and pain should be handled with caution, since further respiratory depression may result. Endotracheal intubation should be considered only in the patient with bacterial pneumonia who fails to maintain an adequate Po_2. Frequent blood gas determinations should be done. Excessive fever should be controlled, particularly in patients with heart disease. Respiratory secretions should be removed with scrupulous attention to sterile technique. Intermittent positive-pressure breathing and humidification should be employed.

Patients with severe bacterial pneumonia should be observed for the development of pulmonary and extrapulmonary complications ranging from sterile pleural effusions to empyema, lung abscess, meningitis, and endocarditis. Meningitis may develop in patients receiving drugs that diffuse poorly into the spinal fluid. Careful attention should be given to the patient's state of consciousness.

HOSPITAL-ACQUIRED PNEUMONIA

Pneumonia that develops in hospitalized patients is more likely to be caused by gram-negative bacilli, staphylococci, or unusual opportunistic microorganisms than is pneumonia acquired outside the hospital. The hospital is a reservoir of these organisms, which replace the normal oral pharyngeal flora of patients with serious illness. Most of these pneumonias are the result of inhalation or aspiration into the lung of organisms present in the upper respiratory tract. Whereas massive aspiration of gastric contents is readily recognized, continued aspiration of lesser amounts of gastric contents or of oropharyngeal secretions is often occult. This is particularly true in the comatose or markedly debilitated patient with impaired cough and glottic reflexes. Inhalation therapy equipment that utilizes reservoir nebulization is readily contaminated with gram-negative bacilli, thus producing aerosols of these organisms. Fortunately, humidifiers will merely saturate gas with water and do not generate bacterial aerosols. The patient with a tracheostomy is particularly in danger from microorganisms transferred by the hands of hospital personnel. Improper suction technique introduces microorganisms or results in trauma to the tracheobronchial tree, providing a site for infection.

Although a number of reports have attempted to characterize the clinical, laboratory, radiographic, and pathologic findings in pneumonia caused by gram-negative bacilli in the absence of isolation of the microorganisms from the blood, it is questionable at this time that a particular pattern is characteristic of a certain microorganism. Diagnosis is particularly difficult in critically ill patients in whom various sources of fever are present. Nonspecific pulmonary infiltrates and cultures of sputum-yielding gram-negative bacilli do not necessarily prove that a patient has pneumonia. Pulmonary infarction, congestive heart failure, uremia, and shock lung must all be differentiated from bacterial pneumonitis. The absence of polymorphonuclear leukocytes from a tracheal aspirate should cause one to question the validity of the culture.

The agents of choice to treat hospital-acquired gram-negative pneumonia are given in Table 18-5 under the particular organism.

ABDOMINAL WOUNDS

In patients with both penetrating and blunt injuries to the abdomen, the peritoneal cavity may be contaminated by the bacterial contents of the small and large bowel. The extent of bacterial contamination varies with the level of intestine involved and the time since injury. The bacterial flora is predominantly anaerobic, including *B. fragilis*, *Peptostreptococcus*, and *Peptococcus* (anaerobic staphylococci). *E. coli* is the most common aerobic organism. Other gram-negative bacilli, such as *Klebsiella* and *Proteus*, account for only a small part of the total flora, and *Pseudomonas* is uncommon.

Antibiotic therapy should begin when the patient is on the way to the operating room. A single agent would not be adequate to cover the afore-mentioned flora. Gentamicin, 1.5 mg/kg every 8 hours; clindamycin, 600 mg every 8 hours; or cefoxitin, 2 gm every 6 hr are possible combinations. Alternative programs have used ticarcillin and an aminoglycoside or chlor-amphenicol rather than clindamycin. The best program is unknown, and each institution will have a preferred one.

Topical irrigation of the abdominal wound with a solution of kanamycin or neomycin is an unwise practice, since such use can lead to respiratory-neuromuscular problems. Copious volumes of sterile saline are just as effica-cious. Placement of adequate drains also plays a significant role.

It is important to remember that a patient in whom peritonitis develops in the hospital or on antibiotics may have a different aerobic flora; *Klebsiella*, *Proteus*, or *Pseudomonas* will be present in larger numbers. They will usually be resistant to ampicillin and cephalothin, and thus these agents would not be first-choice antibiotics.

Continued observation of the patient for signs of local abscess formation is essential. Caution must be used in the interpretation of superficial sur-face wound cultures, since these often fail to reflect the actual infecting agent. Prolonged antibiotic therapy in these infections also is a common cause of superinfection in the ICU patient.

GRAM-NEGATIVE BACTEREMIA

Gram-negative bacilli have become the most common cause of hospital-acquired bacteremia. This syndrome often is the result of manipulations performed within the hospital. Increasingly complex radical surgical proce-dures, immunosuppressive therapy, and measures such as intravenous cathe-terization that provide a route for bacteria to enter the vascular space have contributed to the increased frequency of bacteremia.

E. coli is the most frequent organism, accounting for approximately 35 to 40 percent of cases of gram-negative sepsis. Members of the Klebsielleae, that is, *K. pneumoniae*, *Enterobacters*, and *Serratia*, are second in frequency, accounting for 20 percent. *Proteus* species account for 10 percent, and *Ps. aeruginosa*, for 10 to 15 percent, depending on the type of patient seen in a particular institution. Before 1960, *Bacteroides* bacteremia was infrequent; currently, *Bacteroides* is responsible for 10 percent of cases of gram-nega-tive sepsis. Polymicrobial bacteremia occurs in 5 to 10 percent of the pa-tients.

Microorganisms producing bacteremia within the first 3 to 5 days of hospitalization will be sensitive to many antimicrobial agents. Organisms encountered in patients who have been hospitalized for lengthy periods fre-quently contain R factors that provide multiple resistance to many anti-microbial agents.

Many factors determine which bacterial species will produce a bacteremia: (1) whether the infection was acquired within the hospital or in the community; (2) the type of prior antimicrobial therapy; (3) the site or origin of the bacteremia; and (4) the underlying disease. It is possible to predict a likely etiologic agent from the known anatomic site as well as from certain predisposing types of factors (see Table 18-8).

Currently, it is not possible to detect differences in morbidity and mortality among the various species of gram-negative bacilli, although higher fatality rates are noted, for example, with *Pseudomonas*. However, this is primarily a reflection of the greater frequency of *Pseudomonas* bacteremia in patients with markedly compromised host defense mechanisms. The outcome of gram-negative bacteremia is highly dependent on the host factors that have predisposed to the bacteremia. Patients with known nonfatal disease, that is, those expected to survive 5 years or longer, have survival rates in excess of 85 percent. Patients whose estimated survival is less than 5 years have survival rates in the range of 50 to 60 percent. Those with known rapidly fatal disease, such as acute leukemia, have survival rates of less than 15 percent.

Prevention plays a significant defensive role in treatment of gram-negative bacteremia in the ICU. Unneeded intravenous catheters or indwelling urinary catheters should be removed as soon as possible. Marked attention must be given to tracheostomy sites and to early removal of endotracheal tubes.

INFECTION CONTROL IN THE INTENSIVE CARE UNIT
INTRAVENOUS INFUSIONS
Intravenous therapy is associated with continued risk of septicemia. The critically ill patient in the ICU requires a secure lifeline if he is to survive, but it is a frequent practice to continue the use of indwelling plastic catheters long after they are necessary, needlessly increasing the risk of infection.

Aseptic Technique
If sepsis is to be prevented, the following aspects of care are critical:

1. Hands should be thoroughly washed and care taken not to touch the needle or skin when inserting intravenous catheters. During the placement of hyperalimentation lines, sterile gloves and aseptic technique are required.
2. The site chosen for intravenous placement should be prepared with an adequate solution. Iodine (2% iodine, 70% alcohol) is well tolerated and highly useful. If an iodophor such as Betadine is used, it should not be washed off the skin, since its action is partially dependent on sustained release of iodine. Alcohol (70%) should be used for patients who cannot tolerate iodine. Quaternary ammonium compounds such as Zephiran should not be used.
3. Intravenous catheters should be securely anchored to prevent to-and-fro motion, thus preventing transport of cutaneous bacteria into the puncture wound. Use of a topical antiseptic such as an iodophor should be considered. It is not

TABLE 18-8. Factors Determining the Organisms Involved in Septicemia, with Suggested Antibiotic Programs

Origin	Predisposing Factors	Contributing Underlying Disease	Organisms	Antibiotics*
Genitourinary tract	Indwelling catheters, instrumentation	Prostatic obstruction	E. coli, Klebsiella, Enterobacter, Serratia, Pseudomonas, Proteus	Aminoglycoside or cefoxitin
Gastrointestinal tract Biliary	Cholangitis	Stones, surgery	E. coli, Klebsiella, Bacteroides, streptococci	Clindamycin and gentamicin or chloramphenicol or cefoxitin
Large bowel	Abscesses, diverticulae	Neoplasia, leukemia	Pseudomonas	Ticarcillin and tobramycin
Reproductive system	Surgery, abortion, post partum		Bacteroides, Group B streptococci, enterococci, E. coli	Clindamycin and aminoglycoside or cefoxitin
Respiratory tract	Tracheostomy, ventilatory apparatus, antibiotics		Enterobacter, Klebsiella, Serratia, Pseudomonas, Proteus, E. coli	Aminoglycoside and ticarcillin
Skin	Burns	Leukemia	Pseudomonas, Providencia, Serratia	Ticarcillin and aminoglycoside
Vascular system	Intravenous catheters, foreign bodies, surgery		Pseudomonas, Enterobacter, Serratia, Candida, Staph. epidermidis, enterococci	Depends on suspected species; see above choices

* Amikacin should be the aminoglycoside if there is a high level of resistance in the institution.

established that this will prevent the growth of resistant bacteria and *Candida*, but it is preferred over topical antimicrobial preparations. The infusion site should be covered with a sterile dressing.

4. The date and time of insertion of the intravenous line should be recorded. Cannulas should not be left in place longer than 72 hours; preferably, they should be changed at 48 hours.
5. The infusion site should be inspected daily with aseptic technique with re-application of an iodophor. At the first signs of inflammation or phlebitis, the catheter should be removed.
6. Intravenous containers should be examined before use and discarded if particulate material is present.
7. Fluid should be used as soon as possible. No bottle or bag should be left in place for more than 24 hours. Bottles should be changed every 12 hours if possible. In situations in which a pump delivery system is available, a 0.45- or 0.22-μm filter close to the insertion site should be used.

MANAGEMENT OF SUSPECTED INFUSION SEPSIS
The skin of the insertion site should be cleansed with an adequate antiseptic. The cannulas should be aseptically removed and the tip cut off with sterile scissors and placed in an appropriate transport medium. Any purulence at the site should be cultured with a sterile swab and sent to the laboratory in transport medium. When septicemia appears related to contaminated fluid, 10 to 20 ml of fluid should be aseptically withdrawn from the intravenous line and inoculated into blood-culture bottles.

NOSOCOMIAL INFECTIONS RELATED TO RESPIRATORY CARE EQUIPMENT
The purpose of decontamination or sterilization of inhalation therapy equipment is to eliminate one of the constant bacterial hazards that the patient in the ICU faces. Disposable equipment should be used insofar as possible.

NEBULIZATION EQUIPMENT
Nebulization equipment is the most frequent source of contamination because it is so difficult to decontaminate this equipment adequately. Utilization of 0.25% acetic acid has been a common practice, but failures have been noted with this method, and residual bacterial contamination may occur. Quaternary ammonium compounds, iodophors, and hexachlorophene solutions are not satisfactory decontaminating agents for inhalation therapy equipment. Therefore, the use of ethylene oxide sterilization is recommended.

INTERMITTENT AND CONSTANT PRESSURE BREATHING MACHINES
Surface contamination probably plays a negligible role in the transmission of nosocomial infections. Therefore, the use of standard cleaning solutions for the outsides of intermittent and constant pressure breathing machines is perfectly reasonable. Routine sterilization of the internal parts of this equip-

ment is unnecessary, since most pathogens cannot survive on dry surfaces. Ethylene oxide sterilization should be used where contamination of the machine might create a risk to subsequent patients. Tubing should be replaced every 24 hours.

MAINTENANCE OF IN-USE NEBULIZATION EQUIPMENT

The patient's breathing circuit (i.e., the tubing between the respirator and the patient) ideally should be changed every 8 to 12 hours when used for continuous therapy and every 24 hours when used for intermittent therapy. Only sterile liquids should be nebulized; tap water should not be used. The sterile water or saline used to fill nebulizers should be dispensed aseptically and refrigerated when not in use. Unused portions should be discarded if not used within 24 hours. Reservoirs should be completely emptied and routinely refilled every 12 hours. Fluid in tubing should not be drained back into the reservoir. Unit dose vials should be employed for addition of material to the nebulizer part of the machine. Multiple dose vials are easily contaminated and have been responsible for nosocomial epidemics.

ISOLATION TECHNIQUE

The general guidelines set forth by the Center for Disease Control should be followed. In ICUs that do not have individual rooms with separate air intake and exhaust, we find the following guidelines useful:

1. Strict isolation patients should not be admitted to such an open area. Patients isolated for enteric infections should be admitted only after discussion with the hospital epidemiologist.
2. Patients with primary staphylococcal pneumonia, streptococcal pneumonia, *Pseudomonas* infections, and cavitary tuberculosis need single rooms until they have been on therapy for at least 5 days. Patients with extensive burns should not be placed in general ICUs. They should be cared for in special facilities.
3. During periods of viral pneumonia when influenza, varicella, and measles are seen, such patients' respiratory care should be administered in areas where they will not contaminate the other patients.
4. Patients with viral hepatitis and positive serum tests for hepatitis antigen must be handled with caution, since the virus is transmissible by all secretions as well as by blood. Contamination of staff and other patients is prevented by attention to disposal of materials from such patients.

SURVEILLANCE OF INFECTION

An ongoing program of surveillance of infections in any ICU is vital to its success. The intensive care report form shown in Table 18-3 suggests a possible way of following patients who are in the unit that will allow for effective recognition of potential outbreaks of infection and will encourage the staff to improve their standards in terms of intravenous and respiratory care equipment. All members of the ICU team must remember that attention to hand-washing procedures will significantly decrease infection in the ICU.

PROPHYLACTIC ANTIBIOTICS
The high infection rates encountered in both medical and surgical ICUs may cause physicians to consider the prophylactic use of antibiotics to prevent respiratory, wound, and urinary infections. There is no evidence that systemic antibiotics will decrease such infections if used on every patient. Controlled studies have not shown a benefit from the use of antibiotics in the prophylaxis of infections that occur in cardiac failure, unconsciousness, viral respiratory infections, shock, and cardiac catheterization. Selective use of antibiotics at the time of vascular, cardiac, and certain orthopedic procedures may decrease infection by staphylococci and some gram-negative bacilli. However, experience in surgical units has shown that the incidence of systemic candidiasis is greatest in surgical units utilizing extensive antimicrobial therapy. The topical use of antimicrobials in the treatment of extensive burns is successful if the agents used are not agents that are also used systemically, since topical or oral agents will select a bacterial flora in the unit that will be resistant to the agents most useful for systemic treatment of serious infection.

Donald Silver
Donald Kapsch

19. DIAGNOSIS AND MANAGEMENT OF NONMECHANICAL BLEEDING

Prolonged or excessive bleeding may become life-threatening and therefore must be controlled. Fortunately, most bleeding is controlled by natural defenses or by mechanical means (e.g., ligature, cautery, sutures, tamponade). This chapter will review the mechanisms and management of congenital and acquired causes of nonmechanical bleeding.

COAGULATION MECHANISM
PHYSIOLOGY

The coagulation system is composed of a series of interrelated enzymatic reactions with "biological" feedback amplification which leads to the formation of an insoluble fibrin complex, the stable hemostatic clot. Under most circumstances, intravascular coagulation is associated with activation of the fibrinolytic system, which is responsible for dissolution of the clot when vascular repair has been completed. Thus, actions of the coagulation and fibrinolytic systems serve to preserve vascular integrity and patency. Various disease states or therapeutic maneuvers can disturb this delicate balance between coagulation and fibrinolysis, producing insufficient or disorganized clotting, localized or widespread intravascular coagulation with partial or total consumption of clotting factors, and moderate or excessive activation of the fibrinolytic mechanism.

Twelve clotting factors have been identified—numbered I through XIII, since the original Factor VI is an intermediate product and not a true coagulation factor. Seven factors are proteolytic enzymes; four are cofactors responsible for the facilitation, acceleration, and regulation of the reactions catalyzed by the enzymatic factors; and one, fibrinogen, is converted to fibrin to form the hemostatic clot. Table 19-1 lists the plasma half-lives and blood component sources for the protein coagulation factors. The initiation of the coagulation process can occur by activation of the intrinsic or extrinsic pathways of coagulation (Fig. 19-1). Both pathways produce a common activated clotting factor and share an identical terminal pathway for the production of fibrin from fibrinogen. The prothrombin and activated

Supported in part by U.S. Public Health Service Grant HL-18815.

439

TABLE 19-1. Plasma Half-life and Major Sources for the Protein Coagulation Factors

Factor[a]	Plasma Half-life (hr)	Vitamin K Dependent	Significant Sources		
			Serum	Stored Plasma	Fresh Frozen Plasma
I (fibrinogen)	90	No	No	Yes	Yes
II (prothrombin)	65	Yes	No	Yes	Yes
V (proaccelerin)	15	No	No	No	Yes
VII (proconvertin)	5	Yes	No	Yes	Yes
VIII (antihemophiliac factor A)[b]	10	No	No	No	Yes
IX (antihemophiliac factor B)	25	Yes	Yes[c]	Yes	Yes
X (Stuart-Prower factor)	40	Yes	Yes	Yes	Yes
XI (plasma thromboplastin antecedent)	45	No	Yes	Yes	Yes
XII (Hageman factor)	50	No	Yes	Yes	Yes
XIII (fibrin stabilizing factor)	120	No	No	Yes	Yes

[a] All clotting factors, with the exception of Factor VIII, are synthesized in the liver. Factor VIII appears to be synthesized by the vascular endothelium.
[b] Principal source for clinical use is cryoprecipitated plasma or glycine-precipitated Factor VIII concentrate.
[c] Present as activated Factor IX.

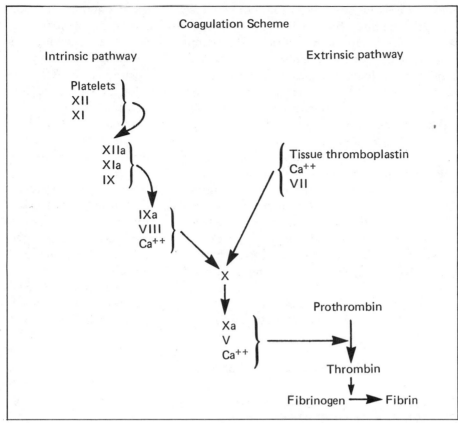

FIGURE 19-1. Schematic representation of the extrinsic and intrinsic coagulation pathways.

partial thromboplastin times may be used to assay the integrity of the extrinsic and intrinsic pathways, respectively.

The intrinsic pathway sequence usually begins when Factor XII is activated by exposure to a foreign substance, such as collagen or vascular basement membrane. Activated Factor XII converts Factor XI to its active form. Activated Factor XI then cleaves a single polypeptide bond of Factor IX to form an active configuration of Factor IX. Activated Factor IX complexes with Factor VIII to bring about activation of Factor X. Thrombin, the product of the reaction catalyzed by activated Factor X, modifies Factor VIII to increase its specific activity and the rate of the reaction producing activated Factor X. There is a phospholipid requirement for the conversion of Factor X to activated Factor X, which is supplied by platelets as Platelet Factor III.

Activated Factor X subsequently complexes with Factor V, calcium, and phospholipid to bring about the conversion of prothrombin to thrombin.

Factor V greatly enhances the rate of conversion of prothrombin. Thrombin catalyzes the hydrolysis of four specific arginyl-glycine bonds of fibrinogen with the liberation of two pairs of fibrinopeptides, A and B. Following this hydrolytic conversion, the fibrin monomers undergo spontaneous polymerization into a loose gel network. Thrombin also activates Factor XIII, the fibrin-stabilizing factor, which catalyzes the formation of peptide bonds between adjacent fibrin monomers and stabilizes the fibrin network.

The extrinsic coagulation pathway is initiated by the conversion of Factor X to its activated form by a complex formed from tissue-derived factor, calcium, and Factor VII. Tissue factor is composed of protein and phospholipid subunits and serves as the reactive surface for the activation of Factor VII and subsequent enzymatic conversion of Factor X to its activated form. After activated Factor X is formed, the coagulation pathway is identical with that described above for the intrinsic system pathway.

Three mechanisms exist to prevent excessive or unnecessary continued formation of fibrin by the coagulation system. Blood flow reduces the local accumulation of activated clotting factors. Activated clotting factors are rapidly removed by hepatocytes and other cells of the reticulonendothelial system. Finally, plasma coagulation inhibitors, primarily antithrombin III, complex with thrombin and activated Factors X, IX, VII, and XI to inhibit their activity. The anticoagulant heparin complexes with antithrombin III as a cofactor and greatly enhances the rate of inactivation of Factors X, IX, VII, XI, and thrombin by antithrombin III.

CLOTTING FACTOR DEFICIENCIES
CONGENITAL DEFICIENCIES
Congenital deficiencies have been described for all of the clotting factors. A congenital deficiency state may be characterized by low levels of production of the clotting factor or the production of a clotting factor that is antigenically similar to the normal factor but without procoagulant activity due to structural alterations. Most heterozygous patients do not manifest bleeding phenomena, since factor concentrations usually remain adequate to provide hemostasis in the absence of severe hemorrhage. Some homozygous patients may also fail to manifest overt bleeding tendencies except when stressed, e.g., with surgery or major trauma, since only 5 to 10 percent of normal factor activity is needed to maintain hemostasis in daily life. Almost all of the congenital clotting disorders involve a single factor deficiency.

Deficiencies of Factors VIII and IX, classical hemophilia and Christmas disease, are the most common congenital deficiency syndromes. Both are sex-linked recessive disorders with affected males and female carriers. Table 19-2 lists the congenital clotting factor deficiency states with their manifestations, inheritance, and incidence. Diagnostic test results and therapy are outlined in Table 19-3.

The congenital disorder von Willebrand's disease affects platelet function and the coagulation mechanism. Patients with this disorder have a quantitative reduction in the circulating levels of Factor VIII and a defect in platelet adhesion, responsible for the prolonged bleeding times noted in these patients. Two separate genetic defects appear to be operative in von Willebrand's disease, since the factor responsible for the correction of the platelet adhesion defect is distinct from Factor VIII coagulant activity. The platelet adhesion defect can be temporarily corrected through the transfusion of fresh frozen plasma or cryoprecipitated plasma fraction. The cryoprecipitate also contributes to an increase in Factor VIII activity through the acceleration of production of Factor VIII, the activity peaking 24 hours after transfusion.

The other congenital factor deficiencies are associated with normal bleeding times, in the absence of administration of platelet-inhibiting agents, since normal platelet function is preserved.

Approximately 7 to 10 percent of hemophiliacs develop alloantibodies to the Factor VIII used in the treatment of their bleeding episodes [17, 19, 21]. These patients should be managed conservatively without Factor VIII replacement for minor bleeding in conjunction with immobilization of the site of hemorrhage to avoid disturbing any formed clot. When use of Factor VIII replacement becomes necessary, immunosuppression with agents such as cyclophosphamide may help, if started early, to reduce the production of the alloantibodies [17]. In the treatment of life-threatening hemorrhage, patients with alloantibodies will require 10,000 units per 12 hours of human or animal lyophilized Factor VIII concentrate in conjunction with antifibrinolytic agents [17]. Failure of this mode of therapy necessitates the use of an activated prothrombin complex and requires comprehensive monitoring to detect the development of excessive intravascular coagulation, which occasionally complicates the use of these concentrates [6, 17, 35]. Partially activated Factor IX concentrate, 1,000 to 2,000 units, has been used successfully in managing bleeding episodes in these patients. This dose is repeated every 4 to 6 hours if bleeding continues [21]. The hemostatic effects associated with the use of Factor IX concentrates in patients with Factor VIII alloantibodies are dependent upon the contamination of these concentrates with minute amounts of activated Factor X. Recent manufacturing advances have almost completely eliminated this contamination in some Factor IX concentrates (e.g., Proplex), although it remains in others [14]. Hemophiliacs with alloantibodies should be managed in conjunction with a hematologist.

If the deficiency is mild and bleeding is not excessive, it is preferable to use cryoprecipitate and plasma in the treatment of Factor VIII and Factor IX deficiencies, respectively. Cryoprecipitate carries less risk of hepatitis transmission than do lyophilized concentrates, which are manufactured from plasma pooled from five to ten thousand donors [21]. Unless the hemorrhage is life-threatening, cryoprecipitate should be used in the man-

TABLE 19-2. Characteristics of the Congenital Coagulation Deficiencies

Deficiency	Manifestations	Inheritance	Incidence
Factor I	Serious neonatal or infant bleeding episodes.	Autosomal recessive affecting both sexes.	<0.5 per million live births.
Factor II	Serious neonatal or infant bleeding episodes.	Autosomal recessive affecting both sexes.	<0.5 per million live births.
Factor V	Mild excessive bleeding early in life—i.e., epistaxis, menorrhagia, prolonged postoperative bleeding.	Highly penetrant autosomal recessive affecting both sexes.	1 per million live births.
Factor VII	Mild to moderate bleeding or purpura.	Autosomal recessive affecting both sexes.	Homozygous form: 1 per 400,000 live births. Heterozygous form more common but may not cause bleeding.
Factor VIII	Neonatal bleeding is unusual. Bleeding becomes manifest at 6–12 mo. Excessive bleeding following dental procedures, hemarthroses, and intraabdominal hemorrhage are common.	Sex-linked recessive with males as bleeders, females as carriers.	Most common congenital coagulation factor deficiency; 1 per 25,000 live births.
Factor IX	Excessive bleeding following trauma or surgery in the male. May cause spontaneous CNS hemorrhage. Hemarthroses are uncommon except in severe cases.	Sex-linked recessive with males as bleeders, females as carriers.	1 per 100,000 live births.

Factor X	Mild bleeding beginning later in life. Hemarthroses can occur but are rare.	Autosomal recessive with equal frequency in males and females.	Homozygous form: 1 per 400,000 live births; heterozygous form: 1 per 500 live births.
Factor XI	Excessive bleeding following trauma or elective surgery, often as a delayed episode.	Autosomal recessive with equal frequency in males and females.	Approximately 1 per million live births in the general population. More common in patients of Jewish ancestry.
Factor XII	Seldom with clinically significant bleeding. Severe deficiency states may be associated with thrombotic episodes.	Autosomal recessive affecting both sexes.	Approximately 1 per million live births.
Factor XIII	Neonatal bleeding is common with cord hemorrhage, echymoses, and hematomas.	Autosomal recessive with equal frequency in both sexes.	<0.5 per million live births.
von Willebrand's disease	Spontaneous epistaxis and easy bruisability in childhood. Gastrointestinal hemorrhage common.	Autosomal dominant with equal frequency in both sexes.	5–10 per million live births.

CNS = central nervous system.

TABLE 19-3. Diagnosis and Therapy of Congenital Coagulation Deficiencies

Deficiency	Diagnostic Tests/Results*	Therapy
Factor I	Plasma fibrinogen concentrations decreased, often undetectable. TT, PT, and APTT markedly prolonged.	Human fibrinogen (Parenogen) 1 gm/10–20 min for active bleeding. Plasma and whole blood may also be used. Minimal level to control bleeding is 60 mg/100 ml. Risk of hepatitis as high as 40% with use of the fibrinogen concentrates.
Factor II	PT prolonged in the presence of normal concentrations of Factors V, VII, X, and XII.	Blood or plasma transfusions; plasma concentrates (Konyne, Proplex) may also be used but carry an increased risk for the transmission of hepatitis.
Factor V	PT and APTT prolonged. APTT is corrected by the addition of normal plasma or normal barium-adsorbed plasma, but not normal serum.	Fresh whole blood, banked blood less than 1 wk old, or FFP. 20 ml FFP/kg body weight every 12 hr recommended if normal renal and cardiac function are present. 20–25% of normal concentrations are adequate for hemostasis.
Factor VII	PT prolonged. Clotting time, prothrombin consumption time, and APTT normal.	Whole blood or FFP transfusion preferred. Plasma concentrates (Konyne, Proplex) may be used but carry an increased risk of hepatitis. 2 units of factor concentrate/kg body weight will increase Factor VII concentrations by 3–4%. 20% of normal levels needed for hemostasis. Treat for 8 days following surgery.
Factor VIII	PT normal; APTT prolonged and not corrected by the addition of normal serum. Clotting times may be normal.	Fresh whole blood, FFP, cryoprecipitate, glycine precipitated Factor VIII concentrate (AHF, Human). 1 unit of Factor VIII/kg body weight will increase plasma levels by 2%. CNS bleeding: 50 units/kg body weight stat., then 40 units/kg/24 hr for 14–21 days. Retropharyngeal and retroperitoneal bleeding: 50 units per kg stat., then 40 units/kg every 12 hr for 3 doses. Surgery: 50 units/kg 1 hr prior to operation; maintain plasma level greater than 60% for 4 days; then 40% for 4 days or until all drains and sutures are out. Maintain 15–20% of

		normal levels for 2 wk following orthopedic procedures. Use of Amicar not indicated except in dental procedures. See text for treatment of patients with Factor VIII alloantibodies.
Factor IX	PT normal; APTT prolonged and corrected by normal serum but not barium-adsorbed normal plasma.	Banked whole blood, plasma, or plasma concentrates (Konyne, Proplex). 1 unit of Factor IX/kg body weight will increase plasma levels by 1½%. Treatment regimens are the same as those outlined for Factor VIII deficiency.
Factor X	PT and APTT prolonged. APTT prolongation is corrected by the addition of normal serum or plasma, but not barium-adsorbed normal plasma.	Banked whole blood, plasma, or serum. Plasma concentrates with Factor X are available but carry an increased risk for the transmission of hepatitis. 15% of normal concentrations are needed for surgery.
Factor XI	PT normal; APTT prolonged and corrected by the addition of normal serum, normal plasma, or barium-adsorbed normal plasma.	Banked whole blood, plasma, or serum. Daily transfusion is suggested for the first 5 days following surgery.
Factor XII	PT and APTT prolonged. Prolongation of the APTT is corrected by the addition of normal serum, normal plasma, or barium-adsorbed normal plasma.	None required.
Factor XIII	PT and APTT normal. Clot is soluble in 5M urea whereas normal clots are not.	Whole blood or plasma transfusion. Frequent transfusions are not necessary due to the 5–7 day half-life of Factor XIII.
von Willebrand's disease	Bleeding time prolonged and platelet adhesiveness as measured by glass bead retention is decreased. APTT may be prolonged due to decreased concentrations of Factor VIII coagulant activity.	Cryoprecipitate is given to maintain the APTT less 100 sec for 7–10 days following surgery. Factor VIII lyophilized concentrates are not recommended; their use has been associated with inadequate hemostasis. Platelet transfusions are not indicated.

TT = thrombin time; PT = prothrombin time; APTT = activated partial thromboplastin time; FFP = fresh frozen plasma; CNS = central nervous system.

* Specific factor assays are available to determine residual activity levels and define the severity of the deficiency state.

agement of children under the age of 3 regardless of the severity of the bleeding, to avoid the high incidence of chronic hepatitis B antigenemia seen with the use of lyophilized Factor VIII concentrates in this age group [21].

Elective surgery can be performed safely in patients with hemophilia and hemophilia-like bleeding disorders if the following precautions are observed: (1) the exact nature of the coagulation defect must be accurately defined; (2) the half-life of the infused therapeutic material must be determined; (3) the plasma must be screened for clotting factor inhibitors; and (4) the anticipated factor replacement needs are available. The surgeon should also be prepared to continue replacement therapy for 2 to 3 weeks postoperatively. The presence of clotting factor inhibitors usually is a contraindication to elective surgery [14, 29].

ACQUIRED FACTOR DEFICIENCIES
Acquired factor deficiency states may be due to deficient production, dilution, or excessive consumption of one or more of the clotting factors.

DEFICIENT PRODUCTION
Impaired hepatic function, such as occurs in hepatitis, cirrhosis, and infiltrative neoplastic lesions, can lead to significant decreases in clotting factor concentrations; clotting Factors II, VII, IX, and X are those most often affected. Diets deficient in vitamin K also may leave the patient with insufficient concentrations of this cofactor for the synthesis of Factors II, VII, IX, and X. Broad spectrum antibiotics, with their alteration of the intestinal flora, can also lead to deficient vitamin K production and absorption. Fat malabsorption may contribute to clotting factor deficiencies because vitamin K is a fat-soluble vitamin.

Bleeding disorders may occur in the neonatal period, especially in the premature, because of low circulating levels of clotting factors from immature protein synthesis in the liver and the absence of vitamin K–producing bacteria in the intestinal tract. The routine oral or intramuscular administration of 1 mg of K_1 to all newborns has practically eliminated this disorder.

DIAGNOSIS. A history of excessive alcohol consumption, previous or concurrent hepatitis, or nutritional deprivation in patients with excessive bleeding should suggest acquired clotting factor deficiencies. Physical examination may demonstrate the stigmata of hepatic insufficiency or evidence of significant weight loss in cases of nutritional deprivation. The prothrombin time (PT) is a sensitive indicator of decreased levels of circulating clotting factors in these cases because the concentration of Factors II, VII, IX, and X is affected early. Low serum albumin concentration levels in patients with liver disease usually indicate depressed hepatic synthesis of all plasma proteins, including clotting factors. Patients with cirrhosis and portal hypertension may have hypersplenism with thrombocytopenia.

MANAGEMENT. Parenteral administration of vitamin K_1 (20–25 mg given slowly intravenously) to patients with adequate hepatic function will correct deficiency states of the vitamin K–dependent factors, usually within 24 hours. Patients with severe hepatocellular disease or in immediate need of correction of their hemostatic abnormalities are best treated with fresh frozen plasma or fresh whole blood. Patients at risk for vitamin K deficiencies, such as newborns or patients undergoing total parenteral nutrition, should be treated with prophylactic parenteral vitamin K_1 (0.5–1 mg intramuscularly (IM) as a single injection in newborns, 2.5–10 mg IM weekly in adults).

EXCESSIVE BLOOD TRANSFUSION

Massive transfusions of banked blood (25–30 units in 24 hr or 5–6 units/ hr) to normal patients, and lesser degrees of blood replacement in patients with depressed clotting factor concentrations, may lead to excessive bleeding through dilution of the labile clotting factors, e.g., Factors V and VIII. Platelet viability and function also suffer during whole blood preservation, and a dilutional thrombocytopenia is frequently associated with transfusion of large volumes of banked blood. Other problems associated with blood transfusion are discussed in the section on whole blood.

DIAGNOSIS. The diagnosis is frequently suggested by the history. If sepsis, shock, transfusion reaction, or other factors can be eliminated as a cause for excessive intravascular coagulation, the massive blood replacement may leave the patient with insufficient amounts of Factor V, Factor VIII, or platelets for hemostasis and bleeding may ensue. Both the PT and partial thromboplastin time (PTT) are prolonged due to deficient concentrations of Factors V and VIII. Platelet counts are depressed, and laboratory evidence of increased fibrinolytic activity is usually absent.

MANAGEMENT. If red cell replacement is also needed, fresh whole blood is the treatment of choice, since it will provide all the deficient clotting factors and viable platelets. If red cells are not needed, the coagulation factors can be provided through the use of fresh frozen plasma, and platelet transfusions can be utilized to provide sufficient numbers ($>30,000/mm^3$) of active platelets. Two to four platelet "packs" and a similar number of units of fresh frozen plasma (see section on blood components) will usually provide adequate coagulation factors and platelets for hemostasis.

DISSEMINATED INTRAVASCULAR COAGULATION

Disseminated intravascular coagulation (DIC) is characterized by acute or chronic intravascular accelerated utilization of clotting factors and platelets and secondary activation of fibrinolysis. If the intravascular coagulation proceeds slowly and the fibrinolytic response maintains vessel patency, the condition may remain unrecognized. If excessive coagulation occurs, clotting factors will be consumed, and bleeding will result. If fibrinolytic activity is insufficient to maintain vessel patency, the microcirculation may be obstructed by thromboses and cellular death or organ death, or both, may occur. The process usually ceases when the procoagulant stimulus is removed.

Intravascular coagulation may be initiated by conditions that: (1) release thromboplastin—especially incompatible blood transfusions, cardiopulmonary bypass, burns, and amniotic fluid embolism; (2) alter blood vessels—e.g., arteriovenous fistula, aneurysm, shock, and rickettsial infections; and (3) result in stasis of blood flow—e.g., giant hemangiomas, shock, pulmonary embolism, and cyanotic heart disease. If the stimulus is excessive or persistent, or both, excessive intravascular coagulation may lead to the depletion of fibrinogen, prothrombin, and Factors V, VIII, IX, X, XII, and XIII. Platelets are decreased in number because platelets aggregate on exposed collagen or are consumed in microthrombi. Secondary fibrinolysis causes thrombolysis and occasionally bleeding, with the production of fibrin degradation products which interfere with fibrin polymerization and lead to the formation of unstable clots. Bleeding may occur if the coagulation factors become sufficiently depressed—e.g., prothrombin less than 10 percent of control, fibrinogen less than 50 mg%, and platelets less than 30,000/mm^3.

DIAGNOSIS. Examination of the peripheral blood smear will demonstrate distorted and fragmented red cells, indicative of a microangiopathic hemolytic anemia. The platelet count is usually decreased below 100,000, and frequently to 20,000 to 40,000 platelets/mm^3. The PT, PTT, and thrombin time are prolonged, and specific coagulation factors are markedly reduced. Fibrin monomers and fibrin degradation products can be detected. Secondary fibrinolysis can be demonstrated with shortened euglobulin and whole blood lysis times.

Secondary fibrinolysis can be distinguished from primary hyperfibrinolysis by the marked depression of clotting factor concentrations *and* platelet counts which characterize excessive intravascular coagulation. The tests of coagulation (e.g., ethanol gelation, protamine paracoagulation) and for fibrin split products are positive during periods of excessive intravascular coagulation.

MANAGEMENT. The underlying cause should be eliminated; i.e., the abscess should be drained, the gram-negative sepsis stopped, the rejected transplant organ removed, and the shock treated. If the underlying cause cannot be eliminated, the coagulation process must be slowed, so that the coagulation factors can be restored and bleeding controlled. Heparin is an effective agent because it slows coagulation and permits restoration of the depleted coagulation factors. Infusion of 500 to 1,000 units of heparin per hour, in adults, should be continued until the platelet count, fibrinogen concentration, and thrombin time return toward normal, the bleeding ceases, *and* the underlying cause is eliminated. Replacement of depleted clotting factors should be undertaken only after heparin therapy has been initiated so that the infused coagulation factors will not contribute to the coagulation process. The secondary fibrinolysis resolves as the intravascular clotting is controlled and only rarely are antifibrinolytic agents, e.g., ϵ-aminocaproic acid, required.

HYPERFIBRINOLYSIS

The fibrinolytic system is one of the body's basic defense systems, existing to restore and maintain patency of blood vessels and other tubular structures which are at risk of being occluded by fibrin. Plasminogen, the inactive precursor of plasmin, is tightly bound to fibrinogen and, when clotting occurs, is incorporated into the fibrin clot. Intravascular fibrin deposition causes a liberation of the intravascular plasminogen activator(s) that convert plasminogen to plasmin, an endopeptidase, which digests fibrin and fibrinogen. Plasmin activity may also be increased through the administration of plasminogen activators such as urokinase or streptokinase. Fibrin is the preferred substrate for plasmin; however, plasmin will nonspecifically digest other components of the coagulation system, i.e., Factors V, VIII, IX, and XI.

Fibrinolysis occurs whenever plasmin is present in amounts greater than can be inhibited by the naturally occurring antiplasmins. Also, α-2-macroglobulin and an α-1-globulin inhibitor, α-1-antitrypsin, inactivate plasmin but at a much slower rate than the specific antiplasmins.

Excessive activation of the fibrinolytic system occurs most often as a response to diffuse intravascular clotting, but may on rare occasions become clinically significant after electric shock, profound hypotension, cardiac arrest, or infusions of activators (e.g., streptokinase or urokinase) or of plasmin-activator combinations (e.g., Thrombolysin). Plasminogen activation can be inhibited through the administration of ϵ-aminocaproic acid or other activator inhibitors [28].

Hyperfibrinolysis may be primary or secondary, with secondary hyperfibrinolysis referring to the fibrinolytic activity that occurs in response to intravascular coagulation. Both primary and secondary hyperfibrinolysis may cause bleeding into body cavities, bleeding around intravenous needles and indwelling catheters, and delayed surgical or traumatic bleeding.

Systemic hypofibrinolysis probably occurs only after the administration of a fibrinolytic inhibitor or during prolonged debilitating illness and may contribute to in vivo thrombus propagation. Local hypofibrinolysis occurs in areas of vascular trauma and may contribute to thrombus propagation and persistence [28].

PRIMARY HYPERFIBRINOLYSIS

Primary hyperfibrinolysis may cause spontaneous bleeding and may be confused with the intravascular coagulation-defibrination syndrome. It is usually associated with conditions causing sudden death (e.g., major trauma, electric shock, massive myocardial infarction, and acute hypoxia) that result in the release of massive quantities of fibrinolytic activators. Primary hyperfibrinolysis is responsible for less than 1 percent of nonmechanical bleeding.

DIAGNOSIS

Clinical and laboratory manifestations are dependent on the amount of fibrinolytic activity. Mild hyperfibrinolysis is often not detected because coagulation studies may be normal, other than increases of fibrin degradation products, and its only manifestation may be delayed or persistent bleeding. Rapid clot lysis or the absence of clot formation may be the manifestations of major hyperfibrinolytic activity, with decreased plasma fibrinogen levels and prolongation of the PT and PTT because of nonspecific proteolysis of clotting factors, principally Factors V, VIII, IX, and XI, by plasmin. The platelet count usually is normal in this disorder.

Laboratory studies will demonstrate shortening of the whole blood lysis time (normal range 90–120 min), euglobulin lysis time (normal range 6–24 hr), reduction of circulating plasminogen, and increased lytic activity of plasma incubated on fibrin plates.

MANAGEMENT

Management is directed primarily toward correcting the underlying defect (e.g., eliminating the hypoxia or hypotension). In most instances, the hyperfibrinolysis resolves as normal conditions are restored. If primary hyperfibrinolysis persists, ε-aminocaproic acid (Amicar) can be given intravenously or orally. The usual dose is 5 gm during the first hour and 1 gm/hr for 6 to 8 hours. If sufficient coagulation factors are present for thrombosis to occur, it is advisable to use small amounts (300–500 units/hr) of heparin simultaneously to prevent intravascular coagulation, since fibrinolysis will be inhibited by Amicar. Rapid intravenous administration of Amicar should be avoided; this has been associated with hypotension, bradycardia, or arrhythmias. It is difficult to prevent primary hyperfibrinolysis, since the initiating event is usually unexpected and frequently not preventable.

SECONDARY HYPERFIBRINOLYSIS

Secondary hyperfibrinolysis occurs much more commonly than primary hyperfibrinolysis, but is a less common cause of bleeding than is the bleeding that accompanies consumption of coagulation factors by excessive intravascular coagulation. The effects of the secondary fibrinolysis may be undetectable or may be excessive and cause active bleeding by lysis of protective clots and by contributing to, through proteolysis, the diminished supply of coagulation factors.

DIAGNOSIS

Secondary hyperfibrinolysis may cause a diffuse oozing or may cause previously "dry" surgical areas to bleed. Increased fibrinolytic activity may be detected by shortening of the euglobulin lysis and whole blood lysis times, decreases in plasminogen, increases in fibrin split products, and increased lysis zones when plasma is placed on fibrin plates. It must be remembered that the fibrinolytic activity is usually secondary to excessive intravascular coagulation, and simultaneous tests of coagulation should be done to establish the relative role of the fibrinolytic process in the bleeding disorder.

MANAGEMENT

Treatment of secondary hyperfibrinolysis should be directed primarily toward the elimination of the cause of the intravascular coagulation. If excessive fibrinolytic activity persists after coagulation has stopped, and the coagulation factors are being restored, Amicar may be utilized in the same manner and with the same precautions as for primary hyperfibrinolysis. Secondary hyperfibrinolysis can be prevented by preventing excessive intravascular coagulation. This can be done by eliminating stasis, protecting the vascular intimal surfaces, and decreasing the propensity for coagulation to occur with anticoagulants such as heparin.

PLATELET DISORDERS

PHYSIOLOGY

Platelets are produced in the bone marrow by megakaryocytes and released into the circulation under the regulation of thrombopoietin. Platelet production can increase to six to eight times the normal amount in response to chronic platelet loss. The normal platelet count is $250,000/mm^3$ plus or minus 40,000. Platelets have an average life span of 9.5 days. Under normal circumstances, two-thirds of the total platelet population are in general circulation and one-third in the spleen. The platelets in the spleen exchange freely with those in the general circulation. Up to 90 percent of the circulating platelets may be found in the spleen during times of hypersplenism and thrombocytopenia. Normal platelet turnover rates are $35,000/mm^3$ plus or minus 4,300 per day.

Platelets contribute to the maintenance of hemostasis by: (1) helping maintain vascular integrity; (2) forming the initial hemostatic plug in response to the interruption of vascular continuity; and (3) accelerating the coagulation cascade through the provision of a reactive surface and the phospholipid requirements of several of the activation reactions of the coagulation factors.

The mechanisms by which platelets help maintain normal vascular integrity remain unknown. The reduction to 10 percent or less of circulating platelets contributes to the migration of red cells through the vascular wall and the formation of petechiae and purpura.

When platelets are exposed to vascular basement membrane and collagen in areas of intimal disruption, platelet adhesion with subsequent aggregation is induced. Platelets release their granule contents during the later stages of aggregation. One of the platelet release products, adenosine diphosphate (ADP), stimulates other platelets to adhere to the growing mass of platelets and to form the initial hemostatic plug. Irreversible fusion of the platelet mass follows thrombin-induced release of additional platelet constituents and the development of a fibrin clot.

Platelets have important roles in the initiation and acceleration of the two coagulation cascades. Platelet membrane adsorbs and transports plasma coagulation factors and provides a surface for their activation. The phospholipid cofactors of several of the reactions of the clotting mechanism are provided by components of the platelet membrane. The fibrin network formed by activation of the coagulation system serves to stabilize the initial platelet hemostatic plug. Contraction of platelet microfilaments in conjunction with the activated Factor XIII leads to clot retraction. Platelet Factor IV, released during platelet aggregation, demonstrates heparin-neutralizing activity.

The template bleeding time provides a reasonable estimate of platelet function. The formation of the initial platelet plug is unimpaired when the concentration of normal platelets is 100,000/mm^3 or more. The bleeding time may be prolonged when fewer platelets are present.

Several tests of platelet function are available: assays of platelet adhesion, aggregation patterns in response to ADP, epinephrine, and collagen; platelet factor III availability, and clot retraction. Unfortunately, these tests are not generally available, are difficult to standardize, and are subject to unexplained variability that makes their interpretation difficult.

Platelet disorders can occur from acquired or congenital causes affecting the numbers of circulating platelets or platelet function. Acquired platelet disorders are far more common than congenital platelet disorders.

CONGENITAL PLATELET DISORDERS
ESSENTIAL THROMBOCYTHEMIA
Essential thrombocythemia is characterized by spontaneous bleeding and thrombosis and is often associated with splenomegaly in patients over 30 years of age. Gastrointestinal bleeding is common, and there is an increased incidence of both arterial and venous thrombosis. Purpura is usually not present. Essential thrombocythemia is a rare disorder. Both sexes are equally

affected. The platelet count is greater than 1 million, and the platelets have bizarre shapes. An associated leukocytosis and an iron-deficiency anemia may be present.

Treatment is by reduction of the platelet count with radioactive phosphorus or alkylating agents such as melphalan or nitrogen mustard. To reduce the ability of platelets to aggregate, aspirin and dipyridamole, alone or in combination, are recommended; 300 mg of aspirin 4 times a day and 50 mg dipyridamole 4 times a day are satisfactory. Anticoagulants may be required to prevent in vivo thrombosis until the platelet count can be reduced. Splenectomy is contraindicated in this disorder since it is often associated with exacerbation of the thrombocythemia, thrombosis, hemorrhage, and death [37].

HEREDITARY THROMBOCYTOPENIA

Five hereditary thrombocytopenic states have been described; all are uncommon. They include the following:

1. *Bernard-Soulier syndrome.* In this syndrome, the platelets are larger than normal and are often decreased in number. The bleeding tendency is not directly related to the thrombocytopenia.
2. *Wiskott-Aldrich syndrome.* This is characterized by thrombocytopenia and reduced levels of the immunoglobulin IgM, which is responsible for the recurrent pyogenic infections and eczema. The platelets are small and have a decreased life span.
3. *Thrombocytopenia with absent radius.* In this condition, the platelets are decreased in number, and the megakaryocytes are abnormal. Other skeletal abnormalities are frequently present in addition to the absent radius.
4. *May-Hegglin anomaly.* In this anomaly, giant platelets are present, with Dohle bodies (areas of basophilic cytoplasm) in the leukocytes. Most patients are asymptomatic, but bleeding can occur.
5. *Hereditary thrombocytopenia resembling idiopathic thrombocytopenic purpura.* These patients, whose symptoms begin in early life, have a positive familial history of purpura. The in vitro assay for antiplatelet antibodies is negative, whereas in idiopathic thrombocytopenic purpura it is often positive.

ABNORMAL PLATELET FUNCTION

THROMBASTHENIA (GLANZMANN'S DISEASE). The signs of thrombasthenia are petechiae, ecchymoses, mucous membrane hemorrhages, and severe anemia. Thrombasthenia occurs early in life; the frequency of bleeding episodes tends to decrease with age. It is rare and inherited as an autosomal recessive trait.

Characteristically, defective clot retraction is associated with a normal platelet count, PT, and PTT. Abnormal platelet morphology is present. The bleeding time may or may not be prolonged. ADP does not induce aggregation in platelet-rich plasma. Platelet adhesiveness is reduced. Platelet transfusions are recommended for treatment, but their effectiveness is variable.

THROMBOCYTOPATHIA. *Thrombocytopathia* is a general term referring to any disorder of platelet function other than thrombasthenia. Patients with these disorders characteristically have prolonged bleeding times in the presence of normal platelet counts. Such disorders are uncommon and await further clinical characterization.

ACQUIRED PLATELET DISORDERS
THROMBOCYTOSIS
A 30 to 100 percent increase in platelets can follow trauma, fractures of the long bones, or surgery. Thrombocytosis commonly occurs 2 to 5 days following splenectomy and usually peaks at 7 to 10 days. Acquired thrombocytosis may also be seen in association with myeloproliferative disorders, such as polycythemia vera and chronic granulocytic leukemia [20, 37]. Thromboembolism may occur with thrombocytosis, but hemorrhagic phenomena are rare unless hemorrhage occurs following thrombosis and secondary necrosis. Occasionally, intravascular coagulation with secondary bleeding may result when the platelet count is increased sufficiently. The incidence of this condition reflects the incidence of the precipitating stress or associated myeloproliferative disorder.

If increased thrombocytosis, with a platelet count greater than 1 million/mm^3 in adults, occurs, one should protect the patient by preventing clotting with heparin or preventing platelet adhesiveness with dipyridamole (100 mg 4 times a day). Children may tolerate platelet counts of up to 2 million/mm^3 (or more) before manifesting symptoms. Thrombocytosis in association with myeloproliferative disorders requires concomitant use of chemotherapy as outlined for essential thrombocythemia.

ACQUIRED THROMBOCYTOPENIA
IDIOPATHIC THROMBOCYTOPENIA
Idiopathic thrombocytopenia (ITP) is most often seen in children and young adults. Less than 10 percent of the cases occur in patients over 40 years of age. Purpura is a hallmark, although excessive bleeding following trauma or surgery may attract attention to a condition that has been present for some time. Familial ITP is rare.

Characteristically, the platelet count is below 60,000/mm^3 (in acute cases, often less than 10,000/mm^3), the bleeding time is prolonged, and the PT, PTT, and clotting time are normal. Studies by Dixon et al. and others have demonstrated increased concentrations of platelet surface–associated immunoglobulins in idiopathic thrombocytopenic purpura [10, 23].

Although platelet transfusions are useful in bleeding crises, they are not routinely used in persistent cases. A limited trial with corticosteroids is advocated, with 60–100 mg of prednisone usually being given daily for 2 weeks. If the number of platelets increases, the dose is reduced 20 mg per week until a 30-mg daily dosage level is achieved. This is gradually reduced to a maintenance level of 10 mg daily. Splenectomy is recommended in patients with splenomegaly, splenic sequestration of platelets documented by platelet scan, or in patients who are unresponsive to the nonoperative management. However, the beneficial effects of splenectomy may be temporary, with ITP recurring in approximately 30 percent of these patients. Work by Dixon et al. has suggested that the duration of the beneficial effect of splenectomy is related to the concentration of platelet surface–bound immunoglobulins, high concentrations being associated with the recurrence of ITP following splenectomy [10].

THROMBOTIC THROMBOCYTOPENIC PURPURA

Thrombotic thrombocytopenic purpura is a rare platelet disorder characterized by microangiopathic anemia, thrombocytopenia, fever, neurological manifestations, and renal abnormalities. The characteristic clinical findings are secondary to occlusions of the microcirculation with a hyaline-like material. Over 400 cases have been reported, and multiple etiologies for this disorder have been proposed. It affects females slightly more often than males and has a peak incidence in the third decade of life. If untreated, it rapidly progresses and is often fatal [5].

Laboratory findings include schistocytes and other evidence of a microangiopathic anemia, marked thrombocytopenia, and renal dysfunction with proteinuria, hematuria, and rising blood urea nitrogen and creatinine. The diagnosis may be established conclusively with a gingival biopsy, which demonstrates occlusion of the microcirculation with hyaline-like material, intimal proliferation, but no evidence of vasculitis.

Management consists of steroids (1,000–2,000 mg of cortisone equivalents/day), and antiplatelet drugs (aspirin 600–1,200 mg/day and dipyridamole 300–400 mg/day), all in equally divided doses. Splenectomy is offered to patients who fail to respond to the steroids and antiplatelet agents. The disorder has been controlled in 70 percent of the patients treated with steroids, antiplatelet agents, and splenectomy [38].

SECONDARY THROMBOCYTOPENIA PURPURA

Thrombocytopenia may occur secondarily to the following: (1) chemical agents, such as chlorothiazide (Diuril), chlorpropamide (Diabinase), tolbutamide (Orinase), chloramphenicol, quinidine, procainamide, and, on rare occasions, heparin; (2) hematopoietic disorders, such as acute leukemia, aplastic anemia, autoimmune hemolytic anemia, pernicious anemia, and those secondary to splenomegaly from any cause; (3) transfusion reactions or multiple transfusions of compatible blood; (4) infections—e.g., gram-negative bacteremia, infectious hepatitis, and Rocky Mountain spotted fever; and (5) excessive intravascular coagulation.

Thrombocytopenia is likely to be responsible for bleeding only if the platelet count is less than 30,000/mm³. Estimates from blood smears are unreliable; quantitative counts should be done by phase contrast microscopy or with the Coulter electronic counter.

Clinical manifestations of secondary thrombocytopenic purpura vary with the precipitating agent or drug. Petechiae and mucosal and cutaneous purpura are present. Occult gastrointestinal bleeding is common.

The primary cause of the thrombocytopenia should be eliminated if possible. If platelets are needed to control hemorrhagic manifestations, transfusion with type-specific platelet (and preferably HL-A cross-matched) concentrates can be utilized. Type-specific and HL-A–cross-matched platelets will minimize the development of alloantibodies, which can significantly shorten the life span of subsequently infused platelets [8].

Prophylactic therapy of thrombocytopenia is aimed at maintaining the platelet count above $30,000/mm^3$. Transfusion of up to 8 units of platelets every 6 to 8 hours may be required to control hemorrhage. Each unit contains the majority of platelets in a unit of whole blood reduced to a volume of approximately 30 to 50 cc of plasma and represents approximately 75×10^9 platelets. When control of the hemorrhage is established, the frequency of transfusion can be reduced. Prophylactic therapy of severe thrombocytopenia may require platelet transfusions every 2 or 3 days until the thrombocytopenia resolves. Treatment of thrombocytopenia secondary to hypersplenism or autoimmune disease will lead to decreased platelet survival times because the transfused platelets are subject to the same destructive forces as the native platelets; thus, platelet transfusions may have to be repeated at more frequent intervals.

Adrenocorticosteroids may increase the platelet count, although the indications for their use remain poorly defined at this time. Splenectomy is frequently indicated when splenomegaly is present or when the cause cannot be treated or removed and bleeding manifestations persist.

ABNORMAL PLATELET FUNCTION

Although many commonly used drugs such as aspirin, antihistamines, and tranquilizers have been demonstrated to alter platelet function as assayed by in vitro platelet function tests, only aspirin, sulfinpyrazone, dipyridamole, and indomethacin have been associated with prolongation of the bleeding time and a clinically significant bleeding diathesis [4, 30]). Acquired platelet dysfunction has also been documented in uremia, chronic liver disease, and hyperglobulinemic states.

Abnormal platelet function is rarely the cause of significant bleeding; however, it may exacerbate existing bleeding, e.g., after trauma or surgery. It is diagnosed when tests for platelet adhesiveness and aggregation are abnormal.

Treatment is directed toward eliminating the underlying causes or stopping the associated drugs and giving platelet transfusions when necessary. It must be noted, however, that the effects of aspirin on the platelet are permanent; normal platelet function returns only when sufficient numbers of new platelets become available for hemostatic purposes. Total recovery may take 9 to 10 days, although functional recovery is usually apparent 1 to 2 days after the drug(s) is stopped.

EXCESSIVE ANTICOAGULATION
HEPARIN
Heparin is the most widely used and reliable anticoagulant available today. It is a negatively charged mucopolysaccharide of 5,000 to 50,000 daltons with a strong negative charge that imparts to it the capability to bind with specific lysine residues of antithrombin III. Heparin has essentially no anticoagulant activity in the absence of antithrombin III and acts principally through an allosteric effector mechanism that mediates a conformational change in antithrombin III and makes the arginine reactive center of this molecule more accessible to binding with the active serine center of thrombin and other serine proteases of the coagulation cascade. Antithrombin III can slowly inactivate the active forms of the serine protease clotting factors; however, in the presence of heparin this reaction is almost instantaneous. The heparin–antithrombin III complex has been shown to inhibit the actions of activated Factors IX, X, XI, and XII in addition to inactivating thrombin and plasmin [36].

Different concentrations of heparin have different modes of action. The minidose heparin regimen appears to be effective primarily through the inactivation of activated Factor X, while larger doses of heparin administered in the therapy of thromboembolic disease interfere with the function of all of the activated serine protease clotting factors.

COMPLICATIONS
The most common complication of heparin therapy is hemorrhage. However, allergic reactions, alopecia, and hyperaldosteronism have also been noted. A rare complication of heparin therapy, heparin-induced thrombocytopenia with associated thromboembolic complications rather than hemorrhage, is now being recognized with increasing frequency [18].

DIAGNOSIS OF BLEEDING FROM HEPARIN
The patient's history usually readily suggests that heparin may be the cause of bleeding. A significant prolongation of the clotting time (>30–40 min), activated partial thromboplastin time (APTT) (>120 sec), or activated clotting time (ACT) (>200 seconds) is usually present. To rule out associated coagulation factor deficiencies or fibrinolysis, thrombin times (TT) and protamine-corrected thrombin times (PCTT) should be done. If the ACT is abnormal and the TT normal, coagulation factor deficiencies exist. If both the ACT and the TT are abnormal and the PCTT is normal, incomplete heparin neutralization is present. An abnormal PCTT, ACT, and TT indicate that a fibrinogen deficiency exists and a workup for DIC should be performed [43].

MANAGEMENT

Bleeding secondary to overanticoagulation with heparin is best managed with discontinuation of the heparin. Its short half-life (1–2 hr) makes the need for heparin neutralization rare. Should heparin reversal be indicated, protamine can be utilized.

When clotting time or APTT is utilized for heparin monitoring, protamine sulfate should be given slowly until the clotting time or APTT returns toward normal. The amount of protamine required depends on the amount of heparin given, the interval between the administration of heparin and protamine, and the status of the patient's renal and hepatic function. It is best to give protamine in repeated small amounts until the coagulation studies return toward normal. The rule of 1 to 2 mg of protamine to neutralize 100 units of heparin is useful if a coagulation laboratory is not available. However, it is best to administer smaller amounts of protamine than thought necessary and to give additional protamine as indicated by the coagulation testing, because excesses of protamine may have an anticoagulant effect, and the too rapid injection of protamine may produce hypotension.

If the ACT method of anticoagulation monitoring is utilized, it may be possible to calculate the amount of protamine needed from a heparin dose response curve. This curve is derived by plotting the ACT versus heparin dose administered for both the control and 5-minute post–heparin-administration samples and joining these points with a straight line. A protamine dose equal to 1.3 times the calculated residual heparin usually provides adequate heparin neutralization [26, 43].

VITAMIN K ANTAGONISTS

Dicumarol, warfarin, and other vitamin K antagonists interfere with the action of vitamin K in the synthesis of Factors II, VII, IX, and X. A vitamin K–dependent carboxylase has been identified which is responsible for the conversion of glutamyl residues on the clotting factor precursors to gamma carboxy-glutamyl residues. This conversion is necessary for the binding of calcium, a necessary cofactor in the reactions catalyzed by the affected clotting factors. Patients receiving vitamin K antagonists produce clotting factor precursors that are antigenically similar to the normal factors, but are without procoagulant activity due to their abnormal calcium-binding characteristics. The reduction of the concentrations of clotting factors that retain normal activity slows clotting by reducing the amount and rate at which thrombin is produced.

DIAGNOSIS OF BLEEDING SECONDARY TO ADMINISTRATION OF VITAMIN K ANTAGONISTS

The prothrombin time is most often utilized to monitor the effects of the vitamin K antagonists. Bleeding often occurs when the PT remains less than 10 percent of the control value (i.e., >25 sec). Prolongation of the PT may occur from an overdose of the prescribed drug or from synergistic effects between the vitamin K antagonists and other drugs. Salicylates, sulfon-amides, indomethacin, quinidine, clofibrate, and other drugs have mild additive effects either through interference with intestinal absorption of vitamin K or through displacement of the vitamin K–antagonistic agents from their plasma carrier proteins, thus increasing their availability to the liver, where they interfere with the synthesis of the vitamin K–dependent clotting factors. It is unlikely that any patient with a PT greater than 30 percent of the control value (or less than 19 sec when the control is 13 sec) will bleed spontaneously or bleed excessively during an operation. Only when the PT is less than 10 percent of the control is excessive or spontaneous bleeding likely to occur.

MANAGEMENT

If bleeding is not life-threatening, clotting abnormalities are best treated by discontinuing the vitamin K antagonists and occasionally by the administration of parenteral vitamin K_1. Giving 25 mg of vitamin K_1 slowly intravenously usually produces a dramatic response within a few hours and returns the PT to normal within 24 hours regardless of the anticoagulant used, provided the patient does not have concomitant hepatic failure. Intramuscular or subcutaneous injections of 5 to 10 mg of vitamin K_1 for the next day or two will usually completely correct the clotting abnormalities induced by the vitamin K antagonists. It must be recognized that rapid and total correction of the anticoagulant state induced by the vitamin K antagonists could contribute to the development of thromboses, and alternate methods of anticoagulation should be considered once hemorrhage is controlled.

If instantaneous correction of the vitamin K–dependent factor deficiency is needed, transfusion with whole blood, fresh frozen plasma, stored plasma, or lyophylized plasma can be used, since the depressed factors are stable. This mode of therapy carries the risk of transmitting hepatitis to the patient. Hepatitis has followed blood or plasma transfusions in as many as 11 percent of patients receiving multiple transfusions. The risk is even higher in patients receiving plasma concentrates and approaches 40 percent in patients receiving fibrinogen infusions [42].

DIAGNOSIS OF BLEEDING DISORDERS
HISTORY

The type of bleeding experienced by the patient, its course, and frequency may help determine the etiology of the bleeding. Prolonged or excessive bleeding with circumcision, tooth extractions, menstruation, trauma, operative procedures, or a history of spontaneous bleeding, chronic iron deficiency anemia, and repeated blood transfusions may be indicative of defects in the hemostatic mechanism. If a family history of bleeding is present, the clinician should try to establish its cause and the pattern of inheritance.

A history of drug therapy with direct or indirect anticoagulants, platelet depressants, broad spectrum antibiotics, or chemotherapy may suggest the etiology of the excessive bleeding. Local or systemic diseases such as leukemia, uremia, collagen vascular disorders, and liver disease may aggravate or even cause a hemorrhagic diathesis.

PHYSICAL EXAM

One should look for the presence and distribution of petechiae, purpura, ecchymoses, jaundice, and hemangiomas. Raised petechiae are most commonly associated with vasculitis, whereas flat petechiae, principally in areas of increased hydrostatic pressure, are usually indicative of thrombocytopenia. Widespread ecchymoses in combination with hematuria and gastrointestinal hemorrhage are common in acquired coagulation defects. Hemarthroses, residual joint deformities, and hematomas secondary to arteriolar bleeding are common sequelae of congenital coagulation factor deficiencies.

Splenomegaly may be associated with thrombocytopenia. Lymphadenopathy or hepatosplenomegaly may indicate the presence of an infiltrative malignancy affecting organs responsible for clotting factor synthesis or platelet production. The stigmata of chronic liver disease, such as ascites and portosystemic collateral channels, should alert one to the possibility of deficiencies in clotting factors synthesized by the liver.

LABORATORY TESTING

The etiology of nonmechanical bleeding can usually be determined by performing a battery of screening tests and, when needed, specific quantitative tests of coagulation and lysis. The screening battery should include the following: fibrinogen concentration; PT, PTT, and TT (if the TT is prolonged, a protamine titration test should be performed); whole-blood lysis time or euglobulin clot lysis time; platelet count (platelet aggregation studies are performed when indicated); and fibrin split product concentrations. The traditional bleeding and clotting times are rarely useful in detecting latent bleeders.

The results of the screening battery (Table 19-4) should permit identification of the various types of bleeding. Specific testing will distinguish between the various acquired and congenital coagulation deficiencies. The whole-blood lysis time and euglobulin lysis time are shortened in both primary and secondary hyperfibrinolysis. If primary lysis is excessive, the coagulation proteins will be lysed and the tests of coagulation prolonged. The main differentiating feature will be a normal platelet count in patients with primary hyperfibrinolysis but a decreased platelet count in those with secondary hyperfibrinolysis.

Low platelet counts may be detected during episodes of thrombocytopenia and DIC. The coagulation factors are markedly decreased during DIC, but they are normal in thrombocytopenia. Significant bleeding is much more common with DIC than with thrombocytopenia.

TABLE 19-4. Results of Screening Battery in Various Nonmechanical Bleeding Disorders

Type of Bleeding Disorder	Fibrinogen Content	Prothrombin Time (PT)	Partial Thrombo-plastin Time (PTT)	Thrombin Time	Lysis Time	Platelet Count	Fibrin Split Products
Congenital coagulation deficiencies	N-A	N-A[a]	N-A[a]	N-A	N	N	N
Disseminated intravascular coagulation	A	A	A	N-A	A	A	A
Decreased platelet number	N	N	N	N	N	A	N
Decreased platelet function[b]	N	N	N	N	N	N	N
Hyperfibrinolysis	N-A	N-A	N-A	N-A	A	N	N-A
Excessive heparin	N	A[c]	A[c]	A[c]	N	N	N
Excessive prothrombinopenic agents	N	A	A	N	N	N	N

A = abnormal; N = normal.

[a] A normal PT and PTT exclude hemophilia and the parahemophilias (except von Willebrand's disease) as a cause of bleeding and indicate that the vitamin K factors are present in adequate amounts. If either the PT or PTT is abnormal, variations of the PTT can be used to determine the specific coagulation defect.

[b] Specific tests of adhesion or aggregation are necessary to define abnormalities of platelet function.

[c] Heparin interferes with most tests of coagulation. If the heparin is "neutralized" with protamine, the PT, PTT, and thrombin time will become normal if the coagulation factors are normal.

463

Normal coagulation factors, normal platelet counts, normal lysis times, and a prolonged TT that is corrected with protamine suggest the presence of excessive heparin. Normal platelets, TT, and lysis times and prolonged PT and PTT suggest depletion of vitamin K–dependent coagulation factors. A normal PT and prolonged PTT suggest that hemophilia or one of the parahemophilias could be the cause of the bleeding.

BLOOD AND BLOOD COMPONENT THERAPY

Blood transfusions have traditionally been utilized to restore the blood volume, increase the oxygen-carrying capacity of the blood, and provide coagulation proteins and platelets. Unfortunately, despite advances in techniques, preservatives, and additives for preserving blood, the limited ex vivo preservability of blood prohibits the acquisition of sufficient quantities of whole blood for all patients' needs. However, blood can be separated into its various components, e.g., (1) cellular—red cells, platelets, and white cells; (2) cryoprecipitate; and (3) cryoprecipitate-poor plasma, which is frequently further divided into components. The components, with appropriate processing, can be stored for long periods of time and thus are available for the needs of patients.

Recent reviews of transfusion practices have suggested that 35 to 50 percent of all transfusions are unnecessary and that only about 1 percent are lifesaving procedures [12]. Complications of blood replacement include transfusion reactions, plasma component sensitization, overexpansion of the intravascular volume, and the risk of the transmission of hepatitis. A thorough knowledge of blood and blood component therapy is essential for safe, effective hemotherapy in trauma and surgical patients.

WHOLE BLOOD

It is likely that the transfusion of whole blood will continue to decline as more and more blood is separated into its components and as physicians realize that their patients do at least as well with transfusions of blood components as they would with whole blood transfusions. Less than 15 percent of the blood transfusions on the surgical service at the University of Missouri Medical Center are whole blood tranfusions.

In addition to the previously mentioned coagulation abnormalities that can be induced by transfusions of large volumes of banked whole blood, progressive alterations of the acid-base status and plasma electrolytes during storage of blood may also adversely affect the recipient of the blood.

Citrate-phosphate-dextrose (CPD) is the anticoagulant-storage solution currently being utilized by most blood banks. Even with CPD and 4° C storage, progressive changes occur in stored blood: (1) the pH falls from 7 at the time of collection to 6.89 and 6.84 at days 14 and 21, respectively; (2) the plasma potassium increases to 10, 20, and 25 mEq/liter at 1, 2, and 3 weeks of storage; (3) 2,3-DPG decreases from 12.5 to 7 and 3.7 μg/gm of hemoglobin by 14 and 21 days of storage; and (4) the plasma ammonia concentration increases from 95 to 255 and 330 mg per 100 ml at storage days 14 and 21 [22]. These changes usually have no effect upon the healthy adult transfusion recipient but may markedly adversely affect the patient with pulmonary, renal, or hepatic insufficiency. Therefore, these patients should receive whole blood that has been stored less than a week or receive red cells only, since the excessive ammonia, potassium, and so on are in the plasma.

The citrate and phosphate in the preservation solution plus the acidotic metabolites that accumulate may contribute to the decline of the pH in the trauma or surgical patients receiving multiple blood transfusions. Rather than administering alkali routinely (e.g., 50 mEq of sodium bicarbonate for each 5 units of blood transfused) during transfusions, it is preferable to monitor the patient's pH frequently and correct it when necessary. Furthermore, the maintenance of the patient's pH near normal helps restore red cell 2,3-DPG and improves oxygen delivery.

Surgeons commonly request whole blood for restoring blood volume. Presumably, their reasoning is that "the patient is bleeding whole blood, which should be replaced with whole blood." Almost without exception, the blood volume can be restored and maintained with red cells plus a crystalloid or colloid. Ringer's lactate, isotonic saline, plasma, fresh frozen plasma, dextran, and even albumin can restore the blood volume. Unless coagulation abnormalities require fresh frozen plasma, we most often use Ringer's lactate with red cells to restore blood volume and hematocrit. Albumin and plasma substitutes are rarely utilized or needed.

The citrate of the CPD solution binds calcium and thus prevents clotting. Excesses of citrate in the transfused blood or blood components can combine with ionized serum calcium. It has been speculated that the excess of citrate (citrate intoxication) could drastically reduce the availability of ionized calcium and thus interfere with muscular, especially myocardial, activity and the ability of blood to coagulate. For these reasons, calcium has been given empirically, usually in a dose of 10 ml of 10% calcium gluconate for each 1,000 ml of blood transfused. However, studies indicate that calcium is never needed in vivo to augment the coagulation mechanism and is only rarely indicated (e.g., after massive transfusions in an acidotic patient, after cardiopulmonary bypass) in patients to improve myocardial contractility [15, 16, 31].

The cool operating room environment and administration of cold blood may be associated with clinically significant hypothermia in the surgical patient [1]. In order to limit this heat loss, it is recommended that warm blood be given to all infants, all debilitated and elderly patients, patients who are undergoing long operative procedures, and patients who receive more than 4 units of blood. A number of blood-warming devices are available. Before any device is used, it should be carefully calibrated to ensure that the warming temperature does not exceed 40° C. When blood is exposed to temperatures a few degrees above 40° C, lysis of cells and coagulation of proteins may occur, with adverse effects upon the recipients of such blood.

The filters included in blood transfusion sets remove large clots and other debris from the blood being transfused. However, these filters have a large pore size (120–170 μ) that permits the infusion of smaller particles. It has been demonstrated that the microaggregates of stored blood may contribute to pulmonary and other organ system dysfunction [11, 34]. Micropore filters have been designed to be added to blood transfusion sets. The authors have found the 40-μ filter (Pall) adequate to remove microaggregates while permitting rapid infusion of large amounts of blood. We recommend that the filter be changed after every second or third unit of blood and be used without exception in all trauma patients, all patients with respiratory insufficiency, and in most other patients who will be receiving more than 3 units of blood.

BLOOD COMPONENTS

The modern blood bank can readily separate a unit of blood into red cells, platelets, cryoprecipitate, and cryoprecipitate-poor plasma. Some of the plasma is frozen as fresh frozen plasma to preserve the coagulation factors; other portions are utilized by the Red Cross or commercial firms to prepare specific plasma fractions, e.g., fibrinogen, albumin, or concentrates of Factors II, VII, IX, and X. The use of these blood components for improving coagulation has been reviewed in earlier sections of this chapter. This section will review red cell preparation, plasma concentrates, and albumin and some of the hazards associated with the transfusion of blood components.

RED CELLS

Red cell packs have an average hematocrit of 70% and, in the absence of continuing hemorrhage, each pack will increase the hematocrit of the recipient 3 to 5 percent. Packed red cells are especially useful for restoring oxygen-carrying capacity in patients with a compromised cardiac reserve because of the reduced volume transfused or in patients with hepatic or renal insufficiency because removal of the plasma reduces the level of potassium, ammonia, and other potentially renal and hepatic toxic metabolites.

The usable shelf-life of red cells in whole blood or packed cells remains 21 days, thus limiting the supply of red cells. It is now possible to freeze red cells and to store them indefinitely at −80° C. Advantages associated with the use of frozen red cells include a reduction in the number of febrile, nonhemolytic transfusion reactions; a marked reduction of transfused microemboli; the ability to stockpile rare blood types and autologous blood for elective surgery; and a reduction in the transmission of disease by transfusion. The observed reduction in posttransfusion hepatitis following the use of frozen red cells appears to be due to dilution of the infectious agent during the washing procedure, since it has been demonstrated that the agent responsible for type B hepatitis is not destroyed by the freezing and deglycerolization process [25]. The freezing of the red cells preserves high energy substrates and 2,3-DPG, thus reducing the oxygen-transport abnormalities noted with the use of regular banked blood.

Frozen red cell suspensions are essentially devoid of leukocytes and platelets. There is controversy regarding the need to transfuse transplant recipients and potential recipients with frozen blood which is leukocyte-poor and not likely to sensitize the patient to transplant antigens. Some studies support the use of leukocyte-poor blood, while others indicate that sensitization with leukocytes may enhance transplant survival [7].

The use of frozen red cells has been hampered by the high cost of processing, the complexity of deglycerolization procedures, and the 24-hour shelf-life of thawed, resuspended red cells [25]. It appears certain, however, that many of these problems will be overcome and that more and more centers for freezing and storing red cells will be developed so that the national supply will be increased, specific blood types will always be available, and leukocyte-poor red cells will be available, if needed.

PLASMA AND PLASMA CONCENTRATES
Plasma and plasma concentrates are utilized to expand the intravascular volume and to correct clotting factor deficiencies. Stored plasma may be used in the treatment of hypovolemia secondary to the loss of the plasma component of the intravascular volume, such as occurs with major burns, and in the treatment of coagulation disorders involving the vitamin K–dependent factors. Fresh frozen plasma should be used to correct acquired deficiencies of the labile clotting factors. The plasma to be transfused should be compatible with the ABO and Rh antigens of the recipient.

Plasma protein fraction is derived from pooled human plasma and is composed principally of albumin and alpha and beta globulins. It contains no clotting factors, gamma globulins, agglutinins, or cellular elements. Because it is heat treated during its processing, it is virtually free of the risk of hepatitis transmission. It is principally used for intravascular volume replacement. Use of plasma protein fraction has been associated in some cases with the production of clinically significant hypotension, thought to be due to the presence of the alpha and beta globulins [3].

Clotting factor concentrates are derived from pooled plasma but are not heat treated; thus, their use is associated with a high incidence of posttransfusion hepatitis.

ALBUMIN
Albumin does not expose the patient to hepatitis and may be utilized to expand the plasma volume and occasionally to treat hypoalbuminemic or hy-

poproteinemic states such as occur during malnutrition, hepatic insufficiency, or the nephrotic syndrome. Albumin may also be used as a plasma binding agent for the removal of toxic agents with exchange transfusions, as in the case of infants with erythroblastosis fetalis [3]. We prefer crystalloid solutions for expanding the plasma volume and rarely use albumin.

PLATELET TRANSFUSIONS

Platelets may be stored at 4° C or at room temperature following their collection. Different temperatures have different effects on platelet survival and function following transfusion. Platelets stored at room temperature will require 24 hours following transfusion to acquire normal in vivo function but have an average life span of 8 to 11 days. Platelets stored at 4° C for up to 18 hours are hemostatically more competent but have an average life span of about 48 hours. This would suggest that the use of platelets stored at room temperature would be most effective in patients requiring prophylactic transfusions, i.e., leukemics and patients with aplastic anemia. Patients with active bleeding would benefit most from the immediate hemostatic competence afforded by the use of platelets stored at 4° C [8].

Recent work with frozen platelets using dimethylsulphoxide (DMSO, 5–7%) and storage at −80° C has been encouraging, the life span of the infused platelet being 8 to 9 days. Frozen platelets have been able to correct aspirin-induced prolongation of bleeding times in healthy volunteers within 24 hours, often within 2 hours, following transfusion of a single platelet unit. Widespread use of frozen platelets awaits determination of their effectiveness in the treatment of bleeding diatheses and development of processing facilities [40].

Use of platelet transfusions is associated with the risk of transmission of infectious diseases such as hepatitis, transfusion reactions, and sensitization to platelet antigens. Immunization against platelet antigens may represent a significant complication of platelet transfusion therapy and reduce the effectiveness of subsequent platelet transfusions.

The matching of platelets for ABO and Rh antigens represents the minimal requirement for platelet transfusions except in extreme emergencies. In addition, HL-A antigens are expressed on the platelet membrane surface. Matching of platelets for HL-A antigens is recommended in patients who are anticipated to receive multiple transfusions to reduce the development of alloantibodies.

BANKED AUTOLOGOUS BLOOD

Use of banked autologous blood for replacement of anticipated blood loss during elective surgical procedures has several advantages. Its use is not associated with hepatitis, isoimmunization to erythrocyte or leukocyte antigens, hemolytic transfusion reactions, or the transmission of other diseases from contaminated blood. As many as 3 units of autologous blood may be obtained from patients scheduled for elective surgery by beginning blood collection 6 weeks before the operation: 2 units of blood are drawn weekly or biweekly after the initial drawing, with readministration of an older unit. The major problem associated with this form of hemotherapy is the logistics associated with the collection and storage of autologous blood, but as this method of blood replacement becomes more widely utilized, this problem should be resolved [24].

AUTOTRANSFUSION

Autotransfusion has received increasing attention for the management of hemorrhage associated with trauma and major vascular procedures [2, 33, 44]. Although it avoids many of the problems associated with massive transfusions of banked blood (e.g., transmission of hepatitis, transfusion reactions, and nonavailability of large quantities of rare blood types), its use may cause significant alterations in coagulation parameters, may irreversibly damage the cellular elements of the blood, and may be associated with pulmonary embolization of microparticulate matter if appropriate additional filters are not utilized. Hemolysis, denaturation or degradation of plasma proteins including coagulation factors, and blood element trauma can be reduced by keeping the aspirating sucker tip below the blood level to prevent an air-fluid interface. Improper use of the Bentley autotransfusion unit has been associated with air embolism [33, 44].

Intraoperative autotransfusion appears to be safe if care is taken to avoid traumatic aspiration of the blood, micropore filters are utilized in the infusion line, and adequate systemic anticoagulation is maintained. Contraindications to autotransfusion include malignancy, fecal or gastrointestinal contamination of the blood, renal or hepatic insufficiency, a wound over 4 hours old, and inability systemically to anticoagulate the patient. Ideal situations for the use of autotransfusion are exsanguinating trauma and vascular procedures where intraoperative blood loss is anticipated to exceed 2 liters [33, 44].

TRANSFUSION REACTIONS

Transfusion reactions vary from mild febrile responses to severe hemolytic reactions with anemia, excessive intravascular coagulation, and renal impairment or failure. Allergic reactions are also encountered in 2 to 3 percent of patients receiving blood transfusions—usually characterized by the development of hives, pruritus, or a diffuse rash, but true anaphylactic reactions may develop on rare occasions.

Febrile reactions represent the most frequently encountered adverse response to blood transfusion therapy. These may be due to minor red cell, white cell, or platelet incompatibilities or a reaction to bacterial or other antigens in the blood. Febrile reactions are usually easily managed by discontinuing the transfusion and administering antipyretic agents. Because it is often impossible to differentiate simple febrile reactions from the initial stages of a hemolytic transfusion reaction or the infusion of bacterially contaminated blood, blood samples should be obtained from the transfusion set and the patient and should be recross-matched and cultured.

Bacteria generally do not propagate in refrigerated blood but upon rewarming the blood, they may multiply rapidly. Blood must be used within 2 hours after removal from refrigeration, and warm blood must not be restored. Blood contaminated during collection may be associated with endotoxemia and a disseminated intravascular coagulation syndrome. After stopping the transfusion and obtaining blood cultures, patients suspected of receiving contaminated blood should be treated with broad spectrum antibiotics, appropriate fluids, and steroids if refractory shock has occurred. These reactions must be treated aggressively and promptly to assure a successful outcome.

Allergic transfusion reactions are generally easily managed by discontinuing the transfusion and administering antihistamines. Blood should be sent for recross-matching and blood from another compatible donor utilized. Anaphylactoid reactions may require use of epinephrine, steroids, and fluid replacement for successful management.

HEMOLYTIC TRANSFUSION REACTIONS

Hemolytic transfusion reactions are the most common of the severe transfusion reactions and occur once in 15,000 to 20,000 transfusions. This reaction usually is brought about by destruction of the transfused red cells by antibodies in the recipient's plasma. Occasionally, the transfused plasma may have high titers of antibodies directed against antigens on the surface of the recipient's red cells. For this reason, cross-matching must demonstrate compatibility of both the cells and serum of the donor and the recipient prior to transfusion. Depending upon the titer of antibody present in the serum of the donor or recipient, hemolytic transfusion reactions may follow transfusion of as little as 25 to 50 ml of incompatible blood or may not be demonstrable until an entire unit has been transfused. The sequelae of a hemolytic transfusion reaction—anemia, hemoglobinemia, excessive intravascular coagulation, and impairment of renal function—are dependent upon the potency and titer of the antibody and amount of blood transfused.

Hemolytic transfusion reactions should be suspected when fever, chills, flushing, headache, nausea, vomiting, or flank pain develop during the transfusion. These symptoms may be followed by hypotension, hemoglobinemia, hemoglobinuria, and unexplained bleeding. These reactions generally occur with the first 20 to 30 minutes of transfusion, and therefore, patients should be closely monitored during this period. Anesthetized or unconscious patients may manifest only tachycardia, hypotension, and unexplained bleeding as the initial findings of a transfusion reaction.

When a hemolytic transfusion reaction is suspected, the transfusion should be discontinued immediately, and the remainder of the transfused blood and a fresh patient blood sample must be tested for compatibility. The urine should be screened for hemoglobinuria. The acute renal failure associated with an acute hemolytic transfusion reaction still carries a 50 percent mortality rate.

Management of a transfusion reaction consists of immediately discontinuing the blood transfusion and counteracting the hypotension and relative hypovolemia with intravenous fluids. Vasoconstrictors will compound the problem of decreased renal blood flow and are not recommended. Treatment with intravenous furosemide (20–80 mg) is recommended to improve renal blood flow and initiate a diuresis; the blood volume must be monitored to prevent the development of a drug-induced hypovolemia. Alkalinization of the urine with intravenous bicarbonate will promote the excretion of hemoglobin and minimize the precipitation of hemoglobin in the renal tubules. The intravascular coagulation usually ceases soon after the transfusion is discontinued and usually is of no consequence. If the intravascular coagulation continues, intravenous heparin may be useful (see the section on management of DIC) [13].

DELAYED TRANSFUSION REACTIONS
Sensitization to donor red cell antigens may follow transfusion by 10 to 14 days, with slow destruction of the transfused erythrocytes as the antibody titer increases. Symptoms may not occur in this reaction; a continuing decrease in the hematocrit 10 to 14 days following transfusion may be the only detectable manifestation. Delayed transfusion reactions may make subsequent cross-matching for other transfusions difficult. However, careful cross-matching must be done to avoid acute hemolytic reactions [32].

POSTTRANSFUSION PURPURA
Posttransfusion purpura is a rare, life-threatening complication that may follow blood transfusion by 7 to 10 days. In this syndrome the recipient's platelets are destroyed by an induced platelet isoantibody. Increased concentrations of platelet-associated IgG have been demonstrated in this disorder. The syndrome can be self-limiting, but management of severe cases may require use of steroids, plasmapheresis, or exchange transfusions to reduce the isoantibody concentration and restore the platelet count [9, 27].

*DISEASE TRANSMISSION BY BLOOD TRANSFUSIONS
AND BLOOD COMPONENT THERAPY*
Disease secondary to a circulating causative agent may be transmitted from an affected donor to a healthy recipient through blood or blood component transfusions. The majority of transmissible diseases may be detected through careful screening of the donor population, but three diseases still create

major problems in their detection and transmission by transfusion. These diseases are malaria, syphilis, and hepatitis. Of the three diseases, hepatitis is the most common and potentially serious disease transmitted by blood or blood component transfusions.

The incidence of posttransfusion hepatitis in a recent large Veterans Administration cooperative study was 11.3 percent, with 20 percent of the cases associated with jaundice and 80 percent anicteric. It is estimated that approximately 120,000 cases of anicteric and 30,000 cases of overt hepatitis occur annually following transfusions, with a mortality rate of 1 or 2 percent to 20 or 30 percent depending on the age, general condition, and associated illnesses of the patient [42].

The major risk factors associated with the development of posttransfusion hepatitis are the use of commercial blood sources, multiple transfusions, and transfusion of blood with detectable hepatitis-associated antigen (HAA) by radioimmunoassay. The overall incidence of hepatitis following transfusion of blood from volunteer donor sources averages 3.5 percent as compared to 6.5 percent following transfusion of a single unit of commercial blood and 27.2 percent in patients receiving 6 to 10 units of commercial blood [41, 42]. For this reason, the use of commercial blood has declined markedly; however, blood obtained from paid donors is still available, but must be labeled as coming from a nonvolunteer source.

The majority of cases of posttransfusion hepatitis are of the non A, non B variety (up to 90% in some series) and are transmitted by an unknown etiological agent. Hepatitis B or HAA positive hepatitis accounts for less than 20 percent of all cases of posttransfusion hepatitis. Although the recently developed sensitive radioimmunoassay for HAA allows for the detection of up to 85 percent of HAA positive infected donors and has decreased the incidence of HAA positive posttransfusion hepatitis, it has not significantly reduced the overall incidence of posttransfusion hepatitis [39, 42].

Prophylactic administration of immune serum globulin (ISG) to patients at high risk for the development of posttransfusion hepatitis has been advocated. Controlled studies have demonstrated beneficial effects associated with the prophylactic use of ISG only in cases involving icteric non–type B posttransfusion hepatitis. No beneficial effects were noted with its use in the prophylaxis of nonicteric or type B hepatitis. Use of hyperimmune globulin with demonstrable hepatitis B antibodies may be of benefit in the prophylaxis of hepatitis following exposure to blood components contaminated with HAA, but conclusive evidence for this is still lacking [39, 41].

The most successful means for the prevention of posttransfusion hepatitis is the judicious use of volunteer blood and blood component transfusions.

EMERGENCY TRANSFUSIONS
In emergency situations type-specific blood may be utilized to treat severe hemorrhage until fully cross-matched blood becomes available. ABO blood

group compatibility must always be respected, but Rh negative blood may be given safely to Rh positive recipients when otherwise compatible. Rh positive blood may be given to Rh negative recipients safely for a few days, but its use is contraindicated in Rh negative women of childbearing age, in previously sensitized Rh negative individuals, or for exchange transfusions in Rh positive infants with hemolytic disease of the newborn.

O negative blood may be lifesaving when type-specific or fully cross-matched blood is not available. Problems associated with the emergency use of O negative blood include the presence of harmful isoantibodies that are present in some type O plasmas. If significant amounts of these antibodies are transfused into a non–group O patient, they may react with the patient's red cells and necessitate continued use of type O blood for transfusion until the antibody titer falls. The harmful effects of the isoantibodies can be reduced through the use of O negative packed red cells rather than whole blood.

The problems associated with emergency transfusions are best managed by prevention—that is, the patient's potential need of hemotherapy should be anticipated whenever possible and cross-matched blood maintained in the blood bank when the need for transfusion is likely to arise.

REFERENCES

1. Boyan, C. P., and Howland, W. S. Cardiac arrest and temperature of bank blood. *J.A.M.A.* 183:58, 1963.
2. Brewster, D. C., Ambrosino, J. J., Darling, R. C., Davison, J. K., Warnock, D. E., May, A. R. L., and Abbott, W. M. Intraoperative autotransfusions in major vascular surgery. *Am. J. Surg.* 137:507, 1979.
3. Buchanan, E. C. Blood and blood substitutes for treating hemorrhagic shock. *Am. J. Hosp. Pharm.* 34:631, 1967.
4. Buchanan, G. R., Martin, V., Levine, P. H., Scoon, K., and Handin, R. I. The effects of "anti-platelet" drugs on bleeding time and platelet aggregation in normal human subjects. *Am. J. Clin. Path.* 68:355, 1977.
5. Bukowski, R. M., Hewlett, J. S., Harris, J. W., Hoffman, G. C., Battle, J. D., Silverblatt, E., and Yang, I. Exchange transfusions in the treatment of thrombotic thrombocytopenic purpura. *Semin. Hematol.* 13:219, 1976.
6. Campbell, E. W., Neff, S., and Bowdler, A. J. Therapy with Factor IX concentrate resulting in DIC and thromboembolic phenomena. *Transfusion* 18:94, 1978.
7. Check, W. Transfusions before transplant? Yes and no. *J.A.M.A.* 240:95, 1978.
8. Curtoni, E. S., and Gabrielli, A. Platelet transfusion. *Hematologica* 61:498, 1976.
9. Dainer, P. M., and Canada, E. D. Post-transfusion purpura and multiple transfusions. *Br. Med. J.* 2:999, 1977.
10. Dixon, R., Roose, W., and Ebberts, L. Quantitative determination of antibody in idiopathic thrombocytopenic purpura. *N. Engl. J. Med.* 292:230, 1975.
11. Gervin, A. S., Mason, K. G., and Buckman, R. F. The source and removal

of microaggregates in aged human blood and human blood components. *Surg. Gynecol. Obstet.* 141:582, 1975.

12. Gibbs, C. E., and Misenhimer, H. R. The use of blood transfusion in obstetrics. *Am. J. Obstet. Gynecol.* 93:26, 1965.

13. Goldfinger, D. Acute hemolytic transfusion reactions—a fresh look at pathogenesis and considerations regarding therapy. *Transfusion* 17:85, 1977.

14. Hilgartner, M. The management of hemophilia. In F. S. Morrison (Ed.), *Hemophilia.* Washington, D.C.: American Association of Blood Banks, 1978.

15. Howland, W. S., Jacobs, R., and Goulet, A. H. An evaluation of calcium administration during rapid blood replacement. *Anesth. Analg.* 39:557, 1960.

16. Howland, W. S., and Schweizer, O. Physiologic compensation for storage lesion of bank blood. *Anesth. Analg.* 44:8, 1965.

17. Jones, P. Developments and problems in the management of hemophilia. *Semin. Hematol.* 14:375, 1977.

18. Kapsch, D. N., Rhodes, G., Adelstein, E., and Silver, D. Heparin induced thrombocytopenia, thrombosis and hemorrhage. *Surgery* 86:148, 1979.

19. Kasper, C. K. Incidence and course of inhibitors among patients with classic hemophilia. *Thrombos. Diathes. Haemorrh.* 30:263, 1973.

20. Laszlo, J. Myeloproliferative disorders (MPD): Myelofibrosis, myelosclerosis, extramedullary hematopoiesis, undifferentiated MPD, hemorrhagic thrombocythemia. *Semin. Hematol.* 12:409, 1975.

21. Lewis, J. H., Spero, J. A., and Hasiba, U. Coagulopathies. *D.M.* 23(9):21, 1977.

22. Limbird, T. J., and Silver, D. Sequential changes in blood preserved with citrate-phosphate-dextrose. *Surg. Gynecol. Obstet.* 138:401, 1974.

23. Luiken, G. A., McMillan, R., Lightsey, A. L., Gordon, P., Zevely, S., Schulman, I., Gribble, T. J., and Longmire, R. L. Platelet-associated IgG in immune thrombocytopenic purpura. *Blood* 50:317, 1977.

24. McKittrick, J. E. Banked autologous blood in elective surgery. *Am. J. Surg.* 128:137, 1974.

25. Meryman, H. T. Red cell freezing by the American Red Cross. *Am. J. Med. Technol.* 41:265, 1975.

26. Mollitt, D. L., Gartner, D. J., and Madura, J. A. Bedside monitoring of heparin therapy. *Am. J. Surg.* 135:801, 1978.

27. Murphy, Z. Z., and Gardner, F. H. Post-transfusion purpura: A heterogeneous syndrome. *Blood* 45:529, 1975.

28. Nilsson, I. M. Coagulation, fibrinolysis, and venous thrombosis. *Triangle* 16:19, 1977.

29. Nilsson, I. M., Hedner, U., Ahlberg, A. S., Anders, L., and Bergentz, S. Surgery of hemophiliacs—20 years of experience. *World J. Surg.* 1:55, 1977.

30. Packham, M. A., and Mustard, F. J. Clinical pharmacology of platelets. *Blood* 50:555, 1977.

31. Perkins, H. A., Snyder, M., Thacher, C., and Rolfs, M. R. Calcium ion activity during rapid exchange transfusion with citrated blood. *Transfusion* 11:204, 1971.

32. Pineda, A., Taswell, H. F., and Brzica, S. M., Jr. Delayed hemolytic transfusion reaction: An immunological hazard of blood transfusion. *Transfusion* 18:1, 1978.

33. Reul, G. J., Jr., Solis, T. R., Greenberg, D. S., Mattox, K. L., and Whisennand, H. H. Experience with autotransfusion in the surgical management of trauma. *Surgery* 76:546, 1974.
34. Rosario, M. D., Rumsey, E., Arakaki, G., Tanoue, R. E., McDanal, J., and McNamara, J. J. Blood microaggregates and ultrafilters. *J. Trauma* 18:498, 1978.
35. Rosen, R., Mikel, T., and Corrigan, J. J. Acquired circulating anticoagulant in classical hemophilia: Treatment with prothrombin concentrate. *Ariz. Med.* 34:340, 1977.
36. Rosenberg, R. D. Biological actions of heparin. *Semin. Hematol.* 14:427, 1977.
37. Rubinowitz, M. J. Thrombocytosis: Practical approach to diagnosis and treatment. *Rocky Mt. Med. J.* 75:261, 1978.
38. Rutkow, I. M. Thrombotic thrombocytopenic purpura (TTP) and splenectomy: A current appraisal. *Ann. Surg.* 188:701, 1978.
39. Schaefer, J. W. Viral hepatitis update 1978. *Rocky Mt. Med. J.* 76:34, 1979.
40. Schiffer, C. A., Aisner, J., and Wiernik, P. H. Clinical experience with transfusion of cryopreserved platelets. *Br. J. Hematol.* 34:377, 1976.
41. Seeff, L. B., Zimmerman, H. J., Wright, E. C., Finkelstein, J. D., García-Pont, P., Greenlee, H. B., Dietz, A. A., Leevy, C. M., Tamburro, C. H., Schiff, E. R., Schimmel, E. M., Zemel, R., Zimmon, D. S., and McCollum, R. W. A randomized double blind controlled trial of the efficacy of immune serum globulin for the prevention of post-transfusion hepatitis. *Gastroenterol.* 72: 111, 1977.
42. Seeff, L. B., Zimmerman, H. J., Wright, E. C., and McCollum, R. W. VA cooperative study of post-transfusion hepatitis, 1969–1974: Incidence and characteristics of hepatitis and responsible risk factors. *Am. J. Med. Sci.* 270: 355, 1975.
43. Vitez, T. S. Intraoperative anticoagulant management. *Contemp. Surg.* 13: 29, 1978.
44. Wall, W., Heimbecker, R. O., McKenzie, F. N., Robert, A., and Barr, R. Intraoperative autotransfusion in major elective vascular operations: A clinical assessment. *Surgery* 79:82, 1976.

SELECTED READINGS

Bowie, E. J. W., and Owen, C. A., Jr. Hemostatic failure in clinical medicine. *Semin. Hematol.* 14:341, 1977.
Gaffney, P. J., and Balkuv-Ulutin, S. *Fibrinolysis: Current Fundamental and Clinical Concepts.* New York: Academic, 1978.
Harker, L. A. *Hemostasis Manual* (2d ed.). Philadelphia: Davis, 1974.
Lewis, J. H., Spero, J. A., and Hasiba, U. Coagulopathies. *D.M.* 23(9), 1977.
Sixma, J. J., and Wester, J. The hemostatic plug. *Semin. Hematol.* 14:265, 1977.

Martin H. Weiss | 20. CRITICAL CARE OF THE NEUROSURGICAL PATIENT

Once cardiopulmonary parameters have been stabilized in the critically ill patient, attention must be logically directed to assessment of the central nervous system (CNS), both brain and spinal cord, since its stability is essential in assuring true recovery. During conditions of normal homeostatic balance, the brain and spinal cord enjoy a biochemically and immunologically privileged status in being isolated from ordinary and even extraordinary variations in metabolic and toxic parameters by the blood-brain and blood–cerebrospinal fluid (CSF) barriers. This privileged status is required for maintenance of the integrity of the excitable membrane potential, which must be carefully regulated if neural function is to be preserved. However, the barriers may be disrupted by external influences impacting directly upon the central nervous system or by systemic influences deviating widely from the norm and thus altering the barriers.

CLINICAL EVALUATION

The clinical evaluation of the patient with central nervous system disorder remains the single most important assessment that can be made to determine the extent of dysfunction and to provide a background upon which an evaluation of therapy may be established. In assessing intracranial function, the following parameters must be considered: level of consciousness, orientation, brain stem/cranial nerve function, motor coordination, motor evaluation of the four extremities, multimodal sensory evaluation, and assessment of normal as well as potential pathological reflexes.

Far and away the most important parameter in assessing any urgent intracranial process in the critically ill patient is evaluation of the level of consciousness. In performing such an evaluation, the examiner should avoid the use of vague terms such as *semicomatose, stuporous, comatose,* or *obtunded.* Although meaningful to that examiner at that particular time, such terms do not describe the patient precisely enough to allow for accurate followup and assessment of therapy. One should accurately describe the patient's reactions with respect to verbalization, eye opening, orientation, and cranial nerve function upon initial evaluation, and the extent of stimulation required to elicit a response. Jennett and Teasdale's [1] Glasgow Coma Score, a standardized coma grading system, is one with which all physicians concerned with the care of patients with marked depression of consciousness should become familiar.

In the awake patient, a degree of confusion as indicated by the orientation evaluation may be the only clue to a disordered metabolic or hypoxic state if this dementia represents a recent change in behavior. It is, of course, important to have historical perspective on the patient's level of mentation before a given ictus, since the dementia may have been long-standing. Brain stem function can frequently be assessed through evaluation of cranial nerves relating to its given levels. The midbrain lends itself best to evaluation by assessment of pupillary status and the conjugate relationship between the globes. One may then evaluate projections from the level of the vestibular nucleus all the way to the third nerve nucleus by performance of ice water calorics. To perform this appropriately, one must first evaluate the patency of the external canal and the integrity of the tympanic membrane. Once any impacted cerumen is removed, the head should be elevated 30 degrees above the horizontal; the lateral semicircular canal is then in a vertical position so as to evoke a maximal response upon stimulation. A small red rubber catheter may be placed in the external canal near the tympanic membrane and filled with cool water (30° C) or small amounts of ice water so as to bathe the tympanic membrane. In the markedly obtunded patient, the conjugate tonic deviation of both eyes toward the side of the cold water stimulation provides evidence of anatomical integrity of the brain stem from the level of the midpons to the third nerve nucleus in the midbrain. The lower brain stem may be assessed by evaluating the integrity of the gag reflex and evidence of swallowing. Medullary compression may also be detected by assessment of vital signs. Slow, shallow respiration, bradycardia, and possible systolic hypertension are classic indexes of medullary dysfunction.

Motor examination provides a reasonable index of localization at all levels of cerebral function. This evaluation should include not only the assessment of power or strength, but also a careful consideration of tone. Hyper- or hypotonicity may clearly point to a frontal or cerebellar lesion, respectively, particularly in the patient lacking cooperation. The sensory examination, on the other hand, generally provides an evaluation of the sophisticated integration of the cerebrum and therein requires an extremely cooperative patient. It is, therefore, of little value in patients who have sustained significant depression of consciousness. In the patient with a depressed level of consciousness, however, all four extremities should be stimulated with sufficient intensity to evoke a motor response; a coincident spinal cord injury may be clinically evident only by the finding of a flaccid paresis in one or more of the extremities.

Assessment of spinal cord injury takes on additional clinical dimensions.

It would be a rare awake patient who failed to complain of significant pain in the vertebral area involved by injury. Pain may also be elicited by careful palpation of the spinal canal. The clinical assessment of the patient's motor, sensory, and reflex responses remains the best index of the extent of spinal cord damage. In the awake patient, sensory modalities—including posterior column functions as evidenced by vibration and position sense, and anterolateral quadrant function as evidenced by pain and temperature sensation—should be meticulously evaluated. Voluntary motion at all joints in a given extremity must also be carefully assessed, as well as all reflexes in each extremity. Perianal sensation and the integrity of both the anal reflex and voluntary contraction of the anal sphincter should be assessed. Total absence of all the above-mentioned parameters (complete sensorimotor areflexic paraplegia) establishes the state of spinal shock, with an extremely poor potential for neurologic recovery. Careful recording of any intact neurologic function provides a basis for optimism about potential recovery as well as a baseline for assessment during the ensuing management.

MONITORING

Monitoring of intracranial parameters provides an index of the status of intracranial physical dynamics as well as alterations in such parameters as effected by therapy. These factors call for continuous on-line monitoring of both intracranial and systemic arterial pressures. While the continuous recording of systemic arterial pressure is well understood, the simultaneous monitoring of intracranial pressure demands additional comment.

Intracranial pressure monitoring is now an accepted part of interventional therapy in the management of patients with severe cranial disorders. Techniques of monitoring intracranial pressure vary from direct cannulation of the lateral ventricles through recording of pressures from the subarachnoid space to recording of pressures measured through the extradural space. Each of these techniques represents an invasion of the cranial vault, although the preservation of integrity of the dura mater by using the extradural space may significantly reduce the potential risk for infection when such monitoring techniques are employed over prolonged periods of time.

A standardized reference to intracranial pressure in terms of millimeters of mercury has been adopted in order to make adequate comparisons of factors considered critical in intracranial dynamics. The generally accepted upper limit of normal for intracranial pressure is 15 mm Hg (approximately 225 mm H_2O), which requires comparison with systemic arterial pressures to determine the adequacy of cerebral perfusion. Because of this relationship, the concept of a cerebral perfusion pressure (CPP) has been derived. The cerebral perfusion pressure expresses the differential between mean systemic arterial pressure and mean intracranial pressure (SAP − ICP). A fall in CPP below 55 mm Hg is associated with significant cerebral ischemia.

The objective of monitoring techniques is to assure maintenance of CPP to provide adequate cerebral circulation.

Spinal cord monitoring has generally revolved about the utilization of somatosensory-evoked responses in an effort to ascertain the physiological integrity of the cord. Experience to date has shown that the utilization of such systems yields no more information than does the clinical examination in an awake patient. A careful and detailed sensory and motor examination in an awake patient appears to document the anatomical and physiological integrity of the cord as well as the utilization of somatosensory-evoked responses. However, this system has value in the operating room when a patient is asleep and spinal cord mobilization is being undertaken, particularly in the treatment for correction of scoliosis.

DIAGNOSTIC TOOLS

The development of computerized tomography (CT) has virtually revolutionized diagnostic capacities for evaluation of intracranial mass lesions. One may also detect the presence of blood in the subarachnoid space secondary to subarachnoid hemorrhage in addition to the extremely important information derived about intracranial mass effects. *Lumbar puncture should be employed only after it has been determined, by noninvasive techniques, that no intracranial mass exists which could result in worsening of the patient's neurologic status subsequent to spinal fluid withdrawal.*

Angiography remains without peer in the diagnosis of intracranial vascular lesions, specifically aneurysms and arteriovenous malformations. The presence of subarachnoid hemorrhage may be suspected from CT examination, but precise definition of the intracranial vascular tree depends upon high-resolution cerebral angiography.

Echoencephalography may provide a reasonable substitute where rapid CT is not readily available. This system allows assessment of the position of the diencephalic midline structures and can yield valuable information with reference to the existence of a supratentorial mass. In experienced hands, this system may also provide information about the width of the cerebral ventricular system and potentially related hydrocephalus. However, the presence of a posterior fossa mass may well be unappreciated using such a system, emphasizing the need for the precision provided by CT.

EVALUATION AND MANAGEMENT OF THE PATIENT WITH A DEPRESSED LEVEL OF CONSCIOUSNESS

Patients with a marked depression in level of consciousness can be readily placed into two general categories: those harboring an intracranial mass and those in whom depression is secondary to metabolic derangement. The clinician must establish, as rapidly as possible, the existence of an intracranial mass lesion, whether this be supra- or infratentorial, since surgical excision of the mass provides the sole modality for resolution of the CNS disorder. Such efforts consequently take on great urgency. The availability of diagnostic equipment will determine the rapidity with which the diagnostic dilemma may be resolved. While preparations are being made for such investigations, however, simultaneous actions can be taken to evaluate and treat disorders arising extrinsic to the CNS that may exert profound influence upon neural function.

Table 20-1 provides a detailed assessment of systemic as well as localized extraneural parameters that may cause profound neuroglial dysfunction even though the sources lie extrinsic to the CNS [2]. Review of these related disorders reveals a number of pertinent laboratory assessments that may be immediately undertaken during the evaluation of the comatose patient. Appropriate blood samples should be procured early in the evaluation of such patients. Once cardiopulmonary parameters appear stable, sufficient blood should be obtained to enable assessment of various metabolic parameters. These should include an immediate arterial sample to evaluate arterial blood gases, as well as serum samples for glucose, calcium, hepatic enzymes, renal substrates, electrolytes, and a toxicology screen to include hypnotics, sedatives, and common narcotics as well as alcohol. Institution of therapy need not await any of these values, but baseline assessment is imperative in order to plan a long-term therapeutic regimen. Once the blood for baseline laboratory studies has been procured, it is reasonable to administer 30 to 50 cc of a 50% dextrose solution intravenously

TABLE 20-1. Metabolic Causes of Stupor and Coma

I. Stupor or coma arising from intrinsic diseases of the neurons or neuroglial cells (primary metabolic encephalopathy)
   A. Gray matter diseases
      1. Jakob-Creutzfeldt disease
      2. Pick's disease
      3. Alzheimer's disease and senile dementia
      4. Huntington's chorea
      5. Progressive myoclonic epilepsy
      6. Lipid storage diseases
   B. White matter diseases
      1. Schilder's disease
      2. Marchiafava-Bignami disease
      3. The leukodystrophies

II. Stupor or coma arising from diseases extrinsic to neurons and glia (secondary metabolic encephalopathy)
   A. Deprivation of oxygen, substrate, or metabolic cofactors
      1. Hypoxia (interference with oxygen supply to the entire brain—CBF normal)

TABLE 20-1. (*Continued*)

    a. Decreased oxygen tension and content of blood
      (1) Pulmonary disease
      (2) Alveolar hypoventilation
      (3) Decreased atmospheric oxygen tension
    b. Decreased oxygen content of blood—normal tension
      (1) Anemia
      (2) Carbon monoxide poisoning
      (3) Methemoglobinemia
  2. Ischemia (diffuse or widespread multifocal interference with blood supply to brain)
    a. Decreased CBF resulting from decreased cardiac output
      (1) Stokes-Adams; cardiac arrest; cardiac arrhythmias
      (2) Myocardial infarction
      (3) Congestive heart failure
      (4) Aortic stenosis
      (5) Pulmonary infarction
    b. Decreased CBF resulting from decreased peripheral resistance in systemic circulation
      (1) Syncope; orthostatic, vasovagal
      (2) Carotid sinus hypersensitivity
      (3) Low blood volume
    c. Decreased CBF due to generalized or multifocal increased vascular resistance
      (1) Hypertensive encephalopathy
      (2) Hyperventilation syndrome
      (3) Hyperviscosity (polycythemia, cryoglobulinemia or macroglobulinemia, sickle cell anemia)
    d. Decreased CBF due to widespread small vessel occlusions
      (1) Disseminated intravascular coagulation
      (2) Systemic lupus erythematosus
      (3) Subacute bacterial endocarditis
      (4) Fat embolism
      (5) Cerebral malaria
      (6) Cardiopulmonary bypass
  3. Hypoglycemia
    a. Resulting from exogenous insulin
    b. Spontaneous (endogenous insulin, liver disease, etc.)
  4. Cofactor deficiency
    a. Thiamine (Wernicke's encephalopathy)
    b. Niacin
    c. Pyridoxine
    d. Cyanocobalamin

B. Diseases of organs other than brain
  1. Diseases of nonendocrine organs
    a. Liver (hepatic coma)

Table 20-1. (*Continued*)

  b. Kidney (uremic coma)
  c. Lung (CO_2 narcosis)
 2. Hyperfunction and/or hypofunction of endocrine organs
  a. Pituitary
  b. Thyroid (myxedema-thyrotoxicosis)
  c. Parathyroid (hypoparathyroidism and hyperparathyroidism)
  d. Adrenal (Addison's disease, Cushing's disease, pheochromocytoma)
  e. Pancreas
 3. Other systemic diseases
  a. Cancer (remote effects)
  b. Porphyria

C. Exogenous poisons
 1. Sedative drugs
  a. Barbiturates
  b. Nonbarbiturate hypnotics
  c. Tranquilizers
  d. Bromides
  e. Ethanol
  f. Anticholinergics
  g. Opiates
 2. Acid poisons or poisons with acidic breakdown products
  a. Paraldehyde
  b. Methyl alcohol
  c. Ethylene glycol
  d. Ammonium chloride
 3. Enzyme inhibitors
  a. Heavy metals
  b. Organic phosphates
  c. Cyanide
  d. Salicylates
D. Abnormalities of ionic or acid-base environment of CNS
 1. Water and sodium (hypernatremia and hyponatremia)
 2. Acidosis (metabolic and respiratory)
 3. Alkalosis (metabolic and respiratory)
 4. Potassium (hyperkalemia and hypokalemia)
 5. Magnesium (hypermagnesemia and hypomagnesemia)
 6. Calcium (hypercalcemia and hypocalcemia)
E. Diseases producing toxins or enzyme inhibition in CNS
 1. Meningitis
 2. Encephalitis
 3. Subarachnoid hemorrhage
F. Disordered temperature regulation
 1. Hypothermia
 2. Heat stroke

CBF = cerebral blood flow; CNS = central nervous system.

over a period of several minutes. Although hypoglycemia is a relatively uncommon source of coma, this administration of glucose carries little risk and may be of great impact in restoring neural function.

Once it has been clearly ascertained that systemic and cerebral perfusion, oxygenation, and substrate availability in the form of glucose are adequate and that no intracranial mass threatens catastrophic distortion of brain substance, then one can proceed to explore the numerous causes of depressed consciousness indicated in Table 20-1. Many of these will require gradual correction, with gradual restoration of neural function paralleling improvement in the underlying metabolic disorder. If intracranial pressure is elevated, with its potential for compromise of adequate cerebral perfusion, then one must turn to the management of persistent intracranial hypertension.

PERSISTENT INTRACRANIAL HYPERTENSION: EVALUATION AND MANAGEMENT

Intracranial pressure above 15 mm Hg indicates an elevation above normal. Transient increases in intracranial pressure do not pose a significant hazard to the patient. However, repeated episodes of intracranial hypertension, particularly in the form of the plateau waves described by Lundberg, as well as persistent intracranial hypertension may well contribute to depressed cerebral metabolic activity in association with impaired cerebral blood flow. Increased intracranial pressure in and of itself may not be an ominous sign in the cerebrum that is otherwise metabolically functioning well. However, in the brain impaired by toxic, metabolic, or traumatic insult, such intracranial hypertension may have disastrous consequences. The need for measures to alter intracranial pressure will, of course, depend upon an accurate measuring and recording of intracranial pressure, followed by measurements to ascertain whether the measures instituted to alter intracranial dynamics have been effective.

When considering the genesis of increased intracranial pressure, it is convenient to think of three separate but interdependent components within the intracranial cavity—the vascular, cerebrospinal fluid, and cerebral parenchymal components. Although each of these obviously affects the others in the interplay that underlies intracranial physical dynamics, one may think of them as individual or independent when attempting to describe a program of therapy designed to decrease intracranial pressure.

Parenchymal causes of increased intracranial pressure relate to swelling of brain substance itself, generally referred to as cerebral edema or compression of such substance by intrinsic or extrinsic masses comprised primarily of tumor, abscess, or hematoma. Without question, any mass lesion demands surgical excision as the effective treatment of increased intracranial pressure. However, diffuse swelling of the brain without focal mass effect provides the setting most desirable for institution of medical management. Brain swelling may be subdivided into two histopathological entities, cytotoxic edema and vasogenic edema. Cytotoxic edema refers to cellular swelling with resultant increase in intracellular volume and decrease in the extracellular compartment. This form of edema relates primarily to ischemic and metabolic disturbances of cerebral parenchyma, at least in their initial phases. Correction of the underlying mechanism (such as improvement in cerebral oxygenation) will inhibit potential extension to unaffected areas but will not necessarily reverse the pathological process that has already taken place. Attack upon this form of cerebral edema has limited potential at the present time. If the blood brain barrier has been spared by the underlying process, then the use of hyperosmotic agents may be effective in reducing cytoplasmic swelling. The generation of serum hyperosmolarity will result in extraction of both extracellular and intracellular fluid because of the osmotic gradient between CNS and serum. This can readily be accomplished by the use of Mannitol administered as ¼ to ½ gm/kg body weight in a rapid bolus. This agent may be utilized for repeated administrations in this relatively low concentration, but higher doses of Mannitol may well result in severe hyperosmolarity, renal failure, and metabolic acidosis. Recent evidence seems to indicate that the loop diuretic, ethacrynic acid, which acts to inhibit bicarbonate-mediated chloride transport in glial cells, may be effective in reducing astroglial swelling. Utilization of this agent in conjunction with periodic infusions of hyperosmotic agents may prove successful in controlling cytoplasmic swelling.

Vasogenic edema, on the other hand, results from a loss of the integrity of the blood brain barrier, with a resultant increase in the extracellular space of brain secondary to leakage of osmotic particles from the intravascular compartment into the extracellular space. This form of cerebral edema may respond to high-potency glucocorticoids, which presumably act by helping to maintain the integrity of the blood brain barrier. For short-term therapy, in the event that pressures are dangerously high, the use of hyperosmotic agents as described above may also be helpful in the reduction of the extracellular compartment of the brain.

Intracranial hypertension can develop as a consequence of expansion of CSF owing either to increased production or decreased absorption. The latter mechanism is by far the more frequent one responsible for accumulation of excess volumes of CSF. The only entity that has been associated with increased production of CSF is the choroid plexus papilloma. This tumor obviously represents a cerebral mass lesion whose treatment is managed by surgical excision. Obstruction of CSF pathways, on the other hand, may produce two different syndromes. The first is dilatation of the cerebral ventricular system (hydrocephalus), which may occur as a consequence of accumulation of excessive volumes of CSF. Evidence indicates that obstruction of CSF pathways is also the most frequent underlying cause of the development of the second syndrome, known as benign increased intracranial pressure or pseudo-tumor cerebri. In this situation the ventricular system is generally normal if not actually reduced in size, but the increase in intracranial pressure can result in retinal ischemia and blindness, demanding prompt and vigorous treatment.

Reduction in intracranial pressure related to aberrant CSF dynamics may be accomplished by the use of a number of pharmacologic agents that have been shown to reduce CSF production. By establishing an osmotic gradient between CSF and serum, Mannitol will reduce the production of CSF as well as decrease the volume of the CSF compartment by causing a water shift from CSF to serum. This mechanism is, of course, a transient event that does not lend itself well to therapeutic efforts of even intermediate duration. A number of additional pharmacologic agents are available, however, to assist in the reduction of CSF production. Diamox, a carbonic anhydrase inhibitor, will reduce CSF production by approximately 50 percent. In addition, the loop diuretics furosemide and ethacrynic acid have both been found significantly to reduce CSF production. Obviously, ethacrynic acid may play a dual role in modifying or modulating intracranial pressure by acting upon CSF production as well as cytotoxic edematous processes. In a superb article, Pollay [3] reviews the numerous pharmacological agents that have been found to reduce CSF production. Reduction of CSF production, however, will have a short-lived effect since, if the defect resides at the absorptive end of the spectrum, pressure may continue to rise as long as any CSF is produced in the face of impaired absorption.

Restoration of normal absorption relies upon surgical intervention. In the presence of a noncommunicating hydrocephalus (obstruction at one or more of the ventricular foramina), relief can be provided only by CSF diversion directly from the ventricular system. This can be accomplished on a temporary basis by the use of an external ventriculostomy system or may be established permanently with insertion of a ventriculo-jugular or ventriculo-peritoneal shunt. If the ventricular system freely communicates with the subarachnoid space, particularly the lumbar subarachnoid space, several additional options are available. Repeated lumbar punctures may be effective in transiently resolving intracranial hypertension due to a temporary process interfering with transmigration of CSF from the subarachnoid space to the venous dural sinuses. CSF is produced at a rate of approximately 500 cc a day so that removal of 20 to 30 cc of CSF is compensated within approximately an hour following removal of this fluid. The effect of the lumbar puncture is dramatic in creating a fistulous communication between the subarachnoid space and the epidural space. This fistulous communication may be enhanced by nursing the patient in a head-up position so as to maximize the hydrostatic gradient between the cranial cavity and the site of the lumbar puncture. Such a position obviously enhances venous return from the head as well as drainage of CSF; these may, either alone or in combination, suffice for the temporary amelioration of increased intracranial pressure. One may increase the temporary drainage of CSF by inserting a lumbar subarachnoid catheter percutaneously through a Touhey needle and allowing constant drainage into an appropriate vehicle. This system permits meticulous control over the amount of drainage but has the liability of potential infection ascending through the externalized catheter; a significant risk of infection would arise if such a drainage system were allowed to remain in place more than 5 days. If prolonged diversion of CSF appears necessary for patient management, insertion of a lumbo-peritoneal shunt or ventricular shunt as described above would be appropriate so as to maximize the benefits of CSF diversion yet minimize the opportunity for secondary infection.

Finally, one must consider the influence of the intracranial vascular component upon intracranial physical parameters. The process of cerebral autoregulation assures relative constancy of cerebral blood flow under varying states of cerebral metabolic activity and systemic arterial pressure variations. This mechanism is dependent upon the reactivity of the cerebral resistance vessels, comprised primarily of the small arterioles and capillaries. If such vessels undergo vasoparalysis, vascular volume will be increased and may, in turn, be reflected in an increase in intracranial pressure. Usually one would not find an increase in intracranial pressure, since an equivalent volume of CSF would be displaced from the intracranial component. However, if such compensation is lost, intracranial pressure will rise. One experiences this constellation of events in the example of malignant systemic arterial hypertension, which breaks through the capacity of cerebral autoregulation to maintain a constant blood flow and therein blood volume.

At the other end of this spectrum, one must be acutely aware of the adequacy of venous drainage. Significant impedance to venous drainage will result in an expansion in the venous compartment, then will be reflected back through the vascular compartment, resulting in overall increase in intravascular volume as well as slowing of cerebral blood flow. One may look at any or all of these mechanisms in an effort to alleviate increased intracranial pressure related to vascular components.

In the absence of arterial hypotension, patients should always be nursed with their heads elevated so as to enhance venous drainage to the heart and minimize the potential for impaired venous drainage. If systemic arterial hypertension is a significant problem (mean arterial pressure greater than 140 mm Hg), then efforts directed primarily at altering cerebral vascular reactivity will be fruitless since autoregulatory phenomena presumably have been lost. In such circumstances, it is imperative to restore normal systemic arterial pressure if the reflected intracranial hypertension is to be lowered. However, too rapid decrease of systemic arterial hypertension may result in a marked depression of cerebral perfusion. As mentioned above, a cerebral perfusion pressure of 75 mm Hg is found under conditions of normal systemic arterial pressure. In lowering systemic arterial pressure, one must be careful not to generate significant cerebral ischemia by lowering systemic arterial pressure without a concomitant fall in intracranial pressure. Intracranial pressure may remain elevated because of secondary cerebral edema processes that require time to abate. In addition, some of the agents used to reduce systemic arterial pressure may significantly affect autoregulatory processes and potentially contribute to sustained intracranial hypertension. In severe cases, one should ideally monitor both systemic arterial pressure and intracranial pressure in order safely to reduce systemic arterial pressure while maintaining adequate cerebral perfusion.

Cerebral autoregulation may be divided into two distinct parts—namely, pressure autoregulation and metabolic autoregulation. Metabolic autoregulation relates to the alteration in carbon dioxide content and hydrogen ion content surrounding the cerebral vasculature. Even in the absence of pressure autoregulation, it may be possible to reduce intracranial pressure and cerebral blood flow by employing hyperventilation techniques. The optimal situation appears to derive from a $PaCO_2$ of approximately 25 to 30 mm Hg, which will maximize the vasoconstrictive effects of hypocarbia without potential superimposed ischemia from excessive vasoconstriction.

Each of these parameters may play an important role in the generation of significant intracranial hypertension. Efforts to control intracranial hypertension should be directed at mechanisms that will reduce parenchymal swelling, decrease cerebral extracellular fluid, decrease CSF production, enhance CSF drainage, and assure an appropriate cerebral blood flow pattern without excessive intracranial cerebrovascular volume.

MANAGEMENT OF ACUTE SPINAL CORD INJURIES

Once the physical examination relevant to spinal cord injury has been performed, appropriate radiographic studies should be made promptly to support the clinical impression and appropriate management should be instituted. Transportation of the patient with a spinal cord injury must be carefully addressed by the attending physician. The area of concern should be immobilized and alignment maintained during any transportation—this, of course, applies to transportation from the site of an accident as well as transportation within a medical facility during the course of diagnostic evaluation. If the patient has an adequate airway, a soft collar may be gently applied without any manipulation of the neck so as to hold the head in alignment if the neck is an area of concern. Under all circumstances, transportation should be on a rigid board or firm stretcher to avoid any undue manipulation. X-ray films should be secured in the anteroposterior and lateral projection, exercising extreme caution in manipulation of the patient. If satisfactory simple x-ray films show no evidence of bony disruption but evidence of spinal cord dysfunction is found on clinical examination, the patient should be managed as a spinal cord injury without overt vertebral subluxation but with the assumption that covert vertebral instability may exist. Radiographic evidence should be sought for paravertebral soft tissue swelling, an index of local spinal trauma. These patients should be nursed, under close supervision, in a facility clearly geared for monitoring neurologic function. We have adopted the policy of nursing these patients in regular hospital beds with "logrolling" manipulation of the patient so as to maintain alignment of the vertebral column. We have found that the use of metal frames for turning patients results in more complications and difficulties than does the use of regular beds.

Once alignment has been determined to be satisfactory in the nondisplaced vertebral column then, after approximately 24 hours of observation, CTs of the suspected area should be secured to provide evidence of any nonvisualized trauma that might result in instability of the spine. Any lack of integrity of the bony vertebral column should be considered an index of instability and should be treated acutely as such. We do *not* advise the implementation of flexion-extension views, particularly in the acute phase, in an effort to assess stability of any area of the spine. Our experience has been that CT provides a valid index of the integrity of the spinal canal. Once the acute phase has resolved (4–5 days), flexion-extension views under medical supervision may be obtained.

If plain x-ray films indicate subluxation or dislocation of vertebral elements, then efforts should be directed at early reduction of the malaligned vertebral components. Several factors come into consideration with respect to the urgency of such maneuvers. In the cervical spine, such efforts should clearly be undertaken initially by the use of traction provided by insertion of skeletal tongs. Weights may be appropriately applied under x-ray guidance in an effort to reduce the unaligned cervical spine. Although weights up to 85 pounds have been applied for cervical traction, one must be acutely aware of the potential for distraction of the spine as well as spinal cord with the application of weight in excess of 35 pounds for injuries involving the lower cervical spine. Lesions involving the upper cervical spine may lend themselves to distraction with even significantly less weight: a rough guide suggests 5 pounds of weight for each level starting at C_1. Radiographic confirmation of spine position should be obtained with each addition of weight. Traction devices are, in general, totally ineffective in reducing dislocated fractures involving the thoracolumbar spine. Such reduction may be accomplished by postural influences while lying in bed, or attempts at open reduction. Considerations for emergency reduction vary with the clinical specialist involved and extend beyond the scope of this discussion, but clearly, acute operative reduction of the spine is rarely necessary in the care of spinal cord injuries.

Several specific parameters are of great import with respect to acute intervention in spinal cord injuries.

Careful attention must be paid to bladder function in the patient with a spinal cord lesion. This will almost always require an indwelling catheter during the acute phases. Control of bladder function will direct the necessary long-term management of the bladder, but overdistension of the urinary bladder is to be avoided, since it can lead to major loss of muscle tone, which will prevent significant bladder recovery. Cervical and high thoracic cord injuries will, in addition, result in significant compromise to pulmonary function because of loss of intercostal innervation. One of the severe early consequences of such an injury is the development of hypoxemia, which must be carefully monitored. Therefore, early and repeated evaluation of arterial blood gases is mandatory, along with twice-daily assessment of vital capacity by respirometer. If evidence of pulmonary insufficiency develops, then nasotracheal intubation should be instituted before the potential for hypoxemic CNS deterioration ensues.

Attention must be carefully directed at repeated evaluation of cardiovascular parameters, particularly in cervical spine injuries. Interruption of the descending sympathetic system in cervical and upper thoracic spine injuries engenders a situation that promotes vascular pooling in the extremities, with the subsequent development of hypotension. Should this occur, vasopressors must be utilized to combat hypotension, along with volume expanders for the patient who has been in bed for some time. The development of a bradycardia, presumably due to unopposed vagal impulses influencing the cardiac mechanism, must also be carefully observed; bradycardia with pulses in the 30s may result in significant organ ischemia. This should be treated with atropine to combat the vagal influences and may require repeated administration.

Minimization of skin breakdown can be accomplished by periodic "logrolling" of the patient and nursing on the so-called egg crate mattress. The potential for development of a decubitus ulcer must be continually recognized, and one must strive to avoid compression at any given site that shows evidence of skin breakdown. Finally, careful attention must be paid to the potential development of thrombophlebitis in chronically bedridden patients without adequate muscle tone. Monitoring of the deep venous system using radio-labeled fibrinogen may detect the early development of deep vein thrombosis. Evidence exists that mini doses of heparin (5,000 units subcutaneously q12h) administered may minimize the potential for such development, and the use of inflatable stockings may further reduce the chance for development of this potentially lethal situation.

TREATMENT OF STATUS EPILEPTICUS

Status epilepticus may be defined as repeated seizure activity without regaining consciousness between attacks. One may also consider prolonged continuous seizure activity in the absence of loss of consciousness as representative of status epilepticus, with particular reference to petit mal epilepsy, myoclonus epilepsy, and epilepsy partialis continua. The last group, however, do not present so urgent a problem since the potential for cardio-respiratory compromise is not so great. The prime intent, therefore, of treatment for status epilepticus is to prevent the development of hypoxemia with its attendant multiple organ system disruption.

Approximately 75 percent of patients with generalized status epilepticus will respond within several hours to a variety of pharmacological regimens employed to abort the seizure activity. However, as many as 25 percent may require up to 3 or 4 days to respond to any of the regimens. Under such circumstances, the patient may well experience the superimposition of iatrogenic or acquired complications in addition to the underlying disorder. Such problems relate specifically to the development of respiratory depression, cardiac arrest, hypotension, prolonged coma, and aspiration pneumonia.

In the approach to the management of a patient with status epilepticus, it is imperative initially to define the patient's vital signs as well as to ascertain that an adequate airway exists. Attempts at insertion of devices such as tongue blades or bite blocks to protect the tongue have frequently resulted in tooth fractures, aspiration, and other problems, so these are generally discouraged. Blood samples should immediately be secured for toxicological screen, including barbiturates, narcotics, phenothiazines, alcohol, and Dilantin. If possible, establish an intravenous line using 5% dextrose in water and administer 50 cc of 50% glucose rapidly along with 100 mg of thiamine. If it is necessary to maintain blood pressure, any of the appropriate pressor agents may be utilized as appropriate; a central venous pressure line or Swan-Ganz catheter may prove invaluable under such circumstances. Fluid balance should be carefully observed, along with evaluation of serum electrolytes.

To suppress seizure activity rapidly, Valium is presently the pharmacological agent of choice. It should be administered intravenously in doses up to 10 mg over a period of 3 minutes. This agent is extremely effective in establishing *short-term* control of seizures. Care must be taken because of the possible development of respiratory depression, hypotension, or cardiac suppression, particularly if the patient had previously been given barbiturates. With the use of Valium, one must be prepared to intubate the patient should evidence of respiratory depression ensue. The greatest liability of this agent is the fact that it is effective in the short-term only and therefore does not provide lasting control of seizures. The initial intravenous 10-mg dose may be repeated in 20 min, since the patient may begin to seize again after the initial effect is dissipated. It is probably wise to supplement Valium with intravenous Dilantin if it is known that the patient has not been previously taking Dilantin.

The administration of intravenous Dilantin must be carefully monitored with an electrocardiogram (ECG), since this may result in the generation of severe cardiac arrhythmias. Dilantin can be administered in doses up to 800 to 1,000 mg intravenously at a rate not to exceed 50 mg per minute in association with constant monitoring by ECG. This regimen, in combination with the initial Valium, should be effective in establishing long-term control as well as cessation of status epilepticus. Once the intravenous Dilantin has been administered, one may resort to daily maintenance levels of 300 mg per day in divided doses either orally or intravenously. Serum Dilantin levels should be secured to determine the adequacy of maintenance therapy.

An appropriate alternative to Dilantin may be the administration of phenobarbital to gain control of recurrent seizures. Phenobarbital can be administered intravenously at a rate of 200 mg per 20 minutes to reach a total dose of 600 to 800 mg. One must, as with Valium, be aware of the potential for respiratory depression and a prolongation of coma due to accumulative effect of this long-acting barbiturate. Therefore, one must be prepared to offer ventilatory as well as cardiovascular support to such patients.

Another alternative, particularly in patients suffering from prolonged seizure activity secondary to alcoholic withdrawal, is the use of paraldehyde. Paraldehyde cannot be sterilized and therefore can only be administered by selected routes. One may administer 6 to 8 cc by the rectum or 4 to 6 cc intramuscularly. A 4% solution of paraldehyde may be administered intravenously up to a total of 8 cc. However, this must be carefully titrated because of the potential development of pulmonary edema with such administration.

Finally, if the above potential regimens should be unsuccessful over a period of 12 to 24 hours, one should consider employing a general anesthetic. This should be done only with the attendance of an anesthesiologist and will require intubation and adequate ventilation. Penthrane administered to a level of Stage III anesthesia appears to be the preferred choice of general anesthetic for uncontrolled status epilepticus, regulated by a competent anesthesiologist.

ACUTE CEREBRAL TRAUMA

The circumstances under which cerebral injuries occur are extremely variable and unpredictable. This section will review those elements of a strategic system that may prove useful in the intensive care setting. The basic objectives can be stated as follows: (1) to provide a milieu that will maximize recovery of cerebral tissue, (2) to recognize or prevent those intra- and/or extracranial complications demanding urgent therapeutic intervention, and (3) to establish a system of priorities for diagnosis and therapy in the best interest of the patient commensurate with resources available.

The reaction of the brain to injury is a dynamic process and, to some degree, follows a predictable pattern of recovery. A departure from this pattern usually provides the first clue to a potential complication. Recognition of ominous clues requires a standard of reference, comprised for the most part of the basic neurological examination. In a setting in which only casual observations have been made and recorded, the most important guideline in the management of the patient with cerebral trauma is frequently lost. Careful consideration of the essentials of the neurological examination relevant to trauma may avoid an unrecognized catastrophic sequence.

Appraisal of the state of consciousness is the single most important component of this examination, since a normal state of cognitive function requires a higher level of integrated performance of neuronal pathways than any other mode of behavior. In a patient with acute posttraumatic encephalopathy, minor fluctuations in the state of consciousness will be observed from examination to examination. Ordinarily, insignificant or minor changes in the factors that alter cerebral metabolism—such as intracranial pressure, cerebral blood flow, or metabolic derangements—may produce some minute-to-minute changes in the conscious state that can be equally perplexing to the experienced and the inexperienced observer. However, the overall trend toward consciousness or unconsciousness appears to be the most critical factor.

One can therefore appreciate the need for explicit details during the course of observations. Terms such as *comatose* have variable meanings to different examiners; therefore, a clear statement of the precise level of consciousness and response to external stimuli is imperative. The only way to avoid misinterpretation of observations is to be certain that all of the evaluation parameters—including assessment of level of consciousness, degree of orientation, specific response patterns, and response to external stimuli—are consistently employed and recorded.

The introduction of the Glasgow Coma Score by Jennett and Teasdale in 1974 made it possible accurately to record important factors relevant to the unconscious patient, whether secondary to trauma or medical disorders. This scoring system, which relates to eye-opening responses, verbalization responses, and motor patterns, has proved extremely helpful in objectively assessing a given degree of coma or unconsciousness so that multiple examiners can interrelate accurately [1].

Funduscopic examination at the outset is generally unremarkable but provides a baseline for evidence of the evolution of intracranial hypertension. One should *never* utilize mydriatics in an effort to visualize the fundus of a patient with a suspected intracranial mass. The importance of the pupillomotor reflex, on the other hand, cannot be overemphasized. In the unresponsive patient, the direct and consensual response of the pupil should be carefully recorded. Loss of either aspect of this response may be a moderately early index of progressive dysfunction of the visual or oculomotor apparatus, particularly in herniation syndromes. Evaluation of facial symmetry is another aspect of the neurological examination that can be made in almost all patients except those with facial trauma extensive enough to produce soft tissue distortion by swelling. If a patient is unresponsive to pain, the symmetry of the grimace may be a useful indication of the integrity of the corticobulbar tract.

In most instances of cerebral injury resulting in posttraumatic encephalopathy of sufficient magnitude to alter the conscious state, detailed sensory testing is not helpful in evaluating the progress of the encephalopathy, but, it is in ascertaining whether an obvious motor deficit is of cerebral, spinal, or peripheral origin. The response to a gross painful stimulus will help to identify an afferent defect due to peripheral nerve, plexus, or root injury. Fine sensory evaluation is not of major consequence in the assessment of the patient with a cerebral injury.

The extent of information obtainable from assessing the motor system depends, of course, upon the state of consciousness. Active motor resistance testing depends upon the patient's ability to understand and willingness to carry out simple commands. In the alert patient without overt motor deficit, one may document with great precision the status of the neuromuscular system. The difficulty arises in the patient who is unresponsive to verbal stimuli. In such a patient, in addition to observing the response to painful stimuli, one must always assess the amount and nature of muscular resistance to passive movement, a process which can be deferred only in the presence of an extremity fracture. The solitary flaccid extremity offering no resistance to passive manipulation should alert the examiner to a lesion involving peripheral nerve or lower motor neuron, whereas a flaccid quadriplegia arouses suspicion of associated spinal cord injury. Although seen in terminal stages, this finding would be unusual as a consequence of head injury. Spasticity, increased resistance to passive motion of the joint noted at the very onset of the movement pattern, is an expression of the exaggerated tendon stretch reflex. Spasticity is a reliable index of a disturbance in the corticospinal system, which may occur at any point between the pyramidal cell in the cortex to the lower motor neuron. Babinski's sign also indicates a disturbance in this pyramidal system, and a change from a normal flexor pattern to the abnormal extensor pattern in Babinski's reflex may be of major significance in following the patient with head trauma.

Decerebrate rigidity does not actually describe rigidity but a posture in which the trunk and extremities reflect an exaggerated state of spasticity in the antigravity (extensor) muscle groups. This posture represents a profound disturbance of conduction in the corticospinal (motor) pathways, the lesion occurring between the red and vestibular nuclei in the brain stem and resulting in uninhibited vestibulo-spinal influences. It may occur as a result of generalized increase in intracranial pressure, compression distortion of the brain stem from direct injury, or a marked shift of the neuroaxis by a mass above or below the tentorium. Although this is a serious or grave sign, it by no means indicates an irreversible situation.

Frequent measurements of the vital signs (blood pressure, pulse, and respiration) provide a highly useful series of observations. The incidence of Cushing's phenomenon (increase in systolic and pulse pressures, slowing of pulse rate) is surprisingly low in supratentorial expanding mass lesions, but its occurrence may point to a possible posterior fossa lesion. Theoretically, a gradual fall and deepening of the respiratory pattern should be the earliest change in vital sign functions, but there is certainly no consistent pattern.

As indicated earlier, the reaction of the brain and, therefore, the clinical behavior of the patient to cerebral injury is not entirely predictable. The primary problem facing the clinician, therefore, is to recognize the remedial intra- and extracranial complications associated with cerebral injury. The classic, typical findings ascribed to extradural and subdural hematomas are rarer in practice than the atypical and partial syndromes.

CLOSED HEAD INJURIES
Closed intracranial injuries are usually categorized as either concussion or contusion. Classic clinical and electrophysiologic criteria may be used to describe these; but absolute correlation of these criteria in a human subject is rare, and they offer the clinician little help in managing any given case of posttraumatic encephalopathy. Immediate posttraumatic encephalopathy can be diagnosed according to the following criteria: Group I, patients rendered unconscious or sustaining a loss of neurologic function for relatively brief periods of time who, upon regaining consciousness, demonstrate no neurologic or behavioral deficits, and Group II, patients who are rendered unconscious for a more prolonged period who demonstrate neurologic or behavioral deficits at the time of evaluation.

Group I patients meet, for the most part, the clinical definition of concussion. When this is the only medical problem, there is little active treatment that the physician need offer other than a period of observation in or near a facility that can provide diagnostic and therapeutic help to manage potential complications. Assuming that ideal circumstances prevail, how long should the patient be kept in the hospital for observation? Almost 100 percent of acute catastrophic intracranial hemorrhagic complications in this group of patients occur within the first 72 hours; 24 hours will cover most instances. Hospitalization is *unnecessary if the patient is asymptomatic* at the time of evaluation. Cerebral edema is virtually nonexistent, at least in a clinically significant form, in Group I patients (concussion). Therefore, if a patient in this category has an alteration in the state of consciousness, complains of increasing headache, or has a discernible progressive neurologic deficit, he or she should be considered to have an intracranial hemorrhage until that diagnosis is excluded.

The foregoing discussion refers only to early management. Chronic subdural hematomas may develop and become evident several weeks or months following injury, along with the more insidious complication of posttraumatic hydrocephalus. Therefore, all of these patients should be seen as outpatients regularly for a minimum of 6 weeks.

Patients in Group II (cerebral contusion) are obviously more severely injured and require hospitalization. The number of variables that affect cerebral function and alter behavior is greatly increased in Group II patients, and therefore, the number of dilemmas in management is correspondingly increased. Many patients who appear to be in Group II at the time of initial evaluation rapidly fall into Group I when the effects of alcohol or other intoxicants have subsided; they can be safely discharged after 24 hours. A toxicology screen is obviously of paramount importance in all patients suspected of head injury, who must be managed in the same way as patients in Group I until they are clearly out of danger. Those showing evidence of progressive neurologic deficit documented along previously described lines demand more definitive diagnostic studies.

In addition to the initial forces of acceleration or deceleration that disrupt the structure and function of brain tissue, the brain tissue itself exerts adverse effects in reacting to the initial injury. This process is commonly ascribed to cerebral edema, but although there is little doubt that edema contributes to cerebral swelling, it is only one component of what is quite likely to be a constellation of complex phenomena only partially understood. The process seems to be most severe between 24 and 48 hours after injury; thereafter, it gradually subsides. The onset may be as early as 6 to 12 hours following injury. This period overlaps the expected time of onset of the surgically remediable hemorrhagic complications of cerebral injury. Time of onset of the decline in performance of the patient's cerebral function therefore provides little help in distinguishing between the two processes. This leads to the question of whether there is a particular pattern of neurologic dysfunction that characterizes one or both of these processes. The answer is clearly no.

Intra-axial cerebral swelling and extra-axial compression by extradural or subdural hemorrhage are frequently concomitant and interrelated. Clinical records too frequently refer only to the presence or absence of localized findings. Their absence, however, is not a reliable diagnostic sign in the evaluation of a potential expanding intracranial mass lesion. The hallmark of any expanding intracranial mass remains the progressive decline in level of consciousness. Thus, documentation of increasing neurologic deficit, in any sphere, should summon further diagnosis and therapy from attending personnel.

DIAGNOSTIC TOOLS
At the point in time when investigation beyond direct bedside observations is required, the clinician's course of action will be greatly influenced by the availability and reliability of diagnostic tools in the institution. Avail-

ability of selected ultrasophisticated diagnostic equipment has been limited by recent legislation, requiring a thoughtful utilization of facilities at hand.

PLAIN FILM RADIOGRAPHY. Conventional radiography of the skull will show the presence or absence of a fracture and provide some indication of whether there is a shift of the brain by the position of the pineal gland when it is calcified. The distribution, presence, or absence of fractures provides little help in diagnosing an intracranial hematoma, although it may be useful in lateralizing extradural hemorrhage. The most significant value of the plain skull radiograph in the assessment of the patient with head trauma is in identifying a depressed skull fracture that cannot be appreciated on clinical examination and in finding of incidental intracranial abnormalities that may have contributed to the original trauma.

ECHOENCEPHALOGRAPHY. Echoencephalography is a rapid, nonhazardous means of plotting the midline position of the brain. Its accuracy is directly related to the skill and experience of the individual doing the study. It must be emphasized that the midline shift can be absent in the presence of bilateral lesions and may be minimal when generalized intra-axial cerebral swelling is present concomitant with lateralized extra-axial hemorrhage.

ELECTROENCEPHALOGRAPHY. Electroencephalography is rarely helpful in the acute traumatic setting.

LUMBAR PUNCTURE. Lumbar puncture is much the same as electroencephalography in assessing the patient with posttraumatic encephalopathy. It provides an indication of intracranial pressure, but the clinical findings are of far greater consequence. The presence or absence of bloody cerebrospinal fluid also does not help in the clinician's decision-making process. It can be argued that the lumbar puncture is contraindicated in the evaluation of an acute posttraumatic encephalopathy, since the release of even a small amount of fluid from the lumbar subarachnoid space may enhance an already existent hemispheric shift due to an intra- or extra-axial hemispheric clot. Therefore, the hazard of lumbar puncture in the presence of possible intracranial mass is rarely justified in the assessment of the acute cerebral injury; its most useful role is in the evaluation of *coma of unknown etiology.*

CT SCANNING. CT equipment provides a rapid, extremely accurate, noninvasive means of defining intracranial pathology. Intracerebral hematomas and significant cerebral distortions can be readily perceived. In addition, with the use of contrast enhancement, a remarkably high percentage of extra-axial clots, both epidural and subdural, can be discerned by this technique. Acute epidural or subdural hematomas, however, may be missed because of their isodense character relative to adjacent bone; one must understand this potential source of false negative evaluation. One additional limiting factor is the risk of movement in the agitated patient, creating the need for general anesthesia in some patients, an undesirable situation in terms of patient management.

CEREBRAL ANGIOGRAPHY. Cerebral angiography has largely been replaced by CT scanning when the latter technique is available within a given institution. However, angiography remains one of the best diagnostic studies in the acute setting for consistent establishment of a preoperative diagnosis. Brachial, carotid, or transfemoral catheter angiography may be employed, depending upon the available facilities. If CT scanning is not readily available, early appropriate angiography may certainly prove to be lifesaving.

EARLY MANAGEMENT

Standard principles of homeostatic support apply to all patients with head injury as well as injuries elsewhere. Assessment of the cardiopulmonary system assumes priority in all circumstances. Airway patency must be uncompromised; endotracheal or nasotracheal intubation, with or without tracheostomy, should be instituted when deemed advisable. When possible, a set of arterial blood gases should be obtained early to corroborate the clinical impression of pulmonary function. In addition, cardiovascular stability should be secured. Once adequate systemic perfusion is assured, a good intravenous system is in place, and drainage of both gastric and urinary systems is operant where deemed advisable, the physician may turn to assessment and initial management of CNS trauma.

Transport of patients with cerebral injuries should be accomplished with the head elevated 30 degrees above the heart in order to maximize venous drainage from the intracranial cavity. This, of course, must be compatible with a stable cardiovascular system, which must assume priority. The initial evaluation also must yield no evidence of vertebral instability; if there should be any question about a potential associated spinal injury, adequate measures to maintain spinal stability must be instituted at the time of initial transport. The physician must always be concerned with the real potential for cervical spine injury in association with any cranial trauma. A good rule is to assume that any trauma severe enough to render a patient unconscious, even momentarily, should be considered severe enough to involve transmission of the axial loading force of the blow to the cervical spine, with possible disruption of the vertebral spinal axis.

Finally, one must consider the utilization of pharmacological adjuvants in the management of such patients. High-potency glucocorticoids are commonly administered in the management of patients with head injuries, although experimental evidence of their efficacy is equivocal at best. The frequently mentioned influence of glucocorticoids in the control of post-traumatic cerebral edema is based upon speculative evidence, and there is some evidence that they may be deleterious. However, *massive* doses of glucocorticoids (methylprednisolone 30 mg/kg given as a loading dose and repeated 6 hr after the initial dose, followed by 250 mg at 6-hr intervals for a period of 48 hr) may significantly improve mortality and/or morbidity from intracranial trauma. Further clinical trials to support this position are pending and hold promise for the care of these patients.

Osmotic agents, such as mannitol or urea, may be utilized in emergencies to buy time to get a patient to the operating room. Owing to their potentially severe metabolic consequences, they are not effective agents for continuous care of such patients. Neurosurgical consultation should be obtained either directly or at least by telephone description before administration of such agents so as not to alter the neurosurgeon's ability to assess the status of the patient. When indicated, mannitol may be administered rapidly in a dose of ½ gm/kg, making sure that a Foley catheter is in place in order to avoid potential bladder overdistension. In the elderly patient, one must be alert to the potential of acute cardiac decompensation secondary to overloading of the intravascular compartment with the hyperosmotic infusion. One can guard against this problem by pretreatment with 40 mg of Lasix prior to the administration of mannitol. If, on the basis of intracranial pressure monitoring, it appears that sustained intracranial hypertension persists in the absence of any surgical intracranial mass, then repeated infusions of ¼ gm/kg of mannitol may be helpful in reducing intracranial pressure while avoiding the severe systemic complications of larger, repeated doses of this hyperosmotic agent.

Evidence is accumulating that barbiturate therapy, with moderately long-acting barbiturates, may be helpful in reducing intracranial pressure. The underlying mechanism is poorly understood, and use of these agents will depend upon the results of further clinical trials prior to their acceptance by the practicing community.

Between 2 and 5 percent of patients with closed cerebral trauma will develop a focal or generalized seizure. This raises the question of prophylactic anticonvulsants in closed head trauma cases. We believe that the potential for drug reaction outweighs the benefits derived and consequently withhold anticonvulsants until the clinical course (a focal or generalized seizure) indicates their need. Should a seizure supervene, however, vigorous efforts must be made to attain therapeutic levels of anticonvulsants to avoid the potential complications of status epilepticus.

In summary, several factors repeatedly appear in the consideration of the assessment and management of patients with acute cranial trauma. First, a precise, recorded neurologic examination should be made as soon as feasible, essentially, as soon as cardiopulmonary systems have been stabilized. Once this has been done and appropriate diagnostic studies have been secured, repeated evaluation of these basic parameters will provide a detailed analysis of any changes in trend that will determine appropriate modifications of therapy. Finally, one must adhere closely to the tenet of introducing some change in therapy, whether medical or surgical, in the face of an increasing neurologic deficit.

REFERENCES

1. Jennett, B., and Teasdale, G. Assessment of coma and impaired consciousness. A practical scale. *Lancet* 2:81, 1974.
2. Plum, F., and Posner, J. (Eds.). *Diagnosis of Stupor and Coma* (2nd ed.). (Contemporary Neurology Series No. 10.) Philadelphia: Davis, 1972.
3. Pollay, M. Formation of cerebrospinal fluid. *J. Neurosurg.* 42:665, 1975.

W. Scott McDougal / 21. RENAL
Robert A. Danielson / DYSFUNCTION

The kidneys play a major role in maintaining the appropriate extracellular fluid (ECF) volume and its proper electrolyte composition. Unfortunately, malfunction of this organ system is not uncommon in the critically ill. It is clear that renal dysfunction in these patients leads to a marked increase in mortality and morbidity. Oftentimes, major malfunctions can only be treated by supportive measures; therefore, the emphasis must be placed on early recognition of impending dysfunction so that preventive measures may be instituted before the dysfunction becomes inevitable. There is considerable evidence to indicate that abnormalities, if corrected early, will result in rapid return of renal function, whereas delays result in a markedly increased incidence of immediately irreversible abnormal renal function. Patients who develop renal failure must then be supported by dialysis until the kidney slowly regains function. Initial signs of renal dysfunction often involve abnormalities of urine flow. Therefore, we have chosen to discuss the subject under two general headings: abnormally low flow or oliguria and excessive flow or polyuria. Note, however, that renal failure may occur despite normal urine flow: the sine qua non of renal dysfunction is an elevated plasma creatinine concentration.

Oliguria is generally defined as a urine flow of less than 400 to 500 ml/day, or less than 20 ml/hr. Polyuria may be defined as urine excretion exceeding 2,400 ml/day or 100 ml/hr. If urine output falls outside 20 to 100 ml/hr, the cause of the abnormality must be identified and corrective measures taken.

In this chapter, the pathophysiology and clinical management of each major category of oliguria and polyuria are discussed. An understanding of the pathophysiologic events leading to oliguria and polyuria forms the basis for correct interpretation of clinical and laboratory observations and for proper therapy.

OLIGURIA
The differential diagnosis of acute oliguria falls into three general pathophysiologic categories: acute postrenal failure, acute prerenal failure, and acute renal failure (ARF). *Acute postrenal failure* is due to obstruction or extravasation of urinary outflow from the urethra, bladder, ureters, or renal pelvis. *Acute prerenal failure* is functional renal insufficiency due to a defi-

cient plasma volume, a deficient cardiac output, or an excessive nitrogen load. *Acute renal failure* is failure of the kidney itself to function. These entities will be discussed in the following section. (*Note:* Hyperkalemia, the most urgent disorder that accompanies any form of oliguria, must be recognized and treated early.)

ACUTE POSTRENAL FAILURE
Acute postrenal failure is defined as obstruction or extravasation of urinary outflow from the urethra, bladder, ureters, or kidneys.

PATHOPHYSIOLOGY
Obstruction of urine flow causes an increase in hydrostatic pressure in the urinary tract proximal to the obstructing lesion. Increased intratubular hydrostatic pressure probably decreases the glomerular filtration rate (GFR) by a fall in the net hydrostatic pressure driving force for filtration. However, glomerular filtration does not cease, even though the obstruction of urine flow may be complete. The tubular fluid that is filtered is partially reabsorbed by the tubules and partially diffuses back into the peritubular and peripelvic lymphatic and venous vessels. On occasion, striking peripelvic extravasation of urine can be demonstrated by intravenous pyelography during acute urinary obstruction.

Morphologic and functional damage to the renal parenchyma may occur. The extent of the damage is correlated with the degree and duration of obstruction, the level of the urinary tract where the obstruction occurs (the more proximal the obstruction, the greater the destruction of renal parenchyma per unit period of time), the nutritional status of the patient, the degree to which renal blood flow is compromised by preexisting disease, and the presence and virulence of associated pyelonephritis [10].

INTRARENAL REGULATION OF GLOMERULAR FILTRATION RATE. The fall in GFR that accompanies severe urinary outflow obstruction may not be due entirely to an increase in tubular fluid hydrostatic pressure but also to a mechanism for the intrarenal regulation of GFR which has been reviewed by Wright [82]. This mechanism involves activation of the intrarenal renin-angiotensin (RA) system by the presence of increased amounts of reabsorbable Na^+ at the macula densa of the distal tubule. Locally, liberated angiotensin II causes constriction of the glomerular afferent arteriole and a fall in GFR.

The intrarenal regulation of GFR may play an important role in many pathophysiologic renal states, including acute postrenal failure, postobstructive diuresis, and acute renal failure. Renin is found in the secretory granules of the juxtaglomerular cells of the juxtaglomerular apparatus [28]. The enzymatic action of renin substrate produces the decapeptide angiotensin I, which has little vasoactive properties until converting enzyme splits off the octapeptide angiotensin II, the most powerful pressor agent known. Within the kidney, angiotensin II causes constriction of the afferent arteriole [61], a reduction in glomerular capillary hydrostatic pressure, and a fall in GFR.

The release of renin can be stimulated by (1) low pulse pressure in the afferent arteriole [77], (2) sympathoadrenergic stimuli [61], and (3) resorbable Na^+ at the macula densa in the early distal tubule (i.e., the proximal portion) [76]. The third stimulus for the release of renin may be involved in the intrarenal regulation of GFR.

This tubular-glomerular feedback mechanism is suggested by the anatomic arrangement of the nephron. Each nephron is arranged so that the early distal tubule is found adjacent to its own glomerulus. The macula densa cells of the early distal tubule are in contact with the juxtaglomerular cells of the afferent and efferent arterioles and the mesangium of the glomerulus. This anatomic complex is the juxtaglomerular apparatus, and it may provide a pathway for tubular-glomerular communication. Functionally, when the macula densa is perfused with a solution containing resorbable Na^+, the single-nephron GFR in that tubule falls; this is called the tubular-glomerular feedback mechanism, and it may cause a low GFR in obstructive uropathy due to increased distal delivery of Na^+. Micropuncture experiments 15 hours after the release of bilateral ureteral obstruction showed the Na^+ concentration in the early distal tubule to be twice as high as control values, demonstrating impaired net Na^+ transport in the proximal tubule and loop of Henle. The increased Na^+ delivery to the macula densa triggers the local RA system to lower GFR.

The renin-angiotensin system may not be solely responsible for the reduction in renal blood flow and hence GFR in postrenal failure. There is accumulating evidence to indicate that the prostaglandins and thromboxanes may also participate in the mediation of this response. A relative absence of the vasodilator prostaglandin may result in unopposed renal vasoconstriction, resulting in a reduction in renal blood flow and thereby a diminished GFR. Moreover, there is limited evidence to indicate that in obstructive uropathy, the thromboxanes, which are known vasoconstrictors, are present in increased concentrations.

ETIOLOGY

The many causes of obstructive uropathy may be grouped under congenital, neoplastic, infectious, traumatic, and other acquired abnormalities. Prostatic enlargement, urethral transection, and strictures are among the common urethral causes of acute postrenal failure. In the bladder, urinary retention may occur for a variety of neurogenic reasons. Ureteral stones or tumor, inadvertently placed pelvic sutures or other ureteral injuries, retroperitoneal fibrosis, or retroperitoneal, bladder, or pelvic malignancies may cause outflow obstruction of the ureters. The ureteropelvic junction may be obstructed by congenital bands, aberrant vessels, neoplasms, infection, strictures, or stones. The differential diagnostic possibilities of acute postrenal failure are many; the foregoing examples are not exhaustive. Most commonly, however, acute postrenal failure is due to problems in the urethra or bladder, since bilateral involvement of both ureters or both kidneys is unusual, provided the patient *has* two kidneys.

Clinical and Laboratory Observations

Frequently, the patient with acute postrenal obstruction or extravasation of urine flow is *anuric*, in contrast with other acute oliguric states. A past history of hesitancy, weak urinary stream, frequency, nocturia, suprapubic pain, or renal colic may precede the acute illness and provide an etiologic clue. A history of recent trauma to the pelvis, back, or abdomen raises suspicion of urinary extravasation.

Physical examination of the patient may reveal the presence of tender kidneys, abdominal or pelvic masses, trauma, a distended bladder, or urethral blood.

A urinalysis may show occult or gross hematuria, while serum blood urea nitrogen (BUN) and creatinine indicate the degree of renal impairment and serve as a baseline to measure therapeutic progress. Renal function studies demonstrate impaired renal concentrating ability and impaired renal Na^+ conservation similar to that seen with acute intrinsic renal failure (Table 21-1).

Management

Catheter drainage of the urinary bladder frequently offers immediate relief of acute postrenal obstruction while narrowing the diagnostic possibilities to the urinary bladder or urethra. (*Note:* One must be certain that the catheter is properly placed and draining freely.) If there is suspicion of acute postrenal obstruction higher in the urinary tract, laminagrams of the kidneys and ultrasonography may be helpful. Ultrasonography has come to play an important role in the diagnosis of acute renal failure. It can be performed at the patient's bedside and therefore is ideally suited for the critically ill patient. The sonographic length of the kidney is calculated and compared to the measured x-ray height of L-2. The normal ratio of normally functioning kidneys is 3.58 ± 0.38. Ratios greater than two standard deviations from normal are considered enlarged and therefore likely to be obstructed. The B mode ultrasonogram also may directly visualize the hydronephrotic system in patients suffering from postrenal failure [67]. In trauma patients, who may undergo surgical exploration for urinary tract injury, it is essential to know that the patient's *other* kidney is present and functioning. Valuable diagnostic information may be obtained by careful catheterization of one ureter and retrograde pyelography. Ureteral catheters may be left in place for a short time to relieve ureteral obstruction until

TABLE 21-1. Laboratory Distinction Between Acute Postrenal, Acute Prerenal, and Acute Renal Failure

Laboratory Determination	Optimal Renal Function	Acute Postrenal Failure	Acute Prerenal Failure	Acute Renal Failure (ARF)
Plasma urea-creatinine concentration ratio	10:1	~10:1	>10:1	~10:1
Urine				
Sodium concentration (mEq/L)	15–40	>40	<20	>30
Potassium concentration (mEq/L)	15–40	Variable	Variable	Variable
Osmolality (mOsm/kg H_2O)	400–600	<400	>400	<400
Specific gravity		~1.010	>1.020	~1.010
Volume (ml/day)	500–2400	<500	<500	Variable
Urine sediment	0–1 RBC 0–1 WBC Occasional hyaline cast No cellular casts	Look for RBCs, WBCs, malignant cells, crystals	Occasional hyaline cast	Tubular epithelial cells and casts, RBCs, free hemoglobin or myoglobin
Urine-plasma concentration ratios				
Urea	20:1	<8:1	>10:1	<4:1
Osmolality*	1.5:1–2:1	<1:1	>1.5:1	<1.1:1

RBC = red blood cells; WBC = white blood cells.

* The single most reliable observation that confirms the diagnosis of oliguric ARF is a urine-plasma osmotic concentration ratio <1.1.

definitive treatment is undertaken; sterile technique is essential. (*Note:* Any modality that introduces infection may initiate pyelonephritis and increase renal parenchymal damage. Frequent urine cultures are advised to identify pathogens and their antibiotic sensitivities so that specific antibiotic treatment may be started early.)

Definitive therapy of postrenal obstruction is directed to the site of obstruction. Immediate surgical procedures for decompression include suprapubic cystostomy, cutaneous ureterostomy, and nephrostomy. Urinary extravasation is relatively harmless for the first 24 to 36 hours. However, evidence of a preexisting urinary tract infection, especially with coliform or *Proteus* organisms, is cause for urgent concern; extravasation under these circumstances requires prompt drainage [52]. The early use of broad-spectrum prophylactic antibiotics in urinary extravasation is advisable to avoid the development of infection in undrained hematomas.

Early relief of postrenal obstruction will avert permanent renal damage, provided infection has been avoided. A dramatic postobstructive diuresis may follow the release of postrenal obstruction within 2 to 24 hours. Impaired renal Na^+ transport throughout the nephron accounts for the massive loss of salt and water despite a low GFR. Preexisting volume overload and elevated BUN may also contribute to the diuresis. Management of postobstructive diuresis requires precise replacement of fluid and electrolyte losses, simultaneously avoiding sustained overhydration on the one hand and hypovolemia on the other.

ACUTE PRERENAL FAILURE
The most common cause of oliguria in critically ill patients is acute prerenal failure. Prerenal failure is defined as functional renal insufficiency [58] due to a deficient plasma volume, cardiac output, or an excessive nitrogen load. In acute prerenal failure the kidney itself is normal; it functions to excrete nitrogenous waste products in an economically small volume of urinary water.

PHYSIOLOGY OF EXTRACELLULAR FLUID VOLUME REGULATION
It is especially important to understand the physiology of ECF volume regulation to distinguish clinical and laboratory findings of functional renal insufficiency from failure of the kidney itself to function (ARF). The physiology of ECF volume regulation is conveniently divided into systemic mechanisms and renal mechanisms. These mechanisms will be discussed briefly and correlated with clinical events and appropriate patient management.

SYSTEMIC MECHANISMS. Extracellular fluid volume regulation, reviewed comprehensively by Gauer et al. [24] and Share and Claybaugh [71] is determined by autoregulation, baroreceptors, volume receptors, and osmotic receptors.

AUTOREGULATION. A modest fall in blood pressure does not *directly* lower renal blood flow (RBF) or GFR. Within a range of 30 mm Hg above or below normal systolic blood pressure, the renal vascular resistance changes directly with blood pressure, so that RBF and GFR are held nearly constant. This phenomenon is called autoregulation. The mechanism by which autoregulation of RBF is achieved is not clear, but it may be due to stretch receptors in the afferent arteriole that reflexly contract with a distending pressure and reflexly relax with a falling pressure [66]. An excessive fall in systemic blood pressure to 60 mm Hg or less cannot be compensated by renal autoregulation, and a fall in RBF, GFR, and urine output occurs. This is a coarse regulatory mechanism seen in shock.

BARORECEPTORS. Nevertheless, renal function can be altered by subtle changes in systemic blood pressure through neurohumoral pathways. A slight fall in arterial blood pressure will decrease vagal afferent impulses from the aortic arch and carotid sinus baroreceptors to allow hypothalamic release of antidiuretic hormone (ADH), increased sympathoadrenergic activity, and increased renin-angiotensin-aldosterone (RAA) activity through sympathetic efferent nerve pathways. These mechanisms act on the kidney to conserve salt and water, thus restoring circulating plasma volume.

Volume receptors. Renal function can also be altered by a 10 percent loss of blood volume; such a loss is insufficient to alter systemic blood pressure. Volume receptors of the low-pressure system in both atria sense a 3-cm water pressure change. A fall in atrial pressure reduces vagal afferent impulses from the subendocardial stretch receptors to allow hypothalamic centers to release ADH from the posterior pituitary. An excellent review of nonosmolar factors affecting renal water excretion has been published by Schrier and Berl [69].

Osmotic receptors. A loss of water in excess of salt causes plasma osmolality to increase. In 1946, Verney [79] first demonstrated the existence of intracranial receptors sensitive to plasma osmotic pressure in unanesthetized dogs undergoing a water diuresis. An injection of hypertonic sodium chloride or dextrose solution into an externalized carotid artery led to prompt interruption of water diuresis. Hypophysectomy blocked, and injections of ADH mimicked, the response to the hypertonic injections. Thus, intracranial osmotic receptors affect the diuresis through modulation of ADH release.

It is apparent that both osmolar and nonosmolar factors regulate ADH release. Arndt [3] studied the competition between osmotic and volume stimuli near threshold for control of ADH secretion. A 6 percent blood volume loss abolished a diuresis that followed an intracarotid injection of distilled water. When blood was retransfused, the water diuresis resumed. Thus, ECF volume stimuli supersede osmotic stimuli in modulating ADH release.

RENAL MECHANISMS. Renal salt and water excretion are modified by four general mechanisms: changes in GFR, RAA activity, third factor, and ADH secretion.

Glomerular filtration rate. A fall in GFR reduces renal salt and water losses. It occurs in response to systemic hypotension outside the range where autoregulation of RBF and GFR can compensate. Glomerular filtration rate also falls in response to a net decrease in opposing hydrostatic and osmotic forces across the glomerular capillary wall, as predicted by Starling's hypothesis. Afferent arteriolar vasoconstriction in response to sympathoadrenergic stimuli or to angiotensin II also reduces GFR.

Renin-angiotensin-aldosterone system. The RAA system, previously described, plays a major role in both normal and pathophysiologic renal function. It is necessary to point out here that angiotensin II is a potent stimulus for aldosterone secretion by the adrenal cortex. Aldosterone restores ECF volume by increasing Na^+ resorption in the distal nephron. Other factors that also stimulate aldosterone secretion include elevated plasma K^+ concentration, adrenocorticotropic hormone (ACTH), and hemodynamic stimuli [40].

Third factor. Third factor is a term applied to mechanisms that alter renal Na^+ excretion other than changes in GFR and aldosterone concentration. A natriuretic hormone has not been conclusively identified. Redistribution of intrarenal blood flow from salt-losing superficial cortical nephrons to salt-conserving juxtamedullary nephrons may play a physiologic role in renal salt and water handling; the intrarenal distribution of blood flow is altered by angiotensin II and sympathoadrenergic stimuli.

Antidiuretic hormone. Antidiuretic hormone permits the kidney to retain water by increasing the water permeability of the collecting duct epithelium. The osmotic pressure driving force that causes the resorption of water from the collecting duct lumen into the medullary tissue is established by active Cl^- transport in the thick ascending limb of the loop of Henle. Medullary hypertonicity is maintained by the countercurrent arrangement of the loops of Henle, vasa recta, and collecting ducts within the renal medulla.

The major solutes contributing to medullary hypertonicity are Na^+, Cl^-, and urea. The presence of concentrated urea in the renal medulla serves two related functions: (1) urea contributes to the osmotic pressure driving force to remove water from the collecting duct lumen, and (2) equilibration of urea concentration across the collecting duct epithelium allows the generation of high urea urinary concentrations. The renal medulla, therefore, achieves the excretion of nitrogenous waste products in an economically small volume of water.

PLASMA UREA-CREATININE CONCENTRATION RATIO. Plasma urea concentration is elevated during extreme oliguria. Increased urea production due to deamination of protein for gluconeogenesis to satisfy hypermetabolic demands in a severely ill patient is partially responsible for the elevated plasma urea concentration. Elevated plasma urea concentration also occurs because of decreased glomerular filtration and increased back diffusion of urea in prerenal failure.

In a physiologically normal kidney, a portion of filtered urea, which circulates within the medulla, diffuses back into the general circulation from the vasa recta and distal tubules [54], contributing to the elevated plasma urea concentration. The plasma urea-creatinine concentration ratio usually exceeds 10 : 1 in acute prerenal failure. In acute intrinsic renal failure, the medullary concentrating mechanism does not function, and the fraction of filtered water excreted is high. Since the renal handling of urea is dependent on tubular water resorption, the fraction of filtered urea excreted should be high in ARF; less back diffusion of filtered urea is expected. The plasma urea-creatinine concentration ratio is about 10 : 1 in ARF, since a failure of filtration alone is largely responsible for the failure of excretion of these two substances.

ETIOLOGY
The patient's history may reveal the cause of plasma volume deficiency. Deficits in plasma volume are commonly due to hemorrhage, acute gastrointestinal losses, excessive insensible losses, inadequate fluid intake, and large third-space losses, such as in pancreatitis, burns, or bowel obstruction.

CLINICAL AND LABORATORY OBSERVATIONS
Physical examination of a patient with acute prerenal failure may reveal signs of hypovolemia, including a rapid pulse, decreased skin turgor, and dry mucous membranes. A measure of central venous pressure (CVP) is low, usually 1 to 2 cm H_2O. Examination of the urine in functional renal insufficiency reveals that the kidney is performing in a physiologically normal manner (Table 21-1): the urine is concentrated with (1) a specific gravity

above 1.020, (2) urine osmolality 400 to 1,200 mOsm/kg H_2O, and (3) a urine-plasma (U/P) osmotic concentration ratio of at least 1.5. The kidney excretes its nitrogenous waste product urea in high concentrations, often exceeding 1,000 mg/100 ml [34]; the U/P urea concentration ratio exceeds 10 [63]. Renal Na^+ conservation is efficient; the urine Na^+ concentration is less than 20 mEq/liter, and the urine Na^+ loss is negligible. Plasma urea and creatinine concentrations are elevated due to hemoconcentration and a diminished GFR, but the ratio of plasma urea to creatinine concentrations is greater than 10 : 1 in prerenal azotemia because of back diffusion of urea from the vasa recta and distal tubules into the general circulation without a proportionate amount of reabsorption of creatinine.

MANAGEMENT

When the present illness and physical findings are consistent with plasma volume depletion, rapid expansion of plasma volume may confirm the diagnosis of prerenal failure while laboratory studies are pending. The type of intravenous fluid given depends on the type of fluid loss incurred. Isotonic losses should be replaced initially with normal saline or Ringer's lactate. Hypertonic dehydration is corrected with 0.45% saline. Whole-blood losses are initially replaced with crystalloid until blood is available. In the first hour or two, 500 to 1,000 ml or more of fluids are infused rapidly (10–15 ml/kg/hr) to reexpand plasma volume and reestablish urine flow. Thereafter, full correction of fluid and electrolyte aberrations is best carried out at a more cautious rate.

A dilemma in managing oliguric postoperative patients often arises in deciding whether or not to give additional fluids. After extensive surgery or trauma, patients in ideal fluid balance gain 1 to 2 kg because of third-space sequestration of fluid and because of normal posttraumatic renal salt and water retention. CVP is not an entirely reliable guide in fluid balance. Usually, the need to give more fluids can be determined by clinical evaluation of the patient. Peripheral or presacral edema is a good sign that the circulating plasma volume compartment is saturated. Pulmonary auscultation and serial chest x-ray studies may reveal early signs of left heart failure that warn against further fluid administration. If uncertainty exists, a Swan-Ganz catheter should be inserted to measure pulmonary wedge pressure, which in turn reflects left atrial pressure. If the pulmonary wedge pressure is less than 15 mm Hg, further fluid may be infused safely.

Patients with heart disease may be oliguric from a low cardiac output. In these patients, the physical findings of congestive heart failure (CHF) and an elevated CVP (>15 cm H_2O) are usually detectable. Improved cardiac output is first obtained by fluid restriction, diuretics, rotating tourniquets, phlebotomy, oxygen, and positive-pressure breathing. If CHF persists after these measures, digoxin may be given, and the blood digoxin concentrations should be monitored by laboratory analysis. The acute use of

TABLE 21-2. Etiology of Acute Intrinsic Renal Failure

Occlusion of renal arteries or renal veins

Arteriolar damage
  Malignant hypertension
  Polyarteritis
  Hypersensitivity angiitis

Disseminated intravascular coagulation (DIC)

Glomerulonephritis
  Lupus erythematosus
  Post streptococcal glomerulonephritis
  Other

Parenchymal damage
  Acute interstitial nephritis
  Acute pyelonephritis
  Papillary necrosis
    Diabetes mellitus
    Nephrosclerosis
    Sickle-cell anemia
    Certain analgesics
  Cortical necrosis
  End-stage renal disease

Hepatorenal syndrome

Vasomotor nephropathy:
  Shock
  Sepsis
  Transfusion reactions
  Crush injury
  Poisons
  Drugs (e.g., gentamicin, kanamycin, cephaloridine,
    methicillin, methoxyflurane)
  Idiopathic

---

digoxin in CHF caused by overhydration is unnecessary, and toxic effects of the drug may be harmful.

When correction of plasma volume deficits and cardiac output fails to restore normal urinary flow and there is no evidence of an excessive exogenous nitrogen load, the ominous diagnosis of acute renal failure must be suspected.

ACUTE RENAL FAILURE

A serious cause of oliguria is acute renal failure (ARF), or intrinsic failure of the kidney itself to function. A list of causes of ARF is presented in Table 21-2.

NOMENCLATURE

The most common form of ARF encountered in the critically ill is the type that follows shock, sepsis, transfusion reactions, and so on. The term *vasomotor nephropathy* was first used for this syndrome in the early part of the century. Changing concepts of the pathophysiology of this entity are reflected in the changing nomenclature: lower nephron nephrosis, crush kidney, and acute tubular necrosis [8]. Recent studies have shown the primary abnormality to be a failure of glomerular filtration; the term *vasomotor nephropathy* has been reintroduced and has the advantage of conveying specific meaning [58]. Nevertheless, in this discussion, we will conform with current usage and retain the more general term *ARF* to refer to the kind of renal failure that follows shock, sepsis, and so on.

The usual course of ARF is one of transient oliguria lasting 8 to 16 days, with a mean duration of 11 days. The oliguric phase is followed by polyuria and a gradual return to near-normal renal function.

The mortality associated with ARF is high. In Vietnam, the U.S. Army reported a 63 to 69 percent mortality; sepsis was the single complication most responsible for death. Associated upper gastrointestinal bleeding carries an 80 percent mortality; jaundice carries a 90 percent mortality [45, 46]. The range of published mortality rates for ARF in civilian surgical patients is 35 to 71 percent [12].

PATHOPHYSIOLOGY

Three hypotheses of the mechanism of oliguria in ARF are (1) tubular obstruction secondary to intraluminal casts or to interstitial edema; (2) increased tubular permeability with associated back diffusion of the glomerular filtrate; and (3) alterations in renal hemodynamics, leading to a failure of glomerular filtration [23]. In experimental animal models of ARF, elevated hydrostatic pressure in the tubular lumen proximal to the casts has not been found. Similarly, increased tubular permeability has not been a constant finding. Micropuncture studies in many experimental models of ARF have shown a low single-nephron GRF. Total renal blood flow is invariably decreased, and the major reduction in RBF is often in the cortical component [30]. There is much circumstantial evidence to implicate the RA system in the initiating phase of ARF, but the specific events that induce and prolong the filtration failure are not yet understood. ARF can be almost totally prevented in experimental models by chronic saline loading [74] or by acute pretreatment with mannitol and saline [80]. The mechanism involved may be the depletion of renin stores *prior to* the renal insult. Currently, tubular permeability, intratubular obstruction, and redistribution of renal blood flow are all thought to contribute to some degree. The magnitude of the effect of each is dependent upon the etiology of the inciting cause [73].

CLINICAL AND LABORATORY OBSERVATIONS

The diagnosis of ARF is suspected after other causes of oliguria have been eliminated, i.e., urinary outflow obstruction, urinary extravasation, and functional renal insufficiency. Plasma volume, CVP, left atrial pressure, and cardiac output are restored to normal with no improvement in renal function in ARF.

Acute renal failure is manifested by oliguria, isosthenuria, and progressive uremia. Laboratory findings are presented in Table 21-1; the laboratory observations reflect severely abnormal renal function. The urine is dilute; the specific gravity is between 1.008 and 1.014, but the specific gravity may be misleadingly high due to the admixture of protein or sugar in the urine. The U/P osmotic concentration ratio is a more reliable index of renal concentrating ability; in ARF it is less than 1.1. The failure to concentrate the urine is reflected by a low U/P urea concentration ratio. Renal handling of Na^+ is impaired; the urinary Na^+ concentration exceeds 30 to 40 mEq/liter. The urine sediment in ARF often contains tubular cells and casts.

Plasma creatinine concentration in ARF increases by 2 to 3 mg/100 ml/day, and the BUN concentration increases by 25 to 35 mg/100 ml/day. In some severe catabolic states the BUN may rise by 60 to 90 mg/100 ml/day [75]. The ratio of plasma urea to plasma creatinine concentrations is less than 10 : 1.

MANAGEMENT

The treatment of ARF is not yet optimal, since there has been no major reduction in the 35 to 71 percent mortality rate in surgical patients. While dialysis has reduced death from overhydration and hyperkalemia, sepsis and gastrointestinal hemorrhage remain difficult to control.

PREVENTION. There are several factors known to predispose patients to the development of ARF. These factors include (1) advanced age, (2) preexisting renal dysfunction, (3) recent exposure to aminoglycosides or other nephrotoxic agents, (4) volume depletion, and (5) myoglobinuria [68]. It is critically important for all patients undergoing surgical procedures to be well hydrated preoperatively. In elective surgical procedures in which large third-space losses or hemorrhage are anticipated, overnight preoperative hydration is beneficial. When the risk of inducing ARF is high, intravenous mannitol during the operative procedure is helpful. Barry et al. [4] reported that in a controlled study of 14 patients undergoing aneurysmectomy of the abdominal aorta, mannitol reduced the expected fall in renal blood flow, GFR, and urine flow when given during the period of aortic clamping (20% mannitol given intravenously at 5.5 ml/min just before and during aortic clamping). In experimental glycerol-induced ARF in rats, combined pretreatment with mannitol and saline "almost totally prevents the development of azotemia" [80]. Prevention is more effective in saving lives of the critically ill than is current treatment of established ARF. In patients who have sustained crush or electric injuries, the potentially nephrotoxic hemochromogen myoglobin is released. It has been shown that the incidence of ARF in patients with myoglobinuria is markedly reduced when a diuresis is maintained. Urine output should therefore be kept at 100 cc/hr until the myoglobin is cleared from the serum.

EARLY DETECTION. Early recognition and prompt treatment of oliguria probably prevent the development of ARF. Certain patients with prerenal failure may remain oliguric despite correction of plasma volume deficits [47]. These patients are oliguric usually less than 50 hours; they have a U/P osmotic concentration ratio of 1.1 to 1.8. They respond to intravenous mannitol (100 ml of a 20% solution infused over 10–30 minutes every 2–3 hours to a maximum dose of 60 gm). In these circumstances, the action of mannitol is not clear. Either it may avert the development of ARF, or it may hasten the onset of diuresis following volume expansion. Mannitol has a vasodilatory effect on the renal vasculature; it also is an osmotic diuretic that may flush nephrons of cell debris and casts, but this latter effect is dubiously beneficial. Mannitol must be used with caution to avoid precipitation of congestive heart failure due to a shift of fluid into the circulating plasma volume compartment. Once the diagnosis of ARF is established by stringent laboratory criteria, mannitol is of no further value.

Early reports about the beneficial effects of furosemide are now regarded with skepticism. Furosemide, 100 to 3,200 mg/day in geometric progression on successive days, was reported to shorten the duration of oliguric azotemia [13]. In a more recent study, however, the need for dialysis was averted by the use of furosemide in only 4 of 49 cases of ARF [12]. Muth [57] reported that furosemide is not of therapeutic value in oliguria except in patients with prerenal failure due to cardiac decompensation.

Nevertheless, many clinicians recommend the use of moderate doses of furosemide in the group of patients with prerenal failure who remain oliguric despite correction of plasma volume deficits. The initial dose of furosemide (usually 80 mg) may be increased up to 320 mg or more, given intravenously. In this circumstance, furosemide may hasten the onset of a diuresis. However, it is difficult to defend this practice in patients who are on potentially nephrotoxic antibiotics, since the combination of furosemide and certain nephrotoxic antibiotics may actually increase renal damage [43, 44]. Both furosemide and ethacrynic acid are associated with ototoxicity. These diuretic agents are particularly dangerous when given mistakenly to ECF volume–depleted patients; the resulting diuresis may cause further volume depletion and shock.

Drugs that are currently being investigated in experimental ARF include dopamine [27], converting enzyme inhibitor, and a competitive antagonist of angiotensin II, 1-sar-8-ala-angiotensin II [59]. As yet, it has not been proved that these agents have a beneficial effect.

TREATMENT OF ESTABLISHED ACUTE RENAL FAILURE. Once a diagnosis of ARF is established, fluid intake is restricted to 400 ml/day plus the volume of other fluid losses. Body weight in an ARF patient in fluid balance will decline 500 gm/day due to protein catabolism. Sodium balance is maintained by quantitatively replacing losses. Frequent serum electrolytes are obtained to monitor Na$^+$ replacement and to detect hyperkalemia.

HYPERKALEMIA. Cardiac dysfunction occurs frequently with a serum K$^+$ concentration in excess of 8.0 mEq/liter; dysfunction is uncommon with a concentration less than 7.0 mEq/liter. Cardiac manifestations of hyperkalemia include bradycardia, hypotension, and cardiac arrest from ventricular fibrillation or standstill. Hyperkalemia interferes with intra-atrial and intraventricular conduction. The sequential electrocardiogram (ECG) abnormalities of increasingly severe hyperkalemia are as follows: tall, peaked T waves, depressed S–T segments, decreased amplitude of R waves, a prolonged P–R interval, P waves that are diminished to absent, widening of the QRS complex, prolongation of the Q–T interval, and finally a sine wave pattern. (*Note:* An initial ECG determines the severity of the hyperkalemia and the urgency of therapy while awaiting return of laboratory serum electrolyte concentrations. The initial ECG serves as a baseline for further evaluation of therapy.)

Moderate hyperkalemia (6.0–7.0 mEq/liter) is treated by withholding K$^+$ administration in any form (it must be remembered that some antibiotics may contribute significant amounts of sodium or potassium) and by correcting existing metabolic or respiratory acidosis. Sodium polystyrene sulfonate (Kayexalate), a cation exchange resin, is given either orally or as an enema; 15 to 60 gm is given in divided doses. Since Kayexalate may cause constipation, sorbitol is also administered. Although oral administration of cation exchange resins is more effective in lowering serum K$^+$ concentration, the rectal route is preferable in patients with alimentary tract dysfunction.

Severe hyperkalemia (>7.0 mEq/liter) should be rapidly controlled with intravenous sodium bicarbonate, and the myocardium can be protected temporarily by the administration of calcium gluconate or calcium chloride. Rarely, it may be necessary to give insulin and glucose (1 unit of regular insulin per 5 gm of glucose), but rebound hypoglycemia could prove fatal. Further control of hyperkalemia is achieved with Kayexalate followed by hemodialysis or peritoneal dialysis if necessary.

A Quinton-Scribner shunt [64] is placed early to control overhydration and hyperkalemic acidosis by hemodialysis when conservative measures are insufficient. Some nephrologists prefer to use percutaneous techniques to cannulate the femoral vessels for short-term dialysis [36]. Sheldon catheters may be placed in the femoral vessels by the Seldinger technique, or a MacIntosh double-lumen catheter may be inserted into the iliac vein through the saphenous vein. Other nephrologists prefer peritoneal dialysis. The choice of route must take into account the safety and comfort of the patient, the experience of the nephrologist, and the expected duration of renal failure.

OTHER THERAPEUTIC MEASURES. Once the diagnosis of ARF is established, the urinary catheter is removed to eliminate a portal of entry for infection. Frequent cultures of sputum, urine, blood, and wounds are obtained. In the absence of specific infection, antibiotics are not recommended, but close observation for sepsis and early specific antibiotic treatment are required.

Roentgenograms of the abdomen with laminagrams of the kidneys (pyelographic visualization of the kidneys is usually not possible) should be obtained in an effort to determine whether or not prior renal disease is superimposed on the acute problem. Ultrasonography can determine renal size and thereby provide information about prior disease. Preexisting renal disease may be demonstrated by unilateral or bilateral small kidneys, which are indicative of vascular or infectious disease. An enlarged renal outline implies either acute renal vein thrombosis or infiltrative lesions, such as myeloma or lymphoma. Renal scans in suspected cases of bilateral renal artery thrombosis may indicate the need for arteriograms.

Since upper gastrointestinal hemorrhage may supervene, contributing to mortality, prophylactic antacid therapy should be used. Aluminum hydroxide is the most desirable antacid in ARF, since it helps to control the hyperphosphatemia of renal failure.

All diet and drug orders must be stopped, and a careful review of each order must be made in the light of absent renal function. The dosage of many therapeutic agents, including digitalis and antibiotics, may need to be adjusted [5, 65].

The timing and frequency of dialysis of patients with ARF are moot. Most centers regularly dialyze these patients 3 times a week as long as the BUN and serum creatinine concentrations continue to increase spontaneously. Kleinknecht and Ganeval [38] and Conger [16] report that preventive dialysis (to keep the BUN less than 70 mg/100 ml and the blood creatinine concentration less than 5 mg/100 ml) reduces mortality, bleeding episodes, and the incidence of major sepsis.

An important approach to improving the survival of ARF may lie in better nutritional management of these patients. Abel et al. [1] report "improved survival in patients with ARF after they had been treated with intravenous essential L-amino acids and glucose." Perhaps combining better nutritional management with more frequent dialyses will result in improved survival in this high-risk group of patients.

If renal function fails to improve spontaneously within 3 weeks, the diagnoses of renal infarction or acute cortical necrosis must be considered. Selective renal arteriograms may demonstrate obstruction of the renal artery and vein or may show loss of cortical blood flow. If a renal biopsy confirms the diagnosis, the patient should be placed on a chronic hemodialysis program. Renal transplantation may be considered if the patient is a suitable candidate.

HEPATORENAL SYNDROME

Hepatorenal syndrome (HRS) is a term that refers to the occurrence of ARF in patients with advanced liver disease. This variety of ARF deserves special comment. The renal failure is manifested by progressive azotemia, oliguria, a concentrated urine with a low urine Na^+ concentration, mild proteinuria, and occasionally hyponatremia. The onset of renal failure in end-stage liver disease frequently marks the terminal stage of the patient's illness [60]. There is no satisfactory treatment for either the renal or the liver failure.

PATHOPHYSIOLOGY. The pathophysiology of HRS is not well understood, but the renal failure appears to be functional and is associated with abnormal renal blood flow. The morphology of kidneys from patients dying with HRS is often normal or shows only minimal changes. Epstein et al. [21] have demonstrated decreased renal blood flow, especially to the superficial cortex, using renal arteriography and xenon washout studies in these patients. Further evidence that the kidneys function normally when the liver malfunction is corrected comes from experiences in transplantation. Kidneys transplanted from a hepatorenal donor to noncirrhotic recipients function normally [39]. Conversely, recovery from HRS following successful liver transplantation has been reported [31].

The functional renal disturbance in HRS has been variously attributed to the following: (1) failure of the liver to detoxify a pressor substance; (2) release of a vasoactive hormone from the damaged liver; (3) abnormal function of the RA system; (4) a decrease in effective plasma volume associated with ascites and splanchnic pooling of blood; and (5) extrarenal diversion of blood through arteriovenous shunts. Clarification of the pathophysiology of the renal failure associated with advanced liver disease must await further studies.

CLINICAL AND LABORATORY OBSERVATIONS AND PATIENT MANAGEMENT. The hepatorenal syndrome usually develops with greatest frequency in patients with the most advanced liver disease; ascites and hepatic encephalopathy are frequently present. The onset of renal failure can occur suddenly without apparent cause but is frequently associated with the use of diuretics, paracentesis, or surgical procedures.

There is no effective treatment for HRS, but the physician must always keep in mind that oliguria in a cirrhotic patient is not always due to the HRS and that other remediable causes, such as urinary obstruction or prerenal failure, may be involved. Therefore, the vigorous diagnostic efforts and treatment of acute oliguria described previously are required in these patients as well.

POLYURIA

The differential diagnosis of polyuria also falls into three general pathophysiologic categories: postrenal, prerenal, and intrinsic renal polyuria (Table 21-3). *Postrenal polyuria* is seen following the release of complete urinary obstruction or in the presence of chronic partial urinary occlusion. *Prerenal polyuria* is caused by insufficient circulating ADH and exogenous or endogenous diuretic agents. *Renal polyuria* is intrinsic renal impairment of the medullary concentrating mechanism due to anatomic disruption from disease, metabolic aberrations affecting ADH-collecting duct interaction, or functional renal derangements.

To diagnose the type of polyuria and manage critically ill polyuric patients properly, it is essential to understand the normal physiology of the renal concentrating mechanism, since disturbances in this function ultimately result in polyuria.

NORMAL RENAL CONCENTRATING MECHANISM

The bulk of the glomerular filtrate (60–70%) is resorbed isotonically from the proximal tubular lumen; 10 to 15 percent is resorbed from the loop of Henle and distal tubular lumen; remaining tubular fluid resorption is modulated in the medullary collecting duct by ADH.

Antidiuretic hormone is synthesized in the supraoptic nucleus of the hypothalamus and transported to the posterior pituitary, where it is stored. Release of the hormone occurs in response to increased plasma osmolality, decreased circulating blood volume, pain, stress, trauma, and anesthesia [26, 70]. Hyposmolar states, plasma volume expansion, and certain drugs (ethanol and nicotine) inhibit ADH release [37]. The hormone circulates to the kidney, where it binds to the collecting-duct cell membrane and activates adenyl cyclase, which facilitates the generation of adenosine $3' : 5' =$ cyclic monophosphate (cyclic AMP) from adenosine triphosphate (ATP). Cyclic AMP activates a protein kinase that is believed to increase water permeability in the collecting duct [29].

The driving force causing water to be resorbed from the medullary collecting-duct lumen is an osmotic pressure difference across the collecting-duct epithelium. Therefore, maintenance of medullary hypertonicity is essential for formation of concentrated urine. Conversely, should the medullary osmotic pressure gradient be dissipated, regardless of the circulating level of ADH, urinary concentration does not occur and polyuria results.

TABLE 21-3. Differential Diagnosis of Polyuria

Postrenal polyuria
  In chronic, partial urinary obstruction
  Following release of complete urinary obstruction (postobstructive diuresis)
Prerenal polyuria
  Insufficient circulating antidiuretic hormone (ADH)
    Suppressed ADH release
      Iatrogenic expansion of extracellular fluid volume
      Compulsive water drinking
      Cerebral lesions causing thirst
    Defects in ADH synthesis (diabetes insipidus)
      Diabetes insipidus associated with tumor, trauma, infection, and
        granulomatous diseases
      Idiopathic diabetes insipidus
      Familial diabetes insipidus
  Diuretic agents
    Inhibitors of renal tubular salt transport
      Diuresis following resolution of cardiac arrhythmias
      Addison's disease, Cushing's syndrome
      Nonosmotic pharmacologic agents
    Extrarenal osmotic diuretics
      Exogenous pharmacologic agents (e.g., mannitol)
      Endogenous diseases of metabolism (e.g., diabetes mellitus, excessive
        protein catabolism)
Renal polyuria (impaired renal concentrating mechanism)
  Anatomic disruption
    Sickle-cell anemia
    Pyelonephritis
    Polyarteritis nodosa
    Polycystic renal disease
    Medullary cystic disease
    Amyloidosis
    Myeloma
    Nephrocalcinosis
    Other
  Metabolic aberrations of ADH: collecting-duct interaction
    Hypercalcemia
    Potassium depletion
    Renal tubular acidosis
    Nephrogenic diabetes insipidus
    Other
  Functional renal derangements
    Acute renal failure, polyuric phase
    Posttransplantation acute renal failure
    Chronic renal failure
    Other

Medullary hypertonicity is established by active transport of Cl^- by the thick ascending limb of the loop of Henle; it is maintained by the counter-current flow arrangement of the loops of Henle, vasa recta, and collecting ducts. Medullary hypertonicity can be abolished by failure of ion transport mechanisms or by washout of medullary solute through rapid flow in either the vasa recta or tubules.

In each of the three broad categories of polyuria to be discussed, one or more elements of the normal renal concentrating mechanism is deranged.

POSTRENAL POLYURIA

Postrenal polyuria occurs during partial chronic urinary obstruction [19] or following release of complete urinary occlusion (postobstructive diuresis), provided that significant parenchymal damage has not occurred. Postrenal polyuria is characterized by excessive water, Na^+, and K^+ losses; decreased maximal tubular resorption of glucose; and decreased renal ability to acidify the urine [7, 20]. As much as 40 percent of filtered water, 30 percent of filtered Na^+, and 140 percent of filtered K^+ may be excreted in the urine [10, 78].

PATHOPHYSIOLOGY

The mechanisms of postobstructive diuresis have been elucidated in experimental animal models [6, 48, 50, 83]. Postobstructive diuresis occurs despite a reduced glomerular filtration rate because of impaired nephron salt and water resorption. A brisk flow of tubular fluid ensues throughout the nephron, resulting in (1) a washout of the medullary osmotic gradient, (2) failure of the medullary concentrating mechanism, (3) an enhanced condition for K^+ secretion, and (4) increased urinary losses of water, Na^+, and K^+.

REDUCED GLOMERULAR FILTRATION RATE. Measurements of GFR and renal blood flow are surprisingly low in postobstructive diuresis; GFR is low despite an increase in glomerular capillary permeability demonstrated by proteinuria, as well as an increased glomerular capillary clearance of horseradish peroxidase (molecular weight 40,000). An analysis of Starling's forces across the glomerular capillary wall suggests that the lowered GFR is a result of a reduced glomerular capillary hydrostatic pressure, since mild elevations in capillary oncotic and proximal tubular hydrostatic pressures are insufficient to explain the reduced filtration. Afferent arteriolar constriction from activation of the intrarenal RA system would account for the reduced GFR. Support for this hypothesis comes from the demonstration of increased adenosine triphosphatase (ATPase) activity and increased renin granularity in juxtaglomerular cells, as well as increased renal-vein concentrations observed after acute ureteral ligation [18, 32, 78]. There is some evidence that the absence of prostaglandins and perhaps the excessive presence of thromboxanes may also be important in reducing renal blood flow during obstruction. The mechanism for intrarenal regulation of GFR is discussed under the pathophysiology of acute postrenal failure (p. 502).

REDUCED RENAL TUBULAR FUNCTION. Tubular salt and water resorption is reduced and permeability increased throughout the nephron in postrenal polyuria. The medullary osmotic pressure gradient is dissipated, and the renal concentrating mechanism fails.

PROXIMAL TUBULE. Within the proximal tubule, decreased ATPase activity in morphologically intact tubular cells implies a reduction in active Na^+ resorption. Histologic evidence for increased tubular permeability comes from observations of widened terminal bars containing electron-microscopic markers. The markers show direct access of tubular fluid to the lateral intracellular spaces through normally tight intracellular junctions. Reduced proximal tubular salt and water resorption, as confirmed by micropuncture studies, appears due to diminished Na^+ resorption as well as to back diffusion of resorbate from the intracellular spaces into the tubular lumen.

LOOP OF HENLE. Similar reductions in Na^+ and Cl^- resorption, coupled with increased epithelial water permeability, occur in the loop of Henle. This functional derangement abolishes the medullary osmotic pressure gradient and thereby cripples the renal concentrating mechanism, leading to increased urinary losses of water and solute.

DISTAL NEPHRON. In the distal nephron, the impaired salt and water transport mechanisms are overwhelmed by the excessive delivery of tubular fluid from the more proximal nephron segments. It is noteworthy that K^+ secretion is greatly enhanced by the rapid flow of dilute tubular fluid through the distal nephron.

Other mechanisms have been proposed to explain the postobstructive diuresis. The roles of ECF volume expansion and solute retention during the period of urinary obstruction have been considered [22, 51, 55]. Extracellular fluid volume expansion and solute diuresis, when present, certainly enhance the diuresis, but the syndrome is seen in patients with volume *contraction* with normal urea loads to the kidney. These observations deny a primary role for ECF volume expansion and urea diuresis in the etiology of postobstructive diuresis.

CLINICAL AND LABORATORY OBSERVATIONS AND PATIENT MANAGEMENT
Clinically, postobstructive diuresis begins 2 to 24 hours after release of urinary obstruction. In these circumstances, the urine specific gravity is below 1.005; the U/P osmotic concentration ratio is less than 1.0; and the U/P urea concentration ratio is often less than 8 (Table 21-1). The urinary

Na^+ concentration exceeds 50 mEq/liter, and the urinary K^+ concentration is over 20 mEq/liter.

The diuresis is self-limiting. Renal Na^+ and K^+ metabolism returns to normal in 48 to 72 hours, while the concentrating defect may persist for 1 to 2 weeks. On occasion, a spectacular diuresis of greater than 10 liters/day with excessive urinary Na^+ and K^+ losses may last for several weeks.

The diuresis is unresponsive to ADH, and the Na^+ transport defect is insensitive to mineralocorticoids. Excessive fluid replacement perpetuates the diuresis and increases urinary Na^+ losses. Generally, 5 gm/100 ml of dextrose in 0.45 gm/100 ml saline can be infused safely until laboratory measurements of urinary Na^+ and K^+ losses are available to guide replacement therapy. The intravenous infusion rate should be adjusted initially to match urine flow, provided the patient is not significantly overhydrated. After 24 hours, the intravenous fluid rate may be decreased cautiously, but ECF volume depletion and dehydration must be prevented. The clinical signs of ECF volume depletion are discussed under clinical and laboratory observations of acute prerenal failure. Therapy to maintain homeostasis of the internal milieu must be continued until adequate renal function returns.

Clinically significant postobstructive diuresis is seen only when the total nephron mass has been obstructed; i.e., unilateral urinary obstruction causes inappropriate water, Na^+, and K^+ losses from that side, but their magnitude is such that routine fluid replacement is usually adequate to manage the patient properly [49].

PRERENAL POLYURIA

Prerenal polyuria is due to insufficient ADH or to exogenous or endogenous diuretic agents; the intrinsic integrity of the renal concentrating mechanism is maintained (Table 21-3). However, if prerenal polyuria is allowed to persist for prolonged periods, washout of the medullary osmotic pressure gradient occurs [2, 17], resulting in a superimposition of renal on prerenal polyuria.

PATHOPHYSIOLOGY AND ETIOLOGY OF INSUFFICIENT ANTIDIURETIC HORMONE

Insufficient ADH activity results either from suppression of ADH release by normal physiologic mechanisms or through failure of ADH production. Physiologic suppression of ADH release is a consequence of ECF volume expansion or of a decrease in plasma osmolality. The more common causes of ECF volume expansion include overadministration of intravenous fluids, compulsive water drinking, and pathologic stimulation of the thirst center. Dilution of plasma osmolality occurs when salt and water losses are replaced with electrolyte-poor fluid. Absent or insufficient ADH production occurs in diabetes insipidus (Table 21-3), which may be an inherited or acquired abnormality.

CLINICAL AND LABORATORY OBSERVATIONS AND PATIENT MANAGEMENT
In the absence of ADH activity, laboratory findings reveal a low urinary specific gravity (<1.005), low urinary osmolality (<200 mOsm/kg H_2O), and a low urinary Na^+ concentration (<25 mEq/liter) [9, 15].

SUPPRESSED ADH RELEASE. Patients with physiologically suppressed ADH release respond to fluid restriction with a fall in urinary flow and a rise in urinary specific gravity and osmolality, provided the polyuric state has not washed out the medullary osmotic pressure gradient. When renal polyuria is superimposed on prerenal polyuria, the response to fluid restriction occurs slowly. In these circumstances, care must be taken to avoid ECF volume depletion and dehydration in the interim. Fluid restriction for several hours will lead to a stable urine osmolality above 250 mOsm/kg H_2O and will not respond to vasopressin administration [53].

DEFECTS IN ANTIDIURETIC HORMONE SYNTHESIS: DIABETES INSIPIDUS. Fluid restriction in patients with diabetes insipidus (Table 21-3) results in unabated renal water loss and progressive hypertonic dehydration. Diabetes insipidus is treated with exogenous vasopressin; several days may be required to reestablish the medullary osmotic pressure gradient before the effects of vasopressin are seen. In the interim, water restriction will cause the urine osmolality to stabilize between 60 and 200 mOsm/kg H_2O. In certain patients with low endogenous ADH production, chlorpropamide is beneficial because it potentiates the action of ADH [42, 56]. In patients with no endogenous ADH, chlorpropamide is ineffective. Until the diuresis of diabetes insipidus is controlled, careful replacement of fluid and electrolytes is required.

PATHOPHYSIOLOGY OF POLYURIA DUE TO DIURETIC AGENTS
The polyuria produced by diuretic agents is caused basically by an increased osmotic content within the nephron, preventing water resorption. The diuretics either inhibit tubular salt transport or impose an extrarenal osmotic load.

INHIBITORS OF RENAL TUBULAR SALT TRANSPORT. Inhibition of Na^+ resorption may be due to nonosmotic pharmacologic agents [69], absence of salt-retaining hormones, renal disease, and cardiac arrhythmias. The solute diuresis that follows conversion of a cardiac arrhythmia, particularly paroxysmal atrial tachycardia, to a normal sinus rhythm appears to be due to inhibition of proximal tubular Na^+ resorption through unknown mechanisms [35]. Formerly, the etiology of the diuresis following correction of a cardiac arrhythmia was ascribed to physiologic suppression of ADH. However, since a solute rather than a water diuresis occurs, other etiologic mechanisms are being considered.

The failure of normal Na^+ resorption in these conditions results in a solute load to the collecting duct. The increased osmotic content of the collecting-duct fluid reduces the osmotic pressure difference between lumen and interstitium and, simultaneously, the driving force for water resorption. If the solute load is of sufficient quantity, polyuria results.

EXTRARENAL OSMOTIC DIURETICS. Osmotic diuresis is a frequent cause of polyuria in the critically ill. The osmotically active substance may be an exogenous pharmacologic agent, e.g., mannitol, or a product of an endogenous metabolic disease, e.g., glucose in diabetes mellitus.

The mechanism by which polyuria occurs with glomerular filtration of nonresorbable solute, such as mannitol, radiographic dyes, and excess urea or glucose, is as follows: the osmotic agent is filtered at the glomerulus in an isosmotic concentration to plasma. In the proximal tubule, Na^+ resorption into the intracellular space sets up an osmotic concentration gradient that leads to isotonic water resorption. However, the nonresorbable osmotic substance within the proximal tubular lumen initially increases in concentration and then balances the Na^+ osmotic concentration in the intracellular spaces. Further water resorption is inhibited. Net Na^+ transport is reduced, due to an increasing Na^+ concentration difference between the proximal tubular lumen and the intracellular spaces. Thus, decreased water resorption indirectly diminishes proximal tubular Na^+ resorption.

Similar inhibition of salt and water resorption in the distal nephron leads to a solute diuresis and dissipation of the medullary osmotic pressure gradient. Thus, even after the osmotic agent is removed, diuresis may continue because of loss of medullary tonicity. In addition to excessive Na^+ and water losses, increased excretion of K^+, Ca^+, phosphate, and magnesium may result in clinically significant deficiencies [25].

RENAL POLYURIA
Renal polyuria results from intrinsic impairment of the renal concentrating mechanism due to anatomic disruption from disease, metabolic aberrations affecting ADH-collecting duct interaction, or functional renal derangements (Table 21-3).

ANATOMIC DISRUPTION
A reduction in renal medullary tonicity due to sickle cell anemia is representative of this group. Increased sickling of erythrocytes may occur in the renal medulla due to hypertonicity, decreased oxygen tension, and decreased pH. The abnormal sickle cell configuration retards blood flow in the medulla and reduces the amount of solute and water removed from the collecting

duct [62]. Complete occlusion of the vasa recta with infarction of the papilla results in permanent alterations [72]. In children, and to a lesser degree in adults, fresh blood transfusions will correct this defect, demonstrating the reversibility of this disease process in its early stages [33]. Urine osmolality and specific gravity vary according to the degree of medullary vascular occlusion. Urinary Na^+ concentrations may be elevated to levels as high as 60 mEq/liter [41]. Treatment is directed at replacing urinary salt and water losses. Exogenous vasopressin has been shown to be mildly effective in increasing urinary concentration.

Alterations that affect the collecting-duct structure (e.g., medullary cystic disease) or alter its permeability by surrounding it with impermeable protein deposits (e.g., amyloidosis [14]) may inhibit the concentrating mechanism sufficiently to produce polyuria.

METABOLIC ABERRATION OF ADH-COLLECTING DUCT INTERACTION

Metabolic alterations in the renal concentrating mechanism are of particular interest, since they may coexist in the critically ill patient. Diagnostic evaluation of polyuric states requires careful evaluation of the serum chemistries and urine pH. Hypercalcemia, prolonged K^+ depletion, and renal tubular acidosis result in polyuria that is rapidly reversed when the primary disorder is corrected. Hypercalcemia initially interferes with the action of ADH on the collecting-duct epithelium; if it is corrected early, there is an immediate reversal of the concentrating defect. However, prolonged hypercalcemia with calcium deposition in the thick ascending limb of the loop of Henle, distal tubule, and collecting-duct epithelia may result in permanent loss of renal concentrating ability.

The mechanism whereby hypokalemia exerts its effect in producing a diuresis is unclear; inhibition of the generation of adenyl cyclase, cyclic AMP, or protein kinase may be responsible. Hypokalemia may also directly inhibit the release of ADH from the posterior pituitary or stimulate hypothalamic thirst centers. Restoration of the K^+ levels in plasma corrects the renal concentrating mechanism [69].

Renal tubular acidosis results in hypokalemia; it is not known whether renal tubular acidosis interferes directly with the concentrating mechanism or whether its effect is mediated by reduced plasma K^+ concentrations. In either case, the renal concentrating mechanism is restored when acidosis and hypokalemia are corrected, provided nephrocalcinosis has not complicated the disease.

In nephrogenic diabetes insipidus, the collecting duct is insensitive to normal or elevated circulating levels of ADH. The urinary findings and response to fluid restriction are similar to those in diabetes insipidus; however, unlike the response in diabetes insipidus, urine osmolality is not affected by vasopressin administration.

FUNCTIONAL RENAL DERANGEMENTS

The pathophysiology of ARF has been discussed previously. In the diuretic phase of ARF, urine osmolality and specific gravity are low. The U/P osmotic concentration ratio is less than 1.1, the U/P urea concentration ratio is less than 4, and the urinary Na^+ concentration exceeds 30 mEq/liter. Sodium, fluid, and, rarely, K^+ losses can be excessive. During the diuretic phase of acute renal failure, urinary salt and water losses must be replaced carefully.

In summary, renal dysfunction often is manifested initially by oliguria or polyuria. Each of these two major categories may be subdivided into postrenal, prerenal, and intrinsic renal abnormalities. It is important to note that uremia may also occur despite normal urine flow; the sine qua non of renal dysfunction is an elevated plasma creatinine concentration. An understanding of the pathophysiology of acute uremia is essential for appropriate patient management.

REFERENCES

1. Abel, R. M., et al. Improved survival from acute renal failure after treatment with intravenous essential L-amino acids and glucose. N. Engl. J. Med. 288:695, 1973.
2. Andriole, V. T., and Epstein, F. H. Prevention of pyelonephritis by water diuresis: Evidence for the role of medullary hypertonicity in promoting renal infection. J. Clin. Invest. 44:73, 1965.
3. Arndt, J. O. Diuresis induced by water infusions into the carotid loop and its inhibition by small hemorrhage. Pfluegers Arch. 282:313, 1965.
4. Barry, K. E., et al. Mannitol infusion. II. The prevention of acute functional renal failure during resection of an aneurysm of the abdominal aorta. N. Engl. J. Med. 264:967, 1961.
5. Bennett, W. M., et al. A practical guide to drug usage in adult patients with impaired renal function. J.A.M.A. 214:1468, 1970.
6. Bercovitch, D. D., et al. The post-obstructive kidney. Observations on nephron function after relief of 24 hours of ureteral ligation in the dog. J. Clin. Invest. 50:1154, 1971.
7. Berlyne, G. M. Distal tubular function in chronic hydronephrosis. Q. J. Med. 30:339, 1961.
8. Berman, L. B. Vasomotor nephropathy. J.A.M.A. 231:1067, 1975.
9. Blom, P. S., et al. Sodium economy in the proximal and distal parts of the nephron studied in patients with diabetes insipidus. Their estimation under normal conditions and after salt restriction, chlorothiazide and a mercurial diuretic. Acta Med. Scand. 174:201, 1963.
10. Bricker, N. S., et al. An abnormality in renal function resulting from urinary tract obstruction. Am. J. Med. 23:554, 1957.
11. Bricker, N. S., and Klahr, S. Obstructive Nephropathy. In M. B. Strauss and L. G. Welt (Eds.), Diseases of the Kidney. Boston: Little, Brown, 1971. Pp. 997–1037.
12. Brown, C. B., et al. Established Acute Renal Failure Following Surgical

Operations. In E. A. Friedman and H. E. Eliahou (Eds.), *Proceedings Acute Renal Failure Conference.* Washington, D.C.: DHEW Publication No. (NIH) 74-608, 1973. Pp. 187–201.

13. Cantarovich, F., et al. Furosemide in high doses in the treatment of acute renal failure. *Postgrad. Med. J.* 47 (Suppl.): 13, 1971.

14. Carone, F. A., and Epstein, F. H. Nephrogenic diabetes insipidus caused by amyloid disease. *Am. J. Med.* 29:539, 1960.

15. Coggins, C. H., and Leaf, A. Diabetes insipidus. *Am. J. Med.* 42:807, 1967.

16. Conger, J. D. A Controlled Evaluation of Daily Dialysis in Post-traumatic Acute Renal Failure. *Abstracts,* The American Society of Nephrology, Nov. 25–26, 1974. P. 18.

17. DeWardener, H. E., and Herxheimer, A. W. The effect of a high water intake on the kidney's ability to concentrate the urine in man. *J. Physiol.* (Lond.) 139:42, 1957.

18. DiBona, G. Effect of mannitol diuresis and ureteral occlusion on distal tubular resorption. *N. Engl. J. Med.* 221:511, 1971.

19. Dorhout-Mees, E. J. Reversible water losing state, caused by incomplete ureteric obstruction. *Acta Med. Scand.* 168:193, 1960.

20. Eiseman, B., et al. Fluid and electrolyte changes following the relief of urinary obstruction. *J. Urol.* 74:222, 1955.

21. Epstein, M., et al. Renal failure in the patient with cirrhosis. *Am. J. Med.* 49:175, 1970.

22. Falls, W. F., and Stacy, W. K. Postobstructive diuresis. Studies in a dialyzed patient with a solitary kidney. *Am. J. Med.* 54:404, 1973.

23. Flamenbaum, W. Pathophysiology of acute renal failure. *Arch. Intern. Med.* 131:911, 1973.

24. Gauer, O. H., et al. The regulation of extracellular fluid volume. *Annu. Rev. Physiol.* 32:547, 1970.

25. Gennari, F. J., and Kassirer, J. P. Osmotic diuresis. *N. Engl. J. Med.* 291: 714, 1974.

26. Ginsburg, M. Production, Release, Transportation and Elimination of the Neurohypophyseal Hormones. In B. Berde (Ed.), *Handbooks of Experimental Pharmacology.* Berlin: Springer, 1968. Pp. 286–371.

27. Goldberg, L. I. Dopamine—Clinical uses of an endogenous catecholamine. *N. Engl. J. Med.* 291:707, 1974.

28. Goormaghtigh, N. Vascular and circulatory changes in renal cortex in the anuric crush-syndrome. *Proc. Soc. Exp. Biol. Med.* 59:303, 1945.

29. Handler, J. S., and Orloff, J. The Mechanism of Action of Antidiuretic Hormone. In J. Orloff, R. W. Berliner, and S. R. Geiger (Eds.), *Handbook of Physiology.* Section 8. Renal Physiology. Washington, D.C.: American Physiological Society, 1973. Pp. 791–814.

30. Hollenberg, N. K., and Adams, D. F. Vascular Factors in the Pathogenesis of Acute Renal Failure in Man. In E. A. Friedman and H. E. Eliahou (Eds.), *Proceedings Acute Renal Failure Conference.* Washington, D.C.: DHEW Publication No. (NIH) 74-608, 1973. Pp. 209–229.

31. Iwatsuki, S., et al. Recovery from "hepatorenal syndrome" after orthotopic liver transplantation. *N. Engl. J. Med.* 289:1155, 1973.

32. Kaloyanides, G. J., et al.   Effect of ureteral clamping and increased renal arterial pressure on renin release. *Am. J. Physiol.* 225:95, 1973.

33. Keifel, H. G., et al.   Hyposthenuria in sickle cell anemia: A reversible renal defect. *J. Clin. Invest.* 35:998, 1956.

34. Kerr, D. N. S.   Acute Renal Failure. In D. Black (Ed.), *Renal Disease*. London: Blackwell, 1972. Pp. 447–452.

35. Kinney, M. J., et al.   The polyuria of paroxysmal atrial tachycardia. *Circulation* 50:429, 1974.

36. Kjellstrand, C. M., et al.   Technique of Hemodialysis. In J. S. Najarian and R. L. Simmons (Eds.), *Transplantation*. Philadelphia: Lea & Febiger, 1972. Pp. 425–445.

37. Kleeman, C. R., et al.   Studies on alcohol diuresis. II. The evaluation of ethyl alcohol as an inhibitor of the neurohypophysis. *J. Clin. Invest.* 34:448, 1955.

38. Kleinknecht, D., and Ganeval, D.   Preventive Hemodialysis in Acute Renal Failure: Its Effect on Mortality and Morbidity. In E. A. Friedman and H. E. Eliahou (Eds.), *Proceedings Acute Renal Failure Conference*. Washington, D.C.: DHEW Publication No. (NIH) 74-608, 1973. Pp. 165–184.

39. Koppel, M. H., et al.   Transplantation of cadaveric kidneys from patients with hepatorenal syndrome: Evidence for the functional nature of renal failure in advanced liver disease. *N. Engl. J. Med.* 280:1367, 1969.

40. Laragh, J. H., and Sealey, J. E.   The Renin-Angiotensin-Aldosterone Hormonal System and Regulation of Sodium, Potassium, and Blood Pressure Homeostasis. In J. Orloff, R. W. Berliner, and S. R. Geiger (Eds.), *Handbook of Physiology*. Section 8. Renal Physiology. Washington, D.C.: American Physiological Society, 1973. Pp. 831–908.

41. Levitt, M. F., et al.   The renal concentrating defect in sickle cell disease. *Am. J. Med.* 29:611, 1960.

42. Liberman, B., et al.   Evidence for a role of antidiuretic hormone (ADH) in the antidiuretic action of chlorpropamide. *J. Clin. Endocrinol. Metab.* 36:894, 1973.

43. Linton, A. L.   Acute renal failure. *Can. Med. Assoc. J.* 110:949, 1974.

44. Linton, A. L., et al.   Protective Effect of Furosemide in Acute Tubular Necrosis and Acute Renal Failure. In E. A. Friedman and H. E. Eliahou (Eds.), *Proceedings Acute Renal Failure Conference*. Washington, D.C.: DHEW Publication No. (NIH) 74-608, 1973. Pp. 71–87.

45. Lordon, R. E.   Acute Renal Failure Following Battle Injury—Mortality, Complications, and Treatment. In E. A. Friedman and H. E. Eliahou (Eds.), *Proceedings Acute Renal Failure Conference*. Washington, D.C.: DHEW Publication No. (NIH) 74-608, 1973. Pp. 109–123.

46. Lordon, R. E., and Burton, J. R.   Post-traumatic renal failure in military personnel in Southeast Asia. *Am. J. Med.* 53:137, 1972.

47. Luke, R. G., et al.   Factors determining response to mannitol in acute renal failure. *Am. J. Med. Sci.* 259:168, 1970.

48. McDougal, W. S., et al.   A Histochemical and Morphologic Study of Postobstructive Diuresis in the Rat. *Abstracts*, The American Urologic Association, May 11–16, 1975.

49. McDougal, W. S., and Persky, L.   Renal functional abnormalities in post-

unilateral ureteral obstruction in man: A comparison of these defects to post-obstructive diuresis. *J. Urol.* 113:601, 1975.

50. McDougal, W. S., and Wright, F. S.   Defect in proximal and distal sodium transport in postobstructive diuresis. *Kidney Int.* 2:304, 1972.

51. Maher, J. F., et al.   Osmotic diuresis due to retained urea after release of obstructive uropathy. *N. Engl. J. Med.* 268:1099, 1963.

52. Mitchell, J. P.   Current concepts; trauma to the urinary tract. *N. Engl. J. Med.* 288:90, 1973.

53. Moses, A. M., and Miller, M.   Urine and plasma osmolality in differentiation of polyuric states. *Postgrad. Med.* 52:187, 1972.

54. Mudge, G. H., et al.   Tubular Transport of Urea, Glucose, Phosphate, Uric Acid, Sulfate, and Thiosulfate. In J. Orloff, R. W. Berliner, and S. R. Geiger (Eds.), *Handbook of Physiology.* Section 8. Renal Physiology. Washington, D.C.: American Physiological Society, 1973. Pp. 589–594.

55. Muldowney, F. P., et al.   Sodium diuresis after relief of obstructive uropathy. *N. Engl. J. Med.* 274:1294, 1966.

56. Murase, T., and Yoshida, S.   Mechanism of chlorpropamide action in patients with diabetes insipidus. *J. Clin. Endocrinol. Metab.* 36:174, 1973.

57. Muth, R. G.   Furosemide in Acute Renal Failure. In E. A. Friedman and H. E. Eliahou (Eds.), *Proceedings Acute Renal Failure Conference.* Washington, D.C.: DHEW Publication No. (NIH) 74-608, 1973. Pp. 245–263.

58. Oken, D. E.   Nosologic considerations in the nomenclature of acute renal failure. *Nephron* 8:505, 1971.

59. Oparil, S., and Haber, E.   The renin-angiotensin system. *N. Engl. J. Med.* 291:446, 1974.

60. Papper, S., and Vaamondo, C. A.   The Kidney in Liver Disease. In M. B. Strauss and L. G. Welt (Eds.), *Diseases of the Kidney.* Boston: Little, Brown, 1971. Pp. 1139–1154.

61. Peart, W. S.   Renin-angiotensin system. *N. Engl. J. Med.* 292:302, 1975.

62. Perillie, P. E., and Epstein, F. H.   Sickling phenomenon produced by hypertonic solutions: A possible explanation for the hyposthenuria of sicklemia. *J. Clin. Invest.* 42:570, 1963.

63. Perlmutter, M., et al.   Urine-serum urea nitrogen ratios. *J.A.M.A.* 170:1533, 1959.

64. Quinton, W. E., et al.   Eight months experience with Silastic-Teflon bypass cannulas. *Trans. Am. Soc. Artif. Intern. Organs* 8:236, 1962.

65. Reindenberg, M. M.   *Renal Function and Drug Action.* Philadelphia: Saunders, 1971.

66. Renkin, E. M., and Robinson, R. R.   Glomerular filtration. *N. Engl. J. Med.* 290:785, 1974.

67. Sanders, R. C., and Jeck, D. L.   B-Scan ultrasound in the evaluation of renal failure. *Radiology* 119:199, 1976.

68. Schrier, R. W.   Acute renal failure. *Kidney Int.* 15:205, 1979.

69. Schrier, R. W., and Berl, T.   Nonosmolar factors affecting renal water excretion. *N. Engl. J. Med.* 292:81, 141–145, 1975.

70. Share, L.   Vasopressin: Its bioassay and the physiological control of its release. *Am. J. Med.* 42:701, 1967.

71. Share, L., and Claybaugh, J. R.   Regulation of body fluids. *Annu. Rev. Physiol.* 34:235, 1972.
72. Statius von Eps, L. W., et al.   Nature of concentrating defect in sickle-cell nephropathy. *Lancet* 1:450, 1970.
73. Stein, J. H., Lifschitz, M. D., and Barnes, L. D.   Current concepts in the pathophysiology of acute renal failure. *Am. J. Physiol.* 234:F171, 1978.
74. Thiel, G., et al.   Micropuncture studies of the basis for protection of renin depleted rates from glycerol induced acute renal failure. *Nephron* 7:67, 1970.
75. Thomson, G. E.   Acute renal failure. *Med. Clin. North Am.* 57:1579, 1973.
76. Thurau, K. J., et al.   Composition of tubular fluid in the macula densa segment as a factor regulating the function of the juxtaglomerular apparatus. *Circ. Res.* 20, 21(Suppl. 2):79, 1967.
77. Vander, A. J.   Control of renin release. *Physiol. Rev.* 47:359, 1967.
78. Vander, A. J., and Miller, R.   Control of renin secretion in the anesthetized dog. *Am. J. Physiol.* 207:537, 1964.
79. Verney, E. B.   Absorption and excretion of water. *Lancet* 2:739, 781, 1946.
80. Wilson, D. R., et al.   Glycerol induced hemoglobinuric acute renal failure in the rat. *Nephron* 4:337, 1967.
81. Witte, M. H., et al.   Massive polyuria and natriuresis following relief of urinary tract obstruction. *Am. J. Med.* 37:320, 1964.
82. Wright, F. S.   Intrarenal regulation of glomerular filtration rate. *N. Engl. J. Med.* 291:135, 1974.
83. Yarger, W. E., et al.   A micropuncture study of postobstructive diuresis in the rat. *J. Clin. Invest.* 51:625, 1972.

SELECTED READINGS

Bricker, N. S., and Klahr, S.   Obstructive Nephropathy. In M. B. Strauss and L. G. Welt (Eds.), *Diseases of the Kidney*. Boston: Little, Brown, 1971. Pp. 997–1037.
Flamenbaum, W.   Pathophysiology of acute renal failure. *Arch. Intern. Med.* 131:911, 1973.
Laragh, J. H., and Sealey, J. E.   The Renin-Angiotensin-Aldosterone Hormonal System and Regulation of Sodium, Potassium, and Blood Pressure Homeostasis. In J. Orloff, R. W. Berliner, and S. R. Geiger (Eds.), *Handbook of Physiology*. Section 8. Renal Physiology. Washington, D.C.: American Physiological Society, 1973. Pp. 831–908.
Papper, S., and Vaamondo, C. A.   The Kidney in Liver Disease. In M. B. Strauss and L. G. Welt (Eds.), *Diseases of the Kidney*. Boston: Little, Brown, 1971. Pp. 1139–1154.
Renkin, E. M., and Robinson, R. R.   Glomerular filtration. *N. Engl. J. Med.* 290: 785, 1974.
Schrier, R. W., and Berl, T.   Nonosmolar factors affecting renal water excretion. *N. Engl. J. Med.* 292:81, 141, 1975.
Wright, F. S.   Intrarenal regulation of glomerular filtration rate. *N. Engl. J. Med.* 291:135, 1974.

Herbert J. Weiss *22. PSYCHOLOGICAL
ASPECTS OF
INTENSIVE CARE*

The development of specially designed intensive care units (ICUs) within
the framework of the general hospital has thrust on the medical and surgical personnel of these facilities the recognition that altered states of consciousness, severe emotional reactions, and accompanying behavior account
for a significant portion of the morbidity regularly encountered in patients
under treatment in these units. The clinical entities to be described and the
general principles elaborated have equal applicability to intensive care programs for cardiac, pulmonary, renal, and suicidal patients, as well as to
the surgical patient and the surgical ICU in particular. Within these unique
settings, conditions may be found that include a broad spectrum of psychological and psychiatric disturbances ranging from overt psychoses to covert,
subtle regressions of a more insidious nature. It is therefore essential to
recognize that the psychological care of the patient cannot be separated
from the concept of total physical care.

The discussion to follow will consider the surgical patient, vulnerability
to stress, and the importance of preparation for the operation and the intensive care that will ensue. The organization and operation of the ICU itself is next considered, with a view to reducing the stress and altering the
morbidity encountered there. Finally, commonly seen disturbances are described, together with specific remedial measures.

THE SURGICAL PATIENT

For most patients, the prospect of undergoing an operation constitutes a
major threat capable of generating psychological reactions out of proportion to the realistic hazard. For the patient, surgery appears always as an
emergency to which he is likely to respond by marshaling all his resources
to combat the sense of attack he feels is imminent. This attack is regularly
visualized, and often verbalized, in terms of his sense of helplessness, immobilization, and total passivity. The reactions to these threats may range
from an intolerable anxiety to depression and apathy and even to a full-
blown psychosis. Nevertheless, it is truly remarkable how well most patients react to an operation, how regularly they contain their fear, pull their
self-control up tight, consciously shut out the many frightening and bewildering stimuli confronting them, and even manage a kind of good humor.

The surgical staff, however, should not be misled by this appearance of composure, particularly if the patient appears to be overstating the case in declaring himself free from worry or in loudly insisting on his total trust and belief in the surgeon. No matter how calm he appears, the element of fear is present—fear of the anesthetic, of disfigurement and mutilation, of helpless dependency, of showing fear, and of not being a "good" patient. Particularly, he is afraid he may die. Although it is true that imagination greatly enhances and distorts reality, there is, in part, a real basis for this dread of surgery, which is never totally imaginary. To overlook these considerations and disregard the psychological significance of undergoing surgery is to invite emotional complications and their somatic expression that prolong and distort convalescence and intensify morbidity.

The preoperative preparation of the patient is best organized around the recognition that the suppression of anxiety before surgery is potentially harmful. The postoperative adjustment is directly related not only to the degree of preoperative anxiety but also to the extent to which it is permitted expression. In particular, this is true of patients who glibly announce a thorough knowledge of what lies ahead and disclaim any need for explanations, and of those patients whose joking declarations and attitudes proclaim the need for an extensive denial to ward off their fears.

More than any other factor, the countering attitude of the surgeon and family physician is crucial in avoiding the inevitable disillusionment and its accompanying emotional disturbance. If the surgeon discourages discussion and questions, dismisses the patient's fears as groundless, minimizes the pain, discomfort, and suffering that is certain to occur, and does not allow the patient an avenue of expression for his anxiety, then the stage is set for a morbid convalescence and a potentially pathologic reaction.

The following points are essential in the preoperative preparation of the patient:

1. *Avoid ambiguity.* The surgical procedure (and the anesthesia) should be explained to the patient in simple, concrete terms. Events to be encountered, the presence of pain and the measures to be used to alleviate it, the nature of the surgical ICU, the use of intravenous fluids, and the like should be described. Patients are likely to be fearful of every unexpected and unexplained event and to interpret such surprising events in morbid terms.

2. *Avoid anonymity.* The surgeon must not be a stranger to the patient. The patient's sense of helplessness will be less frightening if the surgeon is a known person who discusses the procedure in advance, even if he repeats what has been said by the family physician. Similarly, the anesthesiologist should visit the patient beforehand to give a simple explanation of the anesthetic procedure and to allow questions to be asked or anxiety to be expressed. Finally, a visit by the charge nurse of the surgical ICU prior to surgery (or prior to transfer to the unit) will further serve the purposes of explanation and preparation and will allow the patient the opportunity to

express any anxiety. Intensive care units are regularly equated with grave and dangerous outcomes by the patient, often beyond the reality of the particular operation and illness; the preventive aspect of such units in reducing complications and postoperative morbidity is frequently not understood. When such preparation is not possible before the operation, attempts should be made to offer explanations as soon as the patient's condition allows.

3. *Avoid isolation.* Most psychological difficulties encountered in surgery are a direct result of the isolating effect that results from the need of both patient and surgeon to suppress their feelings. In the last analysis, both patient and physician are likely to handle their emotions in whatever manner enables them to carry out what they have to do efficiently. The important task of keeping the lines of communication open should therefore be turned over to other professionals, preferably someone who is exempted from carrying out surgical and nursing procedures. The most natural choice would be the referring physician, who knows the patient best, who is not now in the primary treatment role, and who can now respond more freely to the patient's emotional needs.

THE SURGICAL INTENSIVE CARE UNIT

The surgical patient arriving on the ICU is confronted by a strange land of confusing sights and sounds, staffed by personnel often garbed in mask and gown and intent on carrying out a perpetual series of complex procedures with intricate equipment. The patient's state of mental alertness is likely to be markedly obtunded by the aftermath of the surgery and anesthetic, by the use of postoperative narcotics and sedatives, or by the nature of the illness itself. In this "science-fiction" setting, the patient's tendency to misinterpret and distort events greatly enhances the development of anxiety, restlessness, and agitation. The tendency to use more drugs to calm the agitation may further blur the patient's perceptions, especially in the aged, and thus a cycle is established that grows in intensity. The preoccupation of the caretaking staff with the physiologic and chemical needs of the patient may be at the expense of emotional needs, and a significant period of time may elapse in which little is said to the patient other than perfunctory words of reassurance.

Intensive care units tend to be timeless. Lights are likely to be on constantly, postoperative procedures are carried on at any time, regular mealtimes may be initially eliminated, and family visits are at best perfunctory. The patient—largely mute, physically immobilized, and beset by bewildering, painful stimuli—may see it as a sterile, faceless, timeless world. In short, it is a setting in which confusion, disorientation, and anxiety are prominent. This is coupled with altered physiologic states, in a setting prone to dehumanization and delirium.

Because care of the surgical patient in the ICU is by definition highly specialized and likely to be limited by specialized physical structure and staff available, the following precepts are offered as guides in organization of the service:

1. Mobilize the patient's mental activity as soon as the physical condition allows. Where possible, avoid prolonged periods of sedation and narcosis, uninterrupted use of narcotics or tranquilizers, and prolonged physical restraint. Strive to elevate levels of consciousness, even in the presence of pain. Attempt to orient the patient as to time, place, what is going on now, and what has happened so far. Help to identify the various pains the patient feels and their source. Encourage speech and expression of feelings. Remember that confusion and anxiety add greatly to subjective pain. Do not induce silent submission by excessive reassurance. *Let the patient talk.*

2. Establish a sequence, even if only fragmentary, in which the patient can recognize the passage of time, the passage of day into night. A large visible clock can be a comfort to a patient immobilized by numerous lines, tubes, and equipment. Turn the lights off and on when possible. When feeding begins, attempt to identify a familiar sequence of breakfast, lunch, and dinner, irrespective of the meal's contents.

3. The nursing staff should not be faceless. Identify yourself by name and by your actions with the patient: "I am Pat Jones. I changed your dressing this morning. I am going to help you breathe better now." The surgical staff should follow the same rule. Tell the patient when you are going off duty; tell the patient when you will be back. The next shift should quickly announce themselves to the patient.

4. Explain what you are doing. Advise the patient to expect pain with some procedures and to tell you when the pain is beyond tolerance. Enlist the patient's cooperation; give a feeling that he or she has some control over what is being done.

5. Do not isolate the patient behind screens for prolonged periods of time. If screens are necessary, the patient needs frequent visits and conversation, not merely sedation.

6. The unit should not be sterile, soundless, and devoid of human activities; neither should the staff carry on prolonged, loud discussions or chatter that can be abrasive to the helpless, anxious patient. Avoid technical discussions on treatment programs or patient progress in the patient's presence. If such discussions are unavoidable, tell the patient what you are doing, that it will surely sound confusing and perhaps alarming, that you will explain afterward. *Do not dehumanize the patient by ignoring sensitivities.*

7. If at all possible, provide a staff member whose assignment is devoted to the foregoing measures, who can function as the patient's advocate, who does not carry out procedures on the patient, who can foster a more human relationship in contrast to the inevitable estrangement generated by the sophisticated intensive care that other staff members provide.

8. Do not lock in the unit's staff; give them a room on the unit to which

they can go to momentarily escape their patients, share observations, work off their own feelings, and temporarily reduce the pressure on themselves. Combined conferences among nurses, surgeons, and consultants are essential, not only to enhance the development of technical skills by the staff but also for establishment of morale and a sense of commitment.

Finally, the surgical ICU must not be allowed to develop merely into a momentary way-station designed only to restore or establish a desired state of physiologic-chemical-anatomic balance. It must also function as the initial phase of psychological recovery. To this end, the staff must be alert also for the early signs of pending psychological regression and decompensation.

POSTOPERATIVE PSYCHOPATHOLOGY
LETHARGY

Immediately following surgery, and often for several days, many surgical patients suppress their mental functioning so comprehensively that they fall into a state of lethargy or apathy. Although the mild cases commonly encountered may consist of little more than extreme lassitude and a general lack of interest, when the process goes deeper, the patient may demonstrate an extreme degree of mental and physical sluggishness. Activity and speech may become minimal, and questions may have to be repeated and directions repeatedly emphasized. Such a patient appears to have lost interest even in such basics as appearance, comfort, food, or conversation—indeed, appears oblivious to everything.

Because this apathy occurs frequently, it may go unnoticed or, more regularly, may be seen as part of the reaction to the shock of surgery or a reaction to trauma, anesthesia, lack of nutrition, pain, and so on. Perhaps even the most severe states of apathy may go unrecognized in the surgical ICU as a result of staff attitudes—that is, a tendency to think of all patient reactions as "surgical" in nature and a desire to avoid observation of the patient's anxiety reactions to the whole complex series of events. Such failures of recognition readily arise because of the circumstances that bring a patient to the ICU; the patient may have been admitted directly from emergency surgery or transferred from another division. Accordingly, the surgical staff has had no chance to become acquainted with the patient's normal, premorbid personality.

The importance of a ready recognition of this pathologic state lies in its relation to a developing runaway surge of emotion in which fear and anger are often closely coupled. In other words, a state of panic is developing, and, having no other means available to ward off the breakthrough of these feelings, the patient literally paralyzes mental function into a state almost of stupor as a last-ditch defense maneuver. Such a regression appears to have the structure of a self-developed period of internal rest and recuperation, which is usually self-limited and self-contained.

Because this period of apathy seems to serve a recuperative function, it is important for the surgical staff not to become too active in combating it. It is especially important to establish the nature of the regressive reaction to differentiate it from pathologic depressions and particularly to avoid treatment with psychopharmacologic drugs. Recovery will usually occur within a week and often dramatically follows an encouraging optimistic event, perhaps something as commonplace (to the staff) as the removal of sutures, drainage tubes, or intravenous lines. If, however, the state of apathy persists beyond six or seven days, it is best to urge the patient in a gradual way into increasing activity, especially to care for personal appearance or to perform in a way that will facilitate recovery and eventual discharge. Particularly at these times, it may be enormously helpful to talk with the patient about the suppression of feelings about the danger that he or she has escaped, and to encourage verbalization of previous fears about the operation and the illness; in other words, to encourage the patient to go over and over these events in order to master the acute traumatic experience and its attendant anxiety. It is important to recognize that protracted periods of apathy may signal the approach of a much more severe psychic decompensation, and at this time psychiatric consultation should be resorted to.

DEPRESSION

Because the duration of a stay in an ICU is likely to be short and self-limited, the ICU staff is not likely to see the full development of a major postoperative depression. Rather, the previously described states of apathy and lethargy are more frequently brought to their attention. Nevertheless, it is important for the ICU staff to be alert for the evidence of a depressive reaction, to differentiate it from other pathologic states, and to seek appropriate consultation early. In addition, there is a distinct group of patients whose stay in the ICU is likely to be protracted—for example, patients with burns or with complex metabolic disorders. During such prolonged periods of treatment, the staff has more time to become acquainted with the patient, to observe the development of the depressive process, and to reach some conclusions about its content.

Most postsurgical depressions are reactive depressions, that is, the condition emerges directly from active precipitating factors. The most regularly encountered sources of the reaction stem from the nature of the illness itself, particularly if it is malignant disease, or from the traumatic effects of radical, disfiguring surgical procedures. Central to the emotional state are fear and shock coupled with a persistent anger that has undergone deflection or suppression. As in all depressive reactions, the element of anger is invariably present.

These patients may well resemble those in a state of apathy in that their mental processes appear to be markedly slowed, they are indifferent to their own welfare, uninterested in even brief visits, and apathetic to conversations with the staff, even about their own progress. In addition, one begins to hear from the depressed patient evidence of self-deprecation, self-accusations, and even of guilt. Such patients, when encouraged, may regularly surprise the caretaking staff by repeatedly claiming responsibility for what has happened; that is, the illness is the result of their own neglect, stubbornness, or some other kind of undesirable behavior. They are inclined to insist that surgeons and nurses alike are doing a fine job and offer little or no criticism of all that is going on about them or is being done to them. Rather, they speak disparagingly of themselves and then in rapid progression come to the expressions of hopelessness and pessimism, coupled with frequent statements of their own worthlessness.

By this time, of course, a severe pathologic depression has set in. Prompt detection lies in the staff's alertness to the repeated statements of self-accusation and guilt. In particular, these events are likely to occur when illness is prolonged, recovery slowed, and improvement apparently minimal or nonexistent. Such patients are likely to be concealing considerable anger, often directed at the physician, but their marked dependency on the physician and their essential need for medical care make them unable, because of inner conflict, to express such ambivalent feelings. It is not unlikely, of course, that the depressive process had already been underway prior to the detection of the illness and the operation. However, there can be little question that the eruption of the pathologic state was triggered by the surgical events.

The treatment of these postoperative reactive depressions lies in the recognition of the underlying conflicts, especially about anger. Such patients usually merit psychiatric consultation. It is important for the surgical staff to avoid instituting treatment with antidepressant drugs because there is a tendency to resort to such medication to avoid discussion of the underlying psychological conflicts.

Depression is as ubiquitous as life itself and occurs so regularly in hospital situations as to be considered almost normal; yet such depressions are highly complex psychic events that enormously prolong convalescence, interfere with recuperation, are literally life-threatening, and may even lead to suicidal action. It is commonplace for the surgical staff to take comfort in the familiar cliche that postoperative patients are "too weak to commit suicide," but there is sufficient experience to demonstrate that even such patients may make suicidal gestures or attempts. More important, the nature of the depressive reaction may be so profound that the suicidal risk may persist and even increase following discharge from the ICU and especially on discharge from the hospital.

The observation of a depressive reaction as described calls for more than hearty reassurance, antidepressant drugs, or severely critical lectures telling the patient to "get hold of yourself." Such depressions call for skilled psychiatric consultation and treatment and sometimes even transfer to the psychiatric unit of the hospital as soon as the patient's physical condition will permit.

POSTOPERATIVE PSYCHOSES

The postoperative psychotic reactions encountered in surgical ICUs may be classified into two main groups: (1) organic psychotic reactions that may be a result of disorders of metabolism, electrolyte disturbances, or cerebral vascular circulatory impairment, and (2) functional psychotic reactions, which appear to be responses to the psychological stresses emanating from the underlying disease, the surgery, and the ICU experience itself.

All psychotic reactions have one distinctive finding in common: the patient exhibits a sharp break with reality. The symptomatology may vary from confusion and disorientation to hallucinatory and delusional expression. It goes without saying that immediate detection of the psychotic break, coupled with an early diagnosis of etiology, is essential. The organic psychotic reactions invariably call for immediate correction of the underlying metabolic and physiologic disturbance. The functional psychotic reactions, such as psychotic depressions or acute schizophrenic reactions, require a more protracted and complex mode of treatment. Because of the previously mentioned tendency of the surgical staff to assume that a psychopathologic disturbance in a patient is likely to be "surgical" in nature— that is, as resulting from metabolic and physiologic disturbances—and because patients in the immediate postoperative period are not likely to manifest the subtler aspects of a functional psychotic illness, it is important to stress the need for psychiatric consultation as soon as a psychotic transformation is suspected.

DELIRIUM

CLINICAL SYMPTOMS

Postoperative delirium is an emergency condition that requires immediate diagnosis and rapid treatment. It must be suspected when the patient displays the familiar triad of confusion, disorientation, and memory deficit, coupled with bizarre language, neologisms, slurred speech, extreme restlessness that may mount to combativeness, and disordered behavior, frequently appearing as auditory and visual hallucinations of a paranoid type. Tremor is also likely to be observed, especially in cases of acute alcohol withdrawal (delirium tremens) or abrupt withdrawal of certain drugs, such as barbiturates. If untreated, delirium of this type may be complicated by hyperpyrexia and convulsions, and death may occur in up to 15 percent of the patients seen. Delirium complicates patient management and is associated with prolonged morbidity and mortality.

The surgical staff should have sufficient training and instruction to be able to detect the early signs of acute brain syndromes such as delirium. Establishing the mental status of the patient, checking it two or three times a day as the condition evolves, should be an important part of postoperative observations, and the necessary skill should be developed in the caretaking staff. Where delirium is suspected, patients should be carefully questioned as to their ability to recognize the time, date, and their situation. They should also be asked to carry out certain simple tasks, such as the repetition of short sequences of numbers or serial-seven subtraction. Significant errors in performance may appear early, and the rapid detection and institution of appropriate treatment may do much to prevent the onset of the acute agitation that will rapidly follow.

After the early prodromal signs of confusion and disorientation, an acute stage of tachycardia, sweating, fever, agitation, and hallucination may set in in one to three days. It is important to recognize that the patient may emerge from the delirium state and then relapse into it during the night. The hallucinatory activity is likely to be of a particularly horrifying nature to the patient and is the most common cause of severe injury to such patients because of their frantic attempts to escape the supposed dangers. The most serious complications are hyperpyrexia and convulsions, particularly in patients undergoing alcohol- or drug-withdrawal reactions. Although severe protracted delirium may lead to adrenal exhaustion, the most frequent causes of death in these patients are the severe traumas sustained in efforts to escape supposed dangers, pneumonia, and suicide.

TREATMENT

Treatment for acute brain syndromes of this type is organized around three central points.

First, because the acute delirium is symptomatic of a physiologic disorder resulting from either a metabolic disturbance or biochemical disequilibrium, immediate treatment is necessary to correct the underlying physiologic disturbance. Diagnosis must be established immediately, so that treatment can be instituted and the danger of self-injury and possible residual brain damage reduced.

Second, the use of sedative drugs is essential to control the excessive agitation and impulsivity of such patients, to prevent exhaustion, and to facilitate the required intensive care. If a diagnosis of alcohol withdrawal (delirium tremens) has been established, the most effective drug is chlordiazepoxide HCl (Librium). Dosage schedules vary with the intensity of the agitation but should be from 50 to 100 mg, given intramuscularly every 4 to 6 hours during the first day. Individual patients may require more frequent administration of the drug, or more protracted use may be necessary over a 48-hour period before dosage and frequency can be reduced.

Chlordiazepoxide HCl has been shown to be especially valuable in the treatment of acute delirium tremens because of its anticonvulsant activity. In addition, it is the preferred drug when the use of phenothiazines may be contraindicated because of existing hepatic disease or when possible hypotensive reactions are a hazard. The phenothiazine group of drugs, however, are extremely useful in the management of acute delirium, particularly chlorpromazine, promazine, and thioridazine. If surgical and physiologic conditions contraindicate the use of either chlordiazepoxide HCl or the phenothiazines, paraldehyde, the drug traditionally used in the past, may be resorted to.

Additional elements in the treatment program are restraints, peripheral alimentation, and supplemental doses of thiamine; the use of serum albumin in the management of metabolic changes encountered should be considered. The use of physical restraints must be carefully planned, since there is much evidence that physical restraint may enormously increase the agitation stemming from hallucinatory activity. Nevertheless, the danger of impulsive, out-of-control behavior is such that careful restraints and close observation are essential.

Third, the nature of the intensive care environment may aggravate the symptomatology and behavior of the acute delirium. The timeless nature of the facility, the relative lack of extensive communication with caretaking personnel, the confusing babble of stimulation arising from monitoring equipment, the constant nursing activity with other patients in close proximity, and the frequent nursing and surgical procedures required tend to contribute to the agitation and provide stimuli that the delirious patient readily misinterprets. The best environment is one with relatively little external stimulation, with soft light kept on constantly, and most important, where continuous contact and communication with the patient is carried on in the periods when he is rousable and responsive.

Of particular value are the presence of a familiar person, especially a family member, and constant efforts to orient and reassure the patient and to explain what is occurring. Since most ICUs are unable to provide this type of environment, and because the patient's hyperactivity may prove to be insupportable in terms of the care of other patients, it may be necessary to transfer the patient from the unit to a more appropriate setting. However, it must be pointed out that because the underlying cause of acute delirium is organic in nature and arises from physicochemical disturbances, the correction of these disorders can probably be carried out most expeditiously in the ICU. This factor, coupled with the essential intensive care needed for the patient's surgical state, may outweigh the advantages of a more carefully designed environment. In most cases, early recognition, immediate correction of the underlying disturbance, and appropriate use of sedative medications should make it possible to retain the patient in the ICU.

FUNCTIONAL PSYCHOTIC REACTIONS
Although any of the functional psychoses, such as schizophrenic reactions, manic-depressive psychoses, and paranoid states, may arise in connection

TABLE 22-1. Psychoactive Drugs for the Critical Care Patient

Drug Class	Generic Name	Trade Name	Daily Dose (mg)	
			High	Moderate
Benzodiazepines	Chlordiazepoxide HCl	Librium	150–300	75–150
	Diazepam	Valium	30–60	15–30
	Oxazepam	Serax	75–120	45–75
	Clorazepate	Tranxene	45–90	25–45
Butyrophenone	Haloperidol	Haldol	15–60	6–15
Phenothiazines	Chlorpromazine	Thorazine	300–600	150–300
	Thioridazine	Mellaril	300–600	150–300

with a surgical experience and even present themselves in the ICU, this discussion will be limited to a specific psychotic reaction that appears to be intimately related to the intensive care environment itself. This reaction manifests many of the symptoms of an acute, organic delirium, but does not evolve from a physiologic abnormality. It is thus possible to differentiate two types of postoperative deliria: (1) an organic type, in which the mental impairment of cognitive functions is comprehensive, and (2) a functional, nonorganic type, in which the impairment is selective and restricted. In the second, prominent disorientation and hallucinatory activity are observed, but the patients' recall and performance in mental status evaluation tests are not affected. Patients with the organic type of delirium tend to be drowsy and to have reduced awareness; those with the functional type tend to be overactive and sleepless and to hallucinate actively.

The distinction between these two clinical pictures is of considerable importance in the ICU. It involves distinguishing a syndrome resulting from a physiologic abnormality from one largely caused by the ICU environment itself; that is, monotony, isolation, and sleep deprivation may be the dominant factors in the genesis of the deliriumlike reaction of the latter. Although a great deal of emphasis has been placed on the psychological effects of the ICU environment, it is important to stress that the delirium most commonly seen is of the organic type. However, the fact that rapid mobilization and quick transfer from the ICU are the frequent sequel may be responsible for minimizing the frequency of the environmental type of delirium.

When clinical evaluation of a hyperactive patient demonstrates normal fluid balance, blood gas levels, pH, and so on, and when the mental status examination reveals a selective loss of mental function, a diagnosis of a functional psychosis is in order, and a proper program of sedation and environmental manipulation, as previously described, is required. Care must be taken not to overdiagnose this entity at the expense of the more common organic disorder, in which correction of the underlying physiologic abnormality is crucial.

The hyperactivity and agitation in these patients require immediate treatment with tranquilizing medications, in particular, the phenothiazine group. Table 22-1 is a general guide for achieving rapid control of the disordered behavior.

SELECTED READINGS

Bird, B. *Talking with Patients* (2nd ed.). Philadelphia: Lippincott, 1973.

Friedman, E. H. Symposium: Psychosocial factors in intensive-care nursing. *Heart Lung* 2:355, 1973.

Goldhirsch, H. Post-operative psychosis. *Ohio State Med. J.* 69:375, 1973.

Goldin, M. D. Psychiatric Complications. In *Intensive Care of the Surgical Patient*. Chicago: Year Book, 1971.

Kaim, S. C., et al. Treatment of the acute alcohol withdrawal state: A comparison of four drugs. *Am. J. Psychiatry* 125:1640, 1969.

Katz, N. M., et al. Delirium in surgical patients under intensive care. *Arch. Surg.* 104:310, 1972.

Mays, E. T., et al. Metabolic changes in surgical delirium tremens. *Surgery* 67: 780, 1970.

II / RECENT ADVANCES IN CRITICAL CARE MEDICINE

John E. Brimm
Richard M. Peters

23. APPLICATIONS OF COMPUTERS AND OTHER NEW TECHNIQUES

The history of the development of intensive care gives some hint about the advances that may be expected in the future. One can trace the concentrated use of ventilator support to the severe poliomyelitis epidemic in Denmark in 1952 [4]. Many lives were saved at that time by teams of nurses and medical students who manually ventilated paralyzed children for days. These efforts proved the efficacy of widespread use of artificial ventilation and promoted the development of respirators.

In the middle 1950s, in the early days of open heart surgery, postoperative care required the constant attention of the surgeons and cardiologists. They learned the importance of monitoring the electrocardiogram (ECG), blood pressure, and venous pressure. To monitor these parameters, the original instruments were temporarily brought from either the investigative or the electronic laboratories. Although the laboratory instruments were unstable, complex to operate, and required highly skilled personnel at all times, the importance of electronic monitoring was nonetheless demonstrated. Industry was prompted to develop the present routinely used bedside monitoring instruments.

The effect of the bedside monitoring instruments has been to improve care and free the highly skilled physician from having to be in constant attendance at the patient's bedside. In the future, we will find the same pattern: technology will extend the ability of skilled nurses and physicians to prevent morbidity and mortality. At the same time, it will provide new information to investigators so that they can better understand acute disease and design better forms of therapy.

Technology will contribute through the development of both new sensors to provide new or more reliable information and computer systems to integrate and interpret the vast amounts of information essential to the control of complex therapy in the intensive care unit (ICU). Discussion of technological advances in critical care medicine will focus on five major aspects: the impact of microprocessors, dysrhythmia monitoring, hemodynamic monitoring, respiratory monitoring, and computerized handling and interpreting of data.

THE IMPACT OF MICROPROCESSORS

Today, the issue of whether computers will be used in the ICU is a moot point. Essentially all new instruments—bedside monitors, central stations, cardiac output calculators, intravenous infusion pumps, and others—are being built with integral microcomputers. The development of integrated microcircuits has changed all aspects of instrument and computer design. In the past, instruments were made to take a simple physiologic signal, such as the ECG or the blood pressure wave, and convert it to an electronic signal with a transducer and amplifier combination. The signal could then be fed to a display device, either an oscilloscope or oscillograph. The translation of these simple readings of physiologic signals to useful clinical information required the skill of a trained interpreter.

With the advent of integrated digital logic, however, much more complex instruments, that depend on extensive calculations to provide useful information, can be built. An example is the oximeter. For many years attempts were made to develop a reliable surface sensor to measure arterial oxygenation (i.e., oximetry). These were limited in clinical usefulness because of interference by skin pigments. By increasing the number of wavelengths of light measured, this problem has been largely solved. A microcomputer has been built into the instrument to solve the complex equations resulting from the use of multiple wavelengths of light. The computer converts the pattern of light absorption to what the clinician wants to know, namely, the arterial oxygen saturation.

The inclusion of microprocessors to provide "intelligence" in instruments should have a profound effect on a troublesome limitation of current sensors—their sensitivity to artifact. Artifact is a spurious signal of nonphysiologic origin, such as a noisy ECG from a loose lead. Intelligent monitors should be better able to detect poor signal quality. For example, newer cardiotachometers, heart-rate monitors that process the ECG for the detection of QRS complexes, are far more accurate than their predecessors.

Microprocessor-based instruments will provide at least four other advantages:

1. They will be able to be upgraded without totally redesigning their hardware. By changing memory modules, new signal processing algorithms will be implemented without altering the rest of the instrument. As microprocessor-based dysrhythmia monitors are developed, this capability for evolution will be crucial.
2. Newer instruments will be more reliable and maintainable. Increasing effort is being given toward designing instruments in which single points of failure cannot cause harm to patients. Consequently, instruments will monitor not only patients, but also themselves. Most new instruments provide features for self-testing, which result in improved maintainability.
3. Since a fundamental element of most microprocessors is the capability for communication, newer instruments should be more easily integrated into the

total ICU information system. New intravenous infusion pumps, for example, not only can communicate (to central ICU computer systems) the intravenous volume that has been infused, but also can have the rate adjusted by the computer.
4. Microprocessor-based instruments should be functionally more independent. Functional independence, or modularity, will permit a more rational purchasing policy, particularly in smaller hospitals. Instead of having to choose between a full system or nothing, hospitals will be able to select those instruments or monitors appropriate to their setting.

A controversial aspect of the impact of technology on medicine has been its cost. Surprisingly, the inclusion of microprocessors in instruments does not necessarily result in higher costs. The semiconductor industry is highly competitive; over the last eight years, more and more powerful devices have been produced at constant costs. Instruments which use them have benefited from this counterinflationary trend. Further, since microprocessor-based instruments have lower parts counts, they can be packaged more easily and require smaller power supplies; consequently, they are less expensive to manufacture.

DYSRHYTHMIA MONITORING
Coronary care units proliferated after reports in the early 1960s that their use was associated with reduced mortality following myocardial infarction. Ventricular fibrillation, unless detected and treated promptly, has a high risk of mortality. Experience has suggested that ventricular fibrillation is often preceded by warning dysrhythmias. Thus, the rationale for dysrhythmia monitoring is that, through prompt detection, mortality following myocardial infarction may be reduced by aggressive antiarrhythmic therapy.

Early monitoring was largely dependent on the intermittent surveillance of the ECG waveform on an oscilloscope by trained observers. This visual monitoring was subject to both disruption and boredom. The emergence of minicomputer technology in the late 1960s permitted automated dysrhythmia detection. The problems of dysrhythmia monitoring differ importantly from those of morphologic ECG diagnosis. For monitoring, usually only one lead is analyzed. Because it is sampled for long periods of time in the clinical milieu, signal quality can be plagued by artifact. However, because the signal is sampled for long time periods, important information is available for interpretation in temporal context. In contrast, diagnostic ECGs have little temporal context. They are comprised of 12 leads sampled for 5 to 20 seconds; because a technician supervises data collection, the signal quality is high.

The substitution of a computer for a trained observer has been a technically difficult problem. The wide variety of techniques attempted illustrates that no single, simple approach is satisfactory for the diverse patterns that occur clinically. The fundamental problem is that no absolute pattern of normal can be stored for comparison by the computer. Two basic approaches for classifying beats have been used—correlation and feature extraction. Correlation techniques compare each point of the patient's waveform with that of a known template. Because a patient's QRS morphology may evolve over time, the template must be "learned" for each patient and must be "relearned" as it evolves. Feature extraction techniques characterize each beat based on factors such as the QRS height and duration. Both correlation and feature extraction techniques then utilize timing information for a final waveform classification. The techniques of automated dysrhythmia monitoring have been reviewed by Thomas [13]. Cox [2] pioneered this field with the AZTEC algorithm, which served as the basis for several commercial systems.

Current systems offer an accuracy of over 95 percent in detecting premature ventricular contractions. Analysis techniques are tailored so that few dysrhythmias are missed, at the price that the false positive rates are high. Considerable developmental effort is now being expended to reduce classification errors, and two-lead monitoring systems, which should be more accurate, are on the horizon. A long-standing problem has been the lack of a standardized data base of ECG recordings which could be used for validation of new systems and comparison of existing commercial systems. This data base is now being developed. While controversy exists about the value of automated dysrhythmia monitoring for reducing morbidity and mortality, there is no dispute about the improved accuracy over casual nurse surveillance of an oscilloscope.

HEMODYNAMIC MONITORING

Ideally, cardiopulmonary monitoring would consist of continuous, accurate, noninvasive, and low-cost determination of cardiac output, oxygenation, and various cardiovascular pressures to warn automatically of impending crisis. This ideal has obviously not been achieved, nor is its prospect imminent. However, a profound advance in hemodynamic monitoring occurred with the introduction of the Swan-Ganz flow-directed catheter [12]. It can be used for measuring left and right heart filling pressures, sampling mixed venous blood, and determining cardiac output repetitively using the thermodilution technique. The fundamental importance of this sensor lies in the capability for assessing cardiac function directly, and, if cardiac function is impaired, for evaluating treatment strategy. This capability represents a dramatic improvement over monitoring based on vascular pressures alone.

Cardiovascular pressures—systemic and pulmonary arterial, central venous, and left atrial—can be measured in patients in whom invasive catheters have been inserted. Invasion, of course, always carries the risk of infection; the risks must be weighed against the benefits of the information to be gained. If the risks are warranted, then the measurement of pressures is made at intervals depending on the stability of the patient; the less stable the patient, the more frequent the measurements. The values may be displayed in digitized form by bedside instruments. To provide a record in an ICU without a computer, a nurse must write the values on the patient's chart, taking time from more useful tasks.

To provide warnings of potential problems, alarms are given when parameters exceed preset limits. Limits available on present instruments are sensitive to fast transients and give excessive numbers of false alarms. This often causes the nurse to "disable" the alarm capacity of many monitors. In an effort to overcome the problems of this high/low limit alarm strategy, some investigators have tried to use trends in monitored data, either singly or as multivariate combinations, as more sensitive alarm warnings. Detection of trends requires the use of a computer. However, to date, no one has adequately characterized trends in monitored data either statistically or physiologically for providing reliable early warnings. A partial explanation for the slow progress in trend detection schemes has been their typical utilization of easily monitorable signals, such as the heart rate and systemic arterial pressures. These signals can be profoundly altered by therapy and may be poor reflections of the underlying physiologic state. With the use of afterload control, for example, monitoring of arterial pressure may inform more about the adequacy of treatment than of cardiac function.

In the last decade, commercial computer systems that can read the values of the bedside instruments and store the data have become available. Medical personnel can then recall the information in graphic or alphanumeric form on a television screen. This type of system relieves the nurse of charting functions, but in this role, it serves little more than as an expensive secretary. On the other hand, an example of the computer's potential is a system for automated infusion of blood devised by Sheppard [11] for patients who have undergone cardiac surgery. The system bases the infusion rate on measured chest drainage, urine output, left atrial pressure, systemic pressure, and intermittent determinations of cardiac output. Morgan [6] has found that such automation reduces the total amount of blood needed and cuts down the fluctuations in blood pressure. After a decade's experience, however, this system stands nearly alone as an example of closed-loop control of therapy in the ICU.

The automated control of blood infusion is useful in only a small subset of patients because it requires uniformly highly instrumented patients, reliable actuators, systematized care, and commitment to the concept of closing the loop. A potentially more generally applicable role for computers in the assessment of cardiovascular dynamics is the discarding of measurements with little information content and interpreting of the complex interrelations among various measurements. A simple illustration of a method for interrelating data is the calculation of systemic and pulmonary vascular resistances from various vascular pressures and the cardiac output. The need for data reduction is obvious when one considers the computer's ability to sample multiple pressures every 30 seconds; this amount of data is too much for storage and too much for the clinician to interpret. Algorithms must be developed to scan the data to determine whether or not it has changed significantly and, if not, to discard it. This problem is obviously related to the problem of providing trend alarms.

The more complex automated techniques now being developed for assessing and managing abnormalities of cardiovascular dynamics seem likely to be as commonplace in the future as are bedside monitors today.

ASSESSMENT OF RESPIRATORY FUNCTION

Despite Osborn's description of a system for respiratory monitoring in 1969 [8], two underdeveloped areas of monitoring and testing of acutely ill patients are the assessment of pulmonary function and the provision of alarms for respirator malfunction. Respirator malfunction is a major cause of preventable morbidity and mortality in the ICU. The instruments commercially available for monitoring respirator function have been crude and unreliable. An example has been the lack of a low-cost airflow sensor unaffected by the condensation of water vapor suitable for long-term monitoring. The recent introduction of a stable, variable orifice sensor has changed the prospects for respiratory monitoring substantially [7].

Instruments to assure safe and adequate function of respirators will be most reliable if they are independent of the respirator, using separate sensors and logic. The only practical, reasonably priced sensors available for general use at this time measure airway pressure and expired airflow. To provide safety using these signals, the relation between changes in flow and pressure and inspiratory-expiratory ratio must be assessed for each breath. Microprocessor-based instruments for respirator monitoring have recently become commercially available.

Increasing use of intermittent mandatory ventilation (IMV) has altered the requirements for respirator monitoring. Monitors built into ventilators measure only breaths supplied by the ventilator or, in some instances, a mixture of all breaths. Monitoring of IMV requires evaluation of the relative contribution of spontaneous and ventilator breaths. Osborn and our laboratories have developed automated systems for measuring spontaneous and ventilator rates, tidal volumes, and minute ventilation [1, 7].

Monitoring of airway flow and pressure for patients on controlled ventilation provided some information about their respiratory function through determination of compliance, resistance, and work of breathing; however, it probably informed more about the adequacy of respirator function. In IMV, measurement of lung and chest wall mechanics by analyzing the respirator breaths is unreliable because the pressure generated at the mouth is markedly different, depending on the phase of the patient's breath when the respirator triggers. On the other hand, monitoring of IMV provides novel information about the control of breathing. As patients are weaned from IMV, the pattern of spontaneous compensation for a decreased minute ventilation predicts whether the reduced IMV rate will be tolerated. If the spontaneous alveolar ventilation is insufficient, arterial carbon dioxide tension ($PaCO_2$) will ultimately rise. Thus, by monitoring only airway flow and pressure, which now is little more expensive than ECG or blood pressure monitoring, much useful information for managing patients can be provided.

By adding respiratory gas analyzers, further measurements—end-tidal PCO_2, inspired oxygen concentration, oxygen consumption, CO_2 output, and others—can be added. Two types of respiratory gas analyzers are now available: those that measure concentration of a single gas by using some unique property of the gas, and the mass spectrometer that can measure concentrations of a number of gases. The most commonly used stand-alone gas-measuring devices are the infrared CO_2 analyzer and the various paramagnetic and polarographic oxygen analyzers. These instruments are reasonably reliable, though expensive. Until recently, the mass spectrometer was so expensive and complex to operate that it was not practical for clinical use. The stimulus of the space program has made available mass spectrometers that are clinically useful. They can be used in two ways: the various beds in an ICU can be connected to a single mass spectrometer by plumbing and valving systems, so that each in turn is automatically sampled; or the instrument can be moved from bed to bed for testing individual patients. Either of these methods of sharing instruments is feasible because the time constant for change of respiratory function is long, usually hours. At present, in our ICU, a system has been developed in which signals are transmitted to a computer from a special cart that can be wheeled to the patient's bedside to measure airway flow, pressure, N_2, O_2, CO_2, and He concentrations. Using the sampled data, calculations are carried out, and the results are displayed on a bedside television screen.

Turney [14] has used an approach of a fixed mass spectrometer connected to all beds in the ICU for periodic measurement of end-tidal CO_2 as an indicator of changes in $PaCO_2$. The arterial blood gas is measured and the alveolar-arterial carbon dioxide pressure difference [$P(A-a)CO_2$] determined. Changes in end-tidal CO_2 are then converted by calculator to $PaCO_2$ and the system used as a monitor of $PaCO_2$. The assumption is made that a change in $P(A-a)O_2$ is less likely to occur than a change in $PaCO_2$. The circumstances in which this is a valid assumption must be defined. A further question regards the applicability of end-tidal PCO_2 monitoring to patients on IMV. In IMV, the volume of ventilator breaths is typically much larger than those of spontaneous breaths. Since changes in lung volume and dilutional effects can change end-tidal PCO_2, the reliability of this measurement in IMV needs definition.

Work is progressing on sensors for continuous measurement of arterial

PO_2, PCO_2 and pH [10], although no approach is satisfactory for widespread clinical use yet. Ear oximeters have been made both self-calibrating and drift-free; they are, however, still expensive. Transcutaneous PO_2 monitoring provides a noninvasive method for approximating PaO_2 which has been used in premature infants. In order to ensure adequate perfusion, the skin is heated with an electrode to vasodilate the capillary bed. In adults, however, the measurement is less reliable, particularly during periods of poor perfusion, such as shock.

If surface sensors are perfected, they will not provide a means of measuring central venous oxygen, which is an extremely important parameter in assessing cardiopulmonary function. There are at present a number of intravascular sensors being sold to measure PaO_2 and $PaCO_2$ or arterial oxygen saturation (SaO_2). These instruments are not cost-effective for general use because of their unreliability and the short half-life of the intravascular sensor. It can be anticipated that these shortcomings will be overcome.

Equally important to monitoring respiration is the testing of respiratory function. The widespread use of ventilators has increased the potential for survival of many patients. However, objective measurements to determine the need for ventilatory support are lacking. All too often, patients are removed from the respirator prematurely or kept on it longer than necessary because of the lack of objective criteria.

Assessment of pulmonary function is complex. One cannot measure simple pressures and flows to assess respiratory function as is possible in assessing cardiovascular functions. To evaluate respiratory function accurately, some calculations must be performed on all of the primary signals. For example, failure to appreciate the need for such calculations has resulted in the widespread use of $P(A-a)O_2$ after 20 minutes of 100% oxygen breathing as an index of intrapulmonary shunt and thus of pulmonary function. This simplistic approach ignores the capability of 100% oxygen breathing itself to increase intrapulmonary shunt and the exquisite sensitivity of $P(A-a)O_2$ to arteriovenous oxygen content difference.

Since effective assessment of pulmonary function requires complex, expensive instrumentation for measurement, and complex calculations to derive useful clinical information, analytic instruments must be shared by a number of patients and be interfaced to a computer for calculation of useful parameters of pulmonary function. Such systems are being developed and eventually will become more generally available. The major sensors must measure airflow, O_2, CO_2, indicator gas concentrations, and arterial and venous blood gas partial pressures or contents.

Two specific tests hold promise: measurement of functional residual capacity (FRC) and extravascular lung water (EVLW). In adult respiratory distress syndrome (ARDS), the goal of therapy is to prevent alveolar collapse through the use of positive end-expiratory pressure. Monitoring the effects of therapy can be achieved through serial determinations of compliance or FRC. While methods for measuring FRC have been available in pulmonary function laboratories and in research ICUs, FRC measurements have not been generally available for ICU care. We have developed a simplified helium-dilution technique, using a bag-in-box device for measuring FRC on patients being mechanically ventilated [3].

Lewis [5] has developed a rapid, automated, thermal-dye technique for measuring ELVW. The method is invasive: it requires both a femoral artery and a pulmonary artery catheter. Cold dye is injected into the pulmonary artery and the appearance of each indicator (cold and dye) is measured in the aorta. The theory of the method is that the thermal indicator diffuses into the total water space, both intra- and extravascular, while the dye is confined to the intravascular space. By subtracting the two effects, a measure of EVLW is given. Since ARDS is marked by the accumulation of EVLW, this measurement may be a sensitive sign of impending deterioration.

Evaluation of hemodynamic function became far more objective in the 1970s with the introduction of the Swan-Ganz catheter. A number of developments in respiratory monitoring promise to make the 1980s a decade in which evaluation of respiratory function will become more objective.

DATA HANDLING
To date, most efforts at automating data handling in the ICU have concentrated on collecting and displaying raw data. Realization of the full potential of automation in ICU care will occur only as methods are developed to analyze the multiple types of objective data that are randomly entered in the system. The computer system will bring order out of the chaos by interpreting and refining the data. This will prevent accidents due to failure to recognize significant changes and will improve decision making [9].

To realize these goals, two sets of problems must be dealt with effectively. First, the entry of data into the computer must be complete for all patients in the ICU. Second, the computer must be programmed to put the data in orderly sets and to make correlations and interpretations in order to direct therapy. These goals require improved methods of entering data. An example is the need for a simple way for the nurse to enter into the computer the vital signs of the two-thirds of ICU patients who do not have intravascular catheters. Otherwise, these patients will be without the benefits of automation, and the nurses and physicians will not learn to use the system effectively. The present keyboards used to enter alphanumerics into the computer are too complex for the nurse to use to enter each vital sign. The same type of problem exists in the entry of intake and output data and administered drugs. New input devices to overcome this bottleneck are being developed. If all vital signs, intake-output data, and drugs administered to patients are entered into the computer, the information for patient care will be greatly enhanced. For example:

1. Running totals of the precise cumulative balances of water, Na, K, Cl, CO_2, and so on over any desired period of time are simple calculations for a computer. These cumulative balances over many days can be kept and deficits or excesses reported.
2. Vital signs can be evaluated and trends noted.
3. In the control of respiratory care, predictions about the amount of increase in PaO_2 that will result from change in fraction inspired oxygen concentration (FiO_2) can be made, thus preventing the futile use of high inspired oxygen concentrations in patients with large shunts.

While it might be imagined that automation will make the ICU nurse and physician obsolete, this will not be the case. In the future, as in the past, automation will increase their effectiveness by making it possible for them to concentrate on the care of the patient, not on the acquisition and recording of data. If properly designed, the system will gather information that constantly monitors the patient's condition. Such monitoring can ensure that the level of care does not fluctuate as personnel changes. As well as enhancing care, the system will help in distinguishing those individuals who have the skill to take care of these desperately ill patients from those who need further education.

REFERENCES

1. Brimm, J. E., Janson, C. M., O'Hara, M. R., Patitucci, P. J., and Peters, R. M. An automated testing system for cardiopulmonary function. In *Computers in Cardiology*. Long Beach, Calif.: IEEE Press, 1978. Pp. 335–338.
2. Cox, J. R., Jr., Nolle, F. M., and Arthur, R. M. Digital analysis of the electroencephalogram, the blood pressure wave, and the electrocardiogram. *Proc. IEEE* 60:1137, 1972.
3. Heldt, G. P., and Peters, R. M. A simplified method to determine functional residual capacity during mechanical ventilation. *Chest* 74:492, 1978.
4. Lassen, H. C. A. Preliminary report on the 1952 epidemic of poliomyelitis in Copenhagen. *Lancet* 1:37, 1953.
5. Lewis, F. R., Elings, V. B., and Sturm, J. A. Bedside monitoring of lung water. *J. Surg. Res.* 27:250, 1979.
6. Morgan, A. W., et al. Effects of computer-controlled transfusion on recovery from cardiac surgery. *Ann. Surg.* 178:391, 1973.
7. Osborn, J. J. A flow meter for respiratory monitoring. *Crit. Care Med.* 6:349, 1978.
8. Osborn, J. J., Beaumont, J. O., Raison, J. C. A., et al. Measurement and monitoring of acutely ill patients by digital computer. *Surgery* 64:1057, 1969.
9. Osborn, J. J., Fagan, L. M., Fallat, R. J., Kunz, J. C., McClung, D. H., and Mitchell, R. R. Managing the data from respiratory measurements. *Med. Instru.* 13:330, 1979.

10. Severinghaus, J.   Current trends in continuous blood gas monitoring. *Biotelemetry & Patient Monitoring* 6:9, 1979.
11. Sheppard, L. C., Kouchoukos, N. T., Kurtis, M. A., et al.   Automated treatment of critically ill patients following operation. *Ann. Surg.* 168:596, 1968.
12. Swan, H. J. C., Ganz, W., Forrester, J., et al.   Catheterization of the heart in man with use of a flow-directed balloon-tipped catheter. *N. Engl. J. Med.* 283:447, 1970.
13. Thomas, L. J., Jr., Clark, K. W., Mead, C. N., Ripley, K. L., Spenncr, B. F., and Oliver, G. C., Jr.   Automated cardiac dysrhythmia analysis. *Proc. IEEE* 67:1322, 1979.
14. Turney, S. Z., et al.   Respiratory monitoring: Recent developments in automatic monitoring of gas concentration, flow, pressure, and temperature. *Ann. Thorac. Surg.* 16:184, 1973.

Christopher W. Bryan-Brown

24. OXYGEN TRANSPORT AND THE OXYHEMOGLOBIN DISSOCIATION CURVE

Oxygen transport in the critically ill patient is frequently in precarious balance. The normal adaptive mechanisms that maintain an adequate supply of oxygen to the tissues may become too slow or insufficient to compensate for any deficit when the delivery system is defective. It is therefore essential to assess and correct, when possible, any disorder that may interfere with efficient tissue oxygenation. The normal responses to hypoxia are increased cardiac output, redistribution of blood flow from tissues requiring less oxygen to those tissues with higher oxygen requirements, an increased release of oxygen from hemoglobin, and enhanced erythropoiesis.

The purpose of oxygen delivery to the tissues is to supply the mitochondria with oxygen at a tension in the optimal range of 2 to 20 torr (1 mm Hg = 1 torr). This requires a gradient of 5 to 20 torr between capillary and mitochondrion. For this reason, functional failure is found to develop in many tissues when the venous oxygen tension falls below 20 torr. Those that can function on anaerobic metabolism will continue with lower oxygen tensions. The demand on carbohydrate substrate is 18-fold, and lactic acid production leads to metabolic acidosis. Following shock and severe trauma, both the oxygen delivery system and mitochondrial integrity may be deranged; at a time when there is an increased demand for energy, there is a decreased efficiency of transport and utilization.

NORMAL PHYSIOLOGY

The components of oxygen transport are mechanisms for loading the blood with oxygen and for allocating it to areas where it is needed and at a sufficient tension to diffuse at the necessary rate to keep up with aerobic metabolism in the mitochondria. The physiology of this process consists of adjustments in ventilation, cardiac output, oxygen capacity of the blood, and distribution of flow and the affinity of hemoglobin for oxygen (see Table 24-1).

VENTILATION
Under basal conditions, ventilation and perfusion in the lung are matched, so that about 2.8 liters/M^2 (body surface area) of alveolar ventilation is

TABLE 24-1. Oxygen Transport: Responses to Demand

Responses	Mechanisms
Time Constant: Seconds	
Ventilation ↑	$PaCO_2$ or [H·] acting on CNS respiratory centers
	Severe hypoxia
Cardiac output ↑	Increased venous return due to vasodilation in the tissues with increased metabolism, by hypoxia, elevated [H·] (carbonic or lactic acid), or vasodilator substances (e.g., adenosine)
	Reflex increase in sympathetic tone on capacitance vessels, raising cardiac filling pressure
	Sympathetic stimulation of the myocardium
Redistribution of blood flow to tissues with maximum oxygen extraction	Autoregulation; vasodilation in tissues with greater metabolic activity (see below)
	Increased sympathetic tone, elevating vascular resistance to tissues with low oxygen extraction
Affinity of hemoglobin for oxygen ↓, P_{50} ↑	[H·] ↑ in severe hypoxia (Bohr effect)
Time Constant: Hours	
Affinity of hemoglobin for oxygen ↓, P_{50} ↑	Increase in red cell [2,3-DPG]
	Unsaturated hemoglobin binds more 2,3-DPG, increasing synthesis
	Unsaturated hemoglobin buffers more [H·]; PFK activity ↑, glycolysis ↑
	[H·] ↓, respiratory alkalosis induced by hypoxic drive to respiration
Adjustment of hemodynamics to cope with changed red cell mass, or hypovolemia	Plasma volume expansion from ECF, reducing blood viscosity and returning flow characteristics toward normal
	Adjustment of vascular resistance to control increased cardiac output due to blood volume and viscosity change
	Water and sodium retention adjusted by antidiuretic hormone and aldosterone secretion
Time Constant: Weeks	
Increased red cell mass	Bone marrow stimulated by increased erythropoietin production by hypoxic kidney

[H·] = hydrogen ion concentration; ↓ = decreased; ↑ = increased; CNS = central nervous system; ECF = extracellular fluid; PFK = phosphofructokinase; 2,3-DPG = 2,3-diphosphoglycerate.

adjusted to 3.5 liters/M^2 of cardiac output ($\dot{V}/\dot{Q} = 0.8$). This allows for the most efficient transfer of 140 ml/min/M^2 of oxygen from the atmosphere to the blood. The physiologic mechanism that governs ventilation is not normally oxygen deprivation; rather, it is a positive feedback system that reacts to arterial carbon dioxide tension ($PaCO_2$) and hydrogen ion concentration on the central nervous system chemoreceptors. Thus, the response to both a respiratory and nonrespiratory acidosis is an increase in ventilation that is governed by minute changes in $PaCO_2$ or pH.

The response to hypoxemia is small until there has been a fall in arterial oxygen tension (PaO_2) to at least 50 torr. This is because the sensors (the carotid and aortic bodies) react to reductions in hemoglobin saturation. Under normal conditions, hemoglobin is 85 percent saturated at this level, and the delivery to the tissues is only marginally less efficient. The effect of the increased ventilation on pulmonary function is small; a reduction of the amount of lung with a subnormal $\dot{V}/\dot{Q}$ ratio, an increase of wasted (dead space) ventilation, and a slight reciprocal increase in alveolar oxygen tension due to the washout of carbon dioxide. The consequent respiratory alkalosis temporarily improves the loading of oxygen into the erythrocytes because of the increased affinity of hemoglobin. This may have an adverse effect on the unloading of oxygen in the tissues (see p. 568). During strenuous exercise, the lung can oxygenate five to six times the basal cardiac output, with a 15-fold increase in oxygen uptake.

CARDIAC OUTPUT
Cardiac output does not respond directly to moderate changes in oxygen tension or content. The "available oxygen" or "arterial oxygen transport" is the product of cardiac output and arterial oxygen content. There are various compensatory mechanisms that can adjust oxygen delivery in the tissues, except when the oxygen level is inadequate to maintain normal metabolism.

HYPOXEMIA
Hypoxemia increases sympathetic tone, but this begins to have a marked effect on cardiac output only when the PaO_2 is down to 50 torr. The effect of an increasing metabolism in any tissue is to lower the oxygen tension. There is a greater diffusion of oxygen from the smaller arterioles, diminishing the oxygen tension in the distal part of the arteriolar system and thereby causing vasodilatation. This increases the amount of blood flowing through the tissue and so increases the oxygen delivery and the venous return. Thus, by a system of autoregulation, the cardiac output keeps pace with metabolic activity. Potassium, hydrogen ion (derived from lactic or carbonic acid), and adenosine also have a concomitant vasodilator activity.

REDISTRIBUTION OF BLOOD FLOW
Redistribution of blood flow to deliver oxygen where it is required enables the body to compensate for an increase of 50 percent in oxygen utilization

or a decrease of 30 percent in cardiac output. The main mechanism is the decrease in arteriolar tone in regions where metabolism is increased. When oxygen delivery is diminished, sympathetic activity increases. The initial effect is an increase in the tone of capacitance vessels and increased cardiac filling and output with some tachycardia. Subsequently, the arteriolar tone increases. However, diminished oxygen supply has less effect on autoregulatory tissues; blood is redistributed to the heart and brain, while tissues with a low oxygen requirement, such as skin and resting muscle, get a reduced supply. The splanchnic and renal circulations are markedly reduced, particularly with severe limitations of oxygen supply.

The myocardium has the greatest oxygen extraction of the body's tissues. Normally, it has an arteriovenous oxygen content difference $[C(a-v)O_2]$ of 11 ml of oxygen/100 ml of blood. The coronary sinus blood usually has an oxygen tension of 20 to 25 torr. The heart is working very near hypoxia at all times, and coronary blood flow is increased with the slightest increase in myocardial metabolism. It is controlled by oxygen requirement. The heart receives about 5 percent of cardiac output and 10 percent of oxygen uptake. The brain has a $C(a-v)O_2$ of about 8 ml/100 ml of blood and a venous oxygen tension of 32 to 35 torr. The cerebral circulation is not very sensitive to reduced oxygen tension unless it is below 50 torr. The main regulation is by carbon dioxide. Under basal conditions, the brain gets about 20 percent of the oxygen uptake and 15 percent of the cardiac output.

During hypoxic states, flow is diverted from tissues that have a low oxygen consumption to those that use more. When severe deficits in oxygen delivery occur, they may severely compromise tissues that normally have a moderate oxygen extraction. In the splanchnic area, the pancreas frequently has a proportionately greater reduction in blood flow, which may cause lysosomes to break down and release *myocardial depressant factor*. The kidneys may undergo the syndrome of acute vasomotor nephropathy (i.e., acute tubular necrosis).

HEMATOCRIT

Hematocrit is related to blood viscosity; normally, blood has about twice the viscosity of pure water. In anemia, the oxygen-carrying capacity of the blood diminishes and the viscosity falls, decreasing the resistive forces to cardiac output and allowing an easier venous return. Cardiac output increases, partially compensating for the decreased arterial blood oxygen content. In the experimental setting, if half the normal red cells are replaced with cells filled with methemoglobin (which replace the viscosity but not the oxygen-carrying capacity), the cardiac output increases a trivial amount. If half the red cell mass is replaced by plasma expander (dextran) the cardiac output may nearly double. On the other hand, normovolemic polycythemia greatly increases the resistance to venous return and can reduce cardiac output and arterial oxygen transport.

The ideal hematocrit is far from constant in all conditions. Maximum oxygen delivery to the brain occurs with hematocrits in the range of 45 to 47 percent. Because of reduced viscosity, the health of an ischemic limb may be best served by a hematocrit of 30 percent. Patients in acute respiratory failure have been shown to have a better outcome if the hematocrit is in excess of 40 percent, but other studies have shown that patients with trauma, major surgery, and sepsis may have an optimal mortality rate when the hematocrit is in the range of 33 percent. From the point of view of myocardial oxygenation, the most efficient oxygen delivery for oxygen uptake occurs when the hematocrit is in the range of 40 to 44 percent. In conditions of nonpulsatile blood flow and reduced temperature, such as occurs in extracorporeal bypass, a lower hematocrit than normal improves oxygen delivery. At present, the best that can be offered the critically ill patient with multisystem failure is monitoring of oxygen delivery in relation to hematocrit by testing the system with blood transfusion if the hematocrit is low.

BLOOD VOLUME

Blood volume deficits impair oxygen delivery by decreasing mean circulatory pressure and increasing the resistance to venous return, thus reducing the cardiac output. Oxygen transport can be increased by increasing the blood volume.

In healthy individuals, the hemodynamic changes are adjusted toward normal by changes in peripheral vascular resistance, which keep a balance between the effects of changes in blood volume and viscosity. The blood volume enlarges after normovolemic polycythemia is induced; the plasma volume expands and the viscosity is reduced, returning the flow characteristics and cardiac output toward normal.

NEUROHUMORAL SYMPATHETIC CONTROL

Neurohumoral sympathetic control of cardiac output increases the force of contraction and cardiac rate. The nervous control of redistribution of blood flow has the least effect on the organs with high oxygen consumption. Skin normally gets about 2 percent of the oxygen uptake and a little less than 10 percent of the cardiac output. When the body needs to lose more heat, blood flow is increased through the skin, due to a reflex loss of vasomotor tone. In cardiac failure, strong sympathetic activity can decrease skin blood flow to one-tenth of normal; in cardiogenic shock, with severely reduced myocardial function, gangrene of the extremities can even develop. The difference between skin and core temperature has been used to assess the adequacy of cardiac output.

HEMOGLOBIN CONCENTRATION

Hemoglobin concentration is increased when there is a decrease in arterial blood oxygen content, a reduction of hemoglobin concentration, or an increased affinity of hemoglobin for oxygen. This is sensed in the kidney, which produces erythropoietin when the renal oxygen supply is decreased relative to metabolic demand. Provided there are adequate iron stores, the rate of production of erythrocytes may be doubled. This is too slow an increase to bear much relevance to the treatment of the critically ill. In hypoxic states, when the P_{50} rises ($P_{50} = PO_2$ at which hemoglobin is half-saturated with oxygen), the production of erythropoietin may decline.

HEMOGLOBIN AFFINITY FOR OXYGEN

Hemoglobin affinity for oxygen is altered by various factors, summarized in Table 24-2. The actions of most of these factors combine to maintain a normal oxyhemoglobin dissociation, provided oxygen transport is adequate. Thus, in acute acidosis, hemoglobin unloads more oxygen at a given oxygen tension (PO_2). The higher red cell hydrogen ion concentration decreases phosphofructokinase (PFK) activity, and glycolysis is reduced. Synthesis and concentration of 2,3-diphosphoglycerate (2,3-DPG) fall, and the hemoglobin affinity for oxygen increases toward normal. When there is hypoxia from arterial hypoxemia, anemia, or low cardiac output, the affinity of hemoglobin for oxygen becomes less, thereby facilitating a greater unloading of oxygen at a given PO_2.

OXYHEMOGLOBIN DISSOCIATION

The relation of PO_2 to hemoglobin oxygen saturation (SO_2) is generally described by the oxyhemoglobin dissociation curve (see Figs. 24-1 and 24-3–24-6). The characteristics of this curve ensure that at the wide range of oxygen tensions found in the pulmonary capillary circulation, the hemoglobin will be easily saturated with oxygen. At the oxygen tensions found in metabolically active tissue capillaries (e.g., heart, 23 torr; brain, 32 torr), a slight fall in oxygen tension will release a large amount of oxygen. This property of normal hemoglobin determines the ability of the oxygen transport system to deliver adequate oxygen from the blood to the tissues.

DISSOCIATION CURVE ANALYSIS

Dissociation curve analysis is done either by describing the whole curve or by deriving the PO_2 at which the hemoglobin is half saturated with oxygen (P_{50}). An analysis can refer to the relationship under the conditions of the pH, temperature (T), and base excess (BE) of the patient (i.e., in vivo P_{50}, or P_{50iv}) or under conditions in which pH is 7.4, T is 37° C, and BE is zero (i.e., "standard" P_{50}, or $P_{50(7.4)}$).

The factors used to convert between in vivo P_{50} and standard P_{50} are interdependent variables. An increase in temperature will decrease the effect of hydrogen ion and 2,3-DPG on the hemoglobin molecule and increase the effect of carbon dioxide. Increased 2,3-DPG concentration will increase the effect of hydrogen ion but decrease the effect of carbon dioxide, with which it competes directly as a ligand. Fortunately, for purposes of calculation, the factors are nearest constant in the midsaturation range (30–70%). The Severinghaus factors are frequently used to make approximate in vitro conversions:

$$\Delta \log PO_2 = -0.48 \; \Delta pH$$
$$0.024 \; \Delta T$$
$$0.0013 \; BE$$

Thus, for a given saturation (e.g., 50%), if the blood sample measured pH was 7.10 and the PO_2 was 37.1 torr, the PO_2 at a pH of 7.40 would be 26.6 for the same saturation (see Fig. 24-4). If the temperature of a patient was 39.0° C and the sample was found to have a PO_2 of 26.6 torr at 37.0° C, the PO_2 that would give the same saturation at the patient's temperature would be 29.2 torr. Further, if the same blood sample had a base excess of +10 mEq/liter, and the base excess was corrected to zero, the PO_2 at 37° C would be changed only to 26.8 torr. This last minor correction makes up for changes in oxyhemoglobin dissociation due to carbon dioxide. The P_{50iv} gives information about the adequacy of oxygen transport in the patient, whereas the standard P_{50} tells of changes irrespective of acid-base alterations. Ideally, the red cell pH should be the standard. Normally, this is 0.2 pH units less than whole blood pH, but it may be highly variable in disease states.

HILL EQUATION
Various forms of the Hill equation can be used to linearize the oxyhemoglobin dissociation curve for easier analysis. Although there are more complicated formulas that can give an accurate fit to the whole curve, the Hill equation is acceptable for clinical purposes. The approximation is reasonably accurate between saturation values of 20 and 80 percent (see Fig. 24-1).

$$\log \frac{y}{100 - y} = A(\log x) + B$$

where

$$y = SO_2 \text{ and } x = PO_2$$

$$P_{50} = \text{antilog} \; \frac{-B}{A}$$

A, the slope of the curve, is often given a value of 2.7. If this value is used to calculate P_{50} from a single PO_2, the error is usually less than 1 torr if the SO_2 is between 30 and 70 percent. This is probably as much accuracy as can be achieved in most clinical laboratories by trying to establish

TABLE 24-2. Factors Affecting Hemoglobin Affinity for Oxygen (P_{50})

$P_{50}\uparrow$	$P_{50}\downarrow$	Time Constant	Comment
$[H^\cdot]\uparrow$	$[H^\cdot]\downarrow$	Stat	Bohr effect
$[K_i^\cdot]+[Na_i^\cdot]\uparrow+[Cl_i^\cdot]\uparrow$	$[K_i^\cdot]+[Na_i^\cdot]\downarrow+[Cl_i^\cdot]\downarrow$	Stat	Salt effect; related to intraerythrocyte ion concentration
$T\uparrow$	$T\downarrow$	Stat	
$PCO_2\uparrow$	$\left\{\begin{array}{l} PCO_2\downarrow \\ \text{Carbon monoxide} \end{array}\right.$	Stat Stat	Carbaminohemoglobin has less O_2 affinity Carboxyhemoglobin has very high O_2 affinity
$[H^\cdot]\downarrow$	$[H^\cdot]\uparrow$	Hr	PFK activity inhibited by acidosis; glycolysis and 2,3-DPG synthesis MCHC related to $[H^\cdot]$
Hypoxia or anemia	Hyperoxia	Hr, days	[2,3-DPG]$\uparrow$ when $PO_2\downarrow$ More 2,3-DPG bound to deoxyhemoglobin; activation of PGM; 2,3-DPG synthesis Reaction reduced if compensatory respiratory alkalosis absent Deoxyhemoglobin buffers $H^\cdot$; PFK activated
MCHC$\uparrow$	MCHC$\downarrow$	Stat	?Intraerythrocyte hemoglobin buffers $[H^\cdot]$
Plasma inorganic phosphate $\uparrow$	Plasma inorganic phosphate $\downarrow$	Hr, days	Substrate for ATP and 2,3-DPG
	Storage at 4°C	Days	[ATP], [2,3-DPG], and $[K_i^\cdot]\downarrow$ [2,3-DPG] 20% in 10 days ACD storage CPD storage slows ATP and 2,3-DPG loss

Nucleic acids	Min	Substrate for ATP and 2,3-DPG
		Inosine used in vivo
		Inosine + adenine used in vitro
Thyroxine	Hr	Glycolysis
Propranolol	Min	?Mechanism
Methylprednisolone sodium succinate (high dose)	Min	Mechanisms not established:
		Subnormal $[K_i·]$ ↑ in minutes
		$[H_i·]/[H_p·]$ increased over 30 min
		No constant change of [2,3-DPG] observed
		Effect lasting

$[H·]$ = hydrogen ion concentration; $[H_p·]$ = hydrogen ion concentration; $[H_i·]$, $[Cl_i·]$, $[K_i·]$, and $[Na_i·]$ = intraerythrocyte ion concentrations (hydrogen, chloride, potassium, and sodium); 2,3-DPG = 2,3-diphosphoglycerate; PFK = phosphofructokinase; MCHC = mean corpuscular hemoglobin concentration; ATP = adenosine triphosphate; ACD = acid citrate dextrose; CPD = citrate-phosphate-dextrose.

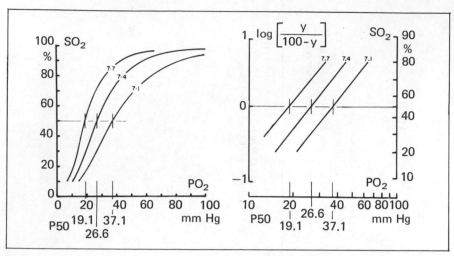

FIGURE 24-1. Hill plot. This is a linear approximation, which has fair accuracy for SO₂ values of between 20 and 80 percent. It is frequently used in estimating position of oxyhemoglobin dissociation curve. Comparison with P_{50} values is given, demonstrating standard curves for three pH values and their linearized versions.

the slope from several samples with different oxygen tensions using polarographic oximetry.

The position of the oxyhemoglobin dissociation curve can be analyzed with the Hill equation:

1. Single point analysis from PO_2 and SO_2.
2. Multiple point analysis (requires special calibration of PO_2 electrode for accuracy).
3. Tonometry with calibrating gases to get accurate PO_2 values. Tonometry gases: oxygen, 2.5 to 5.5 percent (PO_2, 18–39 torr); carbon dioxide, 5.6 percent (PCO_2, 40 torr); nitrogen, balance.

Saturation and pH are measured on 2 to 4 samples of blood tonometered with oxygen mixtures with PO_2 values that straddle the P_{50}, and corrections are made on each PO_2 to standardize the pH and base excess. Values for A and B can be calculated by least squares fit in a linear regression analysis of the data in the Hill equation. From this can be calculated the standard P_{50} and curve positions for any values of pH, base excess, and temperature for calculation of the P_{50iv}.

Points can be measured on 200-μliter divided samples using an Astrup microtonometer. Low PO_2 samples take at least 7 minutes to equilibrate, so 8 minutes of agitation should be used. One limb of the tonometer is used to measure pH, and the other is used to fill a hematocrit tube for saturation measurement in a meter handling microsamples (e.g., Radiometer OSM 1). It is possible to calculate a P_{50} value and slope on 0.51 ml of heparinized blood [2].

For easier handling, 3 to 5 ml can be used for each point. Bubble (e.g., Adam's) tonometers will equilibrate low PO_2 points in 7 to 8 minutes; slower tonometers that do not froth blood take longer. On larger samples, it is also possible to make saturation corrections for carboxyhemoglobin and methemoglobin.

Diluted suspensions of washed red cells in buffered saline solutions exposed to various oxygen tensions in a combined tonometer-spectrophotometer cuvette give the advantages of a small single sample, assurance of equilibration, and negligible pH change. The sample is also easily deoxygenated. The difference due to low PCO_2 is generally ignored in this technique.

Samples can be tonometered, and points established by calculating saturation from measurement of oxygen content and hemoglobin concentration.

Dissociation Curve Analyzers

Dissociation curve analyzers are made for plotting the whole curve. The sample of blood is deoxygenated with nitrogen containing 5% carbon dioxide. This process is sometimes not complete in 30 minutes, which can lead to baseline error. The PO_2 is then recorded while the blood is being saturated with oxygen with 5% carbon dioxide.

Radiometer DCA records on an X-Y-Y' plotter the PO_2 in a sealed chamber above deoxygenated blood and the PO_2 in the sample as it is saturated with oxygen. The fall in pressure in the gas is proportional to the amount of gas moving into the blood sample. The points for SO_2 values of 0 and 100 percent are the X positions at the beginning of the measurement and where the pressure no longer falls in the gas phase. Y is plotted as the PO_2 of the blood and Y' as pH, so that points can be corrected or standardized.

A curve analysis takes 45 minutes to 1 hour to perform. When the hemoglobin is saturated, it becomes more acid. As the system is closed, the PCO_2 will rise, but it usually rises less than 1 torr, so that this will not lead to appreciable error.

Blood can be saturated with increasing oxygen tensions and either continuous or multiple measurements of SO_2, PO_2, and pH plotted.

Samples of blood can be deoxygenated with nitrogen containing 5% carbon dioxide and saturated with 21% oxygen containing 5% carbon dioxide. The deoxygenated and saturated samples are then mixed in precisely measured proportions and the PO_2 is measured. The oxygen content of the mixture is known, since it was all provided by the saturated sample, so the SO_2 can be calculated and a point on the curve established [6].

BELLINGHAM FORMULA

The Bellingham formula [1] calculates the P_{50iv} from most of the factors that are known to be of clinical importance:

$$\log P_{50iv} = \log (26.6 + 0.5 [MCHC - 33] + 0.69 [2,3\text{-}DPG - 14.5])$$
$$+ 0.0013 \, BE + 0.48 [pH - 7.4] + 0.024 (T - 37)*$$

where 2,3-DPG is measured in $\mu mole/gm$ Hb

IN VIVO TEMPERATURE CORRECTION FACTORS

In vivo temperature correction factors should be used to convert the patient's acid-base data measured at 37° C to in vivo values.

The temperature corrections for pH can be approximated by:

$$pH = -0.0146 \, \Delta T$$

A closer value is obtained if the temperature coefficient decrease as the pH falls is taken into account:

$$pH = [0.0065 (7.4 - pH_{37}) - 0.0146] \, \Delta T, \text{ when the pH is measured at 37° C}$$

The change in PCO_2 for a change in temperature is approximated by:

$$\Delta \log PCO_2 = 0.019 (T - 37), \text{ when } PCO_2 \text{ is measured at 37° C}$$

Correction factors of oxygen data generally become less accurate when the saturation is high. The normal factor for temperature change is as follows:

$$\Delta \log PO_2 = 0.031 \, \Delta T$$

When the saturation is greater than 80 percent, the temperature coefficient of oxygen solubility in blood begins to influence the result. If the PO_2 is above 250 torr, $PO_2/\Delta T$ is directly related to it. For saturations above 80 percent, changes can be approximated by the following:

$$\Delta \log PO_2 = \frac{3130 - 62.5 \, Sat + 0.312008 \, Sat^2}{100,000 - 1993 \, Sat + 9.9313 \, Sat^2} \times \Delta T$$

OXYGEN DELIVERY

Oxygen delivery is altered by changes in hemoglobin affinity for oxygen. Figure 24-2 shows the changes in cardiac output needed to maintain a mixed venous PO_2 of 40 torr. The arterial blood is saturated and the oxygen utilization is constant. The changes in P_{50} could be produced by acute pH changes of 7.1 ($P_{50} = 37.1$ torr) and 7.7 ($P_{50} = 19.1$ torr) from the normal values of 7.4 ($P_{50} = 26.6$ torr). A P_{50} value of 19.1 torr could also occur if the 2,3-DPG concentration was 3.7 $\mu mole/gm$ Hb. This sort of value can

* MCHC = mean corpuscular hemoglobin concentration; Hb = hemoglobin.

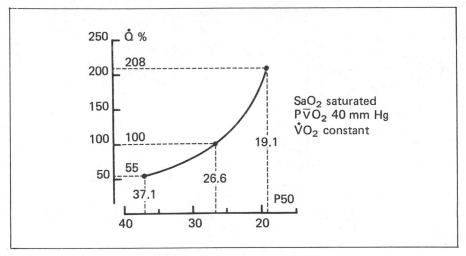

FIGURE 24-2. Change of cardiac output plotted against P_{50}. As P_{50} decreases, a greater cardiac output is needed to maintain $P\bar{v}O_2$ at 40 torr.

be found in patients after massive transfusions of stored acid citrate dextrose blood.

Under normal circumstances the arteriovenous oxygen saturation difference is about 25 percent. Figure 24-3 shows the advantages of a high P_{50} in hypoxic states. The $P_{50} = 37.1$ torr curve shows an ability to drop 25 percent of SO_2 at a higher PO_2 when loaded at PO_2 of 60 torr than does a normal curve when loaded at 80 torr. This advantage would be lost at a loading PO_2 of 50 torr.

The three graphs of Figure 24-3 show that there is a marked difference in PO_2 unloading, with the higher PO_2 value (80 torr) of loading only when the P_{50} is high. When the P_{50} is low, an increase of cardiac output is the only way to make a significant increase in oxygen delivery, since raising the loading tension in the lungs has a negligible effect.

In experimental conditions, the coronary blood flow has been related to increasing hemoglobin affinity for oxygen. Since the coronary circulation initially dilates to the stimulus of hypoxia, it is not surprising to find the flow increasing when the hemoglobin requires lower-than-normal PO_2 levels to release oxygen. Various other, less well-substantiated clinical data would suggest that the response to increased oxygen demand can be a reduction of saturation as well as an increased cardiac output in persons with a high P_{50}. Those with a low P_{50} can respond only with increased cardiac output and have limited exercise tolerance. In various experimental hemodynamic and septic shock models, a high P_{50} is associated with greater survival.

When oxygen delivery becomes less efficient, P_{50iv} is found to increase. It has been difficult to show the clinical relevance of changes of the affinity

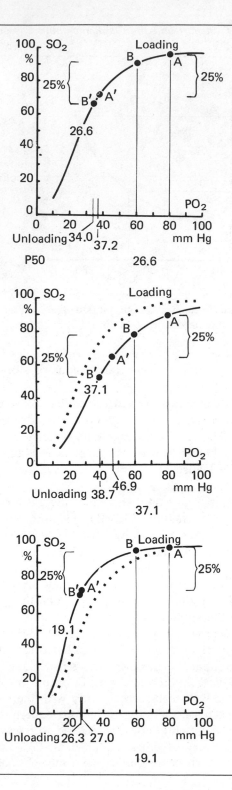

of hemoglobin for oxygen in terms of morbidity or mortality. Neonates with the infant respiratory distress syndrome have been shown to have an improved outcome if they have an exchange transfusion replacing cells filled with fetal hemoglobin for cells containing hemoglobin A. This is a special situation, because of the risk of using high inspired oxygen concentrations in neonates to oxygenate the blood for fear of a retrolental fibroplasia [4]. Patients who have had cardiac surgery who have been on extracorporeal bypass show an improved myocardial performance in- the postoperative period if blood with a higher than normal P_{50} is used in the perfusate [3].

FACTORS AFFECTING THE OXYHEMOGLOBIN RELATIONSHIP
The factors affecting the oxyhemoglobin relationship are summarized in Table 24-2.

HYDROGEN ION CONCENTRATION
Hydrogen ion concentration has a direct effect on the hemoglobin molecule. Oxygen affinity decreases as the hydrogen ion concentration increases (Bohr effect). Figure 24-4 shows three oxyhemoglobin dissociation curves plotted for both saturation and content. An acute pH change from 7.4 (normal) to 7.1 will increase the amount of oxygen released at a PO_2 of 20 torr from two-thirds to over four-fifths, thereby increasing the consumable oxygen. If there is an acute alkalemia to a pH of 7.7, less than half the oxygen will be released at this point.

SODIUM AND POTASSIUM
Sodium, potassium, and chloride ions increase the bonds bridging the chains of the hemoglobin molecule, reducing oxygen affinity (salt effect). Restoration of normal red cell cation concentration causes a rise in P_{50}.

TEMPERATURE
Temperature increases lower hemoglobin oxygen affinity.

FIGURE 24-3. Oxyhemoglobin dissociation curves with P_{50} values of 26.6 (normal), 37.1, and 19.1 torr (normal curve indicated on latter two graphs by dotted line). Effect of a 25 percent decrease in saturation is compared at loading tensions of 80 and 60 torr (A and B) and unloading tensions at A' and B'. Note that curve of a P_{50} of 37.1 is able to unload at a higher tension, even when loaded at 60 torr, than the others loaded at 80\ torr. Also note that an increase in PO_2 from 60 to 80 torr makes no significant change in unloading tension in curve of a P_{50} of 19.1 torr.

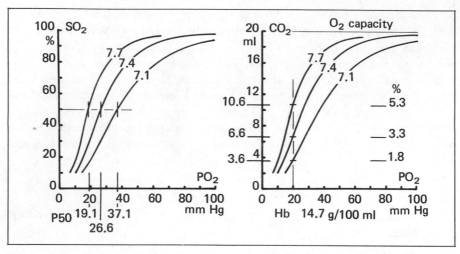

FIGURE 24-4. Oxyhemoglobin dissociation curves plotted for different pH values. Note that at PO_2 of 20 torr, curve 7.7 has over half the oxygen content still bound to hemoglobin (normal 33%). The 7.1 curve has less than one-fifth of oxygen capacity utilized, showing how an increased right shift of curve causes more oxygen to be released at given PO_2.

CARBON DIOXIDE

By forming carbaminohemoglobin, carbon dioxide increases the P_{50}. This is shown whenever blood is acidified by carbon dioxide rather than by direct acidification; the curve shift is about 25 percent greater.

CARBON MONOXIDE

Carbon monoxide has an affinity for hemoglobin 280 times that of oxygen. The occupation of the hemoglobin molecule by carbon monoxide (carboxyhemoglobin) causes both a severe loss of oxygen-carrying capacity and a marked increase in the hemoglobin's affinity for oxygen. Fifty percent carboxyhemoglobin has a P_{50} of 13.3 torr (see Fig. 24-5). This would require over six times the cardiac output required in an anemia with half the normal hemoglobin concentration! The consumable oxygen in the content graph is 2.5 ml at pH 7.4; in a normal man at the absolute limits of hypoxia compatible with survival, this would require at least a 10-liter cardiac output to deliver a minimum of oxygen.

Patients with severe carbon monoxide poisoning are usually hypoxic enough to become acidotic. At a pH of 7.1, the theoretical minimum cardiac output could be reduced by about 45 percent. The correction of acidosis in this type of patient might prove fatal. Alterations of PCO_2 do not affect oxygen affinity with carboxyhemoglobin.

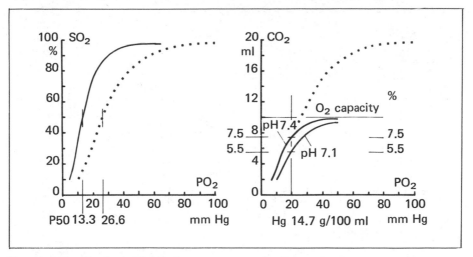

FIGURE 24-5. Oxyhemoglobin dissociation curves (normal, *dotted lines;* 50% carboxyhemoglobin, *solid lines*). Note far left shift of curve (P_{50} = 13.3) and decreased oxygen capacity. Also notice that acute acidosis of pH 7.1 will increase oxygen available at 20 torr (consumable oxygen) by 2 ml/100 ml blood, or 80 percent. This indicates danger of overzealous treatment of acidosis in carbon monoxide poisoning.

INDIRECT EFFECT OF HYDROGEN ION CONCENTRATION

Hydrogen ion concentration also has an indirect effect, which may be related to most of the processes that result in an increased 2,3-DPG concentration. PFK activity is reduced by increasing amounts of hydrogen ion. This inhibition of glycolysis decreases 2,3-DPG synthesis. It has also been found that the MCHC is reduced in acidosis, which also reduces the P_{50}. Thus, after a few hours of acidosis, the oxyhemoglobin dissociation curve can return almost to normal. In alkalosis, there is a reciprocal relation with hydrogen ion concentration and 2,3-DPG production, leading to a normalization of the P_{50}. In the critically ill patient, 2,3-DPG formation may be slowed down, leaving oxygen transport deranged for days.

??IA AND ANEMIA
nd anemia both produce a similar response, causing a right shift
. The reason for this is an increase in 2,3-DPG concentration.
ows a typical change that might be seen in severe anemia
al hemoglobin concentration. The dissociation curve has
left in chronic anemia, with an increase in P_{50} to 31.9
54 percent increase in 2,3-DPG concentration. If
versus tension (PO_2) graph is considered, the

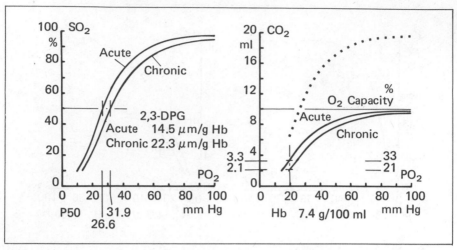

FIGURE 24-6. Oxyhemoglobin dissociation curves plotted for anemia. Increase in 2,3-DPG occurring in chronic anemia has shifted curve to right. In capacity graph (CO_2), hemoglobin affinity for oxygen is decreased 18 percent at 20 torr, indicating additional release of "consumable" oxygen of 1.2 ml/100 ml of blood.

amount of oxygen available at a PO_2 of 20 torr (consumable oxygen) is 1.2 ml/100 ml, or 12 percent more than the oxygen capacity in chronic anemia. If the arterial blood is fully saturated, this would allow for a 10 percent decrease in cardiac output for oxygen delivery at a PO_2 of 40 torr. The graphs in Figure 24-6 are not corrected for arteriovenous acid-base and carbon dioxide changes.

In anemia, there is less hemoglobin to buffer respiratory acid, so the Bohr effect is increased, releasing even more oxygen to the tissues. The increase in 2,3-DPG may be due to the greater affinity of deoxyhemoglobin for 2,3-DPG. Phosphoglyceromutase (PGM) activity is inhibited by 2,3-DPG. As there is less free 2,3-DPG, PGM can convert more 1,3-DPG to 2,3-DPG (Rapaport-Luebering shunt), so that the more time the red cell spends in a low oxygen tension environment, the more the red cell concentration is increased. The problem with this theory is that the 2,3-DPG concentration does not rise as much if the hypoxia-induced respiratory alkalosis i̲ rected or the patient is given acetozolamide to slow down the rat̲ down of carbonic acid. The increase in 2,3-DPG may therefo̲ increased glycolysis, since PFK is activated by the lower h̲ centration. Also, deoxyhemoglobin is a weaker acid t̲ and may buffer more red cell hydrogen ion. Adult̲ respiratory or cardiac failure and children with c̲ high red cell 2,3-DPG concentrations.

MEAN CORPUSCULAR HEMOGLOBIN CONCENTRATION

Mean corpuscular hemoglobin concentration is associated with a decreased hemoglobin affinity for oxygen. This could be due to the increased concentration of intracellular buffer, reducing hydrogen ion concentration, and this would increase 2,3-DPG synthesis. Mean corpuscular hemoglobin concentration and 2,3-DPG concentration rise and fall together in chronic alkalosis and acidosis.

PLASMA INORGANIC PHOSPHATE CONCENTRATION

Plasma inorganic phosphate concentration influences the synthesis of red cell 2,3-DPG and adenosine triphosphate (ATP). This is probably because it is a substrate in the elaboration of these compounds.

EFFECT OF BLOOD STORAGE

Storage of blood in conventional blood banks has long been associated with an increase in hemoglobin affinity for oxygen. This is found in patients who have large transfusions of stored blood (Valtis and Kennedy effect). The normal storage of acid citrate dextrose blood at 4° C reduces the 2,3-DPG level to 20 percent of normal in 10 to 14 days. This by itself would reduce the P_{50} to 18.6 torr, which would require a more than doubled cardiac output to maintain normal oxygen delivery. The levels of ATP and potassium are also reduced. The use of citrate phosphate dextrose has enabled blood to maintain a more normal oxygen affinity longer. Inosine and adenine are also added to blood for storage for this purpose (this technique is still being investigated).

If the respiratory function of stored blood is to be maintained, the red cells have to be deep frozen in glycerol solutions.

NUCLEIC ACIDS

Inosine and adenine can be used to restore and even give supranormal levels of 2,3-DPG in red cells. If the outdated cells are incubated in a medium containing pyruvate, inosine, glucose, and phosphate (PIGP) and then resuspended in a suitable medium for transfusion, this can be achieved (these techniques are still under investigation). If adenine is added to the PIGP, further improvement in respiratory function is marginal, but the ATP concentration is further increased. Recent work suggests that if glucose is not included in the incubating solution, a greater decrease in oxyhemoglobin dissociation occurs [5]. On a preliminary basis, inosine infusions have been used in man.

THYROXINE

Thyroxine has the effect of increasing the P_{50}; this is probably due to increased glycolysis. Increased PGM activity has been related to the state of thyrotoxicosis; decreased activity has been related to reduced thyroid function.

PROPRANOLOL

Propranolol increases the P_{50}, but the mechanism is unclear. Preliminary reports indicate that some β-adrenergic agents may have a weak effect in the opposite direction.

METHYLPREDNISOLONE

Methylprednisolone sodium succinate has been demonstrated to decrease the affinity of hemoglobin for oxygen, especially when it is abnormally high. In high dosage (15–30 mg/kg of body weight), it markedly increases the P_{50} over a half hour to an hour, and the change persists. In patients who have a low red cell potassium concentration, the P_{50} is restored in a few minutes. The red cell pH decreases relative to that of the whole blood for half an hour.

HYPOXIA

The clinical entity of hypoxia is hard to define, since the term is used to describe a number of situations, varying from a lower PaO_2 than would be predicted (without right-to-left intracardiac shunt) to a shortage of oxygen sufficient for the deficit to be made up with significant anaerobic metabolism.

ARTERIAL OXYGEN TENSION

PaO_2 cannot give an adequate picture of hypoxia. It can be normal when the delivery to the tissues is defective because of an inadequate cardiac output, anemia, or the increased affinity of hemoglobin for oxygen. In addition, particularly in hypovolemia, many tissues are poorly perfused due to redistribution.

MIXED VENOUS OXYGEN TENSION

Mixed venous oxygen tension is a more appropriate measure of oxygen delivery than is PaO_2, since it reflects the overall oxygen tension of the blood leaving the tissues. Blood flow through tissues usually varies in relation to metabolism. In pathologic states, the greatest contribution to the mixed venous blood is from the best perfused tissues, and the deficits of other regions with inadequate oxygen may be masked. Since their contribution to the overall amount is small, only a markedly low mixed venous oxygen tension is significant. However, a minor reduction may be masking considerable regional hypoxia.

LACTATE

Lactate measurements may also indicate the adequacy of oxygen transport. A rise in the lactate level may be due to increased anaerobic metabolism.

As a measurement of oxygen transport, however, lactate concentration suffers from the same drawback as mixed venous oxygen tension, in that poorly perfused tissues will not add much to the circulation, and regional hypoxia will not necessarily be detected. The drawback of the lactate-pyruvate ratio is that the levels of both substances rise in the circulation when glycolysis increases. Thus, with β-adrenergic stimulation, lactate and pyruvate appear in greater quantity in the blood; and in β blockade, lactate levels decrease. Even so, serial lactate levels are a good way to observe a patient's progress. The normal is less than 2 mM/liter. Levels of 10 mM/liter are associated with very high mortality.

OTHER SIGNS OF HYPOXIA

2,3-DPG and P_{50iv} increase when the oxygen delivery is poor and may represent an index of prolonged deficit in oxygen delivery. The change is best seen in nondepleted shock patients or in patients with primary cardiopulmonary disease. It may take several days for the P_{50iv} to be spontaneously restored in sick, septic, and acidotic patients.

Clinical evaluation of cerebral function, especially by staff continually at a patient's bedside, may pick up the early changes of cerebral hypoxia (e.g., disorientation, forgetfulness, torpor, confusion, and restlessness). The kidneys may not be able to concentrate urine, and ventricular cardiac arrhythmias may occur.

CLINICAL IMPLICATIONS

The clinical management of the patient with pulmonary and cardiovascular insufficiency and in shock states is dealt with in other chapters. The alteration of the affinity of hemoglobin for oxygen has not been conclusively shown to benefit the outcome of a patient who is critically ill. On the other hand, the efficiency of the circulation in delivering oxygen at a given oxygen tension is decreased when the affinity increases. It is readily inferred that correction of this portion of the oxygen delivery system might add a margin for survival to the patient who would otherwise die because other compensatory mechanisms were inadequate; the clinical implications are therefore largely putative.

There are some helpful therapeutic maneuvers that should be mentioned. Massive blood transfusions will improve oxygen delivery if the blood contains either fresh or rejuvenated red cells. Patients with low flow states who require blood replacement and patients on extracorporeal perfusion should be treated with fresh blood or rejuvenated red cells. Acidosis, unless very acute, should be corrected slowly to allow the P_{50iv} to be maintained. The addition of phosphate to the correction of diabetic ketoacidosis greatly speeds the restoration of red cell 2,3-DPG. Chronic respiratory acidosis should be reduced slowly, once the pH is above 7.3. Plasma phosphate levels should be maintained in all patients on total parenteral nutrition;

2,3-DPG synthesis is dependent on an adequate phosphate concentration. By increasing the P_{50iv}, methylprednisolone sodium succinate may benefit patients in septic shock or after massive blood transfusion, when compensatory mechanisms are failing.

REFERENCES

1. Bellingham, A. J., et al. Regulatory mechanisms of hemoglobin oxygen affinity in acidosis and alkalosis. *J. Clin. Invest.* 50:700, 1971.
2. Bryan-Brown, C. W., et al. Consumable oxygen: Availability of oxygen in relation to oxyhemoglobin dissociation. *Crit. Care Med.* 1:17, 1973.
3. Hechtman, H. B., et al. Importance of oxygen transport in clinical medicine. *Crit. Care Med.* 7:419, 1979.
4. Oski, F. A. Clinical implications of oxyhemoglobin association curve in the neonatal period. *Crit. Care Med.* 7:412, 1979.
5. Valeri, C. R., et al. Biochemical modification and freeze preservation of red blood cells. *Crit. Care Med.* 7:439, 1979.
6. Wilson, R. S., and Laver, M. B. Oxygen analysis. *Anesthesiology* 37:112, 1972.

SELECTED READINGS

Alberti, K. G. M. M., et al. 2,3-diphosphoglycerate and tissue oxygenation in uncontrolled diabetes mellitus. *Lancet* 2:391, 1972.

Bryan-Brown, C. W., et al. Hemodynamic responses and oxygen delivery after methylprednisolone sodium succinate. In T. M. Glenn (Ed.), *Steroids and Shock*. Baltimore: University Park Press, 1974.

Guyton, A. C., et al. *Circulatory Physiology*. Philadelphia: Saunders, 1972.

Kelman, G. R. *Applied Cardiovascular Physiology*. London: Butterworth, 1971.

Lichtman, M. A., et al. Reduced red cell glycolysis, 2,3-diphosphoglycerate and adenosine triphosphate and increased hemoglobin-oxygen affinity during severe hypophosphatemia induced by hyperalimentation. *Ann. Intern. Med.* 74:562, 1971.

McConn, R. 2,3-DPG—What role in septic shock? In B. K. Forscher et al. (Eds.), *Shock in Low- and High-Flow States*. Amsterdam: Excerpta Medica, 1972.

Perutz, M. F. Hemoglobin structure and respiratory transport. *Sci. Am.* 239:92, 1978.

Valeri, C. R., et al. Function of red blood cells. *Crit. Care Med.* 7:357, 1979.

Wade, O. L., and Bishop, J. M. *Cardiac Output and Regional Blood Flow*. Oxford: Blackwell, 1962.

Warren M. Zapol / # 25. CLINICAL APPLICATION OF THE MEMBRANE OXYGENATOR IN REFRACTORY ACUTE RESPIRATORY FAILURE

The membrane artificial lung is an extracorporeal device for exchanging blood gases. By preventing hypoxia and hypercapnia, use of the membrane lung can maintain life while otherwise intolerable pulmonary damage heals. Repair is possible because appropriate levels of extracorporeal support can relieve the patient's lungs of their primary burden of respiratory gas exchange and of the handicaps of conventional therapy: high ventilator pressures and inspired oxygen concentrations.

All membrane lungs gently exchange respiratory gases through thin polymer membranes [5]. Unlike disk and bubble lungs, membrane lungs do not destroy red blood cells and proteins. "Microporous" oxygenators made of membranes containing tiny holes have been used recently to obtain increased gas transfer rates. These devices should not yet be used for long-term (>6 hr) perfusion, since we do not know enough about how they interact with blood or how safe they are [16].

SELECTION OF ADULT PATIENTS FOR EXTRACORPOREAL PERFUSION

Patients for extracorporeal perfusion (ECP) [12] should be carefully selected to have a reversible form of acute respiratory failure. Posttraumatic or "shock" lung [9], Pneumocystis carinii pneumonia, acute pulmonary embolism [4], and newborn meconium aspiration are acute pulmonary diseases from which patients have recovered and survived with ECP. To date, patients selected for perfusion have exhibited severe respiratory distress syndrome with poor compliance, a large intrapulmonary shunt, and bilateral diffuse opacification of chest radiograph [21, 23]. Lungs that have undergone necrosis or severe fibrosis are unlikely to repair during perfusion [19, 20]. Table 25-1 lists known survivors among patients who have had ECP

Supported by a Specialized Center of Research in Adult Respiratory Failure Grant HL 23591, National Heart, Lung, and Blood Institute.

TABLE 25-1. ECP Survivors with Adult[a] Respiratory Distress Syndrome by June 1977

Disease	Survivors
Shock, trauma, fat embolism	7
Cardiac failure (postcardiac surgical myocarditis)	4
Goodpasture's syndrome	3
Pulmonary emboli	2
Drowning, inhalation injury	2
Bacterial pneumonia, septicemia	2
Varicella pneumonia	2
Pneumocystis carinii	2
Influenza viral pneumonia	2
Aspiration pneumonia	1
Total	27[b]

Source: Modified from R. H. Bartlett and A. B. Gazzaniga, Extracorporeal circulation for cardiopulmonary failure. Curr. Prob. Surg. 15:59, 1978.

ECP = extracorporeal perfusion.

[a] Over 10 years of age.
[b] From approximately 190 adult ECP trials.

for primary acute respiratory failure. A randomized prospective study of 90 patients with severe acute respiratory failure showed no increased survival in viral and bacterial pneumonia despite the use of ECP [22].

Early perfusion is essential. Acute respiratory failure of two or three weeks' duration often progresses to extensive fibrosis and destruction of lung tissue [24]. An open lung biopsy is then necessary to determine the anatomic condition of the lungs. Biopsy increases the risk of air leakage, but is necessary if a specific, undefined etiologic agent or process is suspected (e.g., *Pneumocystis carinii*, Goodpasture's syndrome) [11].

Because serious hemorrhagic complications occur in over 20 percent of patients undergoing prolonged ECP, perfusion should be reserved for patients whose condition deteriorates despite maximal medical respiratory therapy. Maximal medical therapy for acute respiratory failure consists of dehydration, intubation, constant-volume mechanical ventilation with at least 10 cm H_2O positive end-expiratory pressure (PEEP), sedation and paralysis, chest physiotherapy, frequent tracheal suctioning, hourly turning, maintenance of normothermia or mild hypothermia (32–37° C), and the administration of antibiotic and cardiotonic drugs when indicated [17]. The patient's condition must be allowed to stabilize for several hours after transfer to the perfusion center. ECP must be considered if the patient's condition continues to deteriorate, and if the patient exhibits progressive hypoxemia despite maximum tolerable PEEP and possibly the following: (1) decreasing compliance (peak ventilator pressure >55 cm H_2O; quasi-static compliance <15 ml/cm H_2O); (2) a need for increasing amounts of cardiotonic drugs to maintain adequate cardiac output; or (3) life-threatening arrhythmias when suctioned [12]. If no contraindications (see later section) are present, membrane lung perfusion should be instituted after informed permission is obtained from the nearest relative.

SELECTION OF CHILDREN FOR PERFUSION
Bartlett has recently reported 16 perfusions for newborn respiratory failure; 9 infants improved and 6 survived. Infants with meconium aspiration syndrome were particularly helped by perfusion. Since requirements for selection of children and techniques are changing, the reader is referred to Bartlett's excellent monograph for further information [1].

CONTRAINDICATIONS TO MEMBRANE LUNG PERFUSION
Contraindications to membrane lung perfusion include active hemorrhage (e.g., gastrointestinal, nasopharyngeal, tracheal, central nervous system), disseminated malignancy, advanced age, chronic pulmonary insufficiency, or major neurological or other organ failure. Major sepsis (e.g., burns over 50% of the body) is a relative contraindication. Renal failure is not a contraindication; concomitant hemodialysis and ECP have been successfully performed [6]. Patients who have undergone recent major surgery or massive trauma can be successfully perfused if given adequate time (12–24 hr) to achieve hemostasis. Marked increases of pulmonary vascular resistance (>3 torr/liter/min) may signal extensive destruction of pulmonary vasculature and a poor prognosis.

THE PERFUSION SYSTEM
An adult extracorporeal perfusion system is shown in Figure 25-1.

CANNULAS
Because membrane lung perfusion requires large extracorporeal blood flows (40–90 ml/kg/min), large-bore drainage cannulas must be used. In adults, we suggest a cannula with a minimal internal diameter (ID) of 6.5 mm. We insert a specially fabricated thin-walled, steel spring–reinforced, segmented polyurethane venous drainage cannula (average adult size 9.50 mm ID, 10.35 mm OD) in the femoral vein* [14]. Proper placement of this cannula must be confirmed radiologically at the time of cannulation (see Figs. 25-2–25-5). Locating the tip of this drainage cannula at the level of the diaphragm for venovenous perfusion ensures minimal blood recirculation and adequate blood flow (3–6 liters/min). The cannula tip can be placed in the right atrium for venoarterial perfusion.

* Available from Mr. Raymond Johnson, 15 Princeton Street, Peabody, MA 01960.

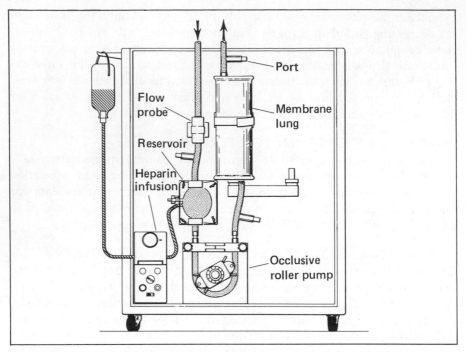

FIGURE 25-1. A simple circuit for clinical membrane oxygenation. (From W. M. Zapol et al., Extracorporeal membrane oxygenation for acute respiratory failure. Reprinted by permission from *Anesthesiology* 46:272, 1977.)

PUMP

We use only filler-free, silicone-coated rubber tubing; 12.7 mm ID for the venous drain line and 9.5 mm ID for other tubing. Blood drains into a 75-ml collapsible servoregulated reservoir bag, which limits blood suction and avoids hemolysis. From the reservoir, blood is nonocclusively pumped by a roller pump using an extended polyurethane pump chamber. This chamber can be safely pumped for periods up to a month without rupture. We do not recommend pumping on polyvinyl chloride tubing for prolonged periods.

MEMBRANE LUNGS

Our group's clinical experience is limited to the filler-free, silicone-coated, spiral-coil membrane lung†; this discussion is limited to that device. We suggest a minimum of 0.5 M² of membrane surface be used per 10 kg of body weight for partial assistance. For total pulmonary failure, a minimum of 1 M² of surface per 10 kg of body weight is required [18].

Judging from our own experience, spiral-coil silicone membrane lungs can withstand 1 atmosphere of transmembrane hydrostatic pressure for

† Available from SciMed, Inc., 13010 County Road 6, Minneapolis, MN 55441.

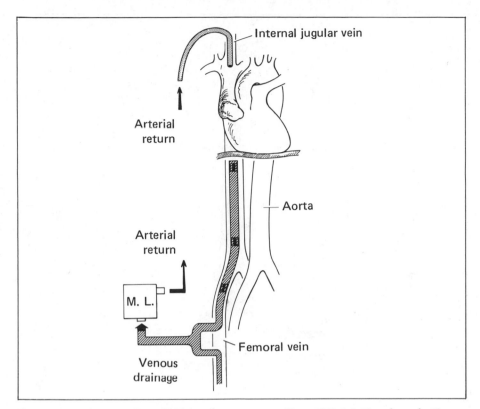

FIGURE 25-2. Venovenous (VV) perfusion route. (From W. M. Zapol et al., Extra-corporeal perfusion for acute respiratory failure: Recent experience with the spiral coil membrane lung. *J. Thorac. Cardiovasc. Surg.* 69:439, 1975.)

prolonged periods without rupture. Since pressure drops across this lung are low (a 75–150 torr drop across a 3.5 M^2 device at 3 liters/min blood flow), it is safe to use a single pump for any perfusion route. The return cannula should be large enough (>6.4 mm ID in adults) not to cause large circuit pressures. Hydrostatic pressures greater than 400 torr are unsafe anywhere in the circuit.

Spiral-coil membrane lungs have been used for clinical perfusion up to 2 weeks without thrombosis or deterioration in gas exchange. If a visible thrombus appears on the clear plastic outflow surface, or outflow saturation falls below 90 percent, the membrane lung should be changed.

We do not use an in-line filter, since the membrane lung itself acts as a filter for large thrombi. We incorporate a cannulating electromagnetic flow probe to measure extracorporeal blood flow. We do not use a heat exchanger. All available heat exchangers expose blood to steel, a very thrombogenic surface. We enclose the extracorporeal apparatus in a vinyl canopy

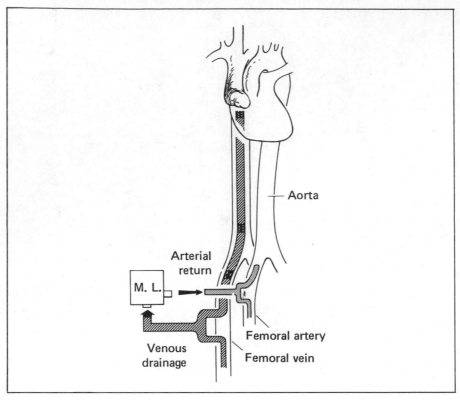

FIGURE 25-3. Venoarterial (VA) perfusion route with femoral artery cannulation and distal aorta return. (From W. M. Zapol et al., Extracorporeal perfusion for acute respiratory failure: Recent experience with the spiral coil membrane lung. J. Thorac. Cardiovasc. Surg. 69:439, 1975.)

and thermoregulate the ambient air temperature. The patient's core temperature is maintained at 32 to 37° C. The extracorporeal priming volume for a 70-kg adult is approximately 1,350 ml. We prime with fresh whole blood with heparin added (4,500 units/liter).

Large-bore Y connectors (12.7 mm ID) occluded by tetrafluoroethylene plugs are placed in the blood tubing to permit replacement of the reservoir and pump chamber or substitution or addition of membrane lungs without stopping perfusion. These access points are a necessity, especially for patients who progress to near-total pulmonary failure. Several silicone tubes (3.2 mm ID, 6.4 mm OD) are bonded to the circuit to allow heparin infusion, rapid volume transfusion, sampling, and pressure monitoring. Since blood cultures are required frequently, and venipuncture sites ooze excessively, a self-sealing latex tube is attached to allow sterile needle puncture for bacteriologic culture. All connecting tubes are continuously flushed with

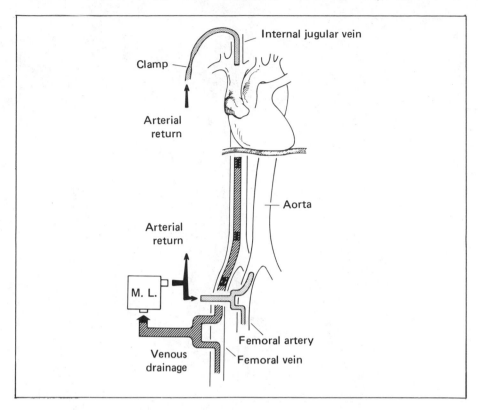

FIGURE 25-4. Mixed venovenous and venoarterial (VVA) perfusion. (From W. M. Zapol et al., Extracorporeal perfusion for acute respiratory failure: Recent experience with the spiral coil membrane lung. *J. Thorac. Cardiovasc. Surg.* 69:439, 1975.)

heparinized saline solution (10 ml/hr). Careful inspection of the circuitry for defects, thrombosis, and other problems should be made every 12 hours during perfusion.

CANNULATIONS
Cannulations can be performed under morphine analgesia (1 mg/kg). Extensive electrocautery is used to achieve hemostasis. The main drainage catheter is placed through the common femoral vein. The distal vein is drained to prevent venous hypertension and oozing. If the proximal common femoral artery is cannulated, a single arteriotomy should be performed and a small catheter placed to provide arterial blood to the distal leg. Femoral venipunctures should be avoided during the care of patients with acute respiratory failure; hematomas make surgery far more difficult. No intramuscular or subcutaneous injections should be permitted. Incisions are

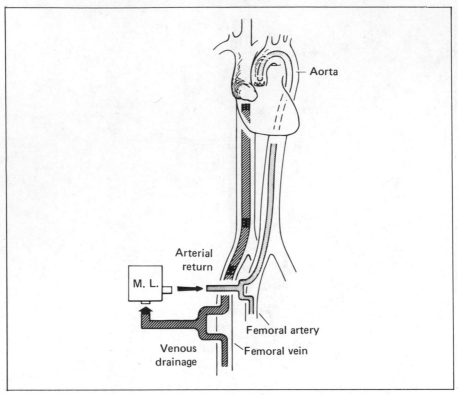

FIGURE 25-5. Venoarterial arch (VA arch) perfusion. (From W. M. Zapol et al., Extracorporeal perfusion for acute respiratory failure: Recent experience with the spiral coil membrane lung. *J. Thorac. Cardiovasc. Surg.* 69:439, 1975.)

closed in layers and the skin sutured. Antibacterial ointment and dry dressings are applied and changed daily. If incision sites bleed over 25 ml/hr, they should be explored.

PERFUSION ROUTES
We have used four perfusion routes (Figs. 25-2–25-5). All require only one blood pump when used with the spiral-coil membrane lung.

VENOVENOUS PERFUSION
We have reported high-flow venovenous (VV) perfusion (Fig. 25-2) in adults and children [20]; VV, or prepulmonary, oxygenation allows the arterial tree to distribute oxygenated blood in a uniform pattern through the left ventricle. Venous blood is drained from the inferior vena cava through the common femoral vein, and oxygenated blood is returned to the superior vena cava. Two incisions (femoral and cervical) are necessary. We

have adapted this technique for use in small children. In an infant weighing only 3.5 kg, the drainage catheter was placed into the right atrium through the right jugular vein; the return cannula was placed in the common femoral vein [19].

VENOARTERIAL PERFUSION (FEMORAL ARTERY RETURN)

Venoarterial (VA) perfusion decreases pulmonary blood flow. If mean pulmonary artery pressure decreases, the blood supply to lung regions with high pulmonary vascular resistance will be reduced, and smaller transcapillary filtration pressures can be expected. Hill et al. [8] have reported that VA perfusion decreases the mean pulmonary artery pressure, but this was rarely observed in our VA or mixed VV and VA perfusions, possibly due to extensive destruction of the lung vasculature. Venoarterial perfusion is always indicated when pulmonary artery pressures are high and right ventricular failure is present.

VA perfusion involves more complex surgery than does VV perfusion (Fig. 25-3), requiring cannulation of the arterial system with a large-bore cannula. In the past, the common femoral artery has been transected and cannulated both proximally and distally. After perfusion, the artery is anastomosed end to end. False aneurysm formation is common 3 to 4 months after perfusion and may necessitate a vein graft. It may be advisable to replace the cannulated segment with a vein graft when bypass is completed.

The major flaw of VA bypass is the inappropriate distribution of arterialized blood. The highest arterial oxygen tensions occur in the region of femoral artery inflow. Oxygenated blood returned to the distal aorta is distributed to the kidneys, mesenteric bed, and lower limbs [13]. In severe acute respiratory failure, we frequently observe the combination of a large cardiac index, intrapulmonary right-to-left shunt greater than 50 percent, and a small arteriovenous oxygen content difference [$C(a-v)O_2$]. In these circumstances, the modest increase in venous oxygen saturation afforded by VA partial perfusion is inadequate to provide sufficiently high arterial oxygen tensions to the heart and brain. Bartlett uses carotid artery return in infant perfusion to improve cerebral oxygenation, and axillary artery return in adults [1].

MIXED VENOVENOUS AND VENOARTERIAL PERFUSION

A modification of the VA technique, mixed venovenous and venoarterial perfusion (VVA) (Fig. 25-4), serves to improve oxygenation of the blood delivered to the heart and brain by returning some oxygenated blood to the superior vena cava. Like VV, but unlike VA perfusion, this technique has the disadvantage of requiring two incisions, femoral as well as cervical. In addition, it requires the insertion of a flow meter to analyze the amount of blood directed to each route.

VENOARTERIAL PERFUSION WITH AORTIC ARCH RETURN

For better distribution of extracorporeal oxygenated blood, we have modified classic venoarterial perfusion by passing the femoral artery cannula to the level of the aortic root (Fig. 25-5). Venoarterial arch perfusion (VA arch) requires an extremely large-bore, spring-reinforced (8.1 mm OD, 7.1 mm ID) cannula to minimize the pressure drop and allow a single roller pump to be used. This cannula allows flows of over 5 liters/min with less than a 75-torr pressure drop. By injecting a bolus of radioactive xenon, we have documented the significant contribution of aortic arch perfusion to cerebral oxygenation [13, 15]. Others have used the right axillary artery for return of bypassed blood. Because this vessel accommodates only a small catheter, high pump pressures are required at large flows, and this increases the mechanical danger of extracorporeal perfusion. In addition, the proximity of the artery to the brachial plexus increases the hazards of local sepsis following prolonged cannulation.

HEMODYNAMIC MONITORING

PRESSURE

Recordings are taken of the right radial or right temporal artery pressure, pulmonary artery pressure, pulmonary capillary wedge pressure, central venous pressure, and the pressure drop across the membrane lung and across the pump.

FLOW

Continuous measurements of perfusion-circuit blood flow are made by a cannulating electromagnetic flow probe. Cardiac output is measured every 6 hours by a modified Swan-Ganz thermodilution method (cold solution is injected through the right ventricular orifice [22]). Urine output is measured hourly through the bladder catheter.

BLOOD GAS TENSIONS

We measure arterial blood gas tensions every hour. Every 12 hours, simultaneous blood samples are taken from pulmonary artery, right radial artery, and across the oxygenator for Van Slyke gas-content measurements. Correlating these measurements with flow and cardiac output measurements, we can precisely define oxygen transport. Every 12 hours, alveolar-arterial oxygen tension difference [$P(A-a)O_2$] is measured. Body temperature is continuously measured to obtain blood gas correction factors. Finally, all indicated blood chemistry measurements for acutely ill patients must be performed as necessary.

RESPIRATORY MANAGEMENT AND MONITORING

Vigorous chest physiotherapy, tracheal suctioning, and frequent postural changes are necessary to foster pulmonary healing. Careful daily fluid input and output computation is vital to patient care. Diuretics may be required to prevent water retention. During perfusion, the FiO_2 is lowered to 0.6 or less. In our experience, PEEP is required for adequate oxygenation during ECP (i.e., 10–15 cm H_2O in patients without bronchopleural fistula). Extracorporeal gas exchange allows us to decrease the tidal volume and lower the peak inspiratory pressure to below 45 cm H_2O, thereby avoiding or reducing the damage of a leaking pneumothorax. When PEEP is discontinued after perfusion begins, complete pulmonary consolidation and a marked decrease in pulmonary compliance rapidly develop.

Because bypass blood can approach the root of the aorta during VA arch perfusion, it is important to determine the precise origin of blood at an arterial sampling site. This information is essential for computing the $P(A-a)O_2$ and the patient's cardiac output. To determine the source of blood at a particular peripheral arterial line (e.g., the left radial artery), dye is injected into the pulmonary artery and dilution curves drawn from the artery. Appearance of a "normal" dye dilution curve indicates an artery is perfused through the left ventricle. We suggest that the simpler technique of thermodilution with right ventricular indicator injection be used for cardiac output determination. It may prove valuable to cannulate both the right temporal artery and the left radial artery to measure cerebral oxygen tensions.

Chest x-ray films are obtained every 12 hours to define changes in the anatomic distribution of disease or to detect a pneumothorax. The latter is treated by careful open placement of a thoracostomy tube with extensive use of electrocautery. Standard pneumotachography yields pressure-volume loops for computation of dynamic compliance. In patients without bronchopleural fistula, functional residual capacity is measured by helium dilution to evaluate lung volume. Radiography, functional residual capacity, and compliance are not affected by changes in extracorporeal blood flow or cardiac output as are the $P(A-a)O_2$ and V_D/V_T and are therefore objective and valuable methods of evaluating lung status during partial ECP.

MANAGEMENT AND MONITORING OF ANTICOAGULATION

We maintain the Lee-White clotting times at about 15 to 20 minutes. Accelerated clotting times are measured hourly using the technique of Hatterslea [7]. We give an initial dose of 100 units of bovine lung heparin per kilogram of body weight immediately preceding insertion of a cannula. Heparin (5,000 units/liter) is added to the extracorporeal priming volume. Additional heparin is administered when the accelerated clotting time is less than 120 seconds. We can maintain this clotting time with 10 to 50 heparin units/kg/hr infused continuously, with the dose modified hourly as necessary.

During perfusion, levels of fibrin split products, Factor VIII, fibrinogen concentration, and prothrombin time are monitored daily. We transfuse fresh-frozen plasma and washed frozen deglycerolized cells for blood replacement to keep the hematocrit about 30 percent. All cellular solutions are filtered through filters with a 40-μm pore size. Despite extensive electrocautery at cannulation sites, minor bleeding occurred during perfusion of several of our patients. Bleeding was readily managed by local pressure, a reduction of the heparin dose, and infusion of platelets. During stable adult perfusion, we usually transfuse 1 to 2 units of whole blood per day. Hemolysis with free hemoglobinemia and red cell sequestration do not appear to be significant during clinical perfusion. Samples for blood studies in these patients often amount to over 500 ml/day. These losses must be carefully documented and blood replaced.

Consumption of platelets due to systemic trauma, pulmonary disease, and extracorporeal treatment of blood is significant [3, 10]. When the platelet count falls below 20,000/mm^3, spontaneous bleeding may occur from cannulation sites and from the gastrointestinal tract, nasopharynx, and trachea. Hemorrhage has ceased with platelet infusions despite platelet counts persisting below 50,000/mm^3. When operations were performed several days prior to perfusion, wound hemorrhage did not occur. At present, only active bleeding can be considered a contraindication to ECP. Upper gastrointestinal hemorrhage during bypass has ceased following iced saline lavage and blood replacement. If hemorrhage continues despite platelet infusion, the clotting time may be lowered to 10 minutes. At this level, in combination with a high blood flow rate, the spiral-coil silicone membrane lung will not clot for many hours.

Platelets are damaged when blood is exposed to silicone-rubber surfaces. To conserve platelets, membrane lungs should be changed and blood exposed to fresh surface areas of membrane only when gas transport is impaired. If disseminated intravascular coagulation develops and the patient consumes plasma coagulation factors, we replace them with fresh-frozen plasma and increase the heparin dose.

WEANING FROM BYPASS

The majority of patients perfused for acute respiratory failure progress to total pulmonary failure with opacification of the chest radiograph and minimal transpulmonary gas exchange [12, 22]. We do not know of any patients who have recovered after more than 12 hours in this condition.

Patients can be weaned from perfusion if they maintain arterial oxygen tensions greater than 50 torr at an F$_I$O$_2$ of 0.6 on 10 cm water PEEP for over 6 hours. During this trial period, bypass flow should be lowered to 500 ml/min but should not be stopped or thrombosis may occur. If the cardiorespiratory system is stable, the perfusion apparatus can be disconnected and heparin infusion discontinued. As soon as possible, all cannulas should be removed and incisions debrided and closed. Attention should be given to the possibility of femoral artery false aneurysm formation in the postperfusion period.

Patients in whom sufficient pulmonary function returns to permit weaning from bypass require constant clinical supervision for many days thereafter. Their severe pulmonary injury usually improves slowly, and they frequently have a constellation of difficult medical and surgical problems. Their nutrition is vital; hyperalimentation should begin during perfusion and continue until sufficient nutrition can be taken by mouth.

The membrane lung has proved to be as limited as such other mechanical assistance devices as the intra-aortic balloon pump and hemodialyzer machine. While each supports a vital body function, it cannot heal the injured organ. Physicians taking care of patients with acute respiratory failure should understand that perfusion is an important tool for maintaining respiration of those who are dying of hypoxemia and hypercapnia.

REFERENCES

1. Bartlett, R. H., and Gazzaniga, A. B. Extracorporeal circulation for cardiopulmonary failure. *Curr. Prob. Surg.* 15:59, 1978.
2. Blake, L. H. Goals and progress of the National Heart and Lung Institute collaborative extracorporeal membrane oxygenation study. In W. M. Zapol and J. Qvist (Eds.), *Artificial Lungs for Acute Respiratory Failure: Theory and Practice.* Washington, D.C.: Hemisphere, 1976. P. 513.
3. Bloom, S., et al. Platelet destruction during 24-hour membrane lung perfusion. *Trans. Am. Soc. Artif. Intern. Organs* 20:299, 1974.
4. Cooper, J. D., et al. Cardio-respiratory failure secondary to peripheral pulmonary emboli. *J. Thorac. Cardiovasc. Surg.* 71:872, 1976.
5. Galletti, P. M. *Heart-Lung Bypass.* New York: Grune & Stratton, 1962.
6. Hanson, E. L., et al. Venoarterial bypass with a membrane oxygenator: Successful respiratory support in a woman following pulmonary hemorrhage secondary to renal failure. *Surgery* 75:557, 1974.
7. Hatterslea, P. G. Activated coagulation time in whole blood. *J.A.M.A.* 196:436, 1966.
8. Hill, J. D., et al. Acute respiratory insufficiency: Treatment with prolonged extracorporeal oxygenation. *J. Thorac. Cardiovasc. Surg.* 64:551, 1972.
9. Hill, J. D., et al. Prolonged extracorporeal oxygenation for acute post-traumatic respiratory failure (shock-lung syndrome). *N. Engl. J. Med.* 286:629, 1972.
10. Hill, J. D., et al. Clinical-prolonged extracorporeal circulation for respiratory insufficiency: Hematological effects. *Trans. Am. Soc. Artif. Intern. Organs* 18:546, 1972.
11. Hill, J. D., et al. Pulmonary pathology in acute respiratory insufficiency: Lung biopsy as a diagnostic tool. *J. Thorac. Cardiovasc. Surg.* 71:64, 1976.
12. Hill, J. D., et al. State of the art: Clinical extracorporeal membrane oxygenation for acute respiratory insufficiency. *Trans. Am. Soc. Artif. Intern. Organs* 24:753, 1978.
13. Kanarek, D., et al. Radionuclide imaging of the distribution of membrane lung perfusion. *Trans. Am. Soc. Artif. Intern. Organs* 20:262, 1974.

14. Kolobow, T., and Zapol, W.   A new thin-walled nonkinking catheter for peripheral vascular cannulation. *Surgery* 68:625, 1970.
15. McEnany, M. T., et al.   Cannulation of the proximal aorta during long term membrane lung perfusion. *J. Thorac. Cardiovasc. Surg.* 70:631, 1975.
16. Murphy, W., et al.   Laboratory and clinical experience with a microporous membrane oxygenator. *Trans. Am. Soc. Artif. Intern. Organs* 20:278, 1974.
17. Pontoppidan, H., et al.   Respiratory intensive care. *Anesthesiology* 46:96, 1977.
18. Ward, B. D., and Hood, A. G.   *Membrane Oxygenator Comparison. Annual Report* (TR-110-002). Salt Lake City: Utah Biomedical Test Laboratory, June 30, 1973.
19. White, J. J., et al.   Prolonged respiratory support in infants with the Kolobow spiral coil respirator. *Mt. Sinai J. Med. N.Y.* 40:173, 1973.
20. Zapol, W., et al.   Clinical membrane lung support for acute respiratory insufficiency. *Trans. Am. Soc. Artif. Intern. Organs* 18:553, 1972.
21. Zapol, W. M., et al.   Extracorporeal perfusion for acute respiratory failure: Recent experience with the spiral coil membrane lung. *J. Thorac. Cardiovasc. Surg.* 69:439, 1975.
22. Zapol, W. M., et al.   Extracorporeal membrane oxygenation for acute respiratory failure. *Anesthesiology* 46:272, 1977.
23. Zapol, W. M., et al.   Extracorporeal membrane oxygenation in severe acute respiratory failure: A randomized prospective study. *J.A.M.A.* 242:2193, 1979.
24. Zapol, W. M., et al.   Pulmonary fibrosis in severe acute respiratory failure. *Am. Rev. Respir. Dis.* 119:547, 1979.

Nathan P. Couch
Jan R. Dmochowski

26. MUSCLE SURFACE pH MEASUREMENT

THEORY OF CATION-SELECTIVE ELECTRODE FUNCTIONS

Since the work of Lord Kelvin, published in 1875, it has been known that glass has electrical conductive properties. Since Cramer's work (1906), it has been recognized that these conductive properties in certain types of glass are affected by hydrogen ion concentration. Over the years, the fabrication of ion-sensitive glass has become progressively more precise, so that electrodes are now available that are suitable for measuring the activity of several ions of biologic importance, including hydrogen, sodium, potassium, calcium, and chloride.

Over the past 15 years, intensive investigation of these glasses has led to a theory, proposed by Eisenman [3], that the ion selectivity depends on cation-exchange phenomena in the glass itself, as well as on its hygroscopicity and durability. A detailed discussion of the physical chemistry of pH electrodes is not, of course, within the scope of this chapter, and the reader is referred to Eisenman's [3] classic work for such a discussion.

Skeletal muscle is a particularly appropriate tissue for continuous monitoring in the critically ill patient because of its low priority in the body economy. When low flow states are developing, it is one of the first tissues to be deprived of oxygen. Because of its high glycogen content and capacity for lactic acid production, as well as its sensitivity to catecholamines, it has the capacity for rapid and dramatic responses. It is also of importance that skeletal muscle makes up 40 percent of the body cell mass.

The measurement of muscle surface pH (pHM) enables continuous monitoring of the balance between oxygen supply and demand in skeletal muscle, because critical reduction of oxygen supply forces a shift in local metabolism to anaerobic glycolysis, increased production of lactic acid, and increased hydrogen ion activity. These changes occur whether oxygen lack is due to hypoxemia or to reduced perfusion.

The surface measurement technique, rather than a percutaneous one, is favored because it minimizes injury to the tissue or to the electrode, standardizes the biologic interface being observed, and avoids the use of needle electrodes, which are not yet easily available.

The surface measurement of hydrogen ion activity is really a measurement of such activity in extracellular fluid. This is a valid approach because it is well established that the hydrogen ion activity of extracellular fluid reflects rapidly and accurately the hydrogen ion activity diffusing through cell membranes.

There are other forms of tissue electrometry for the continuous measurement of tissue potassium ion activity, tissue PO_2, and tissue PCO_2. Although promising, their clinical value remains to be proved.

The measurement of pHM is particularly useful in patients in whom sudden changes in arterial oxygen tension (PaO_2) or arterial carbon dioxide tension ($PaCO_2$) are a threat, or in whom slowly dwindling peripheral perfusion may be undetectable by the measurement of arterial or central venous pressure or of urine volume.

The measurement of pHM in seriously ill patients is of value in the following:

1. In respiratory distress syndromes in which sudden changes of PaO_2 or $PaCO_2$ may occur due to airway obstruction, inappropriate ventilation, or pneumothorax.
2. Where occult bleeding is a threat, i.e., after extensive trauma, including pelvic fractures or solid organ rupture; or after major surgery in which persistent or delayed hemorrhage is possible.
3. In low cardiac output syndrome due to myocardial failure.
4. In monitoring peripheral perfusion during cardiopulmonary bypass [1, 5].
5. In postoperative cardiac surgical patients vulnerable both to continuing hemorrhage and to myocardial failure.
6. In endotoxemia [2].
7. In small infants, in whom blood pressure measurement and blood sampling are very difficult [4].

TECHNIQUES
MATERIALS
The following equipment is needed:

1. An expanded-scale pH meter, battery-powered. The Corning Model 610A (Fig. 26-1) is satisfactory.
2. Right-angle combination glass pH electrode (Fig. 24-1) with 10-foot cord.*
3. Standard buffer solutions of known pH (one with pH 4.0–4.5, and one with pH 6.3–7.6), sterile.
4. Venous cutdown set: scalpel, local anesthetic, two or three hemostats, needle holder, sutures, ligatures, small self-retaining retractor, umbilical tape, gauze squares, adhesive tape.
5. Sterile vacuum drainage system (optional).

METHOD
Before use, the pH electrode and meter are standardized with the buffer solutions according to the instructions of the pH meter manufacturer.

* Instrumentation Laboratories, Lexington, Mass. The 1979 catalogue number is 6300.

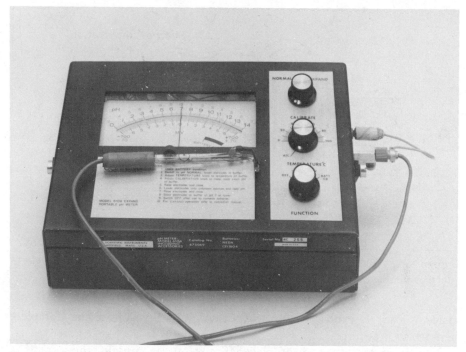

FIGURE 26-1. Right-angle muscle surface pH electrode and pH electrometer (Model 610A Expand Portable pH meter). Electrode shaft is 7 cm long and of combination type. Electrometer is battery-powered. (Courtesy of Scientific Instruments, Corning Glass Works, Medfield, Mass.)

STERILIZATION OF ELECTRODE

The electrode is placed in the tip-down position in a small beaker (20–30 ml) in a larger receptacle (e.g., a cylindrical wire-mesh test tube holder). The entire assembly is wrapped in heavy ·cloth with the plug end of the electrode wire and a plastic cannula protruding a few inches from the package. The inner end of the plastic cannula is in the beaker, and the outer end is fitted with a sterile plug.

After sterilization for 4 hours in ethylene oxide and at least 6 hours before use, the cloth wrapping is opened without contamination of the contents. A small volume of sterile buffer (pH 7.38), enough to immerse the electrode tip, is instilled through the plastic tube into the beaker. Standardization is repeated. The electrode is left immersed in buffer for a minimum of 6 hours until use.

INCISION AND PLACEMENT OF ELECTRODE

After preparation of the skin in the area selected for measuring pHM (usually the anterior midbiceps or the rectus femoris muscle), a 2- to 3-cm in-

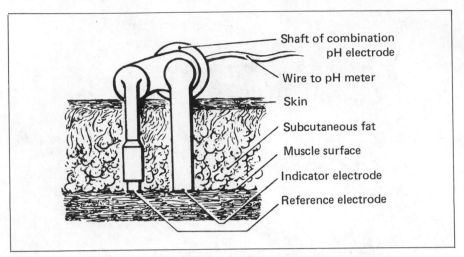

FIGURE 26-2. Enlarged (approximately × 2) end-on, cutaway view of electrode in place on muscle surface. (See text for technical details of placement.)

cision is made to expose the muscle surface at its investing facia. Complete hemostasis is secured.

The tip of the electrode is placed firmly on the muscle, the wound is closed with one or two skin sutures, a small gauze or umbilical tape wick* is placed in each end to draw off delayed ooze, a dressing is applied, and the shaft of the electrode is taped to the skin (Fig. 26-2).

If an electrode with the indicator surface on the side of the shaft is used, it is slid between the subcutaneous fat and the muscle surface, maintaining the contact between the indicator surface and the muscle. When economical and durable needle electrodes become available, the procedure will become even simpler.

RECORDING

The pH readings from the meter can be recorded by hand, continuously on a paper strip, or in a computer system. Digital meters are available, but their convenience does not justify their much greater expense.

RESULTS AND INTERPRETATIONS

Any laboratory test should be interpreted only in the context of other clinical data. The pHM is no exception and should only be used in concert with known or suspected diagnoses, arterial pressure, pulse, central venous pressure, urine flow, PaO_2, $PaCO_2$, arterial blood pH (pHa), and the degree of pulmonary insufficiency.

* A sterile vacuum system may be used instead.

TABLE 26-1. Comparison of Muscle pH with Arterial Blood Gases and pH in Normal and Abnormal States

Condition	pHM	pHa	PaO$_2$	PaCO$_2$
Normal state (unanesthetized)	7.35–7.45	7.35–7.45	Normal	Normal
Low flow state	Decreased (<7.3)	Normal	Normal	Normal
Respiratory acidosis	Decreased	Decreased	Normal	Increased
Respiratory alkalosis	Increased	Increased	Normal	Decreased
Hypoxia	Decreased	Normal or decreased	Decreased	Normal or increased
Metabolic acidosis	Decreased	Decreased	Normal	Decreased
Metabolic alkalosis	Increased	Increased	Normal	Increased

The *normal range* of pHM in unanesthetized human subjects is 7.35 to 7.45, approximately equal to that of pHa. During induction of anesthesia, pHM is often in the range of 7.5 to 7.7, usually because of hyperventilation.

In states of *low flow*, pHM decreases to levels below 7.3. In severe low flow states, pHM can be as low as 6.7. The decrease of pHM often precedes a significant decline of arterial blood pressure [1, 2, 6].

Since, in the *absence* of a low flow state, pHM approximates pHa, pHM is an index of alkalosis or acidosis, whether metabolic or respiratory [7]. For example, if pHM increases to a level higher than normal in a patient on a respirator, an arterial blood gas analysis is indicated. If the pHa is similarly elevated and the PaCO$_2$ lower than normal, a diagnosis of hyperventilation will be confirmed.

Because respiratory disturbances can occur much more abruptly than metabolic pH shifts (and may be lethal), the continuous monitoring of pHM may prove to be more valuable in the former. Experience is still limited, and this concept awaits much further investigation.

Finally, in hypoxia, pHM also declines but at a slower rate than in low flow states or respiratory acidosis.

Table 26-1 summarizes these interpretations.

PITFALLS AND COMPLICATIONS

If there is a rise of pHM above 7.5 when pHa is normal, the pHM is probably false. This is most likely to occur after 24 hours and is due to accumulation of proteinaceous material on the tip or to lack of contact between the electrode and the muscle. The problem is corrected by cleaning the tip with papain or 0.1N HCl or by correcting the position of the electrode.

If the pHm reading is erratic, there is probably a crack in the cation-sensitive glass, and the electrode must be replaced. Erratic behavior of the electrode may also accompany use of the electrocautery. The electrometer should always be turned off at such times.

Failure of the pHm to fall during an obvious low flow state usually indicates that blood has accumulated at the electrode tip. The electrode should be cleaned with a damp sterile sponge, and hemostasis in the wound should be secured.

A low pHm in an obviously well-perfused patient can be due to excessive pressure on the electrode, causing focal ischemia.

Bleeding at the implantation site is always correctable unless it occurs in the presence of a severe coagulation defect. A small vacuum device may keep the wound dry.

Infection is unusual, of minor importance, and easily treated by opening the wound. Electrical hazards are nonexistent where a battery-powered electrometer is used.

REFERENCES

1. Couch, N. P., et al. Muscle surface pH as an index or peripheral perfusion in man. *Ann. Surg.* 173:173, 1971.
2. Dmochowski, J. R., and Couch, N. P. Skeletal muscle hydrogen ion activity in endotoxin shock. *Surg. Gynecol. Obstet.* 131:669, 1970.
3. Eisenman, G. *Glass Electrodes for Hydrogen and Other Cations.* New York: Dekker, 1967.
4. Filler, R. M., et al. Clinical experience with continuous muscle pH monitoring as an index of tissue perfusion and oxygenation and acid-base status. *Surgery* 72:23, 1972.
5. Gazzaniga, A. B., et al. The use of skeletal muscle surface hydrogen ion concentration to monitor peripheral perfusion: Experimental and clinical results. *Surg. Forum* 21:147, 1970.
6. Lemieux, M. D., et al. Surface pH and redox potential of skeletal muscle in graded hemorrhage. *Surgery* 65:457, 1969.
7. Smith, R. N., et al. Effects of acidosis and alkalosis on surface skeletal muscle pH. *Surg. Gynecol. Obstet.* 128:533, 1969.

Manfred Kessler
J. Höper
U. Pohl

27. MONITORING OF LOCAL PO$_2$ IN SKELETAL MUSCLE OF CRITICALLY ILL PATIENTS

An adequate oxygen supply to living tissues can be maintained only by the optimal systemic regulation of a highly organized oxygen transport system. In man this system, which transfers oxygen molecules from the atmosphere to the intracellular oxidases, comprises a long chain of transport mechanisms. The basic principles involved in oxygen transport are diffusion, O$_2$ binding by hemoglobin, and convection. The transport of oxygen to the oxygen-consuming enzymes within the capillary supply unit is achieved by convection and diffusion. The net flux of oxygen from the erythrocytes passing along the capillary to the oxidases is determined by the oxygen tension (PO$_2$) gradient.

The combination of convective and diffusive O$_2$ transport occurring in the capillary supply unit results in a spatial distribution of PO$_2$ in the tissues (Fig. 27-1). Systematic investigations of spatial PO$_2$ fields in tissues of various organs have demonstrated that, under physiological conditions, rather similar non–organ specific PO$_2$ distribution patterns exist [6, 9]. Exceptions are encountered only in the outer cortex of the kidney and probably in the heart. The fact that, despite the variability in organ structure and function, a virtually similar pattern of PO$_2$ distribution is found not only in man, but also in other mammals, indicates that during the course of evolution, the biological systems of man and other mammals have reached an optimal level of functional organization that provides a secure tissue oxygen supply.

From the unexpected similarity of the oxygen distribution curves, we may deduce that the functional organization of the oxygen supply found in the different organs must be achieved by similar mechanisms. The complex functional chain responsible for delivery of oxygen to the tissues can be investigated at various sites. The most relevant information can be obtained by directly measuring the oxygen tension field of tissues (PO$_2$ histogram) by means of PO$_2$-needle [15] or Clark-type [5, 8] electrodes, because there we are measuring at the end of the long transport chain.

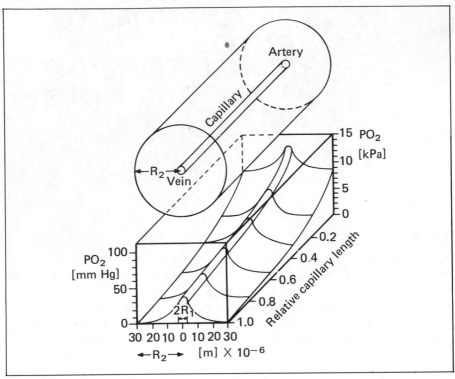

FIGURE 27-1. Three-dimensional PO₂ distribution along a single capillary.

In the research laboratory, tissue PO₂ measurements can be carried out on each organ surface; however, in critically ill patients these measurements are restricted to organs for which the preparation is least invasive. Skeletal muscles satisfy this requirement. In contrast with the intravascular applications of electrodes or catheters, PO₂ measurement at the surface of the skeletal muscle entails a minimal risk of bacterial invasion because living muscle and endothelial cells form an efficient barrier against penetration of germs into the blood.

METHODOLOGY
ELECTRODES
Clark-type, multiwire surface electrodes developed in our laboratories [5, 8] are used for monitoring tissue PO₂ in patients (Fig. 27-2). The electrode consists of 8 platinum wires, each 15 μ in diameter, sealed into glass. An Ag/AgCl electrode serves as a reference electrode. Using 25 μ-thick membranes, a reduction current of 1 to 2 nA/100 torr oxygen partial pressure can be measured.

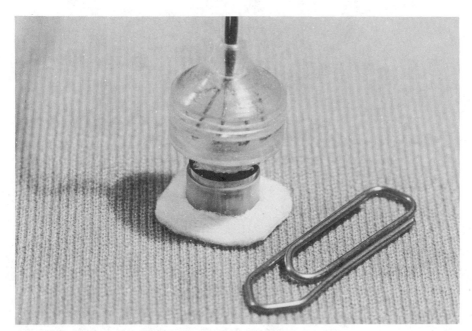

FIGURE 27-2. Multiwire surface electrode for the measurement of PO_2 in tissue.

Each of the 8 wires measures the PO_2 within a hemispherical tissue volume having a radius of about 25 μ. Thus, the local PO_2 within a capillary supply unit can be obtained. Convection error is 2 to 4 percent, and sensitivity drift is approximately 5 percent per hour.

AMPLIFIER SYSTEM AND ON-LINE DATA PROCESSING

For recording the polarographic reduction currents, a multichannel electronic unit has been constructed in our laboratories (Fig. 27-3). The primary circuit with the PO_2 electrode, the polarization voltage, and the current amplifier is galvanically separated from the power supply and the other electronic circuits required for on-line data evaluation. An additional display is provided for the polarization voltage, the electrode current of each PO_2 channel, and the temperature at the measuring site.

For on-line computation, an LSJ 11/03 from Digital Equipment Corporation is used in combination with a Plessey double-density floppy disc drive. For data processing, a FORTRAN program developed on the basis of our experience is available. Before monitoring is started, the electrode must be calibrated. Subsequently, the PO_2 measurement can be initiated and the continuously measured PO_2 values are plotted simultaneously on a graphic

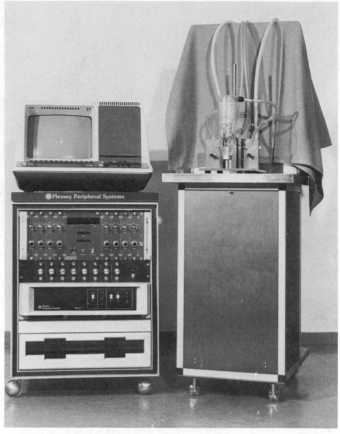

FIGURE 27-3. Set-up for the measurement of tissue PO_2 by multiwire surface electrodes, including the cart for the calibration procedure (*at right*).

display. For a PO_2 histogram, at least 100 values, measured at different sites, are necessary. To obtain this number of values, the electrode has to be moved gently 13 times over the organ surface.

On completion of the measurements, the electrode is recalibrated. Within seconds, the PO_2 histogram is plotted on the screen of the graphic terminal. With the aid of a plotter or printer, the recorded values can be documented. One tremendous advantage of the system is the possibility of achieving immediate information feedback, thus permitting direct monitoring of therapeutic measures.

STERILIZATION AND CALIBRATION
The sterilization of the PO_2 electrode can be accomplished without any problems by using pure ethylene oxide at low pressure in one of the com-

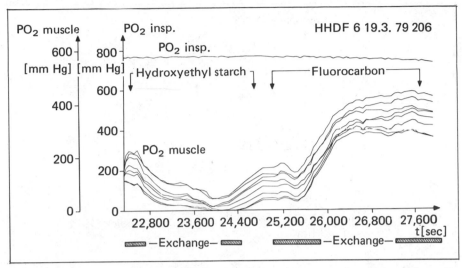

FIGURE 27-4. Original traces of continuous PO₂ measurements performed in the musculus gracilis (dog).

mercially available sterilization units. The calibration unit—consisting of glass chamber provided with a thermostat, sterile gas filters, and needle valves for the adjustment of the gas flow during the calibration procedure—is placed on a small cart and covered with sterile cloths. Practical use of the system in the operating room, as well as in the intensive care unit, has shown that there are no problems with sterility so long as regulations are strictly complied with.

CONTINUOUS MONITORING OF LOCAL PO₂

After calibration, the electrode is coupled to the tissue surface by means of a flange, kept in place by a piece of wet cellophane or wet felt, and continuous measurement of local tissue PO₂ is begun.

In Figure 27-4, an example of continuous monitoring of tissue PO₂ in dog skeletal muscle is shown. After a check run, during which the animal is ventilated with pure oxygen, isovolemic hemodilution with hydroxyethylstarch is performed. The final hematocrit is about 12 percent. At the end of this exchange, the tissue PO₂ values closely approximate initial values. When a steady state has been reached, further isovolemic hemodilution using fluorocarbon solution (Fluosol* DA 35%) is performed. The final hematocrit is about 8 percent. In this experiment it was possible to show, by continuous measurement of tissue PO₂, that tissue oxygenation is maintained by hemodilution with both hydroxyethylstarch and fluorocarbon solution. Owing to the high O₂ solubility of fluorocarbon, skeletal muscle

* Fluosol was kindly provided by Frimmer, Erlangen.

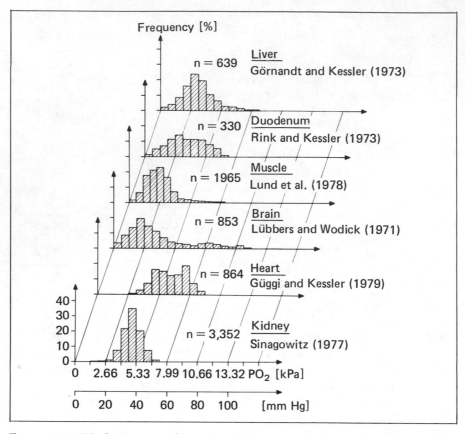

FIGURE 27-5. PO₂ histograms obtained in different organs by various investigators.

PO₂ is even elevated when this is used. This example shows that not only the PO₂ histogram but also the continuous measurement of local tissue PO₂ can provide important information about alterations in local tissue oxygenation.

THE NORMAL PO₂ HISTOGRAM

Systematic studies of the oxygen tension fields in various organs under physiological conditions, performed by various investigators, have revealed the following common features (Fig. 27-5):

1. The PO₂ distribution curves have a similar configuration in all organs with the exception of the outer cortex of the kidney and the heart.
2. The lowest PO₂ values found approach 1 to 2 torr.
3. The modes of the histograms lie below the PO₂ values of the venous blood of the organs. Thus, the venous PO₂ values do not reflect the low PO₂ values of tissue.

The detailed analysis of the biological factors that determine the configuration of the PO_2 histogram provides clear evidence that the following parameters play an important role: (1) capillary length, (2) capillary diameter, (3) the pattern of microflow, and (4) the hemoglobin dissociation curve. The combination of all these factors results in the "normal" PO_2 histogram. Investigations in our laboratories have demonstrated that the tissues contain an oxygen regulating system capable of monitoring cellular oxygen supply and directly modifying local blood flow when cells are threatened by lack of oxygen [3, 4]. Our experiments revealed evidence to suggest that an important element of this system might consist in the monitoring of the local PO_2 by cellular oxidases. These intracellular "signal" oxidases seem to have a threshold, probably of about 3 torr. Owing to the properties of these signal oxidases, an optimal autoregulation of local oxygen supply can be achieved only when some of the tissue PO_2 values approach this threshold. As yet we do not know the principle underlying autoregulation of local oxygen supply of the outer cortex of kidney and the superficial layers of the myocardium.

In this context, it may be of interest that in some patients with high cardiac output (e.g., in the hyperdynamic state), the lowest PO_2 values measured in skeletal muscle are far above this threshold.

The fact that up to 60 percent of the tissue PO_2 values of various organs are lower than the corresponding venous PO_2 values, shows that measurement of the venous PO_2 provides no accurate information about tissue oxygen supply. This discrepancy is caused by the inhomogeneous distribution of the microcirculation ascertainable in all tissues by carrying out measurements of microflow.

To a large extent these inhomogeneities are caused by the difference in the length of the capillaries. In long capillaries with relatively low microflow rates, the blood PO_2 will decrease to a very low level at the venous end, whereas in short capillaries with high microflow rates, a high venous PO_2 is found. Therefore, in short capillaries, a relative perfusion shunt results. The calculation of the mixed venous PO_2, performed in isolated perfused organs and based on the differing O_2 consumption due to different capillary length, is in agreement with the assumed facts [7].

THE PATHOLOGICAL PO₂ HISTOGRAM

At present, local monitoring of the PO_2 histogram is the most accurate technique available for providing an answer to the important question whether the cellular O_2 supply is normal or pathological. The high sensitivity of the method enables one to detect initial disturbances at a time when global hemodynamic parameters or diagnostic techniques for the measurement of tissue homeostasis (e.g., tissue photometry; measurement of microcirculation; measurement of local H^+, K^+, Na^+, and Ca^{2+}; and biochemical parameters) cannot provide comparable information.

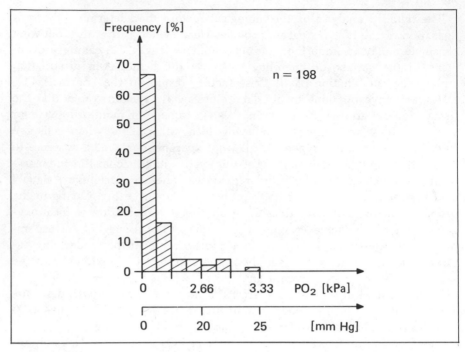

FIGURE 27-6. PO$_2$ histogram obtained in skeletal muscle of dog during hemorrhagic shock.

The causes of alterations in the local O$_2$ supply, as measured by the PO$_2$ histogram, may be subdivided as follows:

1. Local or global low-flow situations that lead to partial tissue hypoxia or anoxia (e.g., hypovolemic shock).
2. Disorders of the microcirculation provoked by a variety of pathogenetic causes—for example, rheological, humoral, inflammatory, immunological (organ transplantation, immune diseases), and vascular sclerosis leading to pathological configuration of the PO$_2$ histograms.
3. Arterial hypoxemia or anemia, inducing partial tissue hypoxia or anoxia.
4. Hyperoxemia-induced disturbances in the pattern of microflow, characterized by a "disintegrated" histogram, either without local hypoxia or combined with local hypoxia.

On this basis, several pathological alterations of the PO$_2$ histogram that may be meaningful during intensive care of critically ill patients will be discussed. Figure 27-6 shows a typical PO$_2$ histogram obtained during acute hemorrhagic shock. The frequency distribution shows a pronounced shift to the left, the histogram containing a high percentage of hypoxic and anoxic PO$_2$ values. Further conclusions about the microflow patterns cannot be drawn from such a histogram because virtually the same dis-

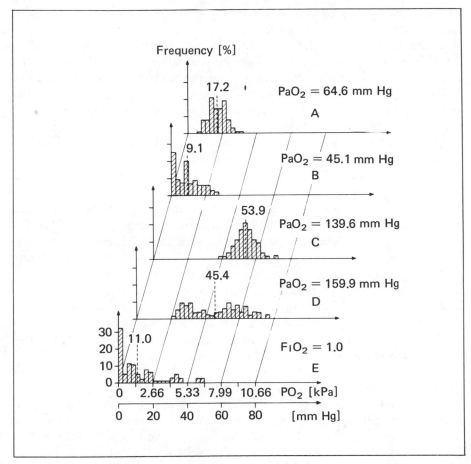

FIGURE 27-7. PO₂ histograms obtained in the m. rectus femoris of patients ventilated mechanically with various FIO₂.

tribution curve is found in deep arterial hypoxemia. Nevertheless, this type of histogram always indicates an extreme, and thus dangerous, state of tissue oxygenation.

In Figure 27-7, a number of typical PO₂ histograms obtained in patients under intensive care can be seen. Figure 27-7A shows the situation of a patient ventilated mechanically with an FIO₂ of 0.5. Even though the arterial PO₂ (PaO₂) achieved by this FIO₂ is only 64.6 torr, a normal PO₂ histogram is obtained. In the same patient, an FIO₂ of 0.3 with a corresponding PaO₂ of only 45 torr had resulted in a deterioration of the oxygen supply to skeletal muscle (Fig. 27-7B). Such a decrease in PaO₂ does not always indicate a deterioration of tissue oxygenation (Kessler et al. [6]). As mentioned above, hyperoxia can give rise to a "distintegration" of the PO₂ histogram, and even hypoxic or anoxic values may be seen. The PaO₂ at which local disturbances of O_2 supply occur seems to be variable and may be lower in critically ill patients.

Figure 27-7C shows the situation in a patient in whom an increase in FIO_2 produced an almost bell-shaped distribution curve, shifted to the right. In our opinion, the homogeneity of the curve does not provide any indication of possible pathological changes in the microcirculation and the resulting tissue oxygenation. In comparison with these findings, in another patient (Fig. 27-7D) ventilation with a comparable FIO_2 which produced a PaO_2 of 160 torr gave rise to a distribution curve with two peaks. This histogram seems to be falling apart. We interpret this type of curve as a disintegrated, normoxic PO_2 histogram caused by incipient disturbances in capillary microflow.

An extreme situation observed during a state of hyperoxia (ventilation of the patient with an FIO_2 of 1.0) is shown in Figure 27-7E. The PO_2 distribution presents a very disintegrated appearance and reveals a high percentage of hypoxic values. When the FIO_2 was decreased to 0.35, an almost bell-shaped PO_2 histogram without hypoxic values appeared spontaneously. Under these conditions, the pathological configuration of the PO_2 histogram is caused by disturbances of microflow. There is evidence that the pathological alterations are induced by a malfunctioning of chemoreceptors of smaller arteries. The relationship which may exist between arterial chemoreceptors and signal oxidases in tissue is still unknown.

CONCLUSION

For an accurate analysis of complex biological systems such as the mammalian oxygen transport chain, it would not seem possible to develop only a single monitoring technique which could provide general information about the biologic "black box" we are dealing with. However, even in such complex systems there will always be areas of particular importance. Any technique permitting the monitoring of a key parameter within such an area will be of considerable significance for analysis.

Experimental experience gained in our laboratories during the past 10 years has clearly shown that—in comparison with results obtained by many global and local monitoring techniques—a knowledge of the spatial PO_2 distribution in tissue as documented by the PO_2 histogram provides valuable information. This is so because the complex transport system is finally linked to the energy-producing system by the intracellular flux of oxygen molecules, determined by the local PO_2.

Owing to the particular significance of cellular oxygen partial pressure as the link between the two complex biological systems, tissue PO_2 can be regarded as truly a key parameter. The possibility of monitoring a particular parameter at a site of high functional relevance is always associated with the risk of overestimating the significance of such a parameter. Therefore, it should be emphasized that disturbances of local oxygen supply to skeletal muscle should primarily be regarded as a warning sign. Hence, in the absence of further information, such disturbances do not permit conclusions to be drawn about the oxygen supply to other organs.

REFERENCES

1. Görnandt, L., and Kessler, M. PO₂ histograms in regenerating liver tissue. In M. Kessler, D. F. Bruley, L. C. Clark et al. (Eds.), *Theoretical and Practical Aspects of Oxygen Supply and Microcirculation of Tissue.* Berlin: Urban & Schwarzenberg, 1973. P. 288.
2. Güggi, M., Kessler, M., Meesmann, W., and Dohse, M. PO₂ measurements of dog myocardium before, during and after coronary occlusion. *Arzneim Forsch,* in press.
3. Höper, J., and Kessler, M. Norepinephrine (NE) induced changes in flow and extracellular activities of Na⁺, K⁺ and Ca²⁺ in isolated perfused liver. *Arzneim. Forsch.* 28:869, 1978.
4. Höper, J., and Kessler, M. Na⁺-dependency of norepinephrine (NE) induced flow changes in isolated perfused rat liver. *Fed. Proc.* 37:3, 1978.
5. Kessler, M., and Grunewald, W. Possibilities of measuring oxygen pressure fields in tissue by multiwire platinum electrodes. *Prog. Resp. Res.* 3:147, 1969.
6. Kessler, H., Höper, J., and Krumme, B. A. Tissue perfusion and cellular function. *Anaesthesiol.* 45:186, 1976.
7. Kessler, M., Lang, H., Sinagowitz, E., Rink, R., and Höper, J. Homeostasis of oxygen supply in liver and kidney. In H. I. Bicher and D. F. Bruley (Eds.), *Oxygen Transport to Tissue.* (Advances in Experimental Medicine and Biology 37A). New York: Plenum, 1973. Pp. 351–360.
8. Kessler, M., and Lübbers, D. W. Aufbau und Anwendungsmöglichkeiten verschiedener PO₂-Elektroden. *Pflügers Arch.* 291:82, 1966.
9. Kessler, M., Lübbers, D. W., Krumme, B. A., Schönleben, K., and Bünte, H. Oxygen tension in different tissues. *Bibl. Anat.* 16:146, 1977.
10. Lübbers, D. W., and Wodick, R. Sauerstofftransport im Warmblüterorganismus. *Umschau in Wissenschaft und Technik* 13:486, 1971.
11. Lund, N. Studies on skeletal muscle surface oxygen pressure fields. Linköping University Medical Dissertations No. 71. Linköping, 1979.
12. Messmer, K., Sunder-Plansmann, L., Jesch, F., Görnandt, L., Sinagowitz, E., and Kessler, M. Oxygen supply to the tissue during limited normovolemic hemodilution. *Res. Exp. Med.* 159:152, 1973.
13. Rink, R., and Kessler, M. Signs of hypoxia in the small intestine of the rat during hemorrhagic shock. In H. I. Bicher and D. F. Bruley (Eds.), *Oxygen Transport to Tissue.* (Advances in Experimental Medicine and Biology 37A). New York: Plenum, 1973. Pp. 505–511.
14. Sinagowitz, E. Die lokale Sauerstoffversorgung der Nierenrinde bei Hydronephrose und Nierenischämie; ihre klinische Bedeutung in der Urologie. Freiburg: Habil-Schrift, 1977.
15. Sinagowitz, E., and Kessler, M. Standardization of producing needle electrodes. In H. I. Bicher and D. F. Bruley (Eds.), *Oxygen Transport to Tissue.* (Advances in Experimental Medicine and Biology 37A.) New York: Plenum, 1973. Pp. 23–27.

Konrad Messmer / # 28. BLOOD SUBSTITUTES

Substitutes replacing all the complex functions of whole blood (e.g., carrier function, clotting function, and immunological defense function) are not yet even on the horizon, despite extensive work in this direction. Homologous blood, even in its optimal state, cannot meet all these functions. The substitute of choice is fresh autologous blood, leading to a revival of interest in the principle of autotransfusion. Autotransfusion is presently used in three different forms: (1) preoperative blood collection and storage [24]; (2) acute preoperative hemodilution [19, 23]; and (3) intraoperative blood salvage and retransfusion by pump systems [7]. These procedures have been shown to reduce the need for homologous donor blood. However, none of them is adequate for all patients undergoing major blood loss due to trauma or surgery.

In order to avoid side-effects from blood components which for the given patient are either inactive or unnecessary, the concept of blood component therapy is now used more extensively. This concept implies the identification of the individual component deficit (oxygen carrier, clotting factors, colloids, immunoglobulins) and selective substitution for the deficiency.

There is general agreement that restoration of the circulating volume is the most important single step in blood replacement therapy; this goal can be achieved sufficiently by infusion of plasma substitutes. However, owing to their dilution of the components of the patient's remaining blood, plasma substitutes have their limits in restoration of blood volume. Clinical studies with pre- and intraoperative normovolemic hemodilution have clearly revealed that surgical patients will tolerate hemoglobin levels of 8 to 10 gm/ 100 ml without risk of hypoxia if a high circulatory blood volume and cardiac output is achieved by the substitute. Increased oxygen demands in the postoperative period (e.g., fever) or coronary disease with inability to augment cardiac output call for a higher proportion of red blood cells [19, 23].

In the following sections, we shall discuss the various clinically available plasma substitutes with special regard to their capacity for restoring volume and efficacy in restoring nutritional blood flow.

PHYSICOCHEMICAL CHARACTERISTICS
OF PLASMA SUBSTITUTES

Plasma substitutes, by definition, aim to replace lost fluid, a colloidal solution containing different proteins. Of these proteins, albumin has the highest concentration and colloid-osmotic power.

Infusion solutions free of colloid molecules can be considered as volume substitutes only because the characteristic features of plasma—namely, the colloid content and, hence, the colloid-osmotic power—are lacking. Circulating volume can be restored by either crystalloid or colloid solutions. Although maintenance of the normal colloid-osmotic pressure (COP) of plasma is not a prerequisite, short-term normovolemia is difficult to establish without significant fluid shifts into other fluid compartments (third space) when COP is allowed to fall to lower values. To achieve and maintain normovolemia exclusively with crystalloids requires volumes 2.5 to 4 times the volume loss; close monitoring of the patient is needed to adjust the infusion speed to the actual hemodynamic status in order to avoid hypovolemia on the one hand and circulatory overloading with pulmonary edema on the other.

Therefore, in view of practicality and safety, we strongly advocate initial replacement of plasma deficits with colloid solutions, which provide predictable, long-lasting volume effects. These depend upon the physicochemical properties of the colloid molecules. Colloidal molecules of a weight below 50,000 pass the glomerular membrane and are rapidly excreted by the kidney [8]. In contrast, albumin, by virtue of its molecular weight of 69,000, is retained in the circulatory system. None of the artificial colloids has the monodisperse form of albumin; the artificial colloidal solutions are polydisperse in nature and thus provide a mixture of different species of molecules, the weights of which are distributed in a gaussian curve.

Hence, the intravascular persistence of artificial colloids depends, first, upon the molecular weight of the majority of molecules and, second, upon the width of distribution of molecular weights. The ratio of average molecular weight ($\overline{M}_w$) to average molecular number ($\overline{M}_n$) indicates the degree of polydispersity (see Table 28-1). Unity of the ratio $\overline{M}_w/\overline{M}_n$ indicates a monodisperse colloid, such as albumin.

The water-retaining capacity or the colloid-osmotic power of colloid solutions depends upon the $\overline{M}_w/\overline{M}_n$ ratio and the colloid content of the solution. Solutions with higher tonicities than plasma will attract water from the interstitial space; these solutions are therefore able to expand the plasma volume—at the expense of the interstitial fluid volume. The effectiveness of colloids in restoring plasma deficits can be predicted from their physicochemical properties; these predictions have been verified in numerous experimental and clinical studies [8, 11, 17]. No plasma substitute should deteriorate the rheologic properties of the blood. Protracted volume loss and shock are characteristically associated with a disturbance of mi-

TABLE 28-1. Artificial Colloids for Plasma Volume Substitution[a]

Colloid and Generic Name	Colloid Content (gm/100 ml)	$\overline{M}_w$	$\overline{M}_w/\overline{M}_n$	Intravascular Persistence	Remarks
Dextran					
Dextran 60[b]	6	60,000	2.0	6	Antithrombotic effect
Dextran 70	6	70,000	1.85	6	Antithrombotic effect
Dextran 40	10	40,000	1.4	2–3	Antithrombotic effect
Starch					
HES 450/0.7	6	450,000	6.3	~6	
HES 40/0.5	6	40,000	2.0	2–3	
Gelatin					
Urea-linked	3–5	35,000	2.3	2–3	Diuretic effect
Modified fluid (MFG)	4	35,000	2.2	2–3	
Oxypolygelatin	5.5	30,000	1.5	2–3	Diuretic effect

HES = hydroxyethylstarch.

[a] Data from literature and manufacturers.
[b] Dextran 60, $\overline{M}_w$ 60,000, available in Germany and Austria; properties nearly identical with those of dextran 70.

crocirculatory flow and with a decrease in blood fluidity. Both microcirculatory flow and blood fluidity seem to be more efficiently improved by colloids than by crystalloids, provided the viscosity of the colloid solution itself does not exceed the viscosity of whole blood [11]. In addition, colloids may provide specific properties, such as the antithrombotic effect of dextran.

NATURAL COLLOIDS

Among the natural colloids, 4% pasteurized protein solution (Plasmanate) and 5% human serum albumin (HSA) are highly suited for plasma volume replacement; both solutions yield a volume effect in vivo that roughly equals the amount of volume infused [8]. These protein preparations are not free from risks: anaphylactoid reactions (immediate and delayed) with severe hypotension may occur [2, 18, 27, 28]. However, the occasional occurrence of adverse reactions does not present a contraindication to routine use. (This statement is valid for all colloids in clinical use today.)

Because of these shortcomings, and for economic reasons (1 gm HSA costs about fifteen times as much as 1 gm dextran), these natural colloids should never be used for *routine* plasma volume replacement; they should be reserved for those hypovolemic patients with significant hypoproteinemia. Also, for the same reasons, routine intraoperative volume replacement with protein solutions cannot be justified. Several authors have addressed the problem whether posttraumatic respiratory insufficiency or acute respiratory distress can be prevented by early administration of HSA; conclusive evidence for superior effects of HSA as compared with artificial colloids in patients without significant hypoproteinemia is not yet available.

ARTIFICIAL COLLOIDS

The literature on artificial colloids contains a number of controversies concerning advantages versus disadvantages of various artificial colloids. The physicochemical properties of the colloids in question are the sole criteria for any comparative judgment. Table 28-1 lists the most important data for the most frequently used artificial colloids. Since the sources, data for $\overline{M}_w$ and $\overline{M}_n$, colloid content, and noncolloidal solutes vary widely for different countries and are matters of change, our discussion will be restricted to representative colloid substitutes (for detailed information, see Gruber [8] and Lutz [17]).

DEXTRANS

Dextrans are high-molecular polysaccharides consisting of glucose molecules connected mainly by 1.6 glucosidic linkages. The clinically used dextrans are obtained by hydrolytic fractionation. Dextran 70 (Macrodex) and dextran 40 (Rheomacrodex) are the most important dextran preparations. The 6% solution of dextran 70 exerts a colloid-osmotic effect—expressed as water-retaining capacity per gram of the nondiffusing polymer (20–25 ml)—higher than that of albumin or plasma proteins. Therefore, dextran 70 seems particularly well suited to be the primary plasma replacement and to maintain intravascular volume over a longer period of time [8, 11, 19].

Dextran 40, with an average molecular weight of 40,000, is available as a 10% solution, which, compared with plasma, is strongly hyperoncotic. For this reason, the initial volume effect of dextran 40 is about twice the volume infused. Owing to the lower $\overline{M}_w$, dextran 40 is more rapidly excreted; 3 to 4 hours after infusion the intravascular volume gain equals about the volume infused. The initial volume gain is due to transcapillary fluid shift at the expense of the interstitial fluid. As a rule, sodium and water should be given in volumes identical with that of dextran 40 in order to avoid dehydration. The colloid-osmotic power drags interstitial fluid into the intravascular space preferentially in the venous part of the microcirculation; for this reason, microcirculatory flow is rapidly restored by dextran 40 infusions because additional hemodilution takes place in the most vulnerable part of the microcirculation, the postcapillary venules. This effect depends upon the colloid-osmotic pressure gradient across the membrane and is thus not specific for dextran 40. Dextran 40 is indicated particularly in patients with protracted shock and with microcirculatory disorders [11].

Dextrans are completely excreted or metabolized after short-term storage in the reticuloendothelial system (RES) and tubular cells. Both dextrans yield antithrombotic properties, which are different from the influence on the clotting mechanism; the latter is observed only when the dose limit of 1.5 gm/kg of body weight per day is exceeded. The antithrombotic properties of dextran are due to a decrease of platelet adhesiveness, depression of factor VIII activity, increased susceptibility of thrombi to fibrinolysis, and blood flow improvement [1, 9]. The literature, mostly European, documents that in addition to their volume effect, both dextran preparations safely prevent postoperative deep venous thrombosis and fatal pulmonary embolism [9, 10]. Besides their effect on blood clotting when the dose limit is exceeded, dextrans, like all other colloids, bear the rare but occasionally fatal risk of anaphylactoid/anaphylactic reactions (see below).

GELATIN
Gelatin is the oldest clinically used colloidal plasma substitute. Three types, differing in source of raw material (collagen) and method of production, are available (Table 28-1).

The major difference between dextran 70 and hydroxyethylstarch (HES) 450/0.7 is the lower average molecular weight of gelatin preparations. For this reason, the intravascular persistence of gelatin is shorter and the initial volume effect is less pronounced when compared with identical volumes of dextran 70. Nevertheless, as shown in animal studies and clinical experience, normovolemia is achieved by infusion of initially higher amounts and can be maintained by more frequent reinfusions. Since no dose limit—apart from the dilutional fall in red cell mass—exists for gelatin, considerable plasma volume replacement can be performed [16]. Lundsgaard-Hansen et al. [16] stress in particular the absence of a specific gelatin effect on the blood clotting mechanism; conversely, however, gelatin has no anti-thrombotic properties (for side-effects, see below).

HYDROXYETHYLSTARCH
HES is manufactured from amylopectin and consists of hydroxyethylated glucose molecules linked by α-1.4 bindings. At present, three preparations are commercially available.

HIGH MOLECULAR WEIGHT HYDROXYETHYLSTARCH (HES 450/0.7)
The average molecular weight of this 6% solution amounts to 450,000 in vitro, and the degree of substitution is 0.7, which means that 7 out of 10 glucose molecules are by hydroxyethyl groups. The initially very large molecules are degraded in vivo by serum α-amylase rather rapidly to molecules in the range of about 70,000 $\overline{M}_w$; thus, the intravascular volume effect is comparable with that of dextran 70. Expansion of plasma volume in excess of the infused volume was not observed in our experiments [13, 20]. Jesch et al. [13] were first to report on the increase in serum α-amylase as a result of starch infusion. While apparently of no pathogenic importance, this effect must be taken into account in patients with increased serum amylase levels so as to avoid the false diagnosis of pancreatitis. The elimination of HES 450/0.7 follows a different pattern when compared with dextran 70/60, since it is stored in the RES cells of the liver for a prolonged time [4, 20]. To circumvent this problem, starch preparations with lower $\overline{M}_w$ and faster elimination patterns are currently under examination [20, 29]. Apart from the dilutional effect, HES 450/0.7 does not influence the clotting system; antithrombotic properties have never been demonstrated.

LOW MOLECULAR WEIGHT HYDROXYETHYLSTARCH (HES 40/0.5)
HES 40/0.5 provides a volume effect comparable with the effect of gelatin preparations. The claim for an intravascular persistence identical with that of dextran 70 has not been corroborated by studies with isovolemic hemodilution [20]. In contrast, whereas the colloid osmotic pressure of the plasma was maintained in the normal range during isovolemic hemodilution with gelatin solution, COP fell significantly with progressing hemodilution by HES 40/0.5.

This starch preparation is therefore not considered a satisfactory colloidal plasma substitute. Serum α-amylase increases in response to infusion of HES 40/0.5 as well; the formation of an HES-amylase complex (macro-amylase) has been demonstrated to cause this phenomenon [14] (for side-effects, see below).

SIDE-EFFECTS OF COLLOIDAL PLASMA SUBSTITUTES

None of the colloids—human serum albumin and plasma proteins in-cluded—is free from the risk of anaphylactoid reactions. The majority of these are mild and affect mainly the skin (flush, erythema, etc.); however, severe reactions, even fatal outcome from cardiac arrest, have been reported over the years. The incidence of adverse reactions is not high when com-pared with other drugs, but the risk of fatal outcome calls for special aware-ness. The incidence of adverse reactions to colloids varies considerably in the literature owing to conceptual differences in the studies; in general, retrospective studies have reported lower figures than prospective, ran-domized trials [27]. The situation can be summarized as follows:

1. Severe adverse reactions with severe hypotension and cardiac arrest have been observed after infusion of HSA and plasma protein solutions, with an overall incidence of <0.1 percent. A clinically applicable prophylaxis is not known.
2. The incidence of dextran-induced anaphylactoid/anaphylactic reactions (DIAR) is from 0.07 to 1.1 percent [10, 28]. Cardiac arrest was observed in a higher frequency with DIAR than with plasma proteins, starch, or gelatin. The re-cently introduced concept of hapten inhibition of DIAR [22] has led to a sig-nificant reduction of the overall incidence of adverse reactions to dextran; life-threatening reactions have been prevented by preinjection of a monovalent hapten-dextran that occupies the binding sites of circulating preformed dextran reactive antibodies [22].
3. The incidence of adverse reactions to gelatin depends upon the type of gelatin preparation. The figures vary from 0.05 to about 10 percent [16, 27, 28]. Life-threatening and fatal reactions have been reported. Prophylaxis by histamine receptor (H_1 and H_2)-antagonists seems possible and is currently under clinical investigation [15].
4. HES has not yet been used to the same extent as dextran and gelatin. The incidence of adverse reactions to HES seems to be around 0.1 percent. Life-threatening reactions do also occur but less often than with dextran 70 [3]. The pathomechanism of these reactions is unknown; therefore, prophylaxis is not possible.

The clinician using colloids has to be aware of the possibility of untoward reactions to the various colloid solutions. However, the low risk of these reactions does not present a contraindication for the use of either colloid.

OXYGEN-CARRYING SUBSTITUTES

Stromafree hemoglobin solution (SFH) and perfluorochemicals (PFC) ap-pear to be the most promising candidates for blood substitutes in the future, if the term *blood substitute* is restricted to oxygen-carrying capacity and volume properties. Preparations of both hemoglobin solution and PFCs have been administered to a few volunteers and to desperately ill patients. However, neither substance is perfected for clinical use at this time.

STROMAFREE HEMOGLOBIN SOLUTION

Hemoglobin solution has been studied more intensively as a blood substitute since Rabiner et al. [26] described their method for preparing hemoglobin solutions without stromal lipid contaminants (SFH). It has been shown [5, 21], however, that SFH, which should raise problems neither in coagulation nor kidney function, still presents two major disadvantages. First, SFH leaves the intravascular space rapidly (with a half-life of 100–140 min) and is thus unable to maintain blood volume over an extended period of time. Second, due to the loss of the red cell membrane and loss of the intraerythrocytic milieu, the affinity of SFH for oxygen is greatly enhanced as compared with intraerythrocytic hemoglobin [5, 21]. SFH is therefore not a useful blood substitute even though its oxygen-carrying capacity is considerably higher than that of the artificial colloids [5].

Several research groups in central Europe and United States have focused on prolonging the intravascular persistence and reducing the oxygen affinity of SFH [5]. SFH is modified to stabilize or to enlarge the tetrameric molecule by intra- or intermolecular bridging. A promising approach to decrease the high oxygen affinity of SFH was described by Benesch et al. [5, 21] and successfully tested in vivo by Jesch et al. [12, 21]. Even though both approaches yielded encouraging results, with prolongation of intravascular persistence and lowered oxygen affinity, a clinically acceptable hemoglobin compound has not yet emerged. Further work is needed in order to determine whether the potential benefits (availability, long-term storage, absence of risk of transmitting diseases, etc.) outweigh the imminent risks (immunogenicity, general and organ toxicity) of chemically modified SFH.

PERFLUOROCHEMICALS

PFCs are solutions of dispersed perfluorocompounds, which became attractive candidates as substitutes for blood by virtue of their ability to dissolve oxygen in quantities comparable with the amount of oxygen bound chemically by hemoglobin. Owing to the linear relation between oxygen content and PO_2 with PFCs, a high oxygen content is achieved only at an FIO_2 of 0.7 to 1.0. Definite proof of the ability of PFCs to carry and to unload oxygen at the tissue level was demonstrated in experiments with total blood exchange for PFC or perfusion of isolated organs with PFC as sole oxygen carrier [6, 25]. To use PFC as a blood substitute, it is mandatory to demonstrate that in conditions where a reduced number of red cells are still circulating, oxygen unloading at the tissue level occurs not only from the red cells but to a significant degree also from PFC. Corresponding experiments with instantaneous measurements of oxygen extraction from the red cell hemoglobin and the circulating PFC remain to be made. With regard to the problem of in vivo storage and elimination, the recently developed compounds (Fluosol-43, Fluosol-DA, Green Cross Corporation, Osaka, Japan) are definitely superior to the former fluorocarbons [25]. However, elimination of the stored material by pulmonary excretion is protracted; the potential sequelae of incorporated PFC have not been explored completely.

Since a high oxygen content in circulating PFC is obtained only with a high F_1O_2 the detrimental effects of high FiO_2 will necessarily limit the use of PFC in patients. Nevertheless, the presently available and forthcoming perfluorocompounds might become useful for organ preservation and for cases of extensive blood loss when no red cells are available.

SUMMARY

Plasma volume replacement is most efficiently and safely achieved with colloidal solutions, providing long-lasting volume and colloid-osmotic effects without deterioration of the blood fluidity. The natural colloids (human serum albumin, pasteurized plasma protein solution), dextran 60/70, and hydroxyethylstarch (HES 450/0.7) fulfill these criteria and are thus most suitable for plasma volume replacement and treatment of hypovolemic shock. Owing to the different physiochemical properties of gelatin, the volume effect of gelatin solutions is less pronounced. Low molecular weight starch (HES 40/0.5) cannot be considered a colloidal plasma substitute.

All colloids carry the risk of occasional anaphylactoid reactions; however, these are not contraindications to their clinical use.

Human protein solutions should be saved for patients needing protein substitution.

Hemodilution resulting from replacement of blood loss by plasma substitutes will not jeopardize the patient's life so long as the hemoglobin concentration does not drop below 8 to 10 gm/100 ml. The contraindications from coronary disease or increased oxygen demands have to be observed.

With regard to volume effect, because of their specific antithrombotic effect and the possibility of their preventing anaphylactoid/anaphylactic reactions by the hapten-inhibition principle, dextran solutions offer definite advantages.

Additional work is necessary before the oxygen-carrying substitutes, stromafree hemoglobin and perfluorochemicals, will be clinically applicable blood substitutes.

REFERENCES

1. Åberg, M., Hedner, U., Bergentz, S. E. Effect of dextran on factor VIII (antihemophilic factor) and platelet function. *Ann. Surg.* 189:243, 1978.
2. Alving, B. M., Hojima, J., Pisano, J. J., Mason, B. L., Buckingham, R. E., Mozen, M. M., and Finlayson, J. S. Hypotension associated with prekalli-

krein activator (Hageman Factor Fragments) in plasma protein fraction. *N. Engl. J. Med.* 299:66, 1978.

3. Beez, M., and Dietl, H. Retrospektive Betrachtung der Häufigkeit anaphylaktoider Reaktionen nach Plasmasteril^R und Longasteril^R. *Infusionstherapie* 6:23, 1979.

4. Boon, J. C., Jesch, F., Ring, J., and Messmer, K. Intravascular persistence of hydroxyethyl starch in man. *Eur. Surg. Res.* 8:497, 1976.

5. DeVenuto, F., Friedman, H. J., Neville, J. R., and Peck, C. C. Appraisal of hemoglobin solution as a blood substitute. *Surg. Gynecol. Obstet.* 149:417, 1979.

6. Geyer, R. P. "Bloodless" rats through the use of artificial blood substitutes. *Fed. Proc.* 34:1499, 1975.

7. Glover, J. L., Smith, R., Yaw, P., Radigan, L. R., Plawecki, R., and Link, W. Intraoperative autotransfusion: An underutilized technique. *Surgery* 80:474, 1976.

8. Gruber, U. F. *Blood replacement.* New York: Springer, 1969.

9. Gruber, U. F. Dextran and the prevention of postoperative thromboembolic complications. *Surg. Clin. North Am.* 55:679, 1975.

10. Gruber, U. F., Saldeen, T., et al. Comparison of the incidence of fatal pulmonary embolism with dextran 70 and low dose heparin prophylaxis. An international multicenter trial. *Br. Med. J.* 280:69, 1980.

11. Gruber, U. F., Sturm, V., and Messmer, K. Fluid replacement in shock. In I. Ledingham, *Shock, Clinical and Experimental Aspects.* Amsterdam: Excerpta Medica, 1976. P. 231.

12. Jesch, F., Hobbhahn, J., Endrich, B., Peters, W., Messmer, K. Improved in vivo oxygen delivery from stromafree hemoglobin by pyridoxilation. *Pflüg. Arch. Europ. Physiol.* 362:R16, 1976.

13. Jesch, F., Kloevekorn, W. P., Sunder-Plassmann, L., Seifert, J., and Messmer, K. Hydroxyläthylstärke als Plasmaersatzmittel. Untersuchungen mit isovolämischer Hämodilution. *Anästhesist* 24:202, 1975.

14. Köhler, H., Kirch, W., Weihrauch, T. R., Prellwitz, W., and Horstmann, H. J. Macroamylasemia after treatment with hydroxylethyl starch. *Eur. J. Clin. Invest.* 7:205, 1977.

15. Lorenz, W., Doenicke, A., Dittmann, I., Hug, P., and Schwarz, B. Anaphylactoid reactions following administration of plasma substitutes in man. Prevention of side-effects of Haemaccel by premedication with H_1- and H_2- Receptor antagonists. *Anaesthesist* 26:644, 1977.

16. Lundsgaard-Hansen, P., and Tschirren, B. Modified fluid gelatin as a plasma substitute. *Prog. Clin. Biol. Res.* 19:227, 1978.

17. Lutz, H. *Plasmaersatzmittel* (2d ed.). Stuttgart: Thieme, 1975.

18. McMillin, R. D., Hood, T. R., and Griffen, W. O. Systemic anaphylaxis secondary to the use of 5% plasma protein fractions. *Am. J. Surg.* 135:706, 1978.

19. Messmer, K. Hemodilution. *Surg. Clin. North Am.* 55:659, 1975.

20. Messmer, K., and Jesch, F. Volumenersatz und Hämodilution durch Hydroxyäthylstärke. *Infusionstherapie* 5:169, 1978.

21. Messmer, K., Jesch, F., Schaff, J., Schönberg, M., Pielsticker, K., and Bonhard, K. Oxygen supply by stroma-free hemoglobin. *Prog. Clin. Biol. Res.* 19:175, 1978.

22. Messmer, K., Ljungström, K., and Gruber, U. F.   Prevention of dextran-induced anaphylactoid reactions by hapten-inhibition. *Lancet* i, 975, 1980.
23. Messmer, K., Ott, E., and Martin, E.   Purpose, means and limitations of hemodilution. *Med. Postgrad. (Tokyo)* 16:1, 1978.
24. Milles, G., Langston, H. T., and Dalessandro, W.   *Autologous transfusions.* Springfield, Ill.: Thomas, 1971.
25. Naito, R., and Yokoyama, K.   *Perfluorochemical blood substitutes "fluosol-43," fluosol DA 20% and 35%.* Technical Information Ser. No. 5. Osaka, Japan: Green Cross, 1978.
26. Rabiner, S. F., Helbert, J. R., Lopas, H., and Friedman, L. H.   Evaluation of stroma-free hemoglobin solution for use as a plasma expander. *J. Exp. Med.* 126:1127, 1967.
27. Ring, J.   Anaphylactoid Reactions. In *Anaesthesiology and Intensive Care Medicine,* Vol. 111. New York: Springer, 1978.
28. Ring, J., and Messmer, K.   Incidence and severity of anaphylactoid reactions to colloid volume substitutes. *Lancet* 1:466, 1977.
29. Thompson, W. L., Bloxham, D. D., and Rudnick, M. S.   New short-persistence hydroxyethylstarch (HES-S). *Intens. Care Med.* 3:206, 1977.

SELECTED READINGS

Artificial Blood.   A symposium sponsored by the Division of Blood Diseases and Resources of the National Heart Lung Inst., NIH, Bethesda, Md., April 1974. *Fed. Proc.* 34:1428–1531, 1975.
Collins, J. A., Litwin, M. S., Lutz, H., Klose, R., Ring, J., Thorén, L., Tschirren, B., Lundsgaard-Hansen, P.   To which extent is the clinical use of dextran, gelatin and hydroxyethylstarch influenced by the incidence and severity of anaphylactoid reactions? *Vox Sang.* 36:39–49, 1979.
Gruber, U. F.   *Blood Replacement.* New York: Springer, 1969.
Jamieson, G. A., and Greenwalt, T. J.   Blood substitutes and plasma expanders. *Prog. Clin. Biol. Res.* 19, 1978.
Lutz, H.   *Plasmaersatzmittel* (3rd ed.). Stuttgart: Thieme, 1980.
Proceedings of Postcongress Symposium. The Xth International Congress of Nutrition. Perfluorochemical Artificial Blood.   Osaka: Igakushoho, 1975.
Ring, J.   Anaphylactoid Reactions. In *Anesthesiology and Intensive Care Medicine,* Vol. 111. New York: Springer, 1978.
Watkins, J., and Ward, A. M.   *Adverse Response to Intravenous Drugs.* New York: Grune & Stratton, 1978.

Stephen M. Ayres | # 29. MASS SPECTROMETRY IN THE CARE OF THE CRITICALLY ILL

In 1923, J. B. S. Haldane, in an essay entitled "Daedalus: or Science and the Future," predicted that biology rather than the physical sciences would dominate the twentieth century. This belief, expressed at a time when important advances in nuclear physics held center stage, appeared natural for a man whose father, John Scott Haldane, was a founder of modern pulmonary physiology. Realizing that measurement of human physiological function was an essential first step in human biology, John Scott Haldane developed a gas analyzer and alveolar sampling technique that enabled him to study alveolar-capillary gas exchange under a variety of environmental conditions, ranging from the bottom of a Scottish coal mine in 1895 to the top of Pike's Peak in 1913.

Since critical care medicine may be regarded as a midcentury flowering of applied human physiology, a discipline requiring rapid on-line acquisition of human physiological data with almost immediate feedback responses in the form of therapeutic interventions, it seems appropriate to look closely at a new measurement technique which is a lineal descendant of Haldane's original gas analyzer. Analysis of physiological and inert gases is the core of cardiopulmonary physiology. Both the Haldane and Scholander gas analyzers and the Van Slyke blood apparatus measured physiological gas concentrations by sequentially removing oxygen and carbon dioxide; the residual gas was considered nitrogen even though almost 1 percent was actually argon. Although it enabled its developers to establish the foundations of modern physiology, this equipment suffered from major drawbacks: analysis was tedious, and continuous sampling obviously impossible.

Continuous gas analyzers for helium and nitrogen were introduced in the early 1940s; analyzers for carbon monoxide and carbon dioxide were developed somewhat later. For the first time, continuous display of expired gas concentrations was possible, permitting dynamic evaluation of alveolar ventilation and its distribution. These new instruments made data collecting considerably less time-consuming, so that efforts could be shifted to mathematical analysis of "wash in" and "wash out" curves, confirming and extending the fundamental concepts of earlier workers who spent long hours with the Haldane apparatus.

The physical gas analyzers were extraordinarily useful but had certain drawbacks: a different analyzer was required for each gas; certain gases, such as oxygen, could not be conveniently analyzed; response times varied from instrument to instrument so that complicated correction factors were necessary; sample sizes were of necessity large, preventing analysis of gases physically removed from blood or other liquids. Clearly, other approaches were necessary.

Before 1920, J. J. Thompson, popularly known as the discoverer of the electron, and his student, F. W. Aston, built instruments that separated positive ions on the basis of atomic or mass weight. Subsequent work led to the development of the magnetic mass spectrometer, an instrument taking advantage of the observation that charged particles moving through a magnetic field are acted upon by perpendicular forces referred to as the Lorentz force. A magnetic mass spectrometer takes neutral molecules, converts a fraction of them into ions, and sends them through a magnetic field. Each ion is subjected to a deflecting force as it moves through the field; the lighter ions are deflected more than the heavier ions, and separation, according to mass, is achieved. Physiologists were quick to appreciate the advantage of rapid sampling of specific gases, and a number of medical applications were suggested by 1950. One of the most important applications was made by West et al. at Hammersmith Hospital in London when they used a newly developed mass spectrometer to serially analyze expired air [23, 24].

Continuous analysis of a number of gases present in expired air has led to convenient techniques for assessing important aspects of cardiac and pulmonary diffusing capacity. Single-breath measurements for residual volume, pulmonary diffusing capacity, pulmonary capillary volume, and pulmonary capillary blood flow were all developed before 1960. Each required measurement of expired concentrations of nitrogen, carbon monoxide, or helium. Usually two samples were obtained, one before and the other following a specified period of breath holding. Johnson et al. [10] combined an infrared analyzer for carbon monoxide, another for acetylene, and a single-channel mass spectrometer capable of measuring helium, oxygen, and carbon dioxide as a means for developing a technique for the simultaneous evaluation of pulmonary capillary blood volume, flow, and diffusing capacity. This complicated array of three gas analyzers and three collection bags provided important data indicating that the increase in diffusing capacity observed with exercise was due to the parallel increase in pulmonary capillary blood flow and volume.

Sackner et al. [21] have refined the techniques developed by Johnson et al. [10] using a mass spectrometer (MGA-1100, Perkin Elmer, Pomona, Calif.) for sampling all test gases and a small digital computer (LINC 8, Digital Equipment Co., Maynard, Mass.) to facilitate data processing. Carbon monoxide and nitrogen both have the same molecular weight and cannot be separated by mass spectrometry. These investigators overcame that problem by using carbon monoxide synthesized from isotopic oxygen, $C^{18}O$. This compound has a mass weight of 30 and is readily distinguished from nitrogen by the mass spectrometer. The continuous recording of acetylene permitted them to measure the initial uptake of acetylene by lung tissue so that diffusing capacity, membrane diffusing capacity, capillary blood volume, pulmonary tissue volume, and cardiac output could all be determined. The continual refinement of single-breath diffusion measurements from Krogh's original method, through Ogilvie et al. [15] and Johnson et al. [10] to Sackner et al. [21], demonstrates the dependence of man's ability to measure his own physiological function on technological advances.

An important use of mass spectrometry is the on-line measurement of expired and end-tidal oxygen, carbon dioxide, and nitrogen tensions. The concept and measurement of alveolar air have vexed physiologists for some time. In fact, there is no single value for alveolar oxygen and carbon dioxide tensions; studies by West [22] and others have emphasized a continuous distribution of alveolar gas tensions, alveolar carbon dioxide tension (P_ACO_2) ranging from 28 torr at the apex of normal man to 42 torr at the base. Capillary blood leaving different lung regions shows similar differences in gas tension; arterial blood is a mixture of all of these regions. A similar average value of alveolar air from different lung regions is needed for evaluation of overall alveolar-capillary gas exchange.

Theoretic considerations suggest that mean arterial carbon dioxide tension ($PaCO_2$) is normally only 1 to 2 torr greater than P_ACO_2; in the Bohr dead space equation, a value for physiological dead space, is obtained by substituting $PaCO_2$ for P_ACO_2. Similarly, substitution of arterial for alveolar carbon dioxide tension in the alveolar air equation permits calculation of mean alveolar oxygen tension (P_AO_2).

Haldane's early efforts centered around the use of expired air samples as indicators of $PaCO_2$ [9]. Haldane-Priestley samples included end-tidal gas obtained after a complete expiration. Subsequent investigators demonstrated that the Haldane-Priestley values were 2 to 3 torr greater when taken at the end of a quiet expiration [18]. Rahn and Otis [19] developed an automatic alveolar sampling device which removed the last few milliliters of each expiration and pooled them for subsequent analysis. Osborn et al. [16] then dramatically changed monitoring techniques in critical care medicine by developing a system using physical gas analyzers and a digital computer. For the first time, they were able continuously to measure ventilatory function and oyxgen consumption in the seriously ill patient.

Modern mass spectrometers permit the continuous measurement of end-tidal samples. Riker and Haberman [20] and McAslan [13] have described systematic approaches to the on-line monitoring of patients during mechanical ventilation. End-tidal oxygen tension is relatively useless because of the large and shifting alveolar-arterial oxygen difference in critically ill patients. End-tidal carbon dioxide tension, however, may be taken as representative of alveolar air and frequently bears a constant relationship to arterial carbon dioxide tension. A rising carbon dioxide tension in end-tidal air suggests decreasing alveolar ventilation. Such measurements are particularly useful in patients receiving positive end-expiratory pressure (PEEP) as the pressure level is varied, hyperventilating patients, and during the transition from mechanical to spontaneous ventilation.

The recent emphasis on separation of ventilatory from oxygenation problems has led to increased interest in continuous end-tidal monitoring. Positive expiratory pressure has been shown to increase functional residual capacity by exerting a continuous distending pressure across the lung; mechanical ventilation is indicated when alveolar ventilation falls and carbon dioxide tension rises. A possible approach to the treatment of the adult respiratory distress syndrome makes use of continuous monitoring and a group of ventilatory techniques. If alveolar carbon dioxide tension is relatively normal, continuous positive airway pressure (CPAP) may be applied to increase oxygenation and end-tidal carbon dioxide tension continuously monitored. Should carbon dioxide tension rise, the patient may then be intubated and ventilated mechanically using the Kirby technique [12] that blends PEEP with intermittent mandatory ventilation (IMV). If alveolar carbon dioxide tension rises again, the rate of machine breaths can be increased.

Riker and Haberman [20] also measured the ratio of dead space to tidal volume (V_D/V_T) by collecting several minutes of expired air and measuring the carbon dioxide concentration. The V_D/V_T ratio is calculated from the Bohr equation

$$V_D/V_T = \frac{PaCO_2 - P\bar{E}CO_2}{PaCO_2}$$

where $PaCO_2$ equals arterial carbon dioxide tension and $P\bar{E}CO_2$ equals expired carbon dioxide tension.

Alveolar-arterial oxygen tension difference during the breathing of 100% oxygen is a measure of the venoarterial intrapulmonary shunt and a precise way of following patients during mechanical ventilation. Alveolar oxygen tension may be approximated by measuring end-tidal oxygen tension and arterial oxygen tension by a platinum electrode technique; both are measured following twenty minutes of ventilation with 100% oxygen.

Several groups have attempted to measure blood gases continuously by sampling through latex toy balloons tied to the end of polyethylene catheters. Brantigan et al. [2] designed a Silastic and a Teflon catheter consisting of a semipermeable membrane mounted over a narrow-gauge, flexible stainless steel tubing. Silastic catheters reach 63 percent of a step change in 25 seconds and can be used for measurement of arterial oxygen and carbon dioxide tensions and for washout of inhaled argon from the arterial blood. The Teflon catheter has a much slower response time and can be inserted in tissue to reflect tissue gas tensions.

The gas- and blood-sampling catheters may be important analytic instruments for a variety of research studies. As gas samplers they are stable, respond rapidly, require extremely small sample sizes, and can provide a continuous readout of changing gas tensions. The membrane cannulae are particularly useful for measuring inert gas tensions in blood or tissue and have the added advantage of not consuming blood, since the gases diffuse across the membrane and move under vacuum into the mass spectrometer.

An ingenious use of the respiratory gas capability is the linkage to computer elements in order to provide an automated approach to exercise physiology. Wilmore [25] continuously measures mixed expired oxygen, nitrogen, and carbon dioxide concentrations during exercise; oxygen consumption, carbon dioxide production, and the respiratory quotient are automatically calculated. The ability to measure nitrogen, rather than calculate it as the difference between total air and the respiratory gases, enabled him to validate the Haldane transformation for the calculation of oxygen consumption [26]. Cardiac output is measured in the automated system by the rebreathing of acetylene or carbon dioxide; whole body density is estimated by helium dilution. These mass spectrometric analytic techniques are an important part of the Human Performance Laboratory at the University of California, Davis.

While the issue of whether the Teflon catheter inserted into tissue measures actual intracellular or interstitial tensions remains unsettled, important observations of changing gas tensions in response to experimental interventions have been made. The actual source of the gas is unimportant in analyzing tissue carbon dioxide appearance, since cellular and extracellular concentrations are identical. The rate of extracellular carbon dioxide accumulation is directly related to intracellular adenosine triphosphate consumption if ischemia is total and washout does not occur. Khuri et al. [11] found that oxygen tension declined about 25 to 35 percent while carbon dioxide tension more than doubled when coronary blood flow was reduced by 50 percent. MacGregor et al. [14] have used intraoperative myocardial carbon dioxide accumulation curves to identify the transition point for the safe termination of ischemic cardiac arrest during open heart surgery.

Our own group [1] and Damman and McAslan [5] have used mass spectrometry to evaluate ventilation and perfusion matching in critically ill patients. Washout of argon from alveolar air reflects the distribution of ventilation; arterial blood washout is a direct measure of the efficiency of gas exchange and is dependent upon total ventilation and the distribution of ventilation/perfusion ratios.

A difficult problem in the critically ill patient is the frequent assessment of alveolar-capillary gas exchange. While alveolar oxygen tension may be calculated from the alveolar air equation, the difficulty in accurately measuring the oxygen concentration of inspired mixtures limits this to patients breathing either room air or 100% oxygen. End-tidal oxygen tension ($P_{ET}O_2$) is easily measured with the mass spectrometer and, together with arterial oxygen tension measurements, may be used to calculate the alveolar-arterial oxygen difference [$P(A-a)O_2$].

The ability to measure the $P(A-a)O_2$ at any level of inspired oxygen tension provides the investigator with a method for separating the various components producing that difference. Farhi and Rahn [7] showed that the effect of the three factors limiting gas exchange—diffusion limitations, variation of alveolar ventilation to capillary blood flow, and venoarterial shunting—varied with the P_AO_2. Diffusion limitations accounted for a large part of the $P(A-a)O_2$ at P_AO_2 below 60 torr; at P_AO_2 between 80 and 100 torr, ventilation/perfusion and venoarterial shunting had similar effects on the difference; at P_AO_2 above 200 torr, the entire $P(A-a)O_2$ was produced by true venoarterial shunting. True venoarterial shunting is conventionally measured during the breathing of 100% oxygen since the P_AO_2 may be readily calculated. The elimination of nitrogen from the inspired air leads to increased alveolar collapse so that values obtained during the breathing of 100% oxygen may be spuriously large. Administration of mixtures containing lower concentrations of oxygen and measurement of $P_{ET}O_2$ and P_AO_2 permit calculation of the true venoarterial shunt while the alveoli are filled with air containing at least 60% nitrogen.

Just as measurements in the critical care unit represent physiological study of the individual under stress, similar measurements during exercise provide assessment of the reserve capacity of normal individuals and those with mild or moderately advanced disease. Wilmore's paper [26] evaluates the use of a mass spectrometer and automatic data-gathering equipment in measuring maximum oxygen uptake during treadmill exercise. An intriguing finding is that a break in the linearity of certain indices derived from expired air coincided with the onset of anaerobic metabolism as indicated by an increase in arterial lactic acid concentration.

Although oxygen delivery to the tissues is a function of blood flow as well as arterial oxygenation, bedside monitoring of cardiac output has lagged behind that of alveolar gas exchange. Douglas and his group [6] applied themselves to that problem with modest success but it was Grollman [8] who developed a practical rebreathing method using acetylene as the test gas. Inert gas methods reflect pulmonary capillary blood flow, and indicator-dilution techniques (indocyanine green or thermal dilution) measure total cardiac output. When venoarterial shunting is minimal, cardiac output and pulmonary capillary blood flows are almost equal; total cardiac output in the critically ill patient could be measured by adding the shunt flow to the pulmonary blood flow determined by an inert gas method.

The ideal gas for measurement of pulmonary capillary blood flow must be soluble in blood, relatively insoluble in lung tissue, and completely removed by the systemic circulation so that recirculation would not occur. Butler [3] has reviewed these criteria and concluded that the ideal gas does not exist.

Acetylene has many of the characteristics of an ideal gas for cardiac output determination and has been used in methods developed by Johnson et al. [10] and Sackner et al. [21]. Continuous recording of either breathing bag or expired acetylene concentration facilitates correction for lung tissue uptake, a correction not possible with discrete sampling because of the rapid equilibration of acetylene with lung tissue. Freon gas has a solubility coefficient close to that of acetylene and has been used by Cotton [4] for measuring pulmonary capillary blood flow in the newborn infant.

The magnetic mass spectrometer was developed some 70 years after Haldane's initial studies with his sampling tube and gas analyzer. Although most of Haldane's concepts, laboriously derived following the analysis of hundreds of individual samples, are probably safe from revision, the availability of a continuous and rapidly responding gas analyzer provides today's investigator with a powerful method for applying these and other physiological concepts to the critically ill patient. What better way would there be, for example, to determine the efficiency of interventions such as PEEP and IMV on alveolar-capillary gas exchange and peripheral blood flows. Even lung water, that most elusive of physiological measurements, may give way to observations based on the instantaneous uptake of acetylene and dimethyl ether [17].

REFERENCES

1. Ayres, S. M. Analysis of ventilation and performance abnormalities by washout in alveolar air and arterial blood continuous measurement of inert gas. *Crit. Care Med.* 4:261, 1976.
2. Brantigan, J. W., Gott, V. L., and Martz, M. N. A Teflon membrane for measurement of blood and intramyocardial gas tensions by mass spectrometry. *J. Appl. Physiol.* 32:276, 1972.
3. Butler, J. Measurement of cardiac output using soluble gases. In W. O. Fenn and H. Rahn (Eds.), *Handbook of Physiology*, Vol. 2, Sec. 3. Washington, D.C.: American Physiological Society, 1965. Pp. 1489.
4. Cotton, E. K. The measurement of effective pulmonary blood flow in the newborn infant using a mass spectrometer. *Crit. Care Med.* 4:245, 1976.
5. Dammann, J. F., and McAslan, T. C. PEEP: Its use in young patients with apparently normal lungs. *Crit. Care Med.* 7:14, 1979.
6. Douglas, C. G., and Haldane, J. S. The regulation of the general circulation rate in man. *J. Physiol. (Lond.)* 56:69, 1922.
7. Farhi, L. E., and Rahn, G. A theoretical analysis of the alveolar-arterial oxygen difference with special reference to the distribution effect. *J. Appl. Physiol.* 7:699, 1955.
8. Grollman, A. The determination of the cardiac output of man by the use of acetylene. *Am. J. Physiol.* 88:432, 1929.

9. Haldane, J. S., and Priestley, J. G. The regulation of lung ventilation. *J. Physiol. (Lond.)* 32:225, 1905.

10. Johnson, R. L., Spicer, W. S., Bishop, J. M., and Forster, R. E. Pulmonary capillary blood volume, flow and diffusing capacity during exercise. *J. Appl. Physiol.* 15:893, 1960.

11. Khuri, S. F., Brawley, R. K., O'Riordan, J. B., et al. The effect of cardiopulmonary bypass perfusion pressure on myocardial gas tensions in the presence of coronary stenosis. *Ann. Thorac. Surg.* 20:661, 1975.

12. Kirby, R. R., Downs, J. B., Civetta, J. M., et al. High level positive end expiratory pressure (PEEP) in acute respiratory insufficiency. *Chest* 67:156, 1975.

13. McAslan, T. C. Automated respiratory gas monitoring of critically injured patients. *Crit. Care Med.* 4:255, 1976.

14. MacGregor, D. C., Wilson, G. J., Holness, D. E., et al. Intramyocardial carbon dioxide tension: A guide to the safe period of anoxic arrest of the heart. *J. Thorac. Cardiovasc. Surg.* 68:101, 1974.

15. Ogilvie, C. M., Forster, R. E., Blakemore, W. S., and Morton, J. W. A standardized breath holding technique for the clinical measurement of the diffusing capacity of the lung for carbon monoxide. *J. Clin. Invest.* 36:1, 1957.

16. Osborn, J. J., Beaumont, J. O., Raison, J. C., et al. Measurement and monitoring of acutely ill patients by digital computer. *Surgery* 64:1057, 1970.

17. Overland, E. S., Ozanne, G. M., and Severinghaus, J. W. A single breath method for determining lung weight and pulmonary blood flow from the differential uptake of two soluble gases. *Physiologist* 18:341, 1975.

18. Rahn, H. The Sampling of Alveolar Gas. In W. M. Boothby (Ed.), *Handbook of Respiratory Physiology.* USAF School of Aviation Medicine, Randolph AFB, Texas, 1954. Pp. 29–37.

19. Rahn, H., and Otis, A. B. Continuous analysis of alveolar gas composition during work, hyperpnea and anoxia. *J. Appl. Physiol.* 1:717, 1948.

20. Riker, J. B., and Haberman, B. Expired gas monitoring by mass spectrometry in a respiratory intensive care unit. *Crit. Care Med.* 4:223, 1976.

21. Sackner, M., Greeneltch, D., Heiman, M. S., et al. Diffusing capacity, membrane diffusing capacity, capillary blood volume, pulmonary tissue volume, and cardiac output measured by a rebreathing technique. *Am. Rev. Respir. Dis.* 111:157, 1975.

22. West, J. Regional differences in gas exchange in the lung of erect man. *J. Appl. Physiol.* 17:893, 1962.

23. West, J. B., Fowler, K. T., Hugh-Jones, P., and O'Donnell, T. V. Measurement of the inequality of ventilation and of perfusion in the lung by analysis of single expirates. *Clin. Sci.* 16:549, 1957.

24. West, J. B., Fowler, K. T., Hugh-Jones, P., and O'Donnell, T. V. Measurement of ventilation-perfusion ratio inequality in the lung by the analysis of a single expirate. *Clin. Sci.* 16:529, 1957.

25. Wilmore, J. H. Mass spectrometry: Application in the exercise sciences. *Crit. Care Med.* 4:230, 1976.

26. Wilmore, J. H., and Costil, D. L. Adequacy of the Haldane transformation in the computation of exercise $\dot{V}O_2$ in man. *J. Appl. Physiol.* 35:85, 1973.

APPENDIXES

1. ABBREVIATIONS, DEFINITIONS, AND NORMAL VALUES

Abbreviation	Definition	Normal Value
BSA	Body surface area	Meters (square)
$\overline{AP}$	Mean systemic arterial pressure	85–95 mm Hg
CVP	Central venous pressure	5–12 cm H_2O
$\overline{PA}$	Mean pulmonary artery pressure	10–17 mm Hg
$\overline{PCWP}$	Mean pulmonary capillary wedge pressure	5–12 mm Hg
CO	Cardiac output	5–6 L/min
CI	Cardiac index	2.5–3.5 L/min/M^2
SVR or TPR	Systemic vascular resistance Total peripheral resistance	900–1,200 dynes $\cdot$ sec $\cdot$ cm^{-5}
PVR	Pulmonary vascular resistance	150–250 dynes $\cdot$ sec $\cdot$ cm^{-5}
HR	Heart rate	60–90 beats/min
SV	Stroke volume	60–70 ml/beat
SI	Stroke index	35–45 ml/beat/M_2
RVSW	Right ventricular stroke work	8–12 gmM/M^2
LVSW	Left ventricular stroke work	51–61 gmM/M^2
CBV	Central blood volume	750–800 ml/M^2
EF	Ejection fraction	0.67
EDV	End-diastolic volume	70 ml/M^2
dp/dt	First time derivative of left ventricular pressure	1,500–1,800 mm Hg/sec (normal value varies with method and equipment)
MTT	Mean transit time Calculated from indicator dilution curve	
	Time from venous injection to peak concentration in artery	13–14 sec
P_AO_2	Mean partial pressure of oxygen in the alveolus	104 mm Hg

Abbreviation	Definition	Normal Value
P_ACO_2	Partial pressure of carbon dioxide in the alveolus	40 mm Hg
PaO_2	Partial pressure of oxygen in arterial blood	Will vary with patient's age and the F_IO_2 on room air: 80–95 mm Hg Hg on 100% O_2: 640 mm Hg
$PaCO_2$	Partial pressure of carbon dioxide in arterial blood	40 mm Hg
$P\bar{v}O_2$	Partial pressure of oxygen in mixed venous blood	Will vary with the F_IO_2, cardiac output, and oxygen consumption from 35–40 mm Hg
$P\bar{v}CO_2$	Partial pressure of carbon dioxide in mixed venous blood	41–51 mm Hg
$P(A-a)O_2$	Alveolar-arterial oxygen gradient	25–65 mm Hg at $F_IO_2 = 1.0$
SaO_2	Percent oxyhemoglobin saturation of arterial blood	97% (air)
$S\bar{v}O_2$	Percent oxyhemoglobin saturation of mixed venous blood	75% (air)
CaO_2	Arterial oxygen content	Will vary with hemoglobin concentration and PaO_2 on air from 19–20 ml/100 ml
$C\bar{v}O_2$	Mixed venous oxygen content	Will vary with CaO_2, cardiac output, and O_2 consumption from 14–15 ml/100 ml
$C(a-v)O_2$	Arteriovenous oxygen content difference	4–6 ml/100 ml
O_2 avail	Oxygen availability	550–650 ml/min/M^2
O_2 "x" ratio	Oxygen extraction ratio	0.25
P_B	Barometric pressure	
$\dot{V}O_2$	Oxygen consumption (STPD[a])	115–165 ml/min/M^2
$\dot{V}CO_2$	Carbon dioxide production (STPD[a])	192 ml/min
R or RQ	Respiratory quotient	0.8
FRC	Functional residual capacity (BTPS[b])	2400 ml
VC	Vital capacity (BTPS[b])	65–75 ml/kg

Abbreviation	Definition	Normal Value
IF	Inspiratory force	75–100 cm H_2O
EDC	Effective dynamic compliance	35–45 ml/cm H_2O females 40–50 ml/cm H_2O males
V_D	Dead space (BTPS[b])	150 ml
V_T	Tidal volume (BTPS[b])	500 ml
V_D/V_T	Dead space to tidal volume ratio	0.25–0.40
$\dot{Q}s/\dot{Q}t$	Right-to-left shunt (percent of cardiac output flowing past nonventilated alveoli or the equivalent)	5–8%

[a] Standard temperature pressure, dry.
[b] Body temperature pressure, saturated.

2. TABLE OF FORMULAS

$\overline{\text{AP}}$ estimate: diastolic pressure plus 1/3 pulse pressure

$$\text{CI (L/min/M}^2) = \frac{\text{cardiac output (L/min)}}{\text{body surface area (M}^2)}$$

$$\text{SVR (TPR) (dynes} \cdot \sec \cdot \text{cm}^{-5}) = \frac{(\overline{\text{AP}} \text{ [mm Hg]} - \text{CVP [mm Hg]}) \times 79.9}{(\text{cardiac output [L/min]})}$$

$$\text{PVR (dynes} \cdot \sec \cdot \text{cm}^{-5}) = \frac{(\overline{\text{PA}} \text{ [mm Hg]} - \overline{\text{PCWP}} \text{ [mm Hg]}) \times 79.9}{\text{cardiac output (L/min)}}$$

$$\text{SV (ml/beat)} = \frac{\text{cardiac output (ml)}}{\text{heart rate}}$$

$$\text{SI (ml/min/M}^2) = \frac{\text{stroke volume}}{\text{body surface area}}$$

$$\text{RVSW (gmM/M}^2) = \text{SI} \times \overline{\text{PA}} \text{ (mm Hg)} \times 0.0136$$

$$\text{LVSW (gmM/M}^2) = \text{SI} \times \overline{\text{AP}} \text{ (mm Hg)} \times 0.0136$$

$$\text{CO}_2 \text{ (ml O}_2/100 \text{ ml blood or vols\%)} = (\text{Hb} \times 1.39) \text{ SaO}_2 + (\text{PaO}_2 \times 0.0031)$$

$$\text{C(a-v)O}_2 \text{ (ml/100 ml or vol\%)} = \text{CaO}_2 - \text{C}\overline{\text{v}}\text{O}_2$$

$$\dot{\text{V}}\text{O}_2 \text{ (ml/min/M}^2) = \text{CI} \times \text{C(a-v)O}_2 \times 10$$

$$\text{RQ} = \frac{\dot{\text{V}}\text{CO}_2}{\dot{\text{V}}\text{O}_2}$$

$$\text{O}_2 \text{ avail (ml/min/M}^2) = \text{CI} \times \text{CaO}_2 \times 10$$

$$\text{CBV (ml/M}^2) = \text{MTT} \times \text{CI} \times 16.7$$

$$\text{O}_2 \text{ "x" ratio} = \frac{\text{C(a-v)O}_2}{\text{CaO}_2}$$

$$\dot{\text{Q}}\text{s}/\dot{\text{Q}}\text{T}(\%) = \frac{\text{CcO}_2 - \text{CaO}_2}{\text{CcO}_2 - \text{CvO}_2} \times 100$$

$$\dot{\text{Q}}\text{s}/\dot{\text{Q}}\text{T}(\%) = \frac{0.0031 \times \text{P(A-a)O}_2}{[\text{C(a-v)O}_2] + (0.0031 \times \text{P(A-a)O}_2)} \times 100$$

Valid only when arterial blood is 100% saturated

$$\text{EDC (ml/cm H}_2\text{O)} = \frac{\text{tidal volume (ml)}}{\text{peak airway pressure (cm H}_2\text{O)}}$$

$$V_D/V_T = \frac{PaCO_2 - P\bar{E}CO_2}{PaCO_2}$$

$$P(A\text{-}a)O_2 \text{ (mm Hg)} = PaO_2 - PaO_2$$

$$\text{Ejection fraction} = \frac{SV}{EDV}$$

$$\text{MTT} = \frac{\int_0^\infty tc(t)dt}{\int_0^\infty c(t)dt}, \text{ where } c = \text{dye concentration and } t = \text{time}$$

3. NOMOGRAMS

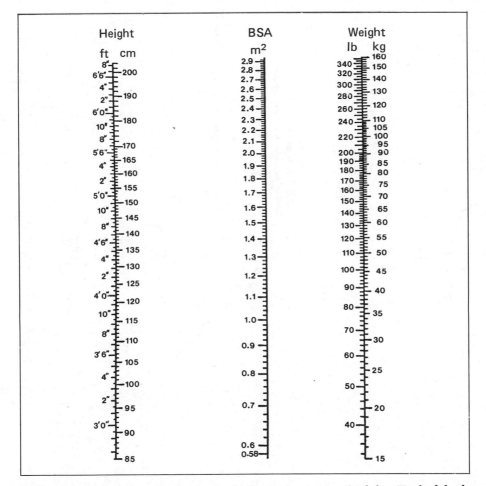

DuBois nomogram for calculating the body surface area of adults. To find body surface of a patient, locate height in inches (or centimeters) on Scale I and weight in pounds (or kilograms) on Scale III and place straight edge (ruler) between these two points. This will intersect Scale II at patient's surface area. (From E. J. DuBois. *Basal Metabolism in Health and Disease*. Philadelphia: Lea & Febiger, 1936. Copyright 1920 by W. M. Boothby and R. B. Sandiford.)

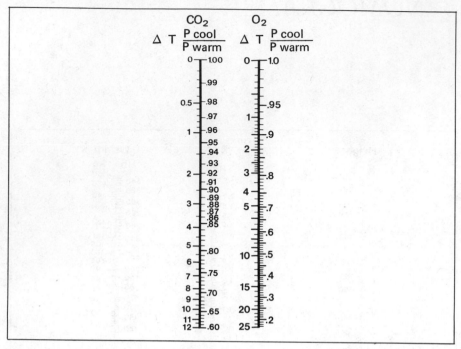

Nomogram for Severinghaus PO_2 and PCO_2 temperature correction factors for blood. These are applicable to either in vitro or in vivo conditions. Factors on right side of the columns are multiplied by the tensions at warmer temperature to correct to cooler temperature. Conversely, factors are divided into tensions at cooler temperature to correct to warmer temperature.

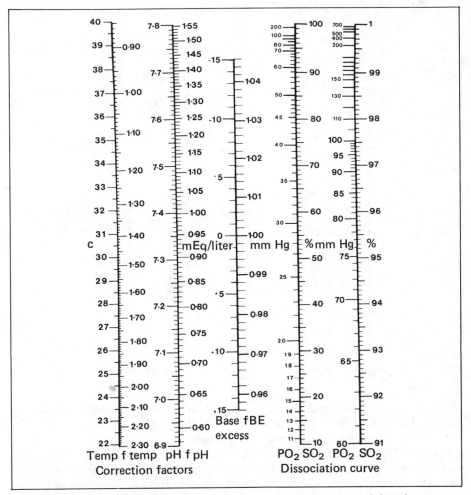

Nomogram for calculating percent oxygen saturation of hemoglobin from measured PO_2. Line charts representing oxyhemoglobin dissociation curve (temperature = 37° C, pH = 7.40, base excess = 0 mEq/L) are on right. Remaining line charts are factors (left to right: temperature, pH, and base excess) by which measured PO_2 should be multiplied before entering standard dissociation curve. (From G. R. Kelman and J. F. Nunn. Nomograms for correction of blood PO_2, PCO_2, pH, and base excess for time and temperature. *J. Appl. Physiol.* 21:1484, 1966.)

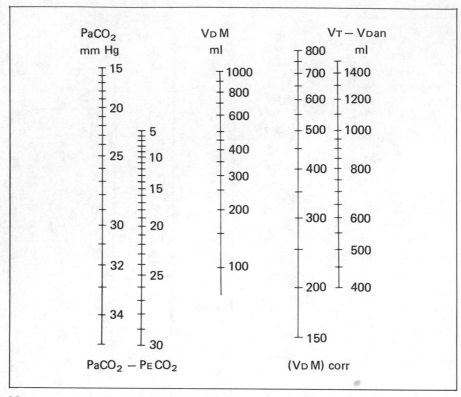

Nomogram for calculating dead space requirement during prolonged artificial ventilation. Mechanical dead space (V_{DM}) required to raise $PaCO_2$ to approximately 40 mm Hg can be predicted from this nomogram. $PaCO_2$ is the observed arterial carbon dioxide tension before introduction of mechanical dead space; V_T is tidal volume, and V_{Dan} is anatomic dead space. For patient with normal pulmonary and circulatory status, line in middle gives required value for V_{DM}. In presence of pulmonary disease or circulatory failure, a correction must be made by connecting points on the ($PaCO_2 - P_ECO_2$) line and V_{DM} line, then extending it to right. Read value on (V_{DM}) correction line. V_{Dan} is two-thirds of body weight (in pounds), plus dead space of tracheostomy tube and ventilator.

Example: A patient is being ventilated at given respiratory frequency with tidal volume of 1,130 ml. $PaCO_2$ is measured and found to be 25 mm Hg. Patient's body weight is 150 pounds; dead space of tracheostomy tube and ventilator is 30 ml. V_{Dan} = two-thirds of body weight + ventilator and tracheostomy dead space = 130 ml. Since V_T = 1,130 ml, $V_T - V_{Dan}$ = 1,000 ml. The two points, 1,000 for $V_T - V_{Dan}$ and 25 for $PaCO_2$ are connected, and we read off the center line that V_{DM} should be 430 ml. Assuming reasonably normal lungs, insertion of dead space of 430 ml should raise this patient's $PaCO_2$ to approximately 40 mm Hg. It is emphasized that respiratory frequency and tidal volume must remain unchanged.

If patient's lung function is not normal, $P\bar{E}CO_2$ is determined also and found to be 10 mm Hg; $PaCO_2 - P\bar{E}CO_2$ is then 25 mm Hg $-$ 10 mm Hg $=$ 15 mm Hg. Connect this point ($PaCO_2 - P\bar{E}CO_2 = 15$ mm Hg) with already obtained VDM of 430 ml; extend connecting line to right and read off corrected VDM (on the line [VDM] corr.). Corrected value is 600 ml. (From K. Suwa et al. A nomogram for dead space requirement during prolonged artificial ventilation. *Anesthesiology* 29:1206, 1968.)

4. DOSES
AND ACTIONS OF
VASOACTIVE DRUGS

Generic and Trade Name of Drug	Intravenous Dose*	Comments
Deslanoside (Cedilanid) Digoxin (Lanoxin)	Will vary with body weight and renal function and whether or not patient has been previously digitalized.	Digitalis has well-established inotropic actions, improving ventricular function. Useful in patients with atrial fibrillation, since it slows AV conduction. Augments force and velocity of contraction. Control ECG should be obtained before initiating therapy. Serum potassium must be monitored, since digitalis toxicity with arrhythmias may occur, particularly in hypokalemia. In these situations K^+, Xylocaine, Dilantin, Pronestyl, Inderal, glucagon, and/or countershock may prove useful. Has mild diuretic effect.
Digoxin	0.50 mg–1.0 mg as an initial dose, with maintenance dose usually 0.125–0.25, depending on above.	
Deslanoside	For very rapid digitalization, 0.8 mg followed by 0.4 mg every 2 hr as needed (up to 2 mg total). Rarely used for maintenance because of rapid dissipation.	Use of this agent in patients with a "normal heart" has been debated, but it appears to have some benefits even in these patients, since critically ill patients may have impairment of contractility secondary to underlying problem (e.g., endotoxin, ? myocardial depressant factor).
Dobutamine (Dobutrex)	2–10 μg/kg/min. On rare occasions, infusion rates up to 40 μg/kg/min have been required.	Dobutamine is a β-adrenergic agonist resulting in inotropic stimulation and peripheral vasodilatation. Some studies suggest that it produces fewer chronotropic and arrhythmogenic effects than does isoproterenol. In patients in shock, because of the vasodilatory effect of dobutamine, the mean arterial pressure should be closely monitored and, in general, not permitted to fall below 50 torr. However, the increase in cardiac output may offset the decrease in systemic vascular resistance so that the arterial pressure may fall little or not at all.
Dopamine (Intropin)	Low dose (<5 μg/kg/min) Moderate dose range (5–30 μg/kg/min)	In low dose range and in low moderate ranges there is an inotropic effect with renal vasodilatation. Immediate

	Dose*	Comments
	High dose range (>30 μg/kg/min) Starting dose, 2–5 μg/kg/min 200 mg in 250 ml = 800 μg/ml 200 mg in 500 ml = 400 μg/ml Do not mix with NaHCO$_3$ solution	precursor of norepinephrine. At upper moderate dose range and in high dose range has actions like norepinephrine. In a small percentage of patients there may be tachycardia even in lower dose ranges. Certain actions not blocked by either α- or β-blocking agents, which has led to postulation of dopaminergic receptor. Less increase in myocardial oxygen demand than with norepinephrine or isoproterenol. Useful in cardiogenic shock and may be used in conjunction with other agents (e.g., sodium nitroprusside, phentolamine) and/or assisted circulation.
Epinephrine	Intravenous route rarely used. If used, drug must be adequately diluted and injected very slowly. IV dose is seldom as much as 0.25 mg. IV infusion of 10–30 μg/min for inotropic effect can be given for short periods of time.	In low doses, primarily β-adrenergic agonist. In higher doses α-adrenergic effects are observed. Will cause increase in heart rate by direct effect on SA node. CVP and pulmonary artery pressure increase with pharmacologic doses. Exhibits both inotropic and chronotropic effects. Decreased systemic vascular resistance when used in small doses.
Isoproterenol (Isuprel)	2–4 μg/min infusion rate is average; should be kept under 10 μg/min. 1–4 mg in 250 ml = 4–16 μg/ml.	Inotropic and chronotropic agent. Causes vasodilatation. Pure β stimulator. Tachyphylaxis may develop. Increases myocardial oxygen demand. Should not be used when heart rate is >120/min, since cardiac arrhythmias may result. During administration, ECG should be monitored, since arrhythmias (PVCs) may result. May be used in propranolol overdose (toxicity). Not recommended in cardiogenic shock because of increased O_2 consumption associated with its inotropic and chronotropic actions.

* Unless otherwise noted.

Generic and Trade Name of Drug	Intravenous Dose*	Comments
Mephentermine (Wyamine)	10–30 mg/1,000 ml 5% D/S or D/W. Rate of infusion determined by response.	Acts as both an α- and β-adrenergic agonist, but major effect appears to be β. Tachyphylaxis may occur with prolonged use. Will increase heart rate, CO, and contractility. Decreases SVR. MAP remains unchanged or is minimally decreased. High doses will cause vasoconstriction. Reported to have antiarrhythmic effects.
Metaraminol (Aramine)	25–100 mg/500 ml 5% D/W by infusion.	Action is primarily indirect (i.e., releases norepinephrine from postganglionic sympathetic nerve endings), and thus its effects are almost identical with norepinephrine's; however, it appears to reduce renal blood flow less. Patients may become refractory to this agent because of norepinephrine depletion secondary to its use. Has some inotropic effect on heart in low dose range. Useful in spinal shock.
Methylprednisolone sodium succinate (Solu-Medrol)	Initially 30 mg/kg body weight given over 15–20 min. If favorable effect is observed, dose may be repeated in 6 hr.	Vasodilator. Inotropic action on heart acts to stabilize lysosomal membranes. May cause hypotension secondary to vasodilatation. Prolonged use may lead to stress ulcer and opportunistic infections. Monitor blood glucose and urine sugar.
Nitroglycerin	10–20 μg/min (increased by 5–10 μg/min Q 5–10 min until desired hemodynamic response obtained)	Reliable, easily controlled, relatively nontoxic. Decreases LV filling pressure more than systemic vascular resistance through significant venodilatation. Also may dilate medium coronary arteries directly. Has application in treating of unstable angina, LV failure, especially when LV filling pressure is markedly elevated and mild ↓ CO present. Useful in control of hypertension in coronary artery bypass surgery. Complications include headache, reversible hypotension and bradycardia.

Norepinephrine Levarterenol (Levophed)	2–4 μg of base per minute is usual dosage. Adjust for desired pressor effect. Inject into a large vein and avoid extravasation.	Primarily α-adrenergic agonist with minimal β-adrenergic effect. Causes intense vasoconstriction (i.e., increased) and thus an increase in blood pressure. Cardiac output is often decreased secondary to reflex bradycardia, which can be blocked with atropine. If α effect is totally blocked (e.g., by phentolamine), an increase in cardiac output is seen. Mean arterial pressure should not be allowed to go above 80 mm Hg. May increase cardiac work secondary to increase in afterload. Tissue necrosis will occur with infiltration; in this event local infiltration with phentolamine may prove useful. Addition of 5 mg phentolamine/4 mg norepinephrine will act to reduce intense vasoconstriction without negating pressor effect. Decreases renal blood flow.
Phentolamine (Regitine)	5 mg slowly.	An α blocker with rapid onset and short duration. Has an antiserotonin property and acts as myocardial stimulant. Used to control hypertension in patients with pheochromocytomas. Its value in shock is not established.
Propranolol (Inderal)	The usual dose is 1–3 mg administered with careful monitoring. The rate should not exceed 1 mg/min. If necessary, a second dose may be given after 2 min. Thereafter, an additional dose should not be given in less than 4 hr. Oral maintenance therapy is in range of 10–40 mg 3–4 times/day and should be begun as soon as possible.	IV administration is reserved for life-threatening arrhythmias. Systemic effects will vary somewhat, depending on sympathetic activity when administered. Has negative inotropic and chronotropic effect and thereby decreases CO. Can precipitate congestive heart failure. Induces bronchoconstriction and thus must be used with caution in patients with bronchial asthma, chronic obstructive lung disease, etc. May induce hypoglycemia secondary to its blockage of epinephrine-induced glycogenolysis. In propranolol toxicity, glucagon, isoproterenol, dopamine, and epinephrine have all been advocated. Some feel glucagon is drug of choice to augment heart under in-

Generic and Trade Name of Drug	Intravenous Dose*	Comments
		fluence of propranolol, since it works through a non-catecholamine mechanism.
		Its major side-effect is acute cardiac failure.
		Its use in patients in shock has been largely experimental, and it is not available for clinical use in shock.
Sodium nitroprusside (Nipride)	50 mg in 500 ml 5% D/W = 100 μg/ml. Average dose 3 μg/kg/min. Range 0.5–8.0 μg/kg/min. Light-sensitive; infusion must be protected from light, and new infusion must be prepared every 4 hr. Use only in D/W.	Arterial vasodilator. Has been found useful in dissecting aortic aneurysm, mitral insufficiency, hypertensive emergencies, and when afterload reduction is desirable (e.g., active myocardial infarction). Potent agent; requires continuous blood pressure monitoring with intra-arterial line.
		When used to reduce afterload in acute myocardial infarction, care must be taken to maintain diastolic pressure at a minimum of 50 mm Hg. In some situations it may be desirable to combine this with intraaortic balloon counterpulsation.
		Hypothyroidism has been reported with prolonged use.
		Major toxicity is due to the accumulation of thiocyanate in the blood; thus, blood thiocyanate levels should be measured with use over 24 hr or in patients with renal failure.
		Rapid onset of action; effect dissipates within 2–3 min following cessation of therapy.
		Extreme caution must be used with this drug, since severe hypotension can occur, further extending infarct size.

SELECTED READINGS

Aviado, D. M.   *Sympathomimetic Drugs.* Springfield, Ill.: Thomas, 1970.

Chatterjee, K., and Swan, H. J. C.   Vasodilator therapy in acute myocardial infarction. *Mod. Concepts Cardiovasc. Dis.* 43(11):119, 1974.

Cohn, J. N.   Indications for digitalis therapy: A new look. *J.A.M.A.* 229:1191, 1974.

Hermreck, A. S., and Thal, A. P.   The adrenergic drugs and their use in shock therapy. *Current Probl. Surg.,* July 1965.

Kones, R. J.   The catecholamines: Reappraisal of their use for acute myocardial infarction and the low cardiac output syndromes. *Crit. Care Med.* 1:203, 1973.

Kones, R. J.   *Cardiogenic Shock: Mechanism and Management.* Mount Kisco, N.Y.: Futura, 1974.

Palmer, R. F., and Lasseter, K. C.   Sodium nitroprusside. *N. Engl. J. Med.* 292:294, 1975.

Tarazi, R. C.   Sympathomimetic agents in the treatment of shock. *Ann. Intern. Med.* 81:364, 1974.

5. CONVERSION FACTORS

TEMPERATURE

Fahrenheit-Centigrade Conversion Table*

° F	°C
93	33.9
94	34.4
95	35.0
96	35.6
97	36.1
98	36.7
98.6	37.0
99	37.2
100	37.8
101	38.3
102	38.9
103	39.4
104	40.0
105	40.6
106	41.1
107	41.7
108	42.2

* Fahrenheit to Centigrade: $°C = (°F - 32) \times 5/9$.
  Centigrade to Fahrenheit: $°F = °C \times 9/5 + 32$.

PRESSURE

1 mm Hg = 1.36 cm H_2O
1 cm H_2O = 0.73 mm Hg

LENGTH

1 inch (in.) = 2.54 cm
1 cm = 0.394 in

WEIGHT

1 pound (lb) = 0.454 kg
1 kilogram (kg) = 2.2 lb
1 grain (g) = 60 mg

INDEX